PESTICIDE CHEMISTRY: HUMAN WELFARE AND THE ENVIRONMENT

Volume 2

NATURAL PRODUCTS

Some Other IUPAC Titles of Interest from Pergamon Press

IUPAC Symposium Series

BENOIT & REMPP: Macromolecules

BRITTON & GOODWIN: Carotenoid Chemistry and Biochemistry

BROWN & DAVIES: Organ-Directed Toxicity — Chemical Indices and Mechanisms

CIARDELLI & GIUSTI: Structural Order in Polymers

FREIDLINA & SKOROVA: Organic Sulfur Chemistry

LAIDLER: Frontiers of Chemistry (Proceedings of the 28th IUPAC Congress)

NOZAKI: Current Trends in Organic Synthesis

ST-PIERRE & BROWN: Future Sources of Organic Raw Materials (CHEMRAWN I)

SHEMILT: Chemistry & World Food Supplies (CHEMRAWN II)

STEC: Phosphorus Chemistry Directed Towards Biology

TROST & HUTCHINSON: Organic Synthesis — Today and Tomorrow

IUPAC Nomenclature Guides

IRVING, FREISER & WEST: Compendium of Analytical Nomenclature

IUPAC: Nomenclature of Inorganic Chemistry & How to Name an Inorganic Substance (2-part set)

RIGAUDY & KLESNEY: Nomenclature of Organic Chemistry

WHIFFEN: Manual of Symbols & Terminology for Physicochemical Quantities and Units

Journals

CHEMISTRY INTERNATIONAL — IUPAC's international news magazine.

PURE AND APPLIED CHEMISTRY — IUPAC's official journal, featuring proceedings of IUPAC conferences, nomenclature rules and technical reports.

INTERNATIONAL UNION OF PURE AND APPLIED CHEMISTRY
(Applied Chemistry Division)

PESTICIDE CHEMISTRY: HUMAN WELFARE AND THE ENVIRONMENT

Proceedings of the 5th International Congress of Pesticide Chemistry, Kyoto, Japan, 29 August - 4 September 1982

Editors-in-Chief

J. MIYAMOTO
Pesticides Division, Sumitomo Chemical Co., Ltd. Takarazuka, Hyogo, Japan

and

P. C. KEARNEY
Agricultural Environmental Quality Institute, US Department of Agriculture, Beltsville, Maryland, USA

Volume 2

NATURAL PRODUCTS

Volume Editors

N. TAKAHASHI
Department of Agricultural Chemistry, University of Tokyo, Japan

H. YOSHIOKA
Sumitomo Chemical Co., Ltd., Takarazuka, Japan

T. MISATO
Institute of Physical & Chemical Research, Wako, Japan

and

S. MATSUNAKA
Kobe University, Japan

PERGAMON PRESS

OXFORD · NEW YORK · TORONTO · SYDNEY · PARIS · FRANKFURT

U.K.	Pergamon Press Ltd., Headington Hill Hall, Oxford OX3 0BW, England
U.S.A.	Pergamon Press Inc., Maxwell House, Fairview Park, Elmsford, New York 10523, U.S.A.
CANADA	Pergamon Press Canada Ltd., Suite 104, 150 Consumers Road, Willowdale, Ontario M2J 1P9, Canada
AUSTRALIA	Pergamon Press (Aust.) Pty. Ltd., P.O. Box 544, Potts Point, N.S.W. 2011, Australia
FRANCE	Pergamon Press SARL, 24 rue des Ecoles, 75240 Paris, Cedex 05, France
FEDERAL REPUBLIC OF GERMANY	Pergamon Press GmbH, Hammerweg 6, D-6242 Kronberg-Taunus, Federal Republic of Germany

First edition 1983

Library of Congress Cataloging in Publication Data

International IUPAC Congress of Pesticide Chemistry (5th: 1982: Kyoto, Japan)
Pesticide chemistry, human welfare and the environment.
(IUPAC symposium series)
At head of title: International Union of Pure and Applied Chemistry. Applied Chemistry Division.
Congress organized by The Science Council of Japan, Pesticide Science Society of Japan, and the Japan Plant Protection Association.
Includes bibliographical references.
1. Pesticides—Congresses. I. Miyamoto, J. (Junshi) II. Kearney, P. C. (Philip C.), 1932- III. International Union of Pure and Applied Chemistry. Applied Chemistry Division. IV. Nihon Gakujutsu Kaigi. V. Nihon Nóyaku Gakkai. VI. Nihon Shokubutsu Bóeki Kyókai. VII. Title. VIII. Series. [DNLM: 1. Pesticides—Congresses. 2. Pesticide—Residues—Congresses. 3. Toxicology—Congresses. 4. Pest control—Congresses. WA 240 P4738]
SB950.93.I57 1982 632'.95 82-24602

British Library Cataloguing in Publication Data

International Congress of Pesticide Chemistry: (*5th: 1982: Kyoto*) Pesticide chemistry.
1. Pesticides. Environmental aspects—Congresses
I. Titlc II. Miyamoto, J. III. Keaney, P. C.
IV.International Union of Pure and Applied Chemistry. *Applied Chemistry Division*
632'.95042 QH545.P4

ISBN 0 08 029219 4 (4 vol set)
ISBN 0 08 029223 2 (volume 2)

In order to make this volume available as economically and as rapidly as possible the authors' typescripts have been reproduced in their original forms. This method unfortunately has its typographical limitations but it is hoped that they in no way distract the reader.

Printed in Great Britain by A. Wheaton & Co. Ltd., Exeter

CONTENTS

Organizing Committee

Chairman: M. Nakajima

Vice Chairman: H. Fukami

Secretary General: T. Misato

Members: T. Endo, M. Eto, T. Fujita, S. Goto, T. Hosotsuji, W. Iida, T. Iwata, A. Kawana, K. Koshimizu, N. Kurihara, S. Kuwatsuka, S. Matsunaka, T. Mitsui, J. Miyamoto, J. Mizutani, K. Munakata, M. Saito, T. Saito, N. Takahashi, S. Takahashi, T. Tanaka, M. Uchiyama, K. Ueki, T. Ueno, I. Yamamoto, K. Yamashita, K. Yasutomi

Scientific Programme Committee

Chairman: J. Miyamoto

Vice Chairman: P. C. Kearney

Members: P. Doyle, N. Drescher, T. Fujita, S. Goto, R. Greenhalgh, D. H. Hutson, S. Kuwatsuka, S. Matsunaka, S. D. Murphy, N. Takahashi

Congress Organizers

The Science Council of Japan
Pesticide Science Society of Japan
Japan Plant Protection Association

INTERNATIONAL UNION OF PURE AND APPLIED CHEMISTRY

IUPAC Secretariat: Bank Court Chambers, 2-3 Pound Way,
Cowley Centre, Oxford OX4 3YF, UK

PREFACE

The Fifth International Congress of Pesticide Chemistry, sponsored by the International Union of Pure and Applied Chemistry, and organized jointly by the National Science Council of Japan, Pesticide Science Society of Japan and Japan Plant Protection Association, was held at Kyoto International Conference Hall in Kyoto, Japan, 29 August - 4 September 1982. The opening of the Congress culminated four years of intensive planning by the Scientific Programme Committee, the Organizing Committee, and a host of internationally recognized scientists dedicated to pesticide chemistry. The main theme of the Congress, **Human Welfare -- Environment -- Pesticides**, was intended to encompass current research topics in pesticide chemistry, not only for increased agricultural production, but also for public health purposes. Xenobiotics other than pesticides were also included. One thousand, six hundred scientists from 55 countries attended the Congress.

Two distinguished scientists, Professor Dr. K. H. Büchel, Bayer AG, Leverkusen, FRG, and Dr. I. J. Graham-Bryce, East Malling Research Station, UK, presented plenary lectures dealing with political, economic and philosophical aspects of pesticide use, as well as future pesticide research for improving human welfare. A number of distinguished invitees also addressed the Congress participants, including the President of IUPAC, Professor S. Nagakura.

Eight main topics were selected as the subjects of the Congress, either because of their timely nature or because the area needs critical review. They included: Synthesis of Pesticides and Growth Regulators; Chemical Structure and Biological Activity; Bioactive Natural Products: Chemistry, Biochemistry and Physiology; Biochemistry of Pests and Mode of Action of Pesticides (including Mechanism of Resistance and Phytotoxicity); Metabolism and Degradation of Pesticides and Xenobiotics; Toxicology of Pesticides and Xenobiotics; Pesticide Residues and Methodology; and Formulation Chemistry. Each main topic included one symposium and several poster-discussion sessions.

Each symposium consisted of several invited presentations, providing the participants with current and provocative overviews on important aspects of the respective topics. Poster-discussion sessions constituted the main body of presentations to the Congress and were intended to cover a wide variety of areas. Each included a few invited papers in addition to the contributed papers. Invited scientists served as leaders during the follow-up discussion after the poster presentations. Overall the Congress was organized into 49 sessions under the eight main topics with 694 submitted papers, including 236 invited papers.

In addition to the eight main topics encompassed by the Congress, three complementary symposia dealing with related subjects were held simultaneously, with 31 invited presentations: Pyrethroid Insecticides -- Biological Activity, Mode of Action, Metabolism and Toxicology; Antibiotics for Agricultural Use; and Herbicides and Plant Growth Regulators for Rice Culture.

The proceedings of the Congress, entitled **Pesticide Chemistry: Human Welfare and the Environment**, comprise four volumes containing over 250 invited papers presented at the symposia, complementary symposia, and poster-discussion sessions. Specifically, the contents are: Volume 1: plenary lectures, synthesis, structure-activity; Volume 2: natural products, complementary symposia; Volume 3: mode of action, metabolism and degradation, toxicology; and Volume 4: residue analysis, formulation chemistry. It is sincerely hoped, by this overview of the present status of chemical and biochemical pest control, that readers gain an appreciation of how pesticide science continues to contribute to human welfare.

Junshi Miyamoto

Philip C. Kearney

PC 2 - A*

BIOACTIVE NATURAL PRODUCTS: CHEMISTRY, BIOCHEMISTRY AND PHYSIOLOGY

RECENT PROGRESS IN RESEARCH ON AGRICULTURAL ANTIBIOTICS IN JAPAN

Noboru Ōtake

Institute of Applied Microbiology, University of Tokyo, Japan

Abstract - The current status and most recent works on agricultural antibiotics developed in Japan are reviewed primarily in connection with the control of plant disease, but also briefly with the livestock disease and promotion of growth.

The use of antibiotics as protectants against plant pathogen was considered a rather novel idea around 1953-1954, however, the discovery since then of blasticidin S (Ref. 1,2,3) and its successful use for control of rice blast disease has stimulated extensive investigations by many research organizations in Japan for new antibiotics effective against various kind of plant disease. As a result, more than twenty new compounds have been developed as protectants against plant pathogen during the past twenty years. In this area, Japan has played a pioneering role in the world in development of antibiotics used specifically for the control of individual plant pathogens. Eventually, in this relatively short time, the term "agricultural antibiotics" was used to refer to such compounds used for the control of pests in the field of agricultural production.

This talk, in which the current status and most recent works on the new antibiotics are reviewed, deals primarily with the control of plant disease, but also refers briefly to compounds used in a broad sense in agrigultural production.

It should be emphasized here that the extensive progress in agricultural antibiotics, in Japan is closely related to the feature of agricultural production namely, type of intensive farming in this country. Therefore, it is natural that in the first instance, a great stimulus to this type of research arose from the need to control the three big pathogens in rice production, namely, rice blight disease caused by *Pyricularia oryzae*, rice sheath blight caused by *Rhizoctonia solani* and bacterial leaf blight caused by *Xanthomonas oryzae*. Inevitably, unless the cost of using antibiotics for disease control will allow a normal profit margin to farmers, their use will be restricted: the success of blasticidin S as the first case indicated that they can economically be used in practice.

It is necessary to consider the background and progress on the discovery of agricultural antibiotics in Japan.

Screening for antibiotics that can be applied in plant disease control is a problem of considerable difficulty. Although screening tests *in vitro* have indicated effectiveness against the target pathogen of a number of antibiotics, *in vivo* tests have usually failed to coroborate the foregoing results. In the past, the screening tests used have consisted of determing the MIC of the antibiotic materials *in vitro* by a disc-plate method against fungal pathogens. The use of usual tests have, in many cases, resulted in the detection of a number of known antifungal antibiotics such as polyene macrolides, antimycins and oligomycins which have no practical value for the use of plant disease control because of their phytotoxicity or instability.

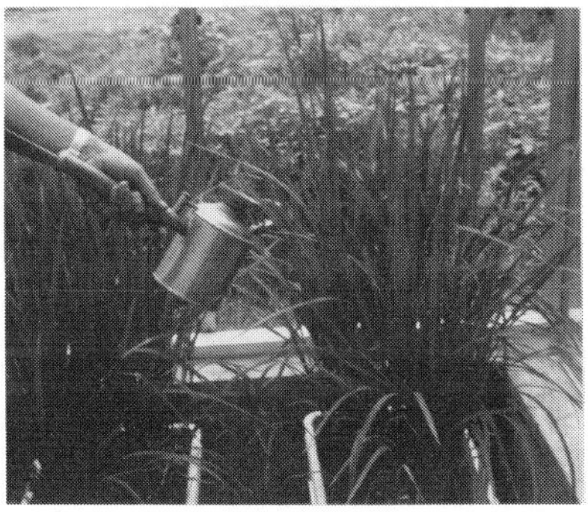

Fig. 1. By use of direct-spray tests of antibiotic samples against rice plants infected with *Pyricularia oryzae*.

It is noteworthy that improvement in screening procedures have been of great importance in discovery of antibiotics having satisfactory effects against target pathogens. For example, blasticidin S was discovered by a direct-spraying method in the green house, shown in Fig. 1, which was developed for the first time by the pioneering researchers, Professors Y. Sumiki and H. Yonehara of Tokyo University in collaboration with Drs. K. Fukunaga and T. Misato of the National Institute for Agricultural Science. In the same way, kasugamycin could never have been discovered by the usual *in vitro* tests because this compound showed only a weak activity against *Pyricularia oryzae* by the plate-assay method, thus, no discernible inhibitory zone was observed. (Ref. 4,5,6)
In practice, considerable amounts of both blasticidin S and kasugamycin are used in treatment of rice blast disease in Japan as well as in Korea and South America.

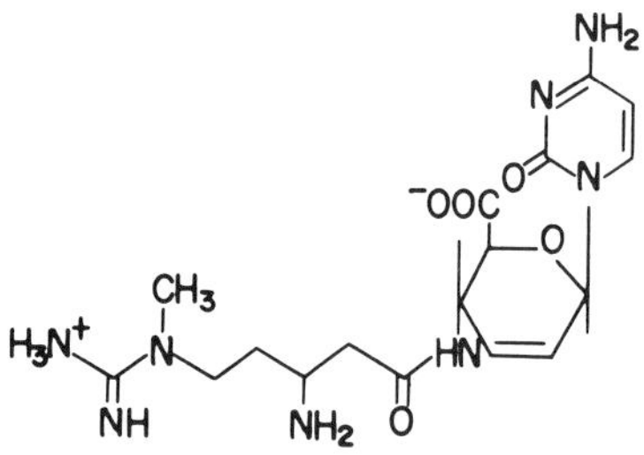

Blasticidin S

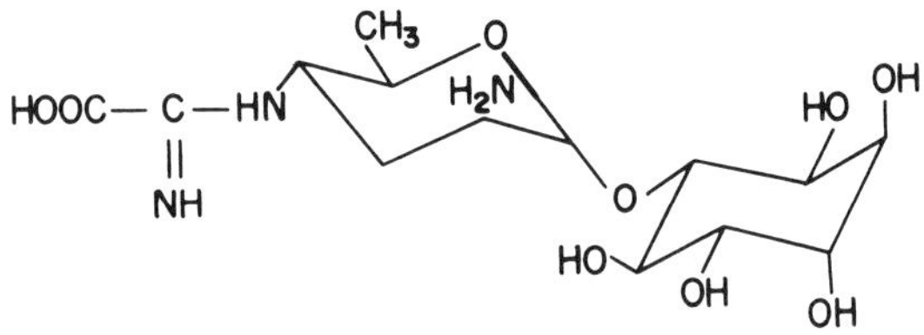

Kasugamycin

Despite the enormous efforts made up to the present time, nothing has been evaluated as better than these two antibiotics as an eradicant against rice blast disease, although a number of new antibiotics have been isolated.
Next, I would like to talk about the control of rice sheath blight. This blight caused by infection with the pathogen *Rhizoctonia solani* is widespread in Japan as well as in various rice cultivating areas of South Asia, and brings about severe economic losses among rice producers.

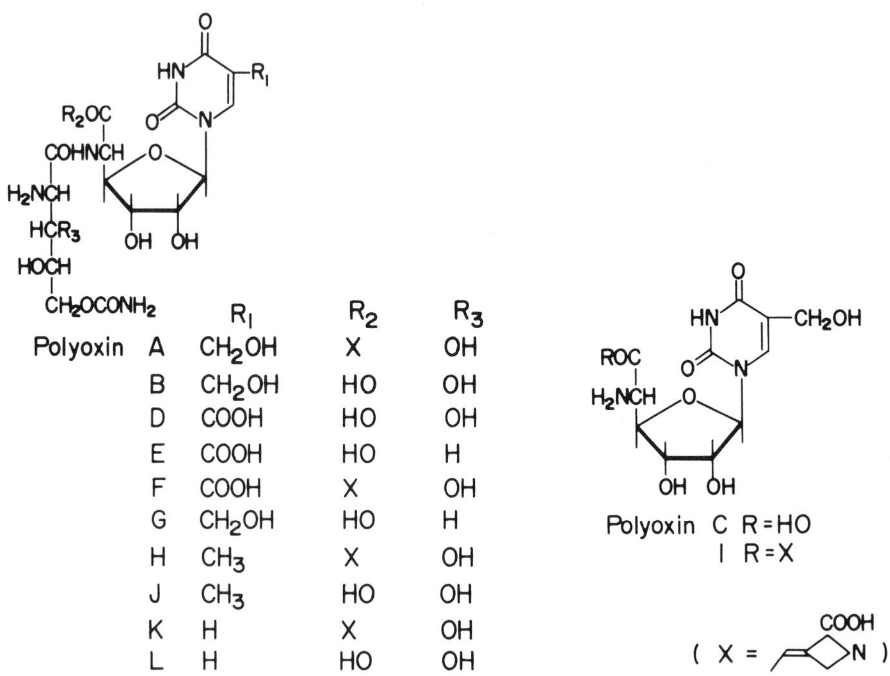

Fig. 2. The Structures of Polyoxin Complex

The first success was attained by the discovery of the polyoxin complex from *Streptomyces cacaoi* var. *asoensis* by Suzuki et al. (Ref. 7,8,9) of the Institute of Physical and Chemical Research, who initiated early attempts to develop control agents for this blight. The polyoxin complex contained a numbered of active components whose structures were shown to be unique nucleosides as depicted in Fig. 2. Among these, polyoxin D has been used in the field as the zinc chelate to control rice sheath blight. Other components will be discussed later such as polyoxin A and polyoxin B, which are also used to control brown spot in tobacco and leaf spot in apple caused by *Alternaria* pathogens.

In 1970, Iwasa et al. (Ref. 11,12,13,14) were led to the discovery of validamycin by direst -spray tests of cultured broths from a strain of *Streptomyces hygroscopicus*. Validamycins drastically reduced sheath blight infections on rice plant and this agent has been used in Japan under the trade name of "validacin". Chemical studies revealed that validamycins were a complex mixture containing a number of active congeners closely related in structure.

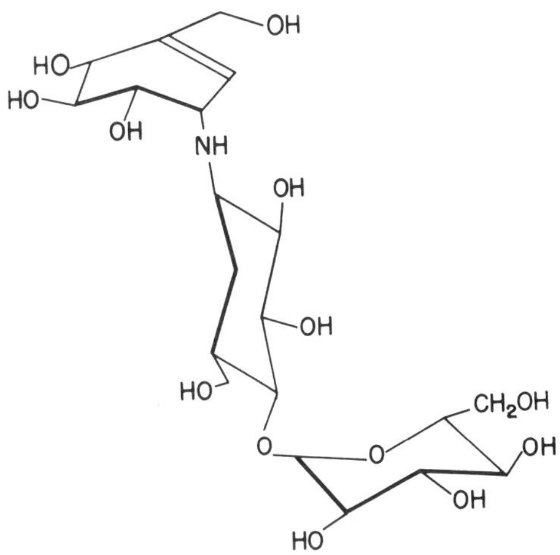

Validamycin A

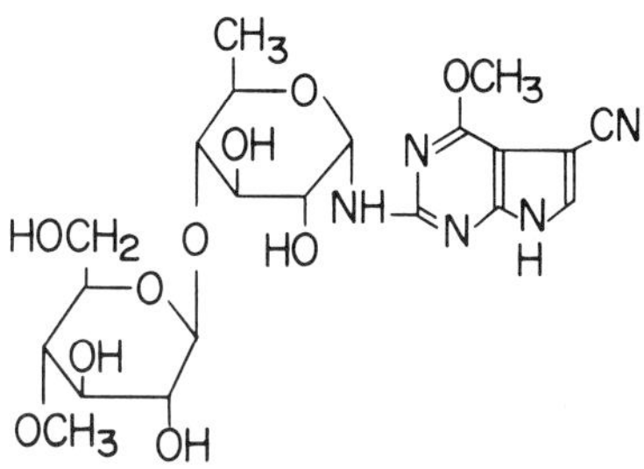

SF-1917

Among these validamycin A is a major component. It is of great interest that validamycins belong to a new class of aminoglycoside antibiotics found for the first time in nature. They are characterized by their very low toxicity and high specificity against a wide range of plant diseases caused by *R. solani* and more than 8700 tons of formulated preparations are used each year in Japan so far.

More recently, Niida et al. (Ref. 16,17) have detected by screening a new antifungal antibiotic SF-1917, produced by a strain of *Micromonospora* sp., which shows very promising effects in control of rice sheath blight. The structure of SF-1917 was shown to belong to an unusual class of nucleoside containing the 7-desazaguanine nucleus. SF-1917 exhibits potent activity against sheath blight disease of rice plants and is in the process of development.

The third blight of rice plant, bacterial leaf blight, is caused by infection with *Xanthomonas oryzae*. This blight causes withering of leaves at the time of fruiting and rice producing areas have been infected by this blight all over the world.

Although various agents were found to be active *in vitro* so far, none of them has been shown

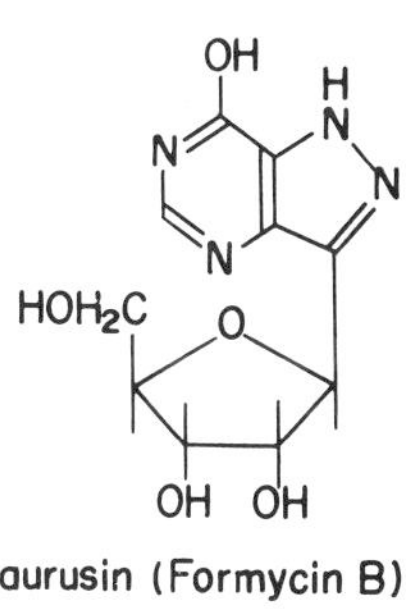

Laurusin (Formycin B)

to be effective both *in vivo* and in the field. Although laurusin (formycin B) were discovered during the search for control agents for this blight, their practical use is not possible due to its toxicity (Ref. 18), thus an antibiotic effective against bacterial leaf blight is still greatly to be desired and earnest efforts to find one continue in many research organizations in Japan.

So far, I have been discussing mainly the diseases of rice plant, but now I wish to extend my comments to diseases of fruit trees, vegetables, various garden and decorative plants. Polyoxin B (Fig. 2) is effective against various kinds of blasts in fruit trees, vegetables and tobacco plant caused by pathogens of the Alternaria species and it is now in commercial use.

Powdery mildew is a troublesome disease which attacks various plants closely involved with our daily life. In the rainy season of early Summer, we can often see rose trees and other Rosa plants covered with white powder: This is actually caused by an *Ascomycetes* fungi, *Sphaerotheca pannosa*, and the artificial cultivation of this pathogen has not yet been achieved.

A substance effective against this fungus was discovered by Iwasa et al. (Ref. 19,20) in mildiomycin. This agent is also a new antibiotic containing the 5-hydroxymethylcytosine nucleus in the molecule. It should be emphasized here that this agent is highly effective against a wide range of powdery mildew in more than 150 kinds of plants including fruit trees, vegetables, wheat etc. Its development as a new agricultural antibiotic is eagerly awaited.

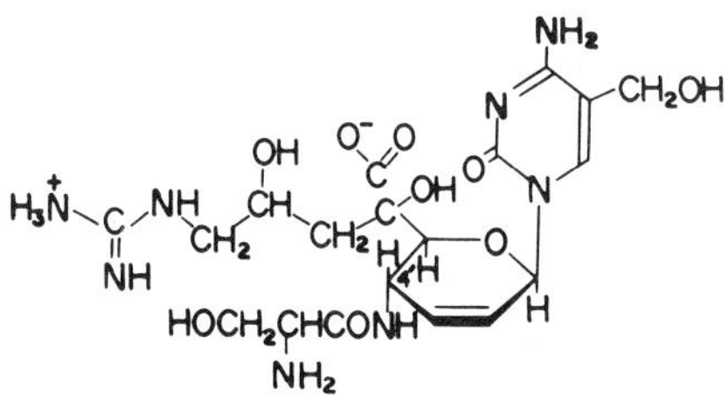

Mildiomycin

It is important to note here that the knowledge we have so far obtained from investigations on the action mechanisms of new antibiotics has revealed to us the presence of many metabolic pathways involving participation by many enzyme systems of which we were previously unaware or which were completely unknown before. These systems can be used as new assay systems, thus leading to further discovery of new compounds. Some examples of such use are discussed below.

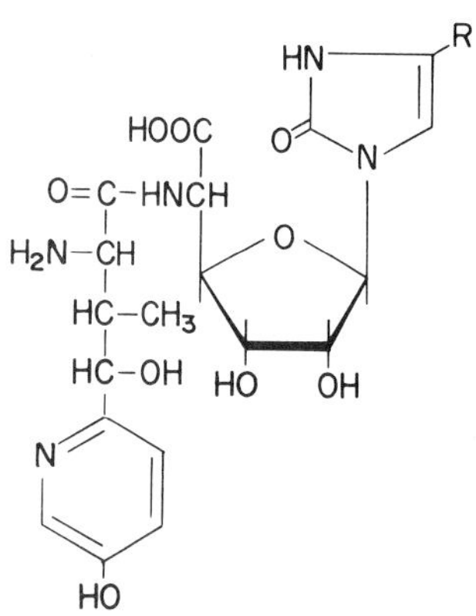

Neopolyoxin A:
Neopolyoxin B:

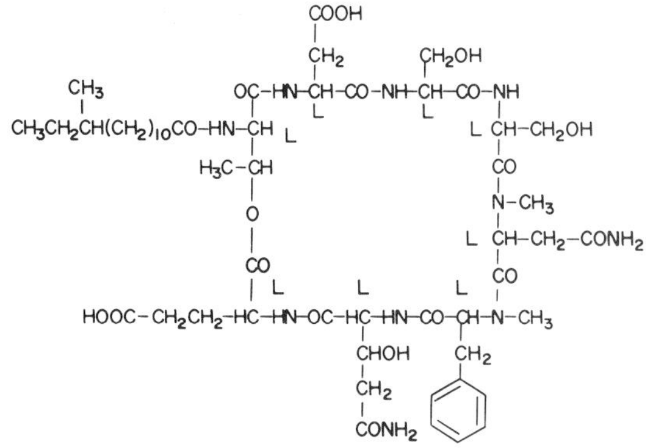

Lipopeptin A

In a search for inhibitors of cell wall biosynthesis, Isono et al. (Ref. 22,23,24,25) have discovered a number of active compounds by using an assay of a chitin-synthetase system. Neopolyoxins are produced by *Streptomyces cacaoi* var. *asoensis* (the same organism as produces polyoxins) and of these, neopolyoxin A is effective against *Sphaerotheca fuliginea* in green house tests. In a similar way, use of a proteo-heteroglycan enzyme system led to the detection and isolation of lipopeptins from *Streptomyces violaceochromogenes*, which showed an effect against powdery mildew in cucumber. Moreover, they have discovered neopeptins recently from a strain of unidentified *Streptomyces* sp., which are also effective against *S. fulginea*. Ōmura et al. (Ref. 26) have discovered irumamycin from *Streptomyces* sp., which was elucidated as a new member of macrolide antibiotics effective against gray mold disease caused by *Botritis cinera*.

Capsimycin discovered by Aizawa et al. (Ref. 27) is active against damping-off of cucumber by *Phytophtora capsisci*. Its structure has been elucidated as a unique polyketide containing the tetramic acid nucleus as chromophore. (Ref. 28)

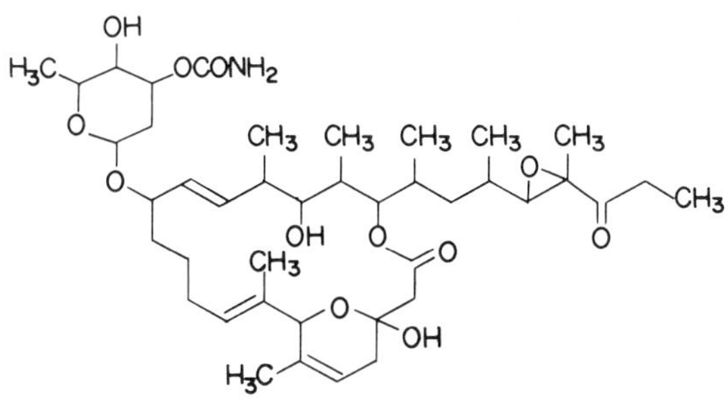

Irumamycin

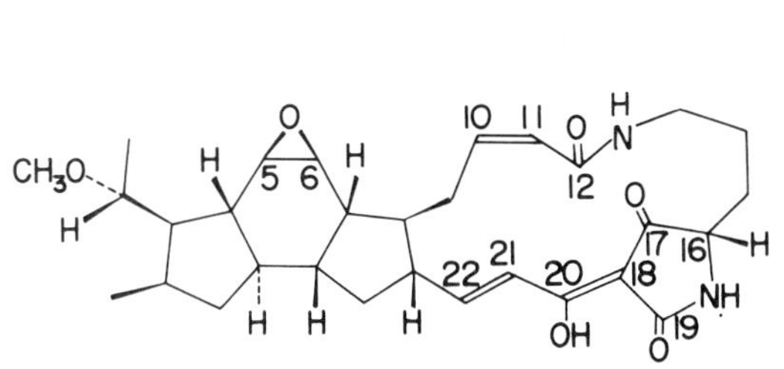

Capsimycin

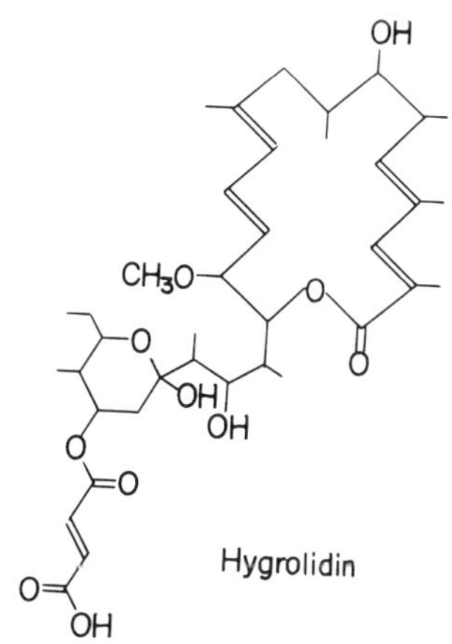

Hygrolidin

Among the damage to fruit trees, apple canker disease caused by invasion of the pathogenic fungi, *Valsa ceratosperma* is one of the most severe economic loss in Japan. We have recently discovered hygrolidin which inhibits germination of the pathogen at a concentration as low as 5 mcg/ml.

Now, I would like to conclude my account with brief examples from the fields of herbicides and control of livestock diseases. Niida et al. (Ref. 30,31) discovered bialaphos produced by a strain of *Streptomyces* sp. The structure of this compound, containing a C-P-C bond is quite uncommon in nature and its strong herbicidal activity holds out some hope of wide application. The mode of action of bialaphos has been shown to involve inhibition of glutamate biosynthesis.

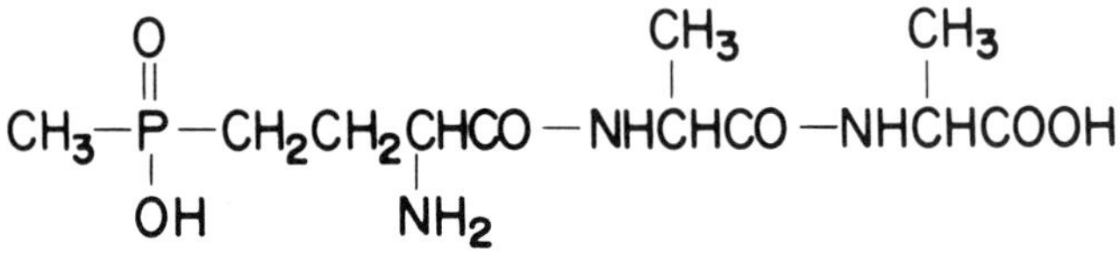

SF-1293 (Bialaphos)

In the area of livestock diseases, coccidiosis of poultly has been troublesome for chicken raisers because of difficulty in controlling it. Miyazaki et al. (Ref. 32,33,34,35) discovered salinomycin produced by *Streptomyces albus*, a substance that is quite unique due to its tricyclic spiroketal ring. This agent is used in practice not only as a coccidiostat but also as growth promotor of ruminant and swine.

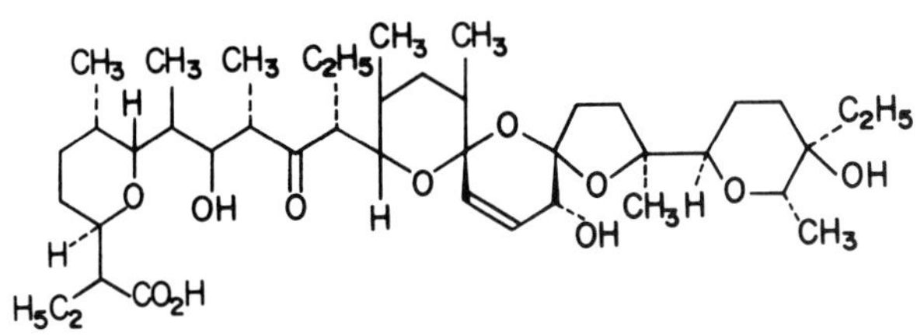

Salinomycin

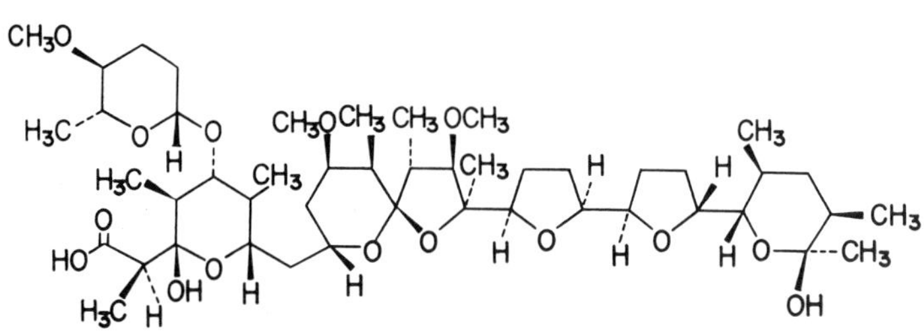

Carriomycin

Since then, discovery of many related compounds such as carriomycin (Ref. 36,37) and cationomycin (Ref. 38) have been reported. These two glycosidated polyether antibiotics which were discovered recently in Japan are characterized by their low toxicity and high anticoccidial activity.

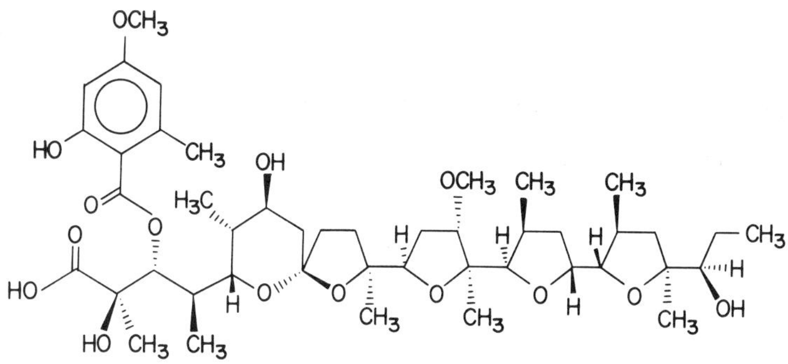

Cationomycin

CONCLUSION

The current status and most recent works on new agricultural antibiotics are reviewed. It is noteworthy that improvements in screening procedures give rise to detection of new compounds of potential value in the control of special diseases such as rice sheath blight, powdery mildew and other blights caused by individual plant pathogens which are classified in the category of diseases difficult to control.

REFERENCES

1. S. Takeuchi, K. Hirayama, K. Ueda, H. Sakai and H. Yonehara, J. Antibiot. 11A, 1 (1958)
2. T. Misato, I. Ishii, M. Asakawa, Y. Okimoto and K. Fukunaga, Ann. Phytopath. Soc. Japan 24, 302 (1959)
3. N. Ōtake, S. Takeuchi, T. Endō and H. Yonehara, Agric. Biol. Chem. 30, 132 (1966)
4. H. Umezawa, Y. Okami, T. Hashimoto, Y. Suhara, M. Hamada and T. Takeuchi, J. Antibiot. 18A, 101 (1965)
5. Y. Suhara, F. Sasaki, K. Maeda, H. Umezawa and M. Ohno, J. Am. Chem. Soc. 90, 6559 (1968)
6. T. Ishiyama, I. Hara, M. Matsuoka, K. Saito, S. Shimada, R. Izawa, T. Hashimoto, M. Hamada, Y. Okami, T. Takeuchi and H. Umezawa, J. Antibiot. 18A 115 (1965)
7. S. Suzuki, K. Isono, J. Nagatsu, T. Mizutani, Y. Kawashima and T. Mizuno, J. Antibiot. 18A 131 (1965)
8. K. Isono, K. Asahi and S. Suzuki, J. Am. Chem. Soc. 91, 7490 (1969)
9. S. Sasaki, N. Ohta, J. Eguchi, Y. Furukawa, T. Akashiba, T. Tsuchiyama and S. Suzuki, Ann. Phytopath. Soc. Japan 34, 272 (1968)
10. J. Eguchi, S. Sasaki, N. Ohta, T. Akashiba, T. Tsuchiyama and S. Suzuki, Ann. Phytopath. Soc. Japan 34, 280 (1965)
11. T. Iwasa, H. Yamamoto and M. Shibata, J. Antibiot. 23, 595 (1970)
12. T. Iwasa, E. Higashide, H. Yamamoto and M. Shibata, J. Antibiot. 24, 107 (1971)
13. T. Iwasa, E. Higashide and M. Shibata, J. Antibiot. 24, 114 (1971)
14. T. Iwasa, Y. Kameda, M. Sai, S. Horii and K. Mizuno, J. Antibiot. 24, 119 (1971)
15. T. Suami, S. Ogawa and N. Chiba, J. Antibiot. 33, 98 (1980)
16. H. Seto, S. Sasaki, N. Ōtake, M. Koyama, Y. Kodama, H. Ogino, Y. Nishizawa, T. Tsuruoka and S. Inoue, Tetrahed. Lett. in press
17. S. Aizawa, T. Hidaka, N. Ōtake, H. Yonehara, K. Isono, N. Igarashi and S. Suzuki, Agric. Biol. Chem. 29, 375 (1965)
18. T. Iwasa, K. Suetomi and T. Kusaka, J. Antibiot. 31, 511 (1978)
19. S. Harada, E. Mizuta and T. Kishi, J. Am. Chem. Soc. 100, 4895 (1978)
20. T. Kusaka, K. Suetomi and T. Iwasa, J. Pesticide Sci. 4, 345 (1979)
21. K. Isono, "Kagaku To Seibutsu" 19, 505 (1981)
22. K. Kobinata, M. Uramoto, M. Nishii, G. Nakamura, K. Isono, Agric. Biol. Chem. 44, 1909 (1980)

23. K. Tsuda, T. Kihara, M. Nishii, Nakamura, K. Isono and S. Suzuki, J. Antibiot. 33, 247 (1980)
24. M. Nishii, T. Kihara, K. Isono, T. Higashijima, T. Miyazawa, S. K. Sethi and J. A. McCloski, Tetrahed. Lett. 21, 4627 (1980)
25. T. Satomi, H. Kusakabe, G. Nakamura, T. Nishio, M. Uramoto and K. Isono, Agric. Biol. Chem. 46, in press
26. S. Ōmura, Y. Tanaka, A. Nakagawa, Y. Iwai, M. Inoue and H. Tanaka, J. Antibiot. 35, 256 (1982)
27. S. Aizawa, H. Akutsu, T. Satomi, T. Nagatsu, R. Taguchi and A. Seino, J. Antibiot. 32, 193 (1979)
28. H. Seto, H. Yonehara, S. Aizawa, H. Akutsu, J. Clardy, E. Arnold, M. Tanabe and S. Urano, Symposium Papers 394, 22nd Symposium on the chemistry of natural products. (1979)
29. H. Seto, H. Akao, K. Furihata and N. Ōtake, Tetrahed. Lett. 23, 2667 (1982)
30. Y. Kondo, T. Shomura, Y. Ogawa, T. Tsuruoka, H. Watanabe, K. Totsukawa, T. Suzuki, C. Moriyama, J. Yoshida, S. Inoue and T. Niida, Sci. Reports of Meiji Seika Kaisha 13, 34 (1973)
31. Y. Ogawa, T. Tsuruoka, S. Inoue and T. Inoue, ibid 42 (1973)
32. Y. Miyazaki, C. Hirose, J. Nagatsu and S. Esumi, J. Antibiot. 27, 814 (1974)
33. H. Kinashi, N. Ōtake and H. Yonehara, Tetrahed. Lett. 49, 4955 (1973)
34. M. Mitani, T. Yamanishi, Y. Miyazaki and N. Ōtake, Antimicrob. Agents Chemother. 9, 655 (1976)
35. K. Itagaki, M. Tsubokura and K. Otsuki, The Jap. J. Veter. Sci. 36, 195 (1974)
36. N. Ōtake, H. Nakayama, H. Miyamae, S. Sato and Y. Saito, J. Chem. Soc. Chem. Comm. 590 (1977)
37. A. Imada, Y. Nozaki, T. Hasegawa, E. Mizuta, S. Igarashi and M. Yoneda, J. Antibiot. 31, 7 (1978)
38. G. Nakamura, K. Kobayashi, T. Sakurai and K. Isono, J. Antibiot. 34, 1513 (1981)

BIOLOGICAL ACTIVITIES AND STRUCTURES OF HOST-SELECTIVE PATHOTOXINS

J. M. Daly*, Y. Kono**, Y. Suzuki** and H. W. Knoche*

*Department of Agricultural Biochemistry, University of Nebraska-Lincoln, Lincoln, Nebraska 68583-0718, USA
**Institute of Physical and Chemical Research, Wako-shi, Saitama 351, Japan

Abstract - Examples of host-specific or -selective toxins (HST) in plant diseases are now well-documented by an increasing number of reports. Knowledge of them is important in formulating theories of disease resistance and its genetics. This knowledge has potential importance to pesticide research because selective toxicity with minimal environmental impact is a major goal in the effective use of pesticide. A limiting factor in studies of HST has been lack of knowledge of their structure. In the last 6 years, elucidation of structures of several HST provides an oppotunity for determining mode of action and the basis of specificity.

INTRODUCTION

Host-specific or host-selective pathotoxins (HST) are metabolites, produced by pathogens causing plant disease, which selectively damage only those crop varieties normally susceptible to the pathogens. Consequently, they play unique roles in the outbreak and severity of plant diseases. There is a strong correlation between microbial pathogencity *in vivo* and the production of HST in culture, as well as between disease susceptibility of the host and sensitivity to toxin. This clearly implies a fundamental role for HST in nature. The destructive epidemics of Victoria blight of oats and Southern corn leaf blight in the USA, as well as the epidemics of apple blotch and black spot of pears in Japan, have their origin in the existence of highly potent molecules with remarkable biologic specificity.

Approximately 15 reasonably-documented instances of HST production by fungal, but not bacterial, plant pathogens have been reported since the first widely recognized report in 1947 (1). The role in plant disease of microbial metabolites from cultures long has been controversial. It is interesting that earlier reports of the occurrence of HST were neglected, probably because of general skepticism about the role of toxins in disease in nature. Reports of new instances of HST have increased markedly in the last 10-15 years, partly because of striking economic losses from diseases in which they involved. Equally important, however, is that rapid development of the science of chemical separations has provided fractions of sufficient purity so that the specific toxicity can be evaluated critically. Although the list still is relatively short, it is expected that it will grow rapidly as research expands.

To date, the existence of HST provides the only clear-cut explanation for two major scientific problems: the remarkable specificity inherent in plant disease and its control by single genes (2). Understanding the chemical basis of this specificity can lead to new methods of plant disease control perhaps by novel forms of genetic engineering, rather than traditional breeding. But HST research also may have profound implications for pesticide development, because a central goal of pesticide research is the development of selectivity in toxicity towards only unwanted species in a mixture of species. General knowledge of the chemistry and host-genetics of HST specificity can have major ramifications in meeting this long-term goal. HST may allow immediate practical applications if they can be demonstrated to be involved in diseases of important weed species. Chemical control of weeds by natural, biodegradable compounds should have minimum impact on the physical and biological environment.

OCCURRENCE AND GENETICS OF HOST SPECIFIC TOXINS

HST are known for 6 genera of fungi, but it is interesting that most of the known HST are produced by only two genera: *Helminthosporium* and *Alternaria*. These are *H. victoriae* (HV) on oats; *H. carbonum* (HC) on corn; *H. maydis*, race T (HMT) on Texas male sterile corn; *H. sacchari* (HS) on sugar cane); *A. kikuchiana* (AK) on pear; *A. mali* (AM) on apple. In addition, pathogenic forms of *A. alternata* on tomato (AAL) and strawberry produce HST for their respective susceptible hosts, while pathogenic forms of *A. citri* produces distinct toxins for rough lemon and for mandarin orange. HST with the same specificity as HMT-toxin affecting Texas male sterile corn is produced by a quite distinct genus, *Phyllosticta maydis* (3, 4). Another well-documented HST is PC-toxin from *Periconia circinata* attacking sorghum. Most HST producing fungi are leaf pathogens which cause necrotic or chlorotic lesions or, as with *H. sacchari* and *H. maydis*, runner lesions or leaf blights at considerable distance from the infected site. *H. victoriae* and *P. circinata*, however, infect roots or stems causing seedling wilting and blights. The symptoms characteristic of naturally infected tissue are reproduced by isolated HST. Thus, diseases involving HST cause economic damage which is disproportionate to the actual amount of pathogenic biomass.

The genetics of host susceptibility to, and pathogen production of, HST has scientific, as well as practical, importance. Current theories of the genetics of specific host-pathogen interactions hold that resistance is a unique event caused by a single dominant gene product of the host which interacts with a single dominant gene product for *avirulence* (not virulence) of the pathogen. There are reasons for questioning these assumptions, particularly since the genetics of HST diseases do not follow this pattern. HST are obviously virulence products which are controlled by single genes. Crosses of *H. carbonum* with *H. victoriae* produced progeny in four equal classes for the respective toxins: neither toxin produced; HC-toxin only; HV-toxin only; both toxins produced by a single strain (5). HMT-toxin is under control of at least one gene and we recently have shown that in the absence of this gene no HMT-toxin is produced, even for near-isogenic strains (6). The inheritance of toxin production by the pathogen is dominant, not recessive, as current theory would expect (7). Further, host susceptibility to HST and disease most usually is inherited as a dominant character, suggesting the presence of a unique substance in susceptible plants which are absent in resistant ones. However, definitive answers to these fundamental questions are dependent on knowledge of structure of HST.

Physiologic Effects

HST cause very rapid (several minutes in some instances) on excised tissues of susceptible plants at very low concentrations (10^{-6} to 10^{-9} M). The dysfunctions induced include ion leakage, growth inhibition, inhibition of respiration, photosynthesis and dark CO_2 fixation, accelerated production of ethylene, etc. Generally, a single toxin (for example, HV) will produce all these effects on a susceptible host. In contrast to other HST, AAL-toxin does not induce rapid ion leakage (8) while HC-toxin promotes uptake, particularly of NO_3^- (9).

It should be noted that all cells and tissue of susceptible plants are affected irrespective of function (i.e., roots, seed, etc.) by HST. Thus, inheritance of susceptibility must entail modification of a basic biochemical systems essential to plants. A basic problem that must be resolved is whether the multiple effects observed are the result of disturbance of a single biochemical target or whether there may be several separate targets (i.e., mitochrondria and chloroplasts) in a single cell.

PRODUCTION AND ASSAY

Although HST have been studied extensively since 1950, an understanding of their chemistry has been obtained only since 1975 when, independently, Okuno et al. (10, 11) and Ueno et al. (12, 13) deduced the structure of AM-toxin, an important advance in the study of plant disease. Factors in production and assay apparently have limited progress in structural determinations.

Production

The existence of a HST sometimes can be inferred from biological aspects of a plant disease, but currently it is considered essential to demonstrate selective host toxicity by fractions obtained from cultures of the pathogen. This procedure imposes several restrictions on the search for HST. Artificial conditions may prevent HST production *in vitro*, or else other metabolites and nutrients may mask their presence during assay. Improvement in separation procedures opens the possibility for the analysis of infected tissue itself, or at least, culture filtrates which have undergone some preliminary purification. Another research restriction has been the general belief that still cultures with high ratios of surface to volume were necessary for optimum production, thus requiring long incubation periods for production. Recently, Van Etten and Daly (14) demonstrated that equivalent production of HV- and HMT-toxin could be achieved in 5-6 days of shake or fermentor cultures as in 3-4 weeks of still culture. Further, interfering residual nutrients were much higher in still production. It is logical that in the past, isolation of HST from culture filtrates has been emphasized as opposed to mycelium since, biologically, HST are significant as extracellular pathogen products. However, over 90% of HMT-toxin obtained in cultures resides in mycelium (6) and this was the chief source for analytical studies by Kono et al. (15-18). Dunkle and colleagues (pers. com.) have also found significant amounts of HC-toxin in mycelium.

Assay

Differential inhibition of root growth of susceptible seedlings has been the most widely used bioassay. In our experience, it can be useful as a semi-quantitative screen in preliminary purifications but is laborious and time-consuming (4 to 5 days per assay). Further, this assay requires large amounts of scarce seed stock which has been removed from production because of disease susceptibility. Thus, use of this assay is not suitable for most current purification procedures, such as monitoring column effluents. In studies of HMT-toxin we have used inhibition of either dark or photosynthetic CO_2 fixation of leaf discs (19) or thin leaf slices (20) and have found these processes to be useful for HV (21) and HS (unpubl.) toxins. Their usefulness probably stems from the fact that both processes are finely regulated by pH or proton flux in the cytoplasm. Thus, any cellular damage, regardless of site, might be expected to be rapidly reflected in altered rates of CO_2 fixation by plant tissues. The assay allows a number of samples to be handled in a short time (3-4 hr) with small amounts of tissue (3-4 mg) and small volumes (0.5 ml) of solutions, using disposable containers to minimize contamination. Leakage of ions often is useful (22) for monitoring isolation and purification but requires more time or labor, and ion leakage can be dependent on the status or handling of tissue (23).

CHEMISTRY

Early work on the structures of HV-, HC- and PC-toxins suggested the presence of cyclic peptide bonds, thus opening the possibility that host specificity could be explained in the same familiar chemical domain as does, for example, enyzme specificity. The first complete elucidation of an HST, that of AM-toxin (10-14), strengthened this possibility since it was shown to be a cyclic tetrapeptide (Fig. 1). However, the sequential elucidation of HMT (15-18), AAL (24, 25) and HS (26, 27) toxins (Figs 2-4) revealed that HST comprise a diverse array of unique structures. The most recent addition to the list, HC-toxin (31), also is a cyclic polypeptide (Fig. 5). The early work with HV- and PC-toxins has not resulted in final elucidation of structure, although a recent report by Wolpert and Dunkle (32) indicates that PC-toxin contains only one amino acid (aspartic) and thus may not be a typical polypeptide. Because of their structural diversity, even though produced by single genus (i.e. Helminthosporium), there are few clues from structure to explain specificity or even to suggest the likely targets in susceptible cells.

For most HST, evidence has been obtained for the existence of several molecular species. It is not always clear whether these are natural products or artifacts created during isolation (15). For AM- and HMT-toxins, this does not appear to be the case. Three species have been chemically characterized for AM-toxin (Fig. 1) and they are products which would be expected as a consequence of cell metabolism of the major toxin species. The order of toxicity is AM-I, AM-III, AM-II. In the case of HMT-toxin (Fig. 2), the species obviously arise during biosynthesis since they differ by 2 carbons and the conversion of a single carbonyl to an alcohol function. Usually, 8-10 components (odd-numbered, linear polyketols, ranging from C_{35}-C_{43}) can be separated by TLC. Unlike the AM mixture, all apparently have the same toxicity and specificity. Similarly, AAL-toxin has 4 species with apparently equal toxicity. Fraction TA (24, 25) contains 1-amino-11,15 dimethylheptadeca-2,4,5,13,14-pentol as a mixture of two esters with tricaballylic acid (Fig. 3). The major component, I, (≅60%) is esterified at the C_{13} position and the minor one, II, at C_{14}. Fraction TB consists of two similar aminopentol esters, but the aminopentol lacks the hydroxyl at C_5. The free aminopentol and tricarballylic acid are very much less toxic than the esters (25).

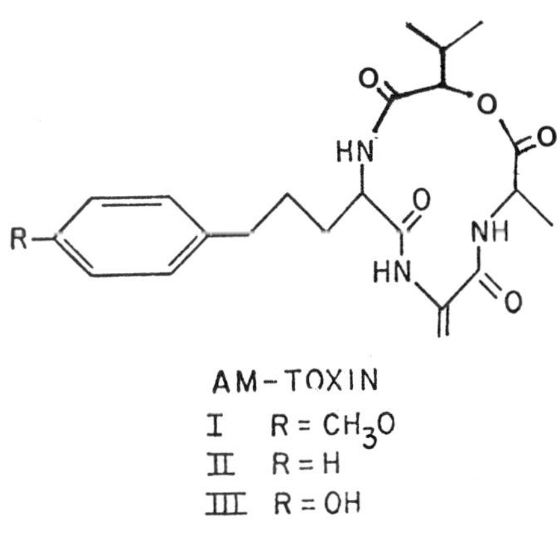

Fig. 1 AM-Toxin. Three molecular species indicated by the appropriate substitution on the aromatic ring.

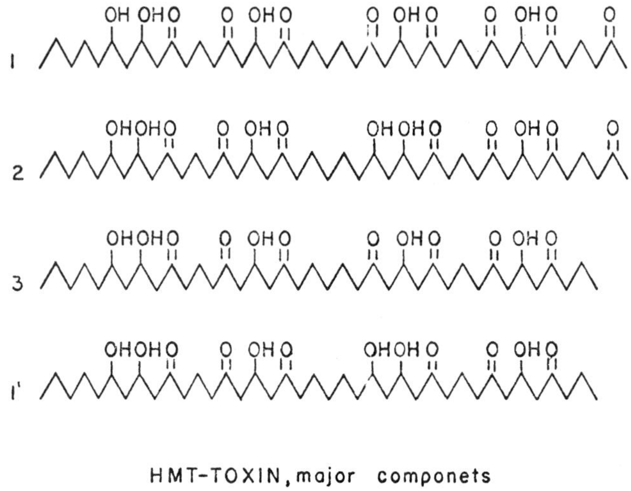

Fig. 2 HMT-Toxin. The four major components of HMT-toxin are shown. The numbers to the left of each structure corresponds to bands observed by thin layer chromatography. Four to six additional molecular species are observed in small quantities.

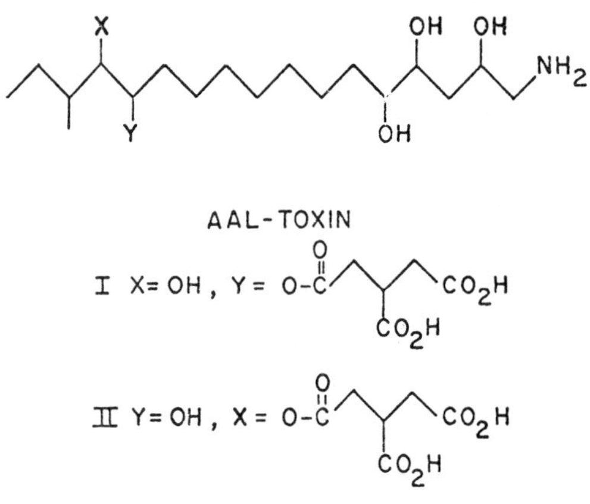

Fig. 3 AAL-Toxin. The two compounds obtained from the TA-fraction of AAL-toxin. The TB-fraction is similar but molecules lack the 5-OH group.

The structure of HS-toxin has been controversial. It was originally proposed to be the monogalactoside of hydroxycyclopropanol (33), but, at best, the evidence indicated only the possible presence of galactose (34). Recently, Livingston and Scheffer (35) reported HS was a pentagalactoside with a terminal sesquiterpene ring (mol wt. 1028). However, the highest m/z observed represented only two galactose units plus $C_{15}H_{21}$. Independently, Macko et al. reported HS-toxin to consist of 3 isomers of mol wt 884. NMR (600 MHZ) studies indicated the structures of Fig. 4 (26, 27). Isomers arise from the location of a double band in the ring. With current isolation methods, the approximate percentages are 56(III), 27(II), 17(I) (Macko, pers. comm.) but their relative biological activities are at present unknown. Purification of HS-toxin led to the interesting finding (35) that culture filtrates of *H. sacchari* also contain a series of related, but non-toxic compounds lacking 1, 2 or 3 galactose moieties. Theoretically, 21 such derivatives are possible and 21 have been observed (Macko, pers. comm.).

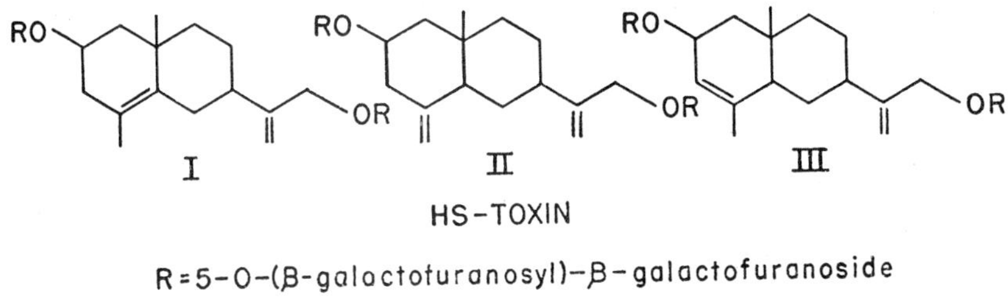

Fig. 4 HS-Toxin. The three isomers of HS-toxin differ only in the position of one double bond.

Pringle and Scheffer (36) first reported isolation from ethanol of crystalline HC-toxin containing several amino acids, including alanine, proline and an amino acid with unusual properties. On the basis of a search of NMR and MS libraries, the group at Michigan State University concluded (28) that the unusual amino acid was 2-amino-9,10-epoxy-8-oxo-decanoic acid (aeo), reported previously in the peptides Cyl-2 (37) and chlamydocin (38). Independently, cooperative work between Purdue University and the University of Nebraska deduced the same structure by decoupling NMR data on HC-toxin and several of its derivatives (30).

For a tetrapeptide of aeo, 2 alanine and 1 proline, there are three possible sequences (Fig. 5). On the basis of EI-MS fragmentation, Leisch et al. believed structure I to be HC-toxin, but rearrangements of cyclic peptides makes sequence assignment by EI-MS equivocable. Hydrolysis of HC-toxin yields ala → ala and pro → ala (not ala → pro) (30, 31). Finally, fast atom bombardment followed by MS-MS analysis (Midwest Regional MS Center, University of Nebraska) demonstrated unequivocally that structure III is correct (30, 31).

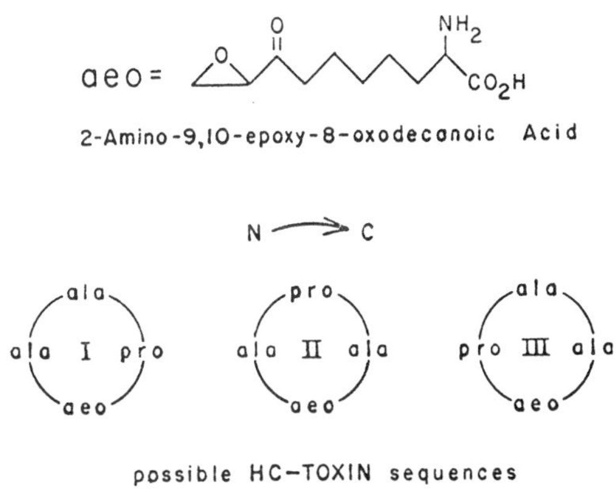

Fig. 5 HC-Toxin. Three possible sequences for HC-toxin are indicated by the cyclic diagram. The direction of the amino group relative to the carbonyl group within an amino acid is clockwise. The structure of an unusual α-amino acid (aeo) is also shown. ala = alanine and pro = proline.

Laboratory Synthesis

Laboratory synthesis of HST should receive more attention in the immediate future for several reasons. Confirmation of structure is one obvious objective. Equally important, synthesis of compounds with the requisitive specificity and toxicity eliminates the possibility that minor contaminants of high biologic activity have not confounded isolation. This is particularly of concern with fungi which produce other minor metabolites of high phytotoxicity. The potent non-specific toxin, tentotoxin, for example, is present in culture filtrates of *A. mali* along with the related AM-toxins. Finally, laboratory synthesis provides an opportunity for extensive structure-activity studies, such as those of Ballio and colleagues and Rich *et al* on the non-specific toxins fusicoccin (39) and tentoxin (41), respectively.

All three AM-toxins have been synthesized and several analogs were tested for biological activity. All analogs were much less active (3-4 fold) than the natural AM-toxins (41). The configuration of HMT-toxin is not usually found in nature because of its length and the presence of oxygen functions which might be expected to result in elimination of H_2O and cyclization to form 5-7 member rings. Suzuki et al (42) used Grignard additions of aldehyde intermediates to di(bromomagnesium) alkanes which resulted in shorter versions (C_{15}-C_{26}) containing the β-polyketol functions of native HMT-toxin (C_{35}-C_{45}). Although synthesis of C_{35}-C_{45} analogs is still underway, the biological activities of the shorter versions is noteworthy (43). Fig. 6 summarizes the activity of analogs on susceptible corn. None were active on resistant corn at concentrations 1000 fold greater (43). Band 3 (Fig. 6) is a natural C_{39} species of HMT-toxin which lacks the terminal methyl ketone of the C_{41} species (see Fig. 1), but which still is as active as the latter (23). Hence, a role for the terminal methyl ketone in either toxicity or specificity can be eliminated. If the native HMT-toxin mixture is reduced by borohydride, there is only a slight loss in toxicity on a weight basis (Fig. 6). The synthetic C_{24} analog (IV) (Fig. 6) is only slightly less active and, suprisingly, a corresponding C_{15} (III) has approximately the same activity as compound IV on a weight basis. It is also interesting that compound I (Fig. 6) is very much less active, suggesting that the terminal ten left carbon atoms of the native toxin, like the methyl ketone at other end of the chain, do not contribute to biological activity. In summary, the β-oxo-oxy-oxo function appears to be the most important one, but on molar basis, chain length appears to make some contribution to toxicity.

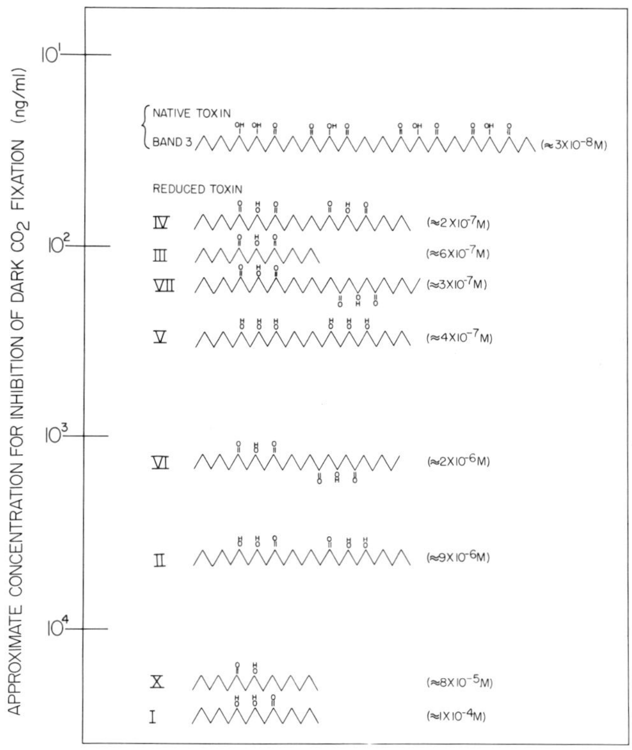

Fig. 6 Structure and activity relationships of one component of HMT-toxin (Native toxin, Band 3) and various synthetic model compounds. The numbers in parentheses indicate the molar concentration of the compound required for 25% inhibition of dark CO_2 fixation.

As far as we are aware, the AM- and HMT-toxins are the only examples of HST for which synthetic analogs have been made. However, the structures of Cyl-2 (37) from *Cylindrocladium scoparum* and chlamadocin (38) from *Diheterospora chlamydospora* have several elements in common with HC-toxin, including the unusual epoxy acid (aeo). In HC-toxin and chlamydocin, the epoxy acid is linked to proline while in Cyl-2 the link is to pipecolic acid, suggesting that the synthetic pathway may be common in a number of fungi. However, HC contains 2 molecules of alanine while Cyl-2 contains methyltyrosine and isoleucine. Phenylanine and α-amino isobutyric acid are the amino acids in chlamydocin. It would be interesting to determine the toxicity and, especially, the specificity of these compounds on corn susceptible to *H. carbonum*.

Biosynthesis

Knowledge of biosynthesis of any HST is lacking so far and no enzymes for their synthesis or degradation have been reported. The lack of knowledge is of some concern because it is logical to assume that biosynthesis of radioactive toxins would provide great advantages in studies of mode of action (i.e. binding) and the fates of HST in resistant, as well as susceptible, hosts. As far as we are aware, there is only one claim (for HS-toxin (44)) that any radioactive plant pathotoxin, either of bacterial or fungal origin, and obtained from biosynthesis has been used to establish a biochemical model of action. This claim has been criticized on a number of grounds (21) and recent studies (45) have failed to confirm the original reports. The central problems in attempting biosynthesis of ^{14}C or ^{3}H HST, are a) the high potencies of pathotoxins and b) the immense dilution of added labelled precursors by the large amounts of organic nutrients (24-37 g/liter) required for good fungal growth and toxin production. For example, HMT is active at approximately 10 ng/ml. To generate statistically sound data for binding studies, a specific activity of 10,000 dpm/ng of HMT-toxin is desirable. This value is only 2 or 3 times less than the specific activity of appropriate, commercially-available labeled precusors, such as acetic acid or glucose. So far, the best ^{14}C-HMT-toxin we have obtained has been 3600 dpm/μg, far below the activity required. This is an additional reason for the need for laboratory synthesis. For HMT-toxin, the data of Fig. 6 is of some interest in this connection. Since compound V is only slightly less toxic than IV, reduction with $Li\,B^{3}H_4$ should lead to biologically active V with a specific activity of greater 20,000 dpm/ng.

MODE OF ACTION

The mode of action of HST has been reviewed in detail recently (21, 45, 46, 47, 48). Although a number of laboratories are actively engaged in such research, we are not aware of any number of recent publications that significantly alter or amplify current theories. Therefore, the following will be only a general summary of these theories.

It is unfortunate that nearly all of the available literature on mode of action of HST preceded the preparation of HST of known purity and structure. It is not possible to know how much the data so obtained were affected by the presence of unrecognized impurities. The presence of impurities in radioactive preparations obtained by biosynthesis make earlier data on HST binding to biochemical targets, or their metabolic fate in tissues, of doubtful significance. It should be noted that much of the literature is devoted to HV-toxin, the first HST discovered in 1947 (1) but still not chemically resolved. Since, 1971, there has arisen considerable literature on HMT-toxin, but most of it before pure preparations were available (15).

With the exception of AAL-toxin, all HST tested appear to cause a change in flux of ions in susceptible, but not resistant, tissues. AM-, HV-, HMT-, PC- and HS-toxins cause efflux of ions. HC causes a initial influx (a), particularly of NO_3^-, but subsequently (24-48 hr) leakage occurs. This has lead to suggestions that the primary site of action for HST is at the plasma membrane. However, definitive biochemical evidence so far is lacking. The most direct evidence is a report that HV-toxin causes rapid bursting (less than 5 minutes) of isolated susceptible protoplasts (49). Indirect evidence consists of the demonstration that ion leakage can be prevented by simultaneous treatment with chemicals presumed to interact with membranes, such as bisulfite, semicarbazide and sulfhydryl reagents. Protection was reversible and led to a postulate that these toxins were interacting with a sulfhydryl-containing membrane protein that was constantly turning over (50).

Another line of evidence advanced to support this picture is the rapid depolarization of plasma membrane by HV-(51), PC-(52) and HMT-(53) toxins and hyperpolarization by HC-(52). However, these early studies should be re-examined because purity of the toxins was not known. A relatively impure preparation of HMT caused rapid depolarization of susceptible cells (53) but pure toxin prepared by the method of Kono and Daly (15) did not produce the same sort of effect (54). Glucose metabolism will cause rapid depolarization of cell membranes and its presence in HST preparations of unknown purity is possible.

The only evidence for a plasma membrane site based on physicochemical methods is that for HS-toxin (44). It was claimed that a toxin-binding protein could be isolated from membrane fractions of susceptible, but not resistant, sugar cane. The protein was thought to be involved in the transport of galactosides (44). The claim has been questioned (21) on several grounds involving the experimental protocols employed. In a recent extension of this work (55), new data are in conflict with the earlier claims. Binding protein was reported from resistant sugar cane, as well species of tobacco and mint. Calculation of the extent of reported binding, however, is unexpectedly high at 4.27 toxin molecules per amino acid residue of protein (21). If such proteins exist in resistant sugar cane, tobacco and mint, it is difficult to see how resistance can be explained on the basis of toxin binding, as originally claimed. A recent, independent study of this problem (45) with purified toxin (35) failed to substantiate the previous claims for HS-toxin binding.

The rapid induction of ion leakage obviously could also be a secondary effect resulting from disturbance of cytoplasmic processes. Dunkle and Wolpert (56) report that symptom production (chlorosis) is independent of the well-documented leakage of ion caused by PC-toxin. Chlorosis develops under conditions where ion leakage is minimal and, conversely, ion leakage can occur in the absence of symptoms. The toxin processes are independent (56). It is not clear, however, whether each process can represent separate sites of action for the PC-toxin.

Where tested, HST will cause inhibition of respiration but usually the inhibition is seen later than other effects, particularly ion leakage. The inhibition of respiration generally has been interpreted as a secondary effect on mitochondria in vivo resulting from plasma membrane damage. As pointed out elsewhere (47), this is a reasonable assumption but not necessarily correct. Better evidence is the fact that mitochondria isolated from susceptible plants are not affected by HV-(57) and PC-(48) toxins.

HMT-toxin, however, causes an apparent uncoupling of mitochondria isolated from susceptible, but not resistant, plants (58). The apparent uncoupling is unusual in that it occurs with certain substrates (NADH), while inhibition of oxidation occurs with others (malate) (59). A mitochondrial target as the primary site is consistent with most, but not all, biological effects of HMT-toxin, but the issue is still unresolved.

It has been argued by Arntzen and colleagues on the basis of indirect evidence that plasma membrane is the primary site for HMT-toxin (60-62). In contrast, damaged mitochondria can be observed in EM photographs of cells without notable damage to the plasma membrane (63). Addition of HMT-toxin to isolated protoplasts in the dark causes a considerable decrease in ATP levels within 30 minutes (64), but this does not happen when protoplasts are kept in the light. The simplest interpretation of these results is that there is an effect only on mitochondria while photosynthesis (i.e., chloroplasts) is unaffected, at least in isolated protoplasts.

The issue is confounded by the fact that HMT-toxin causes necrosis only on leaves exposed to light (19). Further, photosynthetic CO_2 fixation is inhibited, apparently by processes that are separate from other effects (20). This has lead to the suggestion that HMT-toxin may have several independent targets by interfering with energy transduction in membranes (20). Park et al. (65) have also suggested recently that AK-toxin separately affects both chloroplasts and plasma membranes.

The similarities exhibited by most of known HST are not shared by HC-toxin, although it may be affecting membranes (see above), or by AAL-toxin affecting tomato. With AAL-toxin, ion leakage occurs only after several days, when necrosis begins to develop (D. Gilchrist per. comm.). In addition, protection against necrosis was obtained by metabolites associated with aspartate metabolism and pyridine biosynthesis. Preliminary work indicates that the enzyme aspartate transcarbamylase of susceptible, but not resistant, tissues is inhibited in vitro (8). The data are reminescent of the inhibition of ornithine transcarbamylase by the nonspecific bacterial toxin, phaseolotoxin (66).

In summary, the available evidence suggests that HST probably interfere with membrane functions, either at the cell surface or in organelles, except for AAL-toxin. But direct biochemical evidence has not been obtained. This will be possible only when pure HST with suitable radiolabel becomes available.

DISEASE RESISTANCE AND THE NATURE OF HST SPECIFICITY

There are two simple models to explain HST specificity and hence disease resistance. It is possible that HST are metabolized or degraded by resistant tissue. Alternatively, HST may be activated by chemical modification in susceptible, but not resistant, cells. Although attempts have been made to establish the correctness of the first alternative for HV-toxin, the results are ambiguous because of lack of information on structure, which prevents quantitative chemical assessment. For HS-toxin, however, degradation by galactosidases is possible, yielding non-toxic moieties (described above) by cleavage of 1 to 3 galactose units.

As discussed above, the most commonly accepted model holds that specificity is due to the presence in the susceptible cells of a unique site or receptor (i.e., membrane protein) which is not present in resistant cells. There is an additional possibility, however, which has not been considered seriously, but should be in the future. A number of years ago, Wheeler (67) pointed out that both resistant and susceptible cells might contain the same receptor or site, but that resistant tissues had the capacity to heal the initial biochemical lesion caused by HST. The "self-repair" hypothesis could be analogous to the well known "wound" responses of plants to various physical or chemical stress. Evidence for "self-repair" will be difficult to obtain and interpret.

REFERENCES

1. R.P. Scheffer, Physiological Plant Pathology, (C.R. Heitefuss and P.H. Williams, eds) p. 247-269. Springer-Verlag, Berlin (1976).
2. J.M. Daly and I. Uritani (Eds) Recognition and Specificity in Plant Host-Parasite Interactions, Japan Scientific Societies Press, Tokyo.
3. J.C. Comstock, G. A. Martinson and B.G. Gengenback, Phytopathology, 63, 1357-1361 (1973).
4. O.C. Yoder, Phytopathology 63, 1361-1366 (1973).
5. R.P. Scheffer, R. R. Nelson and A.J. Ullstrup, Phytopathology 57, 1288-1291 (1967).
6. K.J. Tegtmeier, J.M. Daly and O.C. Yoder, Phytopathology 72 (In press).
7. J. Leach, K.J. Tegtmeier, O.C. Yoder and J.M. Daly, Physiol. Plant Path. (In press).
8. B.L. McFarland and D.G. Gilchrist, Phytopathology 71, 240 (1981).
9. O.C. Yoder and R.P. Scheffer, Plant Physiol. 52, 513-517 (1973).
10. T. Okuno, Y. Ishita, K. Sawai and T. Matsumoto, Chem. Letts. 635-638 (1974).
11. T. Okuno, Y. Ishita, A. Sugawra, Y. Mori, K. Sawai and T. Matsumoto, Tetrahedron Lett. 5, 335-336 (1975).
12. T. Ueno, Y. Hayashi, T. Nakashima, H. Fukami, S. Nishimia, K. Kohmoto and A. Sekiguchi, Phytopathology 65, 82-83 (1975).
13. T. Ueno, T. Nakashima, Y. Hayashi and H. Fukami, Agr. Biol. Chem. 39, 1115-1122 (1975).
14. J.E. Van Etten and J.M. Daly, Phytopathology, 70, 727-729 (1981).
15. Y. Kono and J.M. Daly, Bioorg. Chem. 8, 391-398 (1979).
16. Y. Kono, S. Takeuchi, A. Kawarada, J.M. Daly and H.W. Knoche, Tetrahedron Letts. 21, 1537-1540
17. Y. Kono, S. Takeuchi, A. Kawarada, J.M. Daly and H. W. Knoche, Agr. Biol. Chem. 44, 2613-2682 (1981a).
18. Y. Kono, S. Takeuchi, A. Kawarada, J.M. Daly and H.W. Knoche, Bioorg. Chem. 10, 206-218 (1981).
19. B.S. Bhullar, J.M. Daly and D.W. Rehfeld, Plant Physiol. 56, 1-7 (1975).
20. J.M. Daly and B. Barna, Plant Physiol. 66, 580-583 (1980).
21. J.M. Daly and H.W. Knoche, Recent Advances in Plant Pathology, (D. Ingram and P.H. Williams, eds.) 1, 83-138 (1982).
22. R.P. Scheffer and R.S. Livingston, Phytopathology 70, 400-404 (1980).
23. G. Payne, H.W. Knoche, Y. Kono and J.M. Daly, Physiol. Plant Pathol. 16, 227-239 (1980).
24. A. Bottini and P.G. Gilchrist, Tetrahedron Letts. 22, 2719-2722 (1981).
25. A. Bottini, J.R. Bowen and P.G. Gilchrist, Tetrahedron Letts. 22, 2723-2726 (1981).
26. V. Macko, K. Goodfriend, T. Wachs, I.A.A. Renwick, W. Acklin and D. Arigoni, Experientia 37, 923-924 (1981).
27. V. Macko, D. Arigoni and W. Acklin, Phytopathology 71, 892 (Abst) (1981).
28. J.M. Liesch, C.C. Sweeley, G.D. Staffeld, M.S. Anderson, D.J. Weber and R. P. Scheffer, Tetrahedron 38, 45-48 (1982).
29. L. Johnson, L.D. Dunkle, M. Pope, H.W. Knoche and J.M. Daly, In preparation.
30. M. Pope, H.W. Knoche, L. Johnson, L. Dunkle and J.M. Daly, In preparation.
31. M. Gross, K. Tomer, F. Crow, D. McCreary, M. Pope and H.W. Knoche, In preparation.
32. T.J. Wolpert and L.D. Dunkle, Phytopathology 70, 872-876 (1980).
33. G.W. Steiner and G.A. Strobel, J. Biol. Chem. 246, 4350-5457 (1971).
34. Y. Kono, H.W. Knoche and J.M. Daly, Toxins in Plant Diseases, (R. Durbin, ed.), p. 221-257, Academic Press, NY (1981)
35. R.S. Livingston and R.P. Scheffer, J. Biol. Chem. 256, 1705-1709 (1980).
36. R.B. Pringle and R.P. Scheffer, Phytopathology 57, 1169-1172 (1967).
37. A. Hirota, A. Suzuki, K. Aizawa and S. Tamura, Agr. Biol. Chem. 37, 955-956 (1973).
38. A. Closse and R. Huguenin, Helvetica Chim. Acta 57, 6061 (1974).
39. A. Ballio, Advances in Pesticide Science (H. Geissbuhler, ed.), p. 366-372, Pergamon Press, Oxford (1979).
40. D.H. Rich, P.K. Bhatnager, R.D. Jasensky, R.D. Steele, T.F. Uchytel and R.D. Durbin, Bioorg. Chem. 7, 207-214 (1978).
41. N. Izumiza, T. Kato, H. Aoyagi, M. Waki and M. Kondo, Synthetic Aspects of of Biologically Active Cyclic Peptides, p. 123-143, Wiley, NY (1979).
42. Y. Suzuki, H.W. Knoche and J.M. Daly, Bioorg. Chem. 11, (In press) (1982).
43. Y. Suzuki, K.J. Tegtmeier, J.M. Daly and H. W. Knoche, Bioorg. Chem. 11, (In press) (1982).
44. G.A. Strobel, J. Biol. Chem. 248, 1321-1328 (1973).
45. M.S. Lesney, R.S. Livingston and R.P. Scheffer, Phytopathology, 71, 889 (1981).
46. O.C. Yoder, Ann. Rev. Phytopathology 18, 103-109 (1980).
47. J.M. Daly, Toxins in Plant Disease, (R. Durbin, ed.), p. 331-394, Academic Press, NY (1981).

48. F. Meehan and H.C. Murphy, Science 106, 270-271 (1947).
49. K.R. Samaddar and R.P. Scheffer, Plant Physiol. 45, 586-590 (1970).
50. J.M. Gardner and R.P. Scheffer, Physiol. Plant Path. 3, 145-157 (1973).
51. A. Novacky and P. Hanchey, Physiol. Plant Path. 4, 161-165 (1974).
52. J.M. Gardner, R.P. Scheffer and N. Higinbotham, Plant Physiol. 54, 246-249 (1975).
53. A. Novacky and A.L. Karr, Regulation of Cell Membrane Activities in Plants, (E. Marre and O. Cifferi, eds.), p. 137-144 (1977).
54. J. Stebbins, A. Novacky and E. Ball, Plant Physiol., (Supp) 67, 76 (1981).
55. D.S. Kenfield and G.A. Strobel, Plant Physiol. 67, 1174-1180 (1981).
56. L.D. Dunkle and T.J. Wolpert, Physiol. Plant Pathol. 18, 315-324 (1981).
57. H. Wheeler and P. Hanchey, Science 154, 1569-1571 (1966).
58. R.J. Miller and D.E. Koeppe, Science 173, 67-69 (1971).
59. G. Payne, Y. Kono and J.M. Daly, Plant Physiol. 65, 785-791 (1980).
60. C.J. Arntzen, D.E. Koeppe, R.J. Miller and J.H. Peverly, Physiol. Plant Path. 3, 79-89 (1973).
61. S.M. Mertz, Jr. and C.J. Arntzen, Plant Physiol. 60, 363-369 (1977).
62. S.M. Mertz, Jr. and C.J. Arntzen, Plant Physiol. 61, 544-548 (1978).
63. H.C. Aldrich, V.E. Gracen, D.W. York, E.D. Earle and O.C. Yoder, Tissue and Cell 9, 167-177 (1977).
64. J.D. Walton, E.D. Earle, O.C. Yoder and R.M. Spanswick, Plant Physiol. 63, 806-810 (1979).
65. P. Park, S. Nishimura, K. Kohmoto, H. Otani and K. Tsujimoto, Can. J. Bot. 59, 301-310 (1981).
66. R.E. Mitchell, Physiol. Plant Path. 14, 1173-1175 (1979).
67. H. Wheeler, Symposium on potential in crop protection, Publication of Cornell Ithaca, NY, p. 9-13 (1969).

LIFE CYCLE REGULATION IN RICE BY ENDOGENOUS PLANT HORMONES

Noboru Murofushi

Department of Agricultural Chemistry, The University of Tokyo, Bunkyo-ku, Tokyo 113, Japan

Abstract - The endogenous gibberellins (GAs) in shoots and ears of the rice plant *Oryza sativa* L., cv. Nihonbare (*japonica*, normal) and cv. Tong-il (a hybrid of *japonica* and *indica*, semi-dwarf), were identified as GA_{19} (major) and GA_1 (minor) by GC-MS, whereas only GA_1 was detected in cv. Tan-ginbozu (*japonica*, semi-dwarf). Marked maxima were observed in the levels of GA_1 and GA_{19} throughout the life cycle of the rice plants, especially in ears at the heading-anthesis stage. The levels of abscisic acid (ABA) in the three cultivars were determined by GC-ECD and a marked maximum was observed in the ears at a ripening stage. The effect of nitrogen fertilizer content on endogenous plant hormones was investigated in Nihonbare: low nitrogen resulted in high ABA and low GA_{19} levels, whereas high nitrogen reversed the levels of ABA and GA_{19}. The endogenous cytokinins in shoots and roots of Nihonbare at a maximal tillering stage were identified as *cis*- and *trans*-zeatin, and *cis*- and *trans*-ribosylzeatin by GC-SIM.

INTRODUCTION

The rice plant is known as one of the most important and productive crops in the world and its life cycle has been extensively investigated from both physiological and agronomical standpoints. However, little is known about the endogenous plant hormones in rice. With the result that the role of endogenous plant hormones in the life cycle of the rice plant has not been clarified. In order to obtain the basic information concerning this problem, we started researches of endogenous plant hormones in rice plants, namely, the identification of the hormones and investigation of the correlation between hormonal levels and physiological phenomena in the life cycle of the rice plant. In addition, the effect of nitrogen status on endogenous levels of plant hormones and growth of rice plants was investigated, because nitrogen content of the fertilizer has a serious effect on the physiology of rice. In this paper, the author summarizes several significant results obtained in the process of the work (1, 2) together with the methodology established for analysis of the endogenous plant hormones.

MATERIALS AND METHODS

Plant materials

Three cultivars of rice plant (*Oryza sativa* L.) were used; cv. Nihonbare (*japonica*, normal), cv. Tan-ginbozu (*japonica*, semidwarf) and cv. Tong-il (a hybrid of *japonica* and *indica*, semi-dwarf, heavy ear). The rice plants were grown in the paddy field of the National Institute of Agricultural Sciences, Konosu, Saitama and growth characteristics were recorded as shown in Table 1 and Fig. 6. Basically, the rice plant has several physiologically important stages, i.e., 3rd-leaf stage (until which plant growth consumes the endosperm), maximal tillering stage, panicle initiation stage (at which internode elongation starts), heading-anthesis stage and maturing stage. The aerial parts were harvested at those stages and ears were harvested several times after heading. In this report, an aerial part means a whole plant without roots, and a shoot means a stem-leaf part. Thus a shoot is the same as an aerial part until an ear grows sufficiently to be cut off with ease.

Extraction

Plant materials harvested were immediately chilled in dry ice-methanol to prevent changes in endogenous plant hormones, especially ABA, and subsequently extracted with methanol using

---

Abbreviations in the text GA, gibberellin; GA_n, gibberellin A_n; ABA, abscisic acid; GC-MS, combined gas-liquid chromatography-mass spectrometry; GC-SIM, combined gas-liquid chromatography-selected ion monitoring; GC-ECD, gas-liquid chromatography using a electron capture detector; HPLC, high performance liquid chromatography; fr wt, fresh weight.

TABLE 1. Characteristics of Nihonbare, Tong-il and Tan-ginbozu (recorded in 1980)

Cultivar		Nihonbare	Tan-ginbozu	Tong-il
Date of panicle initiation		Aug. 4	Aug. 4	Aug. 4
Date of heading		Aug. 22	Aug. 28	Aug. 21
Date of anthesis		Aug. 24	Aug. 30	Aug. 23
Plant height (cm)		114	90	97
Ear length (cm)		21	17	22
Internode length (cm)	I	32	23	38
	II	18	18	11
	III	15	13	11
	IV	8	9	5
Grains/ear		101	84	138
Weight of aerial part (g)		12.3	8.6	17.3
Weight of ear (g)		2.7	2.2	3.6

Internode length I-IV refer to the length of the 1st internode (neck-internode) to the 4th internode. The values such as plant height were those in the final growth stage.

a blender. The methanol extract was concentrated under reduced pressure below 40°C to give an aqueous residue, which was fractionated by solvent partitioning and then subjected to subsequent purification procedures before the analyses of plant hormones, GAs, ABA and cytokinins.

Purification and analysis of plant hormones

Gibberellins. For identification of GAs, an ethyl acetate-soluble acidic fraction was purified by chromatography, monitoring GA activity in each fraction according to Murakami's microdrop method (3) using Tan-ginbozu seedlings. The purified samples were methylated with diazomethane and then trimethylsilylated with bis-*N*,*O*(trimethylsilyl)acetamide-trimethylchlorosilane-pyridine (2:1:1, v/v/v) and analyzed by GC-MS. For quantitative analysis, purified GA_{19} fractions were methylated, trimethylsilylated and subjected to GC-SIM. Quantitative analysis of GA_1 was conducted by the microdrop method with some modifications. Waito-C, a dwarf rice which responds to GA_1 but not to GA_{19}, was used and GA synergist, 4-ethoxy-1-(*p*-tolyl)-s-triazine-2,6-(1H, 3H)-dione, was added to the medium to improve the sensitivity of bioassay (Ref. 4).

Abscisic acid. An ethyl acetate-soluble acidic fraction was purified according to the chromatographic behaviors of authentic ABA and ABA methyl ester. The purified ABA methyl ester fraction was subjected to GC-MS for identification. The quantity of ABA was determined using a gas chromatograph equipped with an electron capture detector, which has high selectivity and sensitivity to ABA methyl ester.

Cytokinins. An aqueous fraction was used for analysis of cytokinins. Purification was performed according to the chromatographic behavior of known cytokinins. *Amaranthus* betacyanin test (5) and soybean callus bioassay were also applied to estimate cytokinin activity in each fraction. Purified cytokinin fractions were trimethylsilylated and subjected to GC-SIM analysis.

The purification and analysis procedures of GAs, ABA and cytokinins in the rice plant are illustrated in Fig. 1 to Fig. 3.

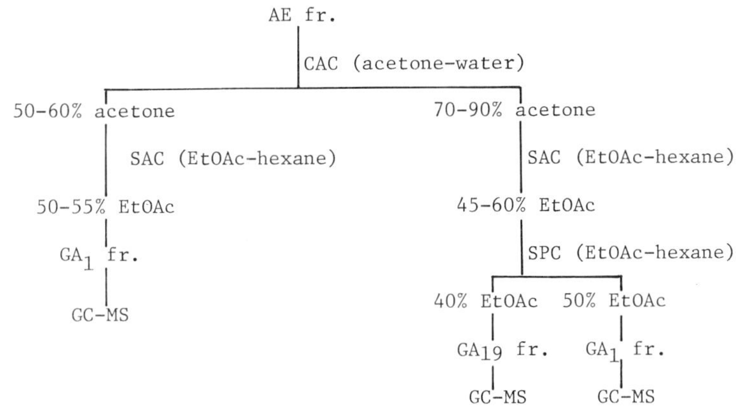

Fig. 1. Purification procedure for identification of GA_1 and GA_{19}. GA fractions were methylated and trimethylsilylated prior to GC-MS analysis. AE fr., ethyl acetate-soluble acidic fraction; CAC, charcoal adsorption column chromatography; SAC, silicic acid adsorption column chromatography; SPC, silicic acid partition column chromatography; EtOAc, ethyl acetate.

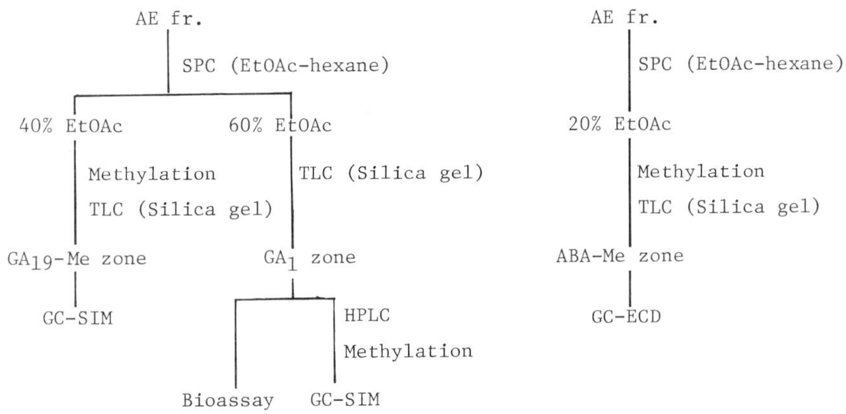

Fig. 2. Purification procedures for quantitative analysis of GA_1, GA_{19} and ABA. Purified samples of GA methyl esters were trimethylsilylated prior to GC-SIM. GA_1-Me, GA_1 methyl ester; TLC, thin layer chromatography.

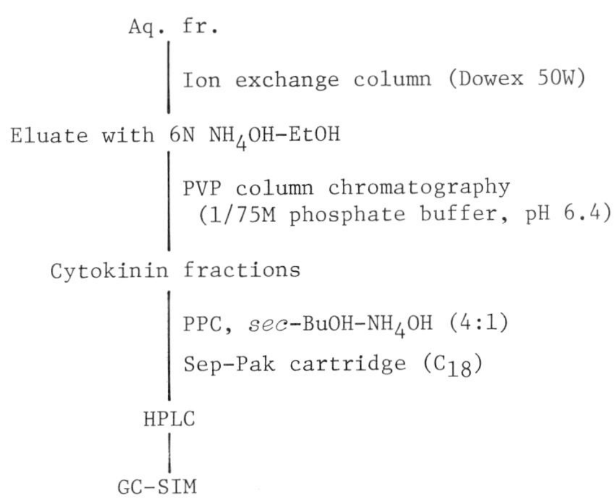

Fig. 3. Purification and identification procedure for cytokinins. Trimethylsilylation was done prior to GC-SIM. PPC, paper chromatography; PVP, insoluble polyvinylpyrrolidone.

RESULTS AND DISCUSSION

Identification of endogenous plant hormones

Gibberellins. The extract obtained from shoots of Nihonbare (9 kg, fr wt) at maximal tillering stage was purified and analyzed by GC-MS, indicating the presence of GA_{19} as a major GA. The identification of GA_{19} in shoots or ears at other stages or in other cultivars was performed by GC-SIM, monitoring the significant peaks in the mass spectrum of methylated trimethylsilylated GA_{19} (m/z 432, 402 and 374). The occurrence of a small amount of GA_1 in shoots and ears in Nihonbare was shown by GC-SIM; no other GAs have been detected in Nihonbare. The same result was obtained in Tong-il. However, Tan-ginbozu was different from the other two. Only GA_1 was identified in the extract from ears but GA_{19} was not detected either in shoots or in ears.

Abscisic acid. ABA was identified easily, compared with other plant hormones, by GC-MS and it was capable of being detected with high sensitivity by GC-ECD. A 10-30 grams of fresh materials was enough for the identification and quantitative analysis of ABA.

Cytokinins. Analysis of endogenous cytokinins was rather difficult. Based on the results of bioassay and chromatographic behaviors of standard cytokinins, several fractions obtained from about 1 kg of plant material were purified by chromatography. As a result, *cis*- and *trans*-zeatin and *cis*- and *trans*-ribosylzeatin were identified in the fractions obtained from aerial parts of Nihonbare at the maximal tillering stage. Other cytokinins, such as isopentenyl adenine, isopentenyladenosine, zeatin ribotide and zeatin glucoside, dihydrozeatin and its conjugates, were either not detected or not pursued for identification due to their low contents and low activity.

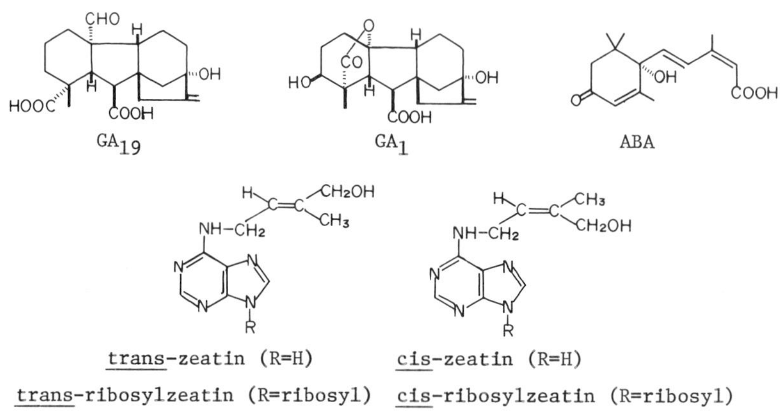

Fig. 4. Identified plant hormones in the rice plant

Seasonal changes of gibberellins and abscisic acid

Gibberellins. The change in GA_{19} level in shoots and ears throughout the life cycle of Nihonbare is shown in Fig. 5: GA_{19} in shoots increases to a peak (ca. 10 μg/kg fr wt) at the tillering stage and decreases rapidly to the heading stage, while the peak level of GA_{19} in ears was observed at the heading-anthesis stage (ca. 15 μg/kg fr wt). Based on the above result, the survey of GA levels in relation to internode elongation and ear development-seed maturation was carried out for the three cultivars, starting from a maximal tillering stage to a full ripening stage. Figs. 6-a and 6-b show the seasonal changes of GA_1 and GA_{19} in Nihonbare and Tong-il, respectively. In shoots of Nihonbare, the level of GA_{19} was high (11.7 μg/kg fr wt) at the beginning of July (maximal tillering stage), then steadily decreased to the panicle initiation stage (ca. 5 μg/kg fr wt). This level was maintained for about 20 days. Two days after heading, GA_{19} was hardly detectable in shoots. In ears of Nihonbare, GA_{19} increased remarkably three days before anthesis, reached the highest level at anthesis (14 μg/kg fr wt) and then rapidly declined to a very low level. The seasonal changes of GA_1 was determined by bioassay, which showed that the pattern of GA_1 fluctuation was similar to that of GA_{19} in both shoots and ears, except that the level of GA_1 was much lower than that of GA_{19}. Early in July, the GA_1 level in shoots (1.6 μg/kg fr wt) decreased steadily. A small peak in GA_1 level was observed at the anthesis stage and after that no GA_1 was detected. In ears, the amount of GA_1 at the anthesis stage reached a maximum which was half that of the GA_{19} level at the same stage.

The changes in GA levels in Tong-il differed somewhat from those in Nihonbare. In shoots,

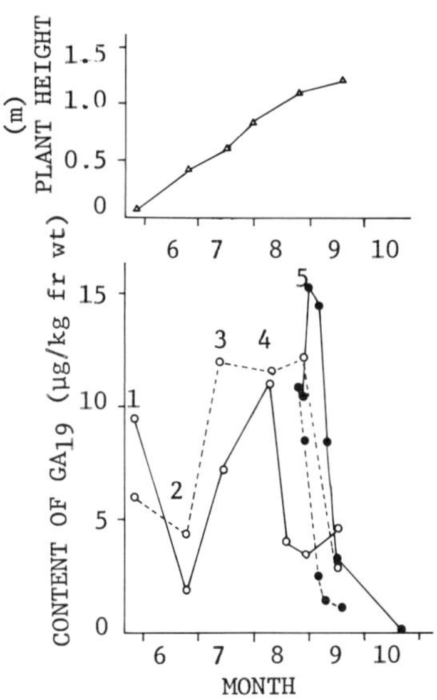

Fig. 5. Seasonal changes of GA_{19} content in Nihonbare. 1, 3rd-leaf stage; 2, 6th-leaf stage; 3, maximal tillering stage; 4, panicle initiation; 5, heading-anthesis; solid curves, record in 1976; broken curves, record in 1977; -o-, GA_{19} in shoots; -•-, GA_{19} in ears.

the GA_{19} level was always lower (ca. 1 μg/kg fr wt) than that in Nihonbare until anthesis and after that GA_{19} was hardly detected. In ears, the change of GA_{19} level was similar to that of Nihonbare. The amount of GA_{19} reached a maximum (15 μg/kg fr wt) at anthesis and rapidly decreased to a very low level within two weeks. The change of the GA_1 level was similar to that of Nihonbare except that the amount in shoots of Tong-il reached maximum in the middle of July.

A very big difference in GAs between Tan-ginbozu and the other two cultivars is observed in that GA_{19} is not detected in shoots or ears of Tan-ginbozu (below ca. 10 ng/kg fr wt) at any stages examined, whereas GA_1 was found and the fluctuation of its level in ears was similar to those of two other cultivars, as shown in Fig. 6-c. However, the GA_1 level in Tan-ginbozu was lower than those in Nihonbare and Tong-il, the maximum in the ears at anthesis being about one fifth of those in the other two cultivars.

GA_{19} shows only a weak growth-promoting activity on Waito-C (dwarf rice), in which the conversion of GA_{19} to GA_1 is supposed to be genetically blocked. On the other hand it promotes the growth of Nihonbare and Tan-ginbozu in which the conversion of GA_{19} to GA_1 probably takes place. By contrast, GA_1 promotes the growth of all three cultivars. This evidence indicates that GA_{19} itself is an inactive GA in the rice plant regardless of its relatively high content, while GA_1, which is a minor GA, may function as an active GA. The striking change in the level of GA_{19} during the life cycle of the rice plant together with the low activity of GA_{19} indicate that GA_{19} may function as a "pool GA". The active GA, possibly GA_1, may actually regulate the growth and development of the plant and its content is regulated by the rate of biosynthesis of GA_{19} and of its metabolic conversion to GA_1.

Although both Tan-ginbozu and Tong-il are dwarf, the patterns of their endogenous GAs are quite different. Basically, the patterns of seasonal changes in GAs in Tong-il are similar to those of Nihonbare, but low content of GA_{19} in shoots may be correlated to its dwarf character. In contrast, the lack of GA_{19} and very low level of GA_1 in Tan-ginbozu can be correlated with its dwarfism. It has been believed that dwarfism in some cultivars, e.g. Tan-ginbozu, might be caused by blocking the biosynthetic pathway of GAs which are under genetic control. The evidences obtained in our experiments indicate that some dwarf cultivars can produce GA(s) although their levels are much lower than those in normal ones.

It is quite interesting to note that high content of GA_1 and GA_{19} in ears at the anthesis stage was observed. This suggests that GAs play some important role in regulation not only of vegetative growth but also of reproductive growth.

Abscisic acid. Quantitative changes in the ABA level showed very similar patterns in the three cultivars. As shown in Fig. 7, their levels were very low (below 10 μg/kg fr wt) in shoots through July and August, which corresponded to the period of internode elongation. In ears, the levels increased rapidly to reach maxima (ca. 250 μg/kg fr wt) 10-15 days after

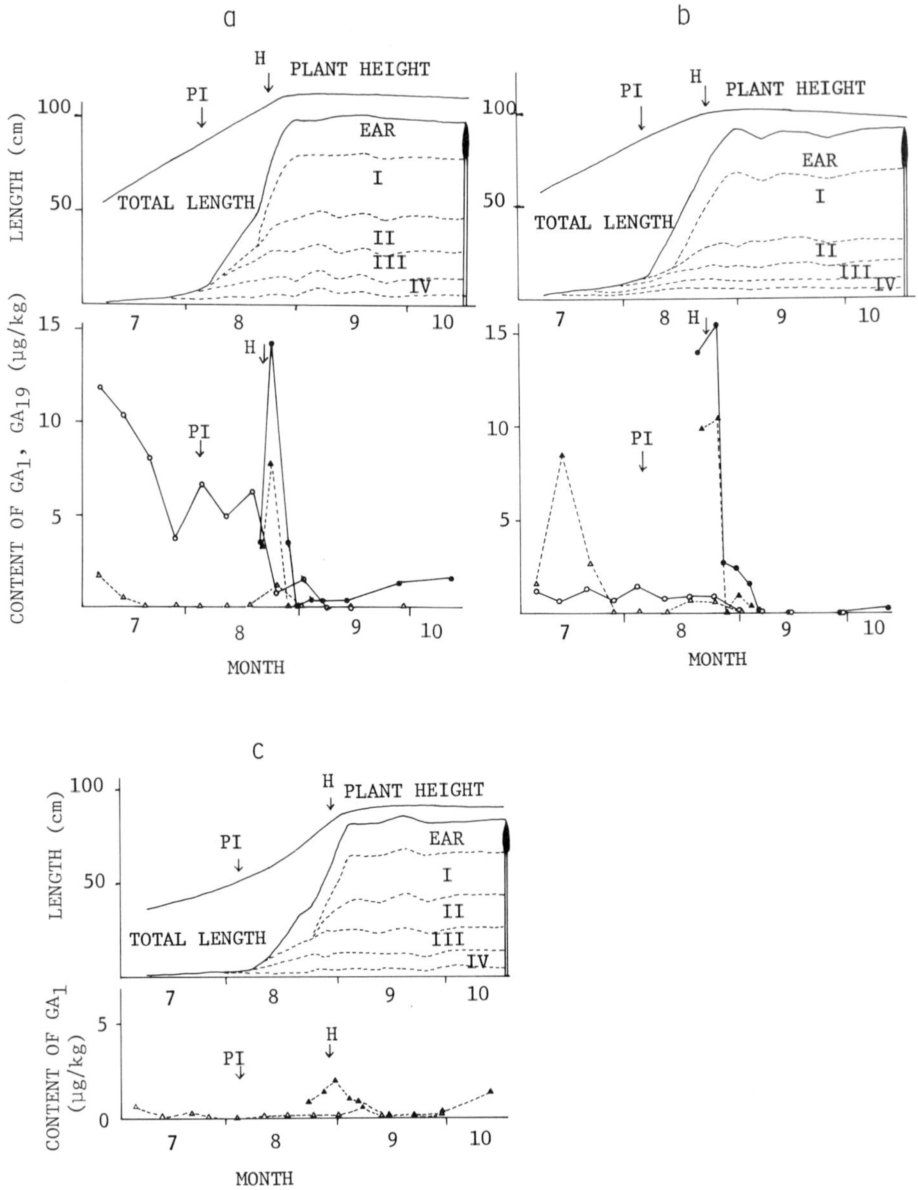

Fig. 6. Growth patterns and seasonal changes of GA_1 and GA_{19} of Nihonbare (6-a), Tong-il (6-b) and Tan-ginbozu (6-c). I, II, III and IV in growth patterns mean 1st, 2nd, 3rd and 4th internode, respectively. PI, panicle initiation; H, heading; —o— , GA_{19} content in shoots; —●—, GA_{19} content in ears; ---△---, GA_1 content in shoots; ---▲---, GA_1 content in ears.

anthesis and then decreased to about 50% of the maxima in the maturation stage. After full maturation, the ABA level was maintained at a fairly high level, being different from the GA level in ears. The only difference among the three cultivars was that ABA levels in both shoots and ears of Tong-il and Tan-ginbozu were a little higher than that in Nihonbare. This result suggests that dwarfism in Tan-ginbozu and Tong-il could be only partially related to the ABA content in shoots. The high content of ABA in ears and its dramatic change in heading-full ripening stage suggest that ABA plays an important role in the regulation of seed dormancy and ripening, as has been discussed in the context of wheat grain maturation by King (6) and Radley (7).

Effect of nitrogen fertilizer on endogenous plant hormones

It is known that rice plants show active elongation under nitrogen rich cultivation conditions. To clarify the relation between nitrogen content in applied fertilizer to paddy field and growth of rice plants, the following investigation was carried out. Nihonbare was grown in paddy fields under various conditions of nitrogen content ranging from 0 to

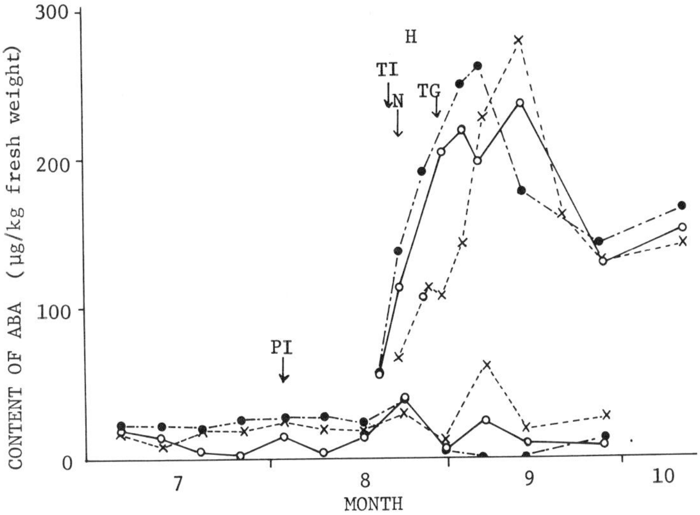

Fig. 7. Seasonal changes of ABA contents in Nihonbare, Tong-il, and Tan-ginbozu. Upper, in ears; lower, in shoots; -o- , Nihonbare (N); -·-●-·-, Tong-il (T); ---x--- , Tan-ginbozu (TG).

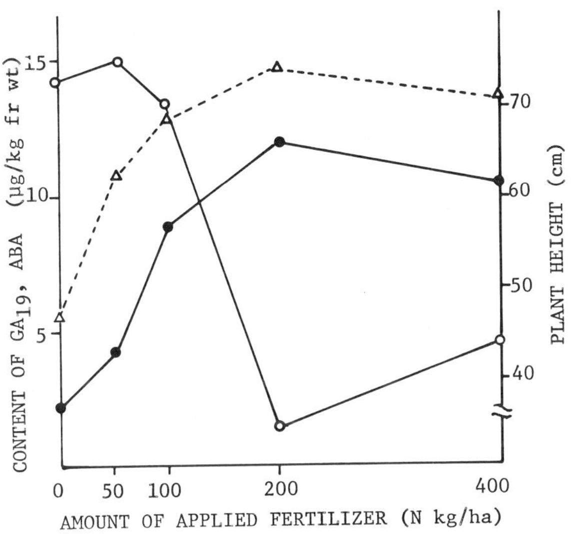

Fig. 8. Effect of nitrogen fertilizer condition on the elongation and the levels of GA_{19} and ABA in Nihonbare. -o-, GA_{19}; -●-, ABA;---Δ---, plant height.

400 kg/ha. The aerial parts were harvested at the maximal tillering stage and the contents of GA_{19} and ABA were determined. As shown in Fig. 8, low GA_{19} level and high ABA level were observed under cultivation condition with low nitrogen content, where the growth of the rice plant was suppressed. On the other hand, increase of nitrogen content caused an increase of the GA_{19} level and decrease of ABA level, where the growth of rice plant was considerably promoted. Further, the excess nitrogen content caused a small suppression of elongation, and this is attributable to the GA_{19} level reaching the upper limit together with the increase in ABA level. A similar result was obtained in Tong-il. These findings suggest that the growth of the rice plant under various cultivation conditions, especially in respect to applied fertilizer, is related to the change of endogenous plant hormonal levels and, as a result, to promotion or suppression of elongation.

As indicated in our studies on the rice plant, this type of investigation affords very valuable information on the relation in higher plants between the change of endogenous hormonal levels and physiological phenomena. On the basis of this information, new techniques might be developed to regulate the growth and development of cultivated plants and to enhance their productivity by exogenous application of chemicals in the agricultural field.

Acknowledgements. - The author express his thanks to Professor N. Takahashi, Dr. S. Kurogochi, Mr. Y. Suzuki and Miss M. Takagi, The University of Tokyo, and Dr. Y. Ota, National Institute of Agricultural Sciences, for their cooperation throughout this work.

REFERENCES

1. S. Kurogochi, N. Murofushi, Y. Ota and N. Takahashi, Planta, 146, 185-191 (1979).
2. Y. Suzuki, S. Kurogochi, N. Murofushi, Y. Ota and N. Takahashi, Plant Cell Physiol., 22, 1085-1093 (1981).
3. Y. Murakami, Bot. Mag. Tokyo, 81, 33-43 (1968).
4. Y. Sato, H. Yamane, N. Takahashi and M. Ogawa, Plant Cell Physiol., 22, 1603-1606 (1981).
5. N.L. Biddington and T.H. Thomas, Planta, 111, 183-186 (1973).
6. R.W. King, Planta, 132, 45-51 (1976).
7. M. Radley, J. Exp. Bot., 32, 129-140 (1981).

ENDOCRINE STRATEGIES FOR INSECT CONTROL

William S. Bowers

Department of Entomology, NYSAES, Cornell University, Geneva, New York, USA

Abstract - Analogs of the insect juvenile hormone III have been successfully applied to the control of several species of insects which are pestiferous in the adult stages. These include insects of economic importance to man and to domestic animals such as mosquitos, manure breeding flies and fleas. However, the juvenile hormone analogs are ineffective for the control of the immature stages of insects which are most important in agriculture through their feeding damage to crops. Thus by the time the juvenile hormone analogs can be effective, the immature stages have already completed their feeding damage. It seemed to me that a method of interfering with the biosynthesis, secretion, or action of the juvenile hormone would be a very useful method of insect control against insects which do their damage as feeding immature stages. Whereas a number of insect hormone mimics have been discovered in plants it seemed possible that plants might be a useful resource to investigate for insect hormone antagonists. Since the juvenile hormones control immature development and adult reproduction, I believed that a juvenile hormone antagonist would be a more suitable endocrine strategy for the control of insects of importance in agriculture. We searched for and discovered two naturally-occurring anti-juvenile hormonal compounds in plants. These anti-hormones (precocenes) induce a lethal, precocious metamorphosis in the immature stages of many insects and also sterilize the adult females.

Through structure optimization, mode of action and metabolism studies, we have found that the precocenes undergo a lethal activation within the corpora allata into selective cytotoxic agents which destroy the endocrine gland. These studies have revealed that the precocenes are acting as suicide substrates for specific enzymes in the insect corpus allatum which is the gland responsible for juvenile hormone production. With the precocenes as a model, we have synthesized additional suicide substrates which are also activated by the same or similar enzymes in the corpus allatum into allatotoxic agents. These and similar approaches may provide new selective biorational methods of insect control.

INTRODUCTION

The use of insecticides to control insect pests of agriculture and vectors of disease has been outstandingly successful. Nevertheless, many important insect pests have become resistant to certain insecticides, while other insecticides have been restricted or eliminated due to our discovery of their environmental hazards. Although many non-chemical techniques are being developed to protect our crops and public health from insects, none are sufficiently successful to eliminate the need for new insecticides. The discovery of drawbacks to certain insecticides has prompted agricultural and public health scientists to reconsider the criteria which must be applied to the development of future insecticides. It is anticipated that insecticides whose mode of action takes advantage of a biochemical, physiological or behavioral difference between vertebrates and invertebrates is highly desirable and, although the development of resistance by insects to chemical methods of control is a fact of natural selection, it is entirely possible that the development of resistance to chemicals affecting fundamental biochemical, physiological or behavioral processes will be very slow. The discovery of insect hormones and their regulation of insect growth, development, reproduction, diapause and behavior provided the first opportunity for agricultural and public health scientists to develop control strategies based upon intrinsically nontoxic chemicals. The following will summarize the development of endocrine strategies for insect control.

JUVENILE HORMONES

Discovery of the insect juvenile hormones

For purposes of insect control the most studied insect hormones are the juvenile hormones. Ito (1) suggested that the corpora allata of *Bombyx mori* might be an endocrine gland. Later Weed-Pfeiffer (2,3) removed the corpora allata from adult grasshoppers and demonstrated that ovarian growth was inhibited. This gave evidence that the corpora allata were involved in stimulating ovarian development. Wigglesworth (4) demonstrated that the corpora allata were necessary for the development of the ovaries in *Rhodnius*. Thomsen (5) related the histological development of the corpora allata with the period of oogenesis in flies and found that extirpation of the corpora allata prevented yolk formation. These experiments repeated over and over in a variety of insects demonstrated that a hormone was produced in the insect corpus allatum which controlled development of the ovaries. Wigglesworth (6) showed that decapitation of immature *Rhodnius* resulted in premature metamorphosis, and when corpora allata of young nymphs were transplanted into last stage nymphs, at the next molt, giant supernumerary nymphs resulted instead of adults. These experiments demonstrated that the corpora allata of immature insects produce a hormone which acts to maintain the immature status, and accordingly this hormone came to be called the juvenile hormone. Many other functions of the juvenile hormone are now well established (Table 1).

Table 1. Principle functions of juvenile hormones

1.	Morphogenesis: Controlled through the regulation of cellular differentiation
2.	Reproduction: Serves as a gonadotropic hormone in females.
3.	Diapause: Regulated by the presence or absence of JH, and in certain species by a specific titer.
4.	Behavior: Regulates production of sex and aggregation pheromones
5.	Caste Formation: Determines morphogenetic and behavioral divisions in many social insects.

Williams (7) found that the ethereal extract of the male Cecropia moth abdomen would prevent the metamorphosis of a variety of insects by topical application or injection into the penultimate stages. It was soon discovered that the hormonally active Cecropia extract would substitute for an active corpus allatum (8). The demonstration by Williams of the juvenile hormone activity in the Cecropia extract by its interruption of normal development, stimulated scientists throughout the world to consider the possibility of using an insect hormone to control insects by interfering with a specific physiological process rather than poisoning with an indifferent protoplasmic toxin.

Chemistry of insect juvenile hormones and the development of juvenile hormone analogs

The excitement generated by Williams' discovery was followed by an intense period of investigation into the chemistry of the juvenile hormones. Although isolation of the natural hormones began soon after Williams' discovery, important chemical information came from a number of sources. Schmialek (9) extracted the faeces of *Tenebrio* and identified two compounds which possessed juvenile hormone activity. These were farnesol and farnesal. Derivatives of farnesol (10), especially its methyl ether and diethyl amine (Fig. 1), were found to be even more active than the isolated compounds, presumably due to their resistance to metabolism within the insect.

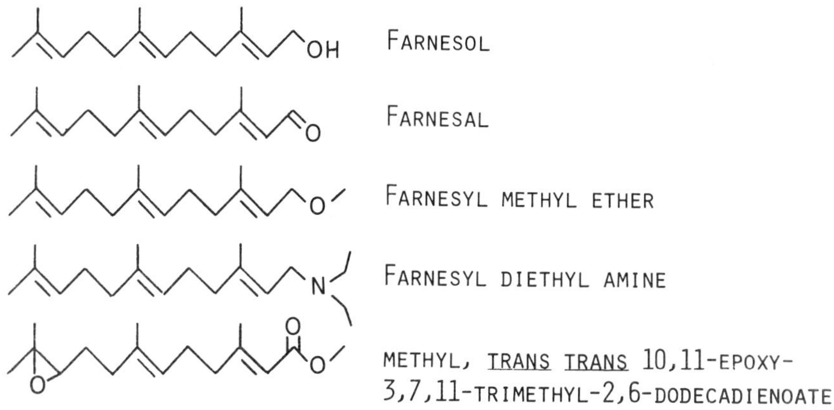

Fig. 1. Natural and synthetic chemicals with juvenile hormone activity.

In my laboratory I began structural modification studies of farnesol to determine the elements of this molecule which were necessary for activity. I found that the hexahydrofarnesol and its methyl ether were quite active and even certain simple saturated alcohols and their methyl ethers were also active, especially dodecyl methyl ether (11). Continuing these studies, and probing the nature of the active substance(s) in the male Cecropia extract I was able to determine enough of the chemical and biological properties of the juvenile hormones to permit the synthesis of trans,trans-10,11-epoxy methyl farnesenate (Fig. 1) which I found to be extremely active in all biological assay systems for juvenile hormone. Since all of the chemical and biological characteristics of this compound seemed to be virtually identical to that of the active substance(s) in the Cecropia extract I predicted that, "this compound will be found to be very similar chemically to the natural hormone when the latter is isolated and characterized" (12). Seven years later Judy et al. (13) demonstrated the authenticity of this compound as a natural juvenile hormone, and it is now clear from numerous studies that this juvenile hormone (Fig. 2, JH III) is the predominant one in insects. Subsequently, Roller et al. (14) and Meyer et al. (15) identified the two juvenile hormones in the Cecropia extract as homologous hormones, and they were called respectively juvenile hormone I and II (Fig. 2).

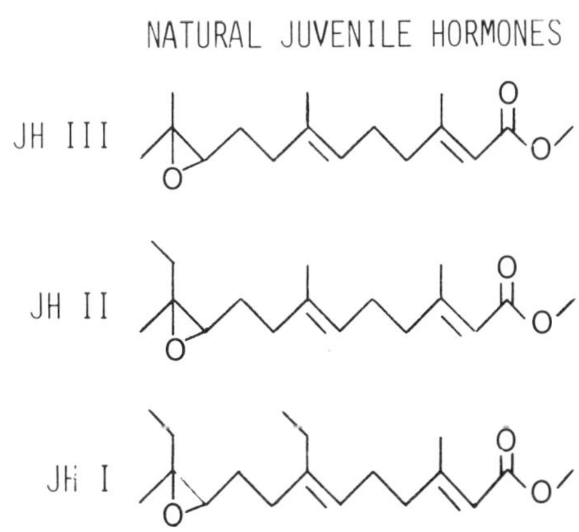

Fig. 2. Natural juvenile hormones.

Although the natural juvenile hormones could be demonstrated to interfere with normal morphogenesis during the ultimate stages of metamorphosis, they were discovered to be very labile in the environment and to be broken down by many insects very quickly. Recognizing that the instability of the juvenile hormones would prevent their application to insect control I tried to stabilize them and increase their activity through the use of insecticide synergists, which are known to protect many insecticides from metabolism.

SYNERGISM EXPERIMENTS	JH ACTIVITY (TENEBRIO TEST)
JH III + SESAMEX	++++
CONTROLS	
JH III	+++
SESAMEX	+

Fig. 3. Discovery of the juvenile hormone activity of an insecticide synergist.

Experiments detailed in Fig. 3 revealed that although a combination of juvenile hormone III and the insecticide synergist sesamex resulted in activity greater than could be anticipated for the hormone alone, control experiments demonstrated that sesamex possessed some juvenile hormone activity. Subsequently several other synergists, both natural and synthetic, were found to possess juvenile hormone activity (Fig. 4, 16).

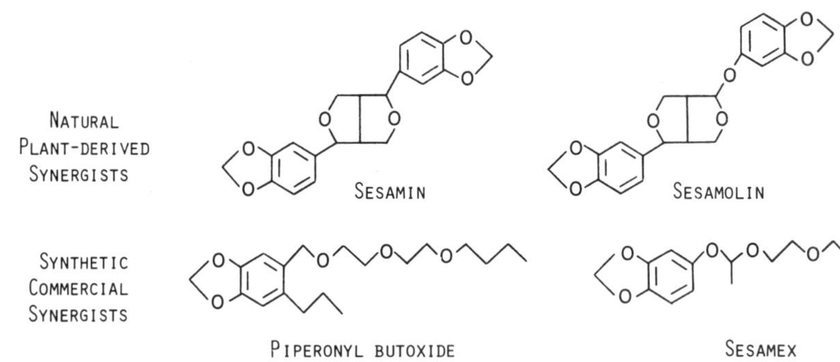

Fig. 4. Natural and synthetic synergists with juvenile hormone activity.

These startling developments suggested that a variety of compounds with little or no relationship chemically to the natural hormones could show juvenile hormone activity. The synthetic synergists, piperonyl butoxide and sesamex, could be imagined to resemble portions of the juvenile hormone molecule and accordingly some derivatives combining features of the synergists and the natural hormones were prepared. Fig. 5 shows the combination of the methylenedioxyphenyl portion of the synergists united with the epoxyfarnesol chain *via* an ether linkage and the resulting increase in activity obtained. Further synthetic optimization of these compounds resulted in the preparation of several hybrid hormone analogs with biological activity and chemical stability much higher than the natural hormones themselves (17-21). These represented the first aromatic compounds with juvenile hormone activity. A great deal of subsequent work in industry resulted in numerous other highly active aromatic analogs. Direct modification of the precursor of juvenile hormone III resulted in some extraordinarily active juvenile hormone analogs especially by the hydrochlorination of methyl farnesenate prepared by Law et al. (22) and Romanuk et al. (23).

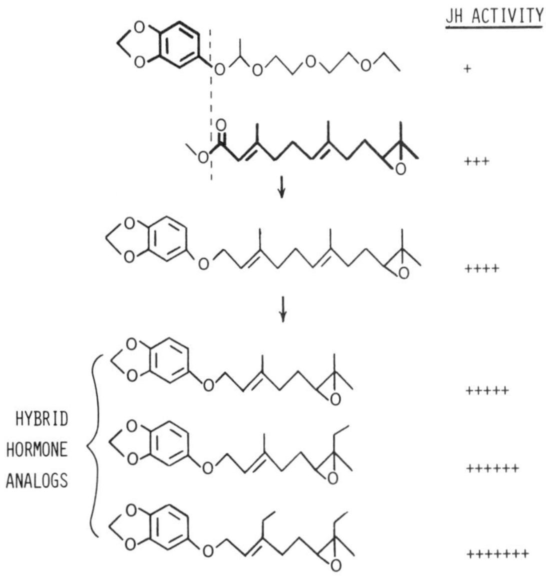

Fig. 5. Chemical hybridization of juvenile hormone III with the insecticide synergist sesamex.

<u>Benefits and deficiencies of juvenile hormone derived insect control agents</u>
A number of stabilized juvenile hormone analogs received extensive testing against agricultural insects and many insect disease vectors. Although the biological activity of the analogs could readily be demonstrated in crop destroying tests, their use did not prevent damage to the crops. In most agricultural situations it is the immature insect stages which do damage through their feeding. Treatment of crops with juvenile hormone analogs could be shown to inhibit normal development of insects and eventually result in their death, but the lethal action of excess juvenile hormone affects only the ultimate stages of development when the insect is undergoing metamorphosis. Thus, the effectiveness of these hormones comes too late to protect the crop from feeding damage. In some cases the hormone forced the pest insect into an extra immature molt resulting in a larger supernumerary stage, which although it never reached adulthood continued to feed and damage the crop far longer than it would have without exposure to excess juvenile hormone. In the latter case, damage to the agricultural crop was even greater than would have occurred without any treatment. The use of juvenile hormone analogs in plant protection is very clearly limited. On the other hand, many insect vectors of disease, which are important during the adult stage, are easily controlled by juvenile hormone analogs. Mosquitoes have been shown to be very sensitive to a variety of hormone mimics and Zoecon Corporation concentrated their efforts on the development of hormone analogs for the control of mosquito larvae. They have successfully developed and marketed an analog of juvenile hormone III which is called "ALTOSID" or methoprene (24). A second analog "ENSTAR" has now been registered for the control of certain greenhouse insects (Fig. 6).

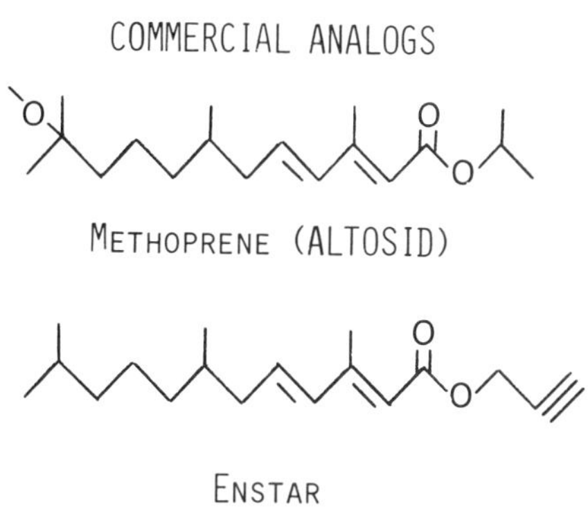

Fig. 6. Registered commercial products based upon juvenile hormone.

Table 2 summarizes the commercial products based on juvenile hormone analogs and their targeted species.

Table 2. Commercial products based on JH analogs

Pest species	JH analog	Product name
Mosquitoes	Methoprene	ALTOSID
Manure breeding flies	"	"
Cigarette beetle	"	KABAT
Pharaoh ant	"	PHAROGONE
Fungus gnat	"	APEX
Fleas	"	PRECOR
Greenhouse Homoptera	Enstar	ENSTAR

ANTI-JUVENILE HORMONES

Rationale for insect juvenile hormone antagonists

The discovery and application of the juvenile hormones to insect control represents an important break with traditional methods of insecticide development, where indifferent toxicants were discovered from the screening of miscellaneous industrial byproducts. The development of insect growth regulators which are intrinsically non-toxic even to insects, but which interrupt specific aspects of their development can be seen originating as fruits of fundamental biological and biochemical research. The safety and specificity of the hormone analogs is very encouraging and has set a precedent to which future efforts can be compared. Notwithstanding the useful actions of juvenile hormone analogs to control public health pests, the lack of utility in plant protection as noted above stimulated new thinking about alternative endocrine related strategies for the control of the immature stages whose feeding damage is most important in agriculture. Early studies in insect physiology, principally those of Bounhiol (25) and Fukuda (26), demonstrated that extirpation of the corpora allata from early larval stages of the commercial silkworm, Bombyx mori resulted in precocious metamorphosis of these tiny larvae into minature adults. These results demonstrated that the induced absence of juvenile hormone during an early insect developmental stage could be followed by premature adult development. Since the immature stages of insects are the agriculturally important ones, some method of preventing the biosynthesis, secretion or action of the juvenile hormones would stop the development of the damaging stages and induce them to undergo precocious maturation. Since the juvenile hormone is also necessary for the development of ovaries in most insects, reproduction would be impossible. Clearly a chemical method of allatectomy would be a superior approach to insect control in agricultural situations. Since compounds with insect juvenile and molting hormone activity had been discovered in plants (27,28,29) I wondered if plants might also have developed strategies to interfere with the production of juvenile hormone. Accordingly, I began to extract plants and test the extracts against insects, assaying in a variety of biological tests for the induction of precocious metamorphosis and/or sterilization. Eventually, I found such activity in the organosoluble extract of the plant Ageratum houstonianum. By contact, feeding or fumigation with these compounds a variety of paurometabolous insects would undergo precocious metamorphosis, eliminating several of their immature stages, and adults were sterile.

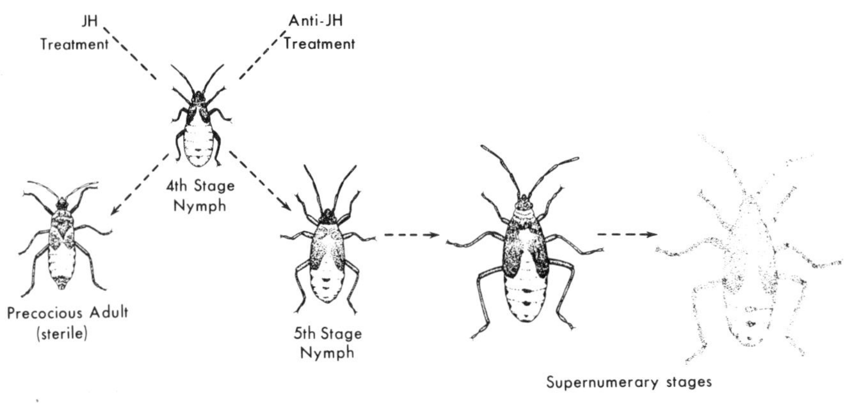

Fig. 7. Contrasting effects of excess juvenile hormone and anti-juvenile hormone on the ultimate stage(s) of insect development.

A few holometabolous species were also sterilized by contact treatment. We isolated and identified the compounds in <u>Ageratum</u> and found them to be simple substituted chromenes (30,31).

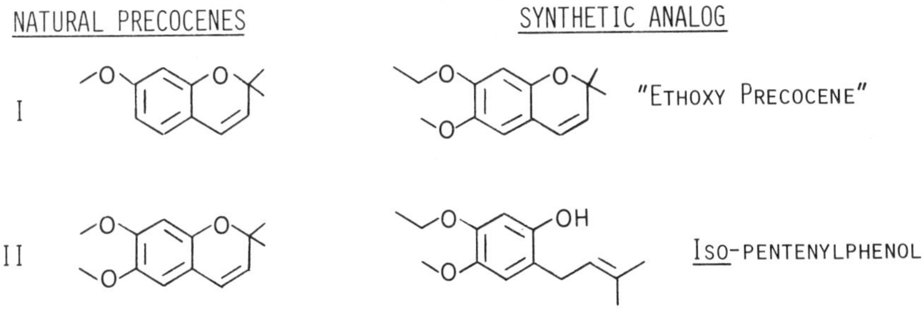

Fig. 8. Natural precocenes with a highly active analog "ethoxy precocene" and a non-chromene anti-JH.

These simple chromenes (Fig. 7) were called "precocenes" because of their ability to induce precocious metamorphosis. We were able to develop useful synthetic procedures to the natural compounds (30-33) which also allowed us to optimize the natural structures through the synthesis of analogs (34). One of the most active analogs shown in Fig. 7 is called "ethoxy precocene". These facile synthetic methods made available to many investigators samples of the precocenes and an immense base of data has now been accumulated on additional biological activities of these compounds (35-39).

<u>Mode of action of the precocenes</u>
Our earliest approach to the mode of action of the precocenes involved observations of the corpora allata in normal and precocene-treated insects. We found (40) that the allata of precocene-treated insects became very shrunken and small, and we believed that the secretion of juvenile hormone from the corpora allata had somehow been turned off. We suspected that precocene might be acting upon the brain to turn off the corpus allatum. However, in a subsequent study we found that surgical denervation of the corpora allata did not prevent the effects of precocene. This result ruled out the brain as the primary side of precocene action (41). Concurrently, we were synthesizing analogs of the precocene and investigating their structure-biological activity relationships. We found that the double bond of the chromene ring was absolutely necessary to activity (34). Metabolism studies with radiolabeled precocene gave several significant metabolites, especially the 3,4-dihydrodiol (42). The abundance of the dihydrodiol suggested an epoxide intermediate. We were unsuccessful in isolating the epoxide intermediate, but finally succeeded in synthesizing the epoxide of precocene II under strictly anhydrous conditions (43). By a similar method Jennings and Ottridge (44) prepared the epoxide of precocene I and Hamnett et al. (45) demonstrated the extreme lability of precocene I epoxide. These studies indicated that the precocene epoxides were highly reactive with nucleophilic substrates. Brooks et al. (46) discovered that the methylenedioxy analog of precocene II inhibited the anti-juvenile activity of precocene II. This demonstrated that the methylenedioxyphenyl portion of the precocene analog inhibited the enzymes necessary to the epoxidation of precocene II. This was fairly direct evidence for a reactive epoxide mode of action. At the present time it appears that the precocenes are oxidized within the insect corpus allatum, and the resulting epoxides react with cellular elements bringing about destruction of the allatal cells. Histological studies by Unnithan et al. (47), Liechty and Sedlak (48), and Schooneveld (49,50) confirmed the cytotoxic action of precocenes on the corpora allata. Pratt et al. (51) demonstrated the incorporation of radiolabeled precocene I into macromolecular components of the corpora allata of <u>locusta</u> <u>in</u> <u>vitro</u>. The oxidative biotransformation of the precocenes into cytotoxic agents reveals a very subtle plant defensive strategy against insect attack. Heretofore, similar mechanisms have been described for certain fungicidal components in plants where simple aromatic substrates are oxidized into alkylating agents called quinone methides (52,53). We synthesized some simple substituted <u>iso</u>-pentenylphenols which we imagined might be oxidized into suicide substrates and discovered that they possessed anti-juvenile hormone activity on insects very similar to the precocenes (54). Metabolism and mode of action studies in progress will explain their specific mode of action. The discovery of compounds in plants with the unique ability to derange the insect endocrine system may provide the molecular models for the development of useful strategies for insect control based upon selective perturbation of insect-specific physiological processes.

REFERENCES

1. H. Ito, Bull. Imp. Tokyo Sericult. Coll. 1, 63 (1918).
2. I. G. Weed, Proc. Soc. exp. Biol. 34, 883 (1936).
3. I. G. Weed-Pfeifer, J. Exp. Zool. 82, 439 (1939).
4. V. B. Wigglesworth, Quart. J. Micr. Sci. 79, 91 (1936).
5. E. Thomsen, Vidensk. Medd. Naturh. Foren. Kbk. 106, 320 (1942).
6. V. B. Wigglesworth, Quart. J. Micr. Sci. 77, 191 (1934).
7. C. M. Williams, Nature 178, 212 (1956).
8. D. H. Chen, W. E. Robbins and R. E. Monroe, Experientia 18, 577 (1980).
9. P. Schmialek, Z. Naturforsch. 16(b), 461 (1961).
10. P. Schmialek, Z. Naturforsch. 18(b), 513 (1963).
11. W. S. Bowers and M. J. Thompson, Science 142, 1469 (1963).
12. W. S. Bowers, M. J. Thompson and E. C. Uebel, Life Sci. 4, 2323 (1965).
13. K. J. Judy, D. H. Schooley, L. L. Dunham, M. S. Hall, B. J. Bergot and J. B. Siddall, Proc. Natl. Acad. Sci. (Amer.) 70, 1509 (1973).
14. H. Roller, K. H. Dahm, C. C. Sweeley and B. M. Trost, Angew. Chem. 79 190 (1967).
15. A. S. Meyer, H. A. Schneiderman, E. Hanzmann and J. H. Ko, Proc. Natl. Acad. Sci. (Amer.) 60, 853 (1978).
16. W. S. Bowers, Science 161, 895 (1968).
17. W. S. Bowers, Science 164, 323 (1969).
18. J. H. Fales, O. F. Bodenstein and W. S. Bowers, J. Econ. Entomol. 63(4), 1231 (1970).
19. W. S. Bowers, in "Naturally Occurring Insecticides", p. 307 Marcel Dekkar, Inc., NY (1971).
20. W. S. Bowers, Bull. Wld. Hlth. Org. 44 381 (1971).
21. W. S. Bowers, Bull. Soc. Ent. Suisse 44, 115 (1971).
22. J. H. Law, C. Yuan and C. M. Williams, Proc. Natl. Acad. Sci. (Amer.) 55 (1966).
23. M. Romanuk, K. Slama and F. Sorm, Proc. Natl. Acad. Sci. (Amer.) 57, 349 (1967).
24. C. K. Henrick, G. B. Staal and J. B. Siddall, J. Agric. Food Chem. 21, 354 (1973).
25. J. J. Bounhiol, C. R. Acad. Sci. (Paris) 205, 175 (1937).
26. S. Fukuda, J. Fac. Sci. Tokyo Univ. 6, 477 (1944).
27. W. S. Bowers, H. M. Fales, M. J. Thompson and E. C. Uebel, Science 154, 1020 (1966).
28. W. S. Bowers and R. Nishida, Science 209, 1030 (1980).
29. K. Nakanishi, M. Koreeda, S. Sasaki, M. L. Chang and H. Y. Hsu, Chem. Commun. 915 (1966).
30. W. S. Bowers, in "The Juvenile Hormones", p. 394 Plenum Publ. Corp., NY (1976).
31. W. S. Bowers, T. Ohta, J. S. Cleere and P. A. Marsella, Science 193, 542 (1976).
32. T. Ohta and W. S. Bowers, Chem. Pharm. Bull. 25(9), 2788 (1977).
33. F. Camps, J. Coll, A. Messeguer, M. A. Pericas, S. Ricart, W. S. Bowers and D. M. Soderlund, Synthesis 725 (1980).
34. W. S. Bowers, Pontif. Acad. Sci., Scripta Varia. 41, 129 (1977).
35. W. S. Bowers, in "Insect Biology in the Future, p. 613 Academic Press (1980).
36. W. S. Bowers and D. M. Soderlund, in "Regulation of Insect Development and Behavior" p. 307 Wroclaw Tech. Univ. Press (1981).
37. C. Tarrant, E. W. Cupp and W. S. Bowers, Trans. Roy. Soc. Trop. Hyg., in press (1982).
38. W. S. Bowers, Ent. Exp. et. Appl. 31, 1 (1982).
39. W. S. Bowers, in "1st Japanese/USA Symp. on IPM 60 (1981).
40. W. S. Bowers and R. Martinez-Pardo, Science 197, 1369 (1977).
41. W. S. Bowers and J. R. Aldrich, Experientia 36, 362 (1980).
42. T. Ohta, R. J. Kuhr and W. S. Bowers, Agric. & Food Chem. 25, 478 (1977).
43. D. M. Soderlund, A. Messeguer and W. S. Bowers, Agric. Food Chem. 28, 724 (1980).
44. R. C. Jennings and A. P. Ottridge, Chem. Comm. 920 (1979).
45. A. F. Hamnett, A. P. Ottridge, G. E. Pratt, R. C. Jennings and K. M. Stott, Pestic. Sci. 12, 245 (1981).
46. G. T. Brooks, G. E. Pratt and R. C. Jennings, Nature 281, 570 (1979).
47. G. C. Unnithan, K. K. Nair and W. S. Bowers, J. Insect Physiol. 23, 1081 (1977).
48. L. Liechty and B. J. Sedlak, Gen. Comp. Endocrin. 36, 433 (1978).
49. H. Schooneveld, Cell Tissue Res. 203, 25 (1979).
50. H. Schooneveld, Gen. Comp. Endocrin. 40, 360 (1980).
51. G. E. Pratt, R. C. Jennings, A. F. Hamnett and G. T. Brooks, Nature 284, 320 (1980).
52. L. Jurd and G. D. Manners, J. Agric. Food Chem. 28, 183 (1980).
53. L. Jurd, K. Stevens and G. D. Manners, Phytochem 11, 2535 (1972).
54. W. S. Bowers, P.H. Evans, P. A. Marsella, D. M. Soderlund and F. Bettarini, submitted for publication (1982).

INSECT SEX PHEROMONES AND INTEGRATED PEST MANAGEMENT: PROBLEMS AND PERSPECTIVES

Yoshio Tamaki

Division of Entomology, National Institute of Agricultural Sciences, Tsukuba, Ibaraki 305, Japan

Abstract - Despite continuing researches and practical application of a few sex pheromones, a variety of problems remain to be solved before establising the status of sex pheromones in integrated pest management (IPM). Methods of chemical characterization of active components of a sex pheromone has been improved remarkably, but biological techniques for monitoring and specifying active components are poorly established, resulting in slow progress in the development of pheromonal materials for IPM. Rapid development of materials for a whole pest complex in a particular crop is highly desirable for experimentation on the use of pheromones in IPM. Basic knowledge for forecasting the time of occurrence and the population density is lacking for most insect species. Detailed analysis of population dynamics, including adult stage, is required for each target pest species. This knowledge is also basic for utilization of pheromonal materials for direct control. It should be noted that the use of pheromones is a preventive method of pest outbreaks. Integration of the preventive method with other control measures including insecticides will contribute to the establishment of IPM.

INTRODUCTION

Sex pheromones have been isolated and identified for more than 120 species of insects, and investigation have been undertaken on use of these pheromonal chemicals for pest management. However, a variety of problems remains to be solved before sex pheromones can be used in integrated pest management (IPM). Chemical identification of the active compounds is apparently an important part of the study of sex pheromones and a prerequisite for the use of sex pheromones in IPM. However, identification is only part of the total system for establising sex pheromone application in IPM. Most of the problems remaining are concerned with ethology and ecology of each target species. In this paper the author discusses some of these problems with special reference to several pest insects in Japan.

ISOLATION AND IDENTIFICATION

For identification of pheromonal compounds, the active chemical(s) should be purified and isolated using a particular biological activity monitored by an appropriate bioassay method. The procedures for sex pheromone identification generally progress in the following manner: confirmation of the presence of sex pheromone in the target insect species, establishment of a bioassay method to monitor the pheromone titre of various fractions, establishment of conditions for collecting or extracting active materials to maximize the recovery of pheromonal compounds, purification and isolation of each pheromonal component, structural analysis of isolated compounds, synthesis of compounds of suggested structure, comparison of chemical characteristics between the synthetic and the isolated compounds, and then comparison of biological activity between the synthetic and the isolated compounds, or comparison with live insects under natural conditions. Thus, isolation studies on pheromonal chemicals consists of at least two different scientific disciplines, chemistry and behavioral biology. Coordination of these two diciplines is crucial for successful identification of pheromonal chemicals. In the case of several insect species, chemical structures originally reported by one research group were challenged by a subsequent research group and some of the original structure have been retracted. These examples are the oak leafroller moth, *Archips semiferanus* (1), the false condling moth, *Cryptophlebia leucotreta* (2), the codling moth, *Laspeyresia pomonella* (3), the gypsy moth, *Lymantria dispar* (4), the pink bollworm moth, *Pectinophora gossypiella* (5), and the American cockroach, *Periplaneta americana* (6). Although these errors are suggestive of the difficulty of pheromone identification, much of the explanation can be traced to imbalanced cooperation between chemists and biologists; much more effort has been concentrated on chemical techniques than on biological techniques such as behavioral assays.

Chemical and analytical method have improved significantly in the last 10 years. Improvements in methods of extracting and collecting pheromones, in purification techniques and micro-chemical analysis, and in analytical equipment such as IR, NMR, and GCMS have made isolation and identification of pheromonal compounds easier. Though the amounts of pheromones vary with species, one virgin female of most lepidopterous species produces 1 to 100 ng pheromone. We need only 10 to 100 individuals for identifying compounds with simple structure. In particular cases, analysis on the glandular extract from only a single female can provide a great deal of useful information (7).

In contrast to chemical techniques, there are still some difficult problems with the biological techniques required to monitor pheromonal activity of compounds. Since isolation of pheromonal compounds is monitored with a bioassay method, biological activity of the isolated compounds depends entirely on the particular method of bioassay. Mating behavior of insects usually consist of a sequence of behavioral components in both male and female. Of these, only a part is usually adopted as criterion for a bioassay. Sex pheromones which are isolated and identified, based on these bioassay do not necessarily indicate the complete pheromonal system of the insect. There are many examples of pheromone identification in which the identified compound(s) is not competitive with virgin female under field conditions.

TABLE 1. Sex pheromones of important pest insects on agricultural crops in Japan and their application in the field

Species	Compounds**	Application***	References
Rice plant			
Chilo suppressalis	Z11-16Ald; Z13-18Ald	C	11,12
Naranga aenescens	Z9-14Ac; Z9-16Ac; Z11-16Ac	M	13
Sesamia inferens	Z11-16Ac		14
Vegetable and upland farming crops			
Spodoptera litura	ZE9,11-14Ac; ZE9,12-14Ac	M, MT, C	29
Leucania separata	Z11-16OH; Z11-16Ac		20
Leucania loreyi	Z11-16Ac; Z9-14Ac		20
Mamestra brassicae	Z11-16Ac		21
Agrotis ipsilon	Z7-12Ac; Z9-14Ac		16
Agrotis segetum	Z5-10Ac, Z7-10Ac	M	17
Amathes c-nigrum	Z7-14Ac		18
Ostrinia furnacalis	Z12-14Ac; E12-14Ac		22
Phthorimaea operculella	EZ4,7-13Ac; EZZ4,7,10-13Ac	M	23,24,25
Brachmia macroscopa	E11-16Ac		19
Plutella xylostella	Z11-16Ac; Z11-16Ald; Z11-16OH*	M, C	26,27
Acrolepia alliella	Z11-16Ac*; Z11-16Ald*; Z11-16OH*	M	15
Popillia japonica	(R,Z)-5-(1-decenyl)dihydro-2(3H)-furanone	M	28
Fruit trees			
Grapholitha molesta	Z8-12Ac; E8-12Ac; Z8-12OH	M, MT, C	35,36
Adoxophyes orana fasciata	Z9-14Ac; Z11-14Ac	M, MT, C	30
Archippus breviplicanus	E11-14Ac; Z11-14Ac	M	31
Carposina niponensis	(Z)-7-eicosen-11-one (Z)-7-nonadecen-11-one	M, MT, C	32
Conopia hector	ZZ3,13-18Ac*; EZ3,13-18Ac*	M, MT, C	33
Conopia tenuis	ZZ3,13-18Ac	M	34
Pseudococcus comstocki	2,6-dimethyl-3-acetoxy-1,5-heptadiene	M	39
Pseudaulacaspis pentagona	(Z)-3,9-dimethyl-6-isopropenyl-3,9-decadienyl propanoate		38
Planococcus citri	2,2-dimethyl-3-(1-methylethenyl)-cyclobutanemethyl acetate		37
Tea			
Adoxophyes sp.	Z9-14Ac; Z11-14Ac; E11-14Ac; 10Me-12Ac	M, MT, C	40,41
Homona magnanima	Z11-14Ac; Z9-12Ac; 11-12Ac	M, MT, C	42

* These compounds have not been confirmed as sex pheromones but these are quite competitive with virgin female in their attractancy.
** Z11-14Ac indicates (Z)-11-tetradecenyl acetate; Ald is aldehyde; OH is alcohol.
*** M is monitoring; MT, mass trapping; C, communication disruption.

Behavioral bioassays, based on a sexual stimulation and orientation, require large numbers of insets, and can become a serious limitation for identification studies. An electroantennogram (EAG) technique has been widely used in pheromonal identification and this was improved by direct coupling with a capillary GC (8). Although these EAG techniques require only a small number of insect to monitor some of the pheromonal compounds, they still possess major limitations. Some minor components can not be detected by these methods, and all the EAG active compounds are not necessarily the pheromonal components (9, 10). Conclusions derived by EAG studies should be always confirmed by behavioral investigation. We need, therefore, a simple behavioral bioassay method which requires relatively small numbers of test insects and yields reliable information on the biological activity of test compounds.

SEX PHEROMONES OF PEST INSECTS ON AGRICULTURAL CROPS IN JAPAN

Sex pheromones or sex attractants have been identified for various important pest insects on agricultural crops in Japan and researches for their application for IPM are now in progress (Table 1). These consist of 3 Lepidoptera on rice, 12 Lepidoptera and 1 Coleoptera on vegetables and upland farming crops, 6 Lepidoptera and 3 Homoptera on fruit trees, and 2 Lepidoptera on tea. Of these, compounds for *Acrolepia alliella* on green onion, *Conopia hector* on peach, and *Conopia nenuis* on persimmon are sex attractants, because the presence of each compound in virgin females has not yet been verified in respective species. Several species are subject of reinvestigation or more detailed investigation for chemical characterization, because their compounds are not competitive with virgin females under natural conditions. These include *Sesamia inferens*, *Leucania separata*, *Mamestra brassicae*, *Brachmia macroscopa*, *Agrotis ipsilon*, *Amathes c-nigrum*, and *Ostrinia furnacalis*. The attractiveness of the synthetic sex pheromone of the two scale insects, *Pseudaulacaspis pentagona* and *Planococcus citri* has not yet been evaluated in Japan. All the other species are now the subject of active investigations on the use of synthetic pheromonal chemicals for IPM, and commercial formulations for monitoring use are available in Japan for 10 species such as *Spodoptera litura*, *Plutella xylostella*, *Acrolepia alliella*, *Grapholitha molesta*, *Adoxophyes orana fasciata*, *Adoxophyes* sp., *Homona magnanima*, *Archippus breviplicanus*, *Carposina niponensis*, and *Conopia hector*. One formulation for mass trapping has been registered with the Ministry of Agriculture, Forestry, and Fisheries (MAFF) for the control of *Spodoptera litura* on upland farming crops.

EARLY STAGE DETECTION OF INTRODUCED FOREIGN PEST INSECTS

Recent developments in transportation, with the resulting expansion in international movements of peoples and commodities, have increased the possibility of accidental introduction of various important foreign pest insects. Insects and diseases detected on imported plants in Japan numbered 185,714 in 1978. Even for selected important insects, 6 Diptera, 5 Coleoptera, and 1 Lepidoptera were detected 146 times in 1979 on various plant materials imported from 14 countries (Yokohama Plant Quarantine Station, MAFF). Although these data apparently indicate the importance of plant quarantine, we are always threatened with the accidental introduction and establishment of foreign important pest insects. Recent typical examples of the establishment of introduced pests in Japan are the greenhouse whitefly, *Trialeurodes vaporariorum*, since 1974 (51), the rice water weevil, *Lissorhoptrus oryzophilus*, since 1976 (52), and the southern yellow thrips, *Thrips palmi*, since 1980 (53). The rice water weevil in Japan is parthenogenetic type, and the other two species are of extremely high reproductive potential. These characteristics are favorable for their establishment after the introduction to a new areas.

TABLE 2. Examples of important foreign insect pests of which introduction could be detected by sex pheromone traps

Species	Compounds*	References
Estigmene acrea (saltmarsh caterpillar)	*ZZ*9,12-18Ald; *ZZZ*9,12,15-18Ald; *ZZ*3,6-*cis*-9,10-epoxy-21Hy	43
Spodoptera frugiperda (fall armyworm)	*Z*9-14Ac; *Z*9-12Ac	44,45
Heliothis zea (corn earworm)	*Z*11-16Ald; *Z*9-16Ald	46,47
Laspeyresia pomonella (codling moth)	*EE*8,10-12OH	48,49
Anarsia lineatella (peach twig borer)	*E*5-10Ac; *E*5-10OH	50

* *ZZ*9,12-18Ald indicates (*Z*,*Z*)-9,12-octadecadienal; Ac, OH, and Hy show acetate, alcohol, and hydrocarbon.

Identification of sex pheromones has been mostly concerned with lepidopterous insects. Plant quarantine staffs in Yokohama Plant Quarantine Station, MAFF, recently listed foreign insect pests of prime importance, whose introduction into Japan is to be avoided. Of the 6 lepidopterous species in this list, the sex pheromones of 5 have been isolated and identified (Table 2). Routine trapping systems for these species are apparently valuable for early detection of their introduction. International cooperation and exchanges of information will be desirable for the establishment of routine monitoring systems for these and other insects.

FORECASTING THE TIME OF CONTROL ACTION BY SEX PHEROMONE TRAPS

The sex pheromone trap is a convenient and powerful tool for population survey of pest insects, not detected by routine light traps such as *Grapholitha molesta*, *Carposina niponensis*, and *Conopia hector*. Details of early season occurrence of *Spodoptera litura* were impossible to detect by the routine light trap, but are now easily followed by a trap baited with a synthetic sex pheromone. Sex pheromone formulations and traps for monitoring use for these and other pest insects in Japan are commercially available.

Forecasting the time of pest occurrence is a prerequisite for IPM. This requires for the reduction of the amount of insecticides and for improving the efficacy of an insecticide application. Seasonal trapping of a target pest species with traps baited with synthetic sex pheromone (pheromone traps) has been routinely conducted with various insects. A typical example is the case of *Grapholitha molesta*. This insect occurs 3 to 6 times a year in Japan. By using three years trapping data, Tanaka & Yabuki (54) found a relationship between the rate of development for one generation (V) and mean temperature (t), V=0.27t-3.01. An observed developmental zero and a total effective temperature were thus calculated as 11.1°C and 383.7 degree-days from the field trapping data. Occurrence times after the 2nd flight season were well estimated by using these data except for mid-summer season when the temperature exceeds 28°C, the upper limit for the development of this species. By correcting the effective temperature during the seasons exceedomg 28°C, occurrence peaks from summer to autumn generations coincided well with the calculated dates (54). Thus sex-pheromone traps can be utilized to forecast the time of occurrence of *G. molesta* in Japan.

Another example is the case of *Adoxophyes orana*. Minks & DeJong (55) predicted the hatching of larvae based on sex-pheromone trap observations of the preceding moth flight and temperature recordings during embryonic development of the eggs. This model was designed for quick calculation of the stage of egg development as a percentage of total development; when the cumulative percentages exceeds 100, hatching can be expected. This method has been successfully applied to the Japanese subspecies, *A. orana fasciata* (56). The most effective date of insecticide spray for this species was found to be just after the cumulative percentages exceeded 100 for the egg layed at the time of peak trap catches. For this species, developmental zero and total effective temperature for the egg stage were calculated as 6.98°C and 115.24 degree-days, respectively (56).

The method of total effective temperatures, based on seasonal pheromone trap data and temperature recordings, may be applicable to various other insects to determine the timing of insecticide spray. For successful application of this method the date of peak trapping should truely reflect the maximum density of adults in the field. This is unfortunately not necessarily the case. Some unknown factors affect the temporal pattern of trapping. *Spodoptera litura*, an important pest of upland farming crops such as sweet potato and taro plant in southwestern Japan, occurs 5 times from April to November and populations increase dramatically from generation to generation. Miyahara *et al.* (57) analysed the relationship between the timing of male trapping and of female oviposition on taro plants, using traps baited with virgin females. Egg masses are found on taro plants from July to early November in Chikugo district, representing the largest oviposition peaks by 3rd generation moths between late August and early September. Their four-years results apparently indicate that the date of 50% oviposition is 4 to 10 days earlier than that of 50% male capture by the virgin female traps except for 1975. A similar phenomenon is also seen in other parts of southwestern Japan (58). The reason is not clear, but we can't use trapping data directly for determination of the optimum timing for insecticide spray. The delay in peak capture of males is probably due to competition between trap and wild females. Nakamura (59), using a simulation model, indicated that an even larger delay is expected under higher population density. Another possible reason for this phenomenon is the influx of males from outside the experimental field; *S. litura* is a typical polyphagous species and a strong flier. Influx of male moths from a large population outside may seriously affect the trap catches in the field of target crop. Influx or a short distance migration is one of the central problems awaiting solution in various phases of sex-pheromone application.

FORECASTING THE POPULATION LEVEL BY SEX PHEROMONE TRAP

Use of pheromone trap records for estimating the level of forthcoming outbreaks of target insect is expected to be an important measure in IPM in making decision to spray insecticide. For this purpose, relationships between the trap catch of adult insects during a definite period and the rate of injury caused by the larvae of subsequent generations must be elucidated. Unfortunately, trap catches do not necessarily indicate the population density of the adult stage in the strict sense. Numerous factors influencing not only traps but also responding insects, often adversely affect relationships between the trap catch and adult population density. Although these factors are the target of detailed investigations, it may be impossible to analyse all the factors for each pest species. For this reason, correlations between trap catches and appropriate values indicating population density or damages are often analysed directly.

Sugino (60) indicated that pheromone trap records in the spring can be utilized to estimate the rate of damage in the autumn in the case of S. litura. There is a good correlation (r^2= 0.85 to 0.99) with trap catches between May-June and August-September. Then, the trap catches in August-September correlate well with the area of occurrence of damage by this insect (r^2=0.86 to 0.91). This method is useful to forecast the damage for areas of more than several thousands hectares.

For estimation of the control threshold density of this species in a smaller area, pheromone traps have also proven to be a convenient tool. Nakasuji & Kiritani (61) constructed an empirical system model to forecast the yield of taro by means of the number of males caught by pheromone traps. Parameters used are number of moths caught by a trap per day, number of egg masses per 100 plants, egg mass size (489.9 for July, 672.6 for August), duration of egg stage (2 days), hatchability (94.5% for July, 81.1 for August), developmental period from the hatch to the 4th instar (T=9.9 days), and survival rate (log S = -0.140T). In the case of taro plant, the injury threshold density is 4.8 larvae of 4th instar per square meter. This model indicated that the control threshold for S. litura on taro plant is 190 males/trap/day in July generation and 160 males/trap/day in August generation in this particular district, Kochi. Although the parameters used in this model varies with circumstances and should be determined on each crop of respective locations, there is a need for this type of approach with other pest insects using pheromone traps in IPM. Further improvements of this model will be attained by the analysis of factors influencing the trap catches, because the correlation coefficient between trap catches and egg masses is not so good in this case (r^2=0.513). Analysis of the temporal differences between trap catches and oviposition, the short distance migration of adult males, and seasonal variation of trapping efficiency, will greatly improve the model.

In general, the following items should be studied for the use of sex pheromone trap for monitoring population level.

1) seasonal stability of attractant lure
2) trap structure for stable trapping efficiency
3) trap location for stable trapping effciency
4) influx or short distance migration of adult insects
5) optimum trap density or distribution of traps in and around the target area
6) correlation between trap catches and oviposition in each generation
7) construction of a system model indicating a relation between trap catches and control threshold density

MASS TRAPPING

Mass trapping or trap-out is one of potential method of applicating sex pheromones to direct control of pest insects. As a part of research project of MAFF, Japan, on integrated pest control during the period of 1971 to 1975, mass trapping of Spodoptera litura by synthetic sex pheromone was suggested as an effective technique on which further investigation should be concentrated. A pilot mass trapping project on S. litura, funded by MAFF, was conducted in 1977 and 1978. Area covered by this project was 1,947 ha of 14 prefectures: trap density was 2 to 3 per hectare. Results of these mass trapping trials were comparable with those on S. littoralis in Israel (62). In the case of Tokushima prefecture, 720 ha was covered by pheromone traps. Trapping treatment suppressed the damages on taro plant less than 10% in more than 96% of the treated areas, though about 45% of check areas were found to be 31 to 51% damage (63). Further investigation of trap density and mating rate of tethered females indicated that effective suppression of mating was obtained by more than 20 traps per hectare in soybean field in September, the season of maximum population density (64).

The feasibility of mass trapping by sex-attractant traps was also proven on the smaller tea tortrix moth, Adoxophyes sp., an important pest of tea plant. Negishi et al (65,66) found that (Z,E)-9,12-tetradecadienyl acetate and 11-methyl (Z)-9,12-tridecadienyl acetate are good synergists of the major components of the sex pheromone of this species. Results of mass trapping in very small plots of tea field using this attractant lure have been reported by Shimada (67) and Negishi et al. (68). These trials used 600 to 700 m^2 plots and trap density of 5 to 7 per 100 m^2. In the trial of Kumamoto Tea Experiment Station (67), the efficacy of mass trapping was apparent in the 1st and 2nd flight seasons, the injury of the treated plot being 50 to 60% of that of the check plot, respectively. Another experiment also indicated that the amount of infested leaves in the mass-trapped plot were 26 and 11% of that of the check plot for 1st and 2nd flight seasons, respectively (68). Since the check plots in these experiments were treated by routine insecticide spray, the control effect of mass trapping is very pronounced.

Effect of mass trapping depends on the population density of adults in the field. Negishi (69) and Ohtaishi & Horikawa (70) compiled the results of 13 mass trapping trials on the smaller tea tortrix moth. Mean number of males per trap in these trials could be used as a criterion of population levels in each trial. When the population is lower than 100 males/trap, the larval density or leaf damage in the next generation was effectively suppressed below 50% of conventional treatment by insecticide spray. Analysis of 11 trials revealed that there is an apparent correlation between the number of males per trap and percentage control (r2=0.83) (Fig. 1). Attractant lure used in these mass trapping is a mixture composed of Z9-14Ac, Z11-14Ac, ZE9,12-14Ac, and 11Me-Z9,12-13Ac. The sex pheromone of this species is now known to be a four component mixture of Z9-14Ac, Z11-14Ac, E11-14Ac, and 10Me-12Ac (41), and a particular formulation of this four-component mixture is more potent than the above mentioned attractant mixture (71). Therefore, this synthetic pheromone would be more effective than the synthetic attractant in mass trapping of this species.

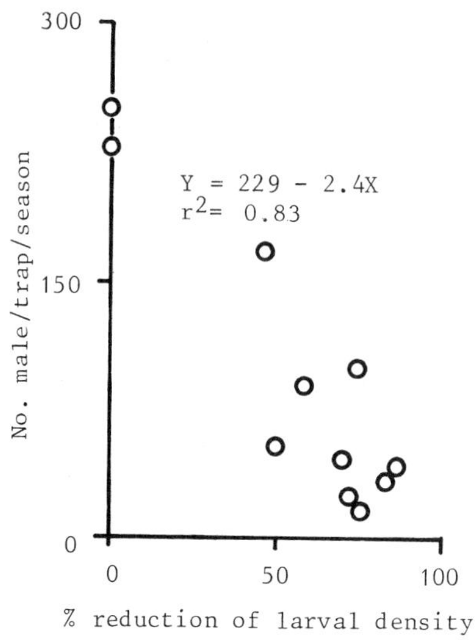

Fig. 1. Relationship between the number of males caught by traps in mass-trapping treatments for Adoxophyes sp. and percentage of reduction of larval density. For details see text.

In addition to adult population density, the size of experimental plot would seriously affect mass trapping. Influx of gravid females from outside the plot adversely affects the results of mass trapping. Flight distance or flight range of gravid females should be determined for each target species, though this is not known for most species so far investigated. In these cases, flight distances of male insects could be used as a valuable information. On the other hands, trap density in an experimental plot can be decided based on the information of active spece of pheromone trap. About 50 to 60 m has been proposed as an active space for S. litura (72) and 5 to 10 m for Adoxophyes sp. (73) based on the recovery of marked males released at various distances from pheromone traps. These results indicate that minimum trap densities for S. litura and Adoxophyes sp. are 4 and 400 per hectare, respectively.

Release and trapping of marked insects and analysis of the resulting data are often impossible because of shortage in insects available for release and insufficient data constructing simulation model. In this case, the active space of a pheromone trap could be estimated by analyzing the interaction of traps separated by various distances. Based on this method, Ohbayashi (74) suggested that the active space of the sex pheromone trap for the diamondback moth is between 3 to 5 m.

For application of the mass trapping method following items should be evaluated in general.

1) pheromone formulation for optimum attraction
2) trap structure for optimum catch and for easy handling
3) trap location for optimum catch
4) minimum area of mass trapping plot
5) trap density and distribution pattern of trap in and around the plot
6) determination of threshold density of adults for the success of this method

COMMUNICATION DISRUPTION

Another application of sex pheromones for direct control of pest insects is disruption of sexual communication between males and females during the mating behavior. In general, a synthetic sex pheromone is evaporated and evenly distributed in the air in and around the habitat of target insect. The feasibility of this method was verified for the first time on Trichoplusia ni by Shorey et al. (75). Thereafter, many trials were conducted on various pest insects, and led to the development of the first commercial disruptant, Gossyplure H.F. or Nomate PBW for the pink bollworm moth, Pectinophora gossypiella, by Conrell Co. Ltd., USA.

Mechanism of communication disruption by sex pheromones is not yet known. Male confusion by a number of pseudo-females emitting pheromone, habituation in central nervous system, adaptation in pheromone receptor sites, or combination of these seem to operate in disruption of communication by sex pheromone in the field. Fundamental studies on the mechanism of communication disruption are required for developing effective disruptant and for establishing effective application method. Initial studies on S. litura in Japan showed that an efficient disruptant is the minor component of the sex pheromone, ZE9,12-14Ac (76). However, later work showed that the sex pheromone itself, a binary mixture of the major and the minor components, ZE9,11-14Ac and ZE9,12-14Ac, is a better disruptant than either component alone in a larger experimental plots (77). Pheromone mimics are also promising candidates for disruptants. An example in Japan is the case of Chilo suppressalis. (Z)-5-Hexadecene, a structural mimic of the major component of the sex pheromone, Z11-16Ald, of this insect showed high activity in the field. Evaporation of the alkene at a rate of 87.5 g/ha from dispensers distributed as 1 x 1.5 m grid in 0.2 ha plot caused about 50% reduction of injury to rice stems compared with check plots (78). For this species Z9-14-formate and Z11-16-formate are also potential disruptants (97). These approaches to find effective substitutes as disruptant will be necessary, especially in the case of unstable pheromones.

When we consider a pest insect complex on a particular agricultural crop, high species specificity of sex pheromone is an inconvenient characteristics, because specific pheromone formulation must be developed for each species. However, it may be possible to develop a common disruptant for multiple species. Recent progress in pheromone chemistry has made clear that taxonomically related species uses a common "key" compound as pheromonal component (80). The "key" compound or its combination with other additives could be used as a common disruptant for the the pest complex. Efficacy of such type of common disruptant has been evaluated on the two tortricid moth species attacking tea plant (70,81). Z11-14Ac is a common pheromonal component for Adoxophyes sp. and Homona magnanima, the two important leaf feeders of tea plant (41,42), and this compound is a good common disruptant for both species.

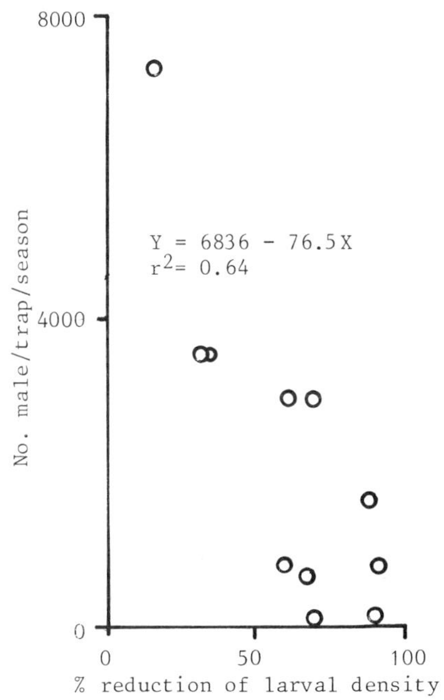

Fig. 2. Relationship between the number of males caught by a monitoring trap in a check plot for disruption trial on Adoxophyes sp. and percentage of reduction of larval density.

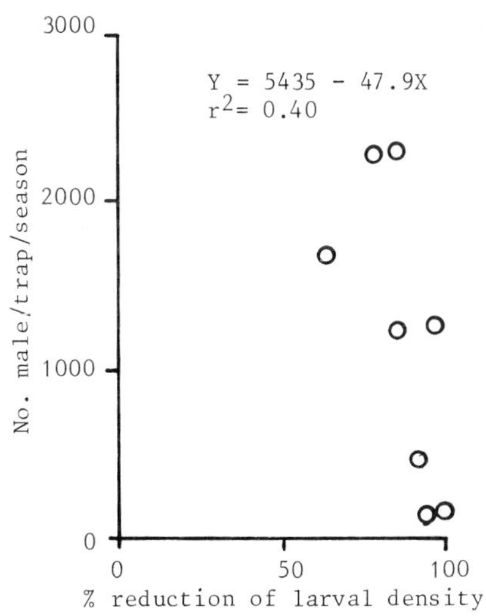

Fig. 3. Relationship between the number of males caught by a monitoring trap in a check plot for disruption trial on Homona magnanima and percentage of reduction of larval density.

In addition to the chemical nature of the disruptant, there are other factors affecting the communication disruption. Most are the same as in the case of mass trapping. Population density of adult insects seems to be an important factor affecting the efficacy of the disruptant. Fig. 2 indicates the relationship between numbers of males caught by monitoring traps in check field (Y) and percentage reduction of larval density (X) in 11 trials of communication disruption on Adoxophyes sp. by a synthetic sex pheromone or its component, Z11-14Ac. Percentage reduction of larval density, was calculated by 100 - (100 x Ta x Cb)/(Tb x Ca), where T is number of damaged tea leaves or larvae per unit area of treated plot before (Tb) and after (Ta) the application, C is the same values in check fields before (Cb) and after (Ca) the experiment. There is a significant correlation between X and Y ($r^2=0.64$). This means that the percentage of control correlates inversely with adult population density. Trials of communication disruption on the another tortricid moth, *Homona magnanima*, attacking tea plant, indicated a similar relationship between the adult population density and the efficacy of treatments; analysis on 8 trials showed a weak correlation between the number of males caught by traps in check plot and percentage of control ($r^2=0.40$) (Fig. 3). The influence of adult density on the control effect seems to be smaller in *Homona* than in *Adoxophyes*. Disruption of pheromonal communication was suggested to be easier in *Homona* than in *Adoxophyes*.

The apparent relationships between adult density and control effect of communication disruption are only noticed in the first flight season for the both species. No apparent relation was found between the density and the effect in other flight seasons; unknown factors other than adult density may greatly affect the control efficacy after the 2nd flight season. The effect of communication disruption is generally low in the 2nd and the 3rd flight seasons especially for *Adoxophyes*. Detailed analysis is awaited for these seasonal variation of disruption effect.

For application of the communication disruption method the following items should be evaluated in general.

1) disruptant chemical or a mixture of chemicals
2) formulation of disruptant
3) application method of disruptant
4) minimum area of treatment
5) determination of threshold density of adults

POSSIBLE ROLE OF SEX PHEROMONE IN IPM

The control efficiency of sex pheromones is often compared with that of insecticides. The control field in pheromone application is usually sprayed with conventional insecticides. Thus, the results are directly compared with conventional insecticide spray. These comparisons between pheromone and insecticide often lead to inappropriate evaluation of the possible role of sex pheromones in IPM. It is not necessary to consider pheromones as substitutes for insecticides. The two approaches have different characteristics and can be used to complement each other. Insecticides immediately kill the larvae attacking crops, but sex pheromones suppress the mating of adults and lower the larval density of the next generation. Insecticides have a wide spectrum of activity, which often affects beneficial insects, but pheromones are extremely specific in their activity. Insecticide can be applied in very small area, but pheromone is necessary to be applied over a wide area.

Although insecticide and pheromone are mutually complementary in their use, sex pheromones would be especially effective for pest insects of a weak flight ability and narrow host range. In addition, the effect of delayed mating on reproduction differs with species. Those species in which reproduction is seriously affected by delayed or suppressed mating are preferable targets for pheromone application. Because of the high specificity of sex pheromones, treatment of a whole pest complex on a target crop is an important problem of pheromone application. Furthermore, pheromone application must be generally applied over a wide area for the control of adult behavior. However, in the particular conditions of intensive agriculture in Japan, many varieties of agricultural crops are distributed over a small area. Thus, multiple pest insects on various crops would become the targets of pheromone application in a wide area.

Efficiency and limitations in the use of sex pheromones have not yet been fully evaluated for any pest insects in Japan. Correct evaluation of the possible role of sex pheromones for pest control will be conducted only by an experimental IPM. Simple comparison between insecticide and pheromone is not necesssrily enough for their final evaluation. A medium or large scale experiment on IPM is desirable for a particular model crop. In this case, the sex pheromone may be used in combination with other control measures such as microbial agents and insecticides. Detailed monitoring of population density based on sex-pheromone traps in each field will become an important technique for the selection and timing of control measures to be used. Mass trapping itself has a use in fine monitoring of target insects and acts as a control measure suppressing or delaying the population build up under the conditions of low population density. This technique could be utilized as a kind of preventive method of the outbreak of particular key pest on the crop. The mass trapping data will provide us with information on the time and location of necessary additional control measures. Pheromonal disruptants, microbial agents, insecticides, and others are the components of the additional measures, and either one or their combination will be selected based on various factors such as population level of the pest insect and characteristics of each control measure.

Acknowledgement - The author is indebted to Dr. N. Takahashi for his reading the draft.

REFERENCES

1. L.B. Hendry, J. Jugovich, L. Roman, M.E. Anderson and R.O. Mumma, Experientia 30, 886 (1974).
2. J.S. Read and F.L. Warren, Chem. Comm. 792 (1968).
3. L.M. McDonough, D.A. George, B.A. Butt, J.M. Ruth and K.R. Hill, Science 177, 177 (1972)
4. M. Jacobson, M. Beroza and W.A. Jones, Science 132, 1011 (1960)
5. W.A. Jones, M. Jacobson and D.F. Martin, Science 152, 1516 (1966)
6. M. Jacobson, M. Beroza and R.T. Yamamoto, Science 139, 48 (1963)
7. J.A. Klun, J.R. Plimmer, B.A. Bier-Leonhardt, A.N. Sparks and O.L. Chapman, Science 204, 1328 (1979)
8. H. Arn, E. Städler and S. Rauscher, Z. Naturforsch. 30c, 722 (1975)
9. W.L. Roelofs, Crop Protection Agents, ed. N. McFarlane, p. 147-165, Academic Press, London (1977)
10. Y. Tamaki, Chemical Ecology: Odour Communication in Animals, ed. F.J. Ritter, p. 169-180, Elsevier, Amsterdam (1979)
11. B.F. Nesbitt, P.S. Beevor, D.R. Hall, R. Lester and V.A. Dyck, J. Insect Physiol. 21, 1883 (1975)
12. K. Ohta, S. Tatsuki, K. Uchiumi, M. Kurihara and J. Fukami, Agric. Biol. Chem. 40, 1897 (1976)
13. T. Ando, K. Kishino, S. Tatsuki, H. Nakajima, S. Yoshida and N. Takahashi, Agric. Biol. Chem. 41, 1819 (1977)
14. B.F. Nesbitt, P.S. Beevor, D.R. Hall, R. Lester and V.A. Dyck, Insect Biochem. 6, 105 (1976)
15. R. Sato, K. Yaginuma and K. Kumakura, Jap. J. Appl. Ent. Zool. 23, 115 (1979)
16. A.S. Hill, R.W. Rings, S.R. Swier and W.L. Roelofs, J. Chem. Ecol 5, 439 (1979)
17. S. Wakamura, Appl. Ent. Zool. 13, 290 (1978)
18. Y. Hirai, Proc. Symp. Insect Pheromones and Their Applications, p. 165, Japan Plant Protection Association, Tokyo (1976)
19. C. Hirano, H. Muramoto and M. Horiike, Naturwiss. 63, 439 (1976)
20. S. Takahashi, M. Kawaradani, Y. Sato and M. Sakai, Jap. J. Appl. Ent. Zool. 23, 78 (1979)
21. Y. Hirai, H. Kimura, K. Kawasaki and Y. Tamaki, Appl. Ent. Zool. 13, 136 (1978)
22. T. Ando, O. Saito, K. Arai and N. Takahashi, Agric. Biol. Chem. 44, 2643 (1980)
23. W.L. Roelofs, J.P. Kochansky, R.T. Cardé and G.G. Kennedy, Life Sci. 17, 699 (1975)
24. C.J. Persoons, S. Voerman, P.E.J. Verwiel, F.J. Ritter, W.J. Nooijen and A.K. Minks, Ent. Exp. Appl. 20, 289 (1976)
25. R. Yamaoka, H. Fukami and S. Ishii, Agric. Biol. Chem. 40, 1971 (1976)
26. Y. Tamaki, K. Kawasaki, H. Yamada, T. Koshihara, N. Osaki, T. Ando, S. Yoshida and H. Kakinohana, Appl. Ent. Zool. 12, 208 (1977)
27. T. Ando, T. Koshihara, H. Yamada, M.H. Vu, N. Takahashi and Y. Tamaki, Appl. Ent. Zool. 14, 362 (1979)
28. J.H. Tumlinson, M.G. Klein, R.E. Doolittle, T.L. Ladd and A.T. Proveaux, Science 197, 789 (1977)
29. Y. Tamaki, H. Noguchi and T. Yushima, Appl. Ent. Zool. 8, 200 (1973)
30. Y. Tamaki, H. Noguchi, T. Yushima, C. Hirano, K. Honma and H. Sugawara, Kontyu 39, 338 (1971)
31. H. Sugie, K. Yaginuma and Y. Tamaki, Appl. Ent. Zool. 12, 69 (1977)
32. Y. Tamaki, H. Honma and K. Kawasaki, Appl. Ent. Zool. 12, 60 (1977)
33. K. Yaginuma, M. Kumakura, Y. Tamaki, T. Yushima and J.H. Tumlinson, Appl. Ent. Zool. 11, 266 (1976)
34. Y. Tamaki, T. Yushima, M. Oda, K. Kita, K. Kitamura, S. Yabuki and J.H. Tumlinson, Jap. J. Appl. Ent. Zool. 21, 106 (1977)
35. W.L. Roelofs, A. Comeau and R. Selle, Nature 224, 723 (1969)
36. A.M. Cardé, T.C. Baker and R.T. Cardé, J. Chem. Ecol. 5, 423 (1979)
37. B.A. Bier-Leonhard, D.S. Moreno, M. Schwarz, J. Fargerlund and J.R. Plimmer, Tetrahedron Let. 22, 389 (1981)
38. B.A. Bierl-Leonhard, D.S. Moreno, M. Schwarz, H.S. Forster, J.R. Plimmer and E.D. Devilbiss, Life Sci. 27, 399 (1980)
39. T. Negishi, M. Uchida, Y. Tamaki, K. Mori, T. Ishiwatari, S. Asano and K. Nakagawa, Appl. Ent. Zool. 15, 328 (1980)
40. Y. Tamaki, H. Noguchi, T. Yushima and C. Hirano, Appl. Ent. Zool. 6, 139 (1971)
41. Y. Tamaki, H. Noguchi, H. Sugie, R. Sato and A. Kariya, Appl. Ent. Zool. 14, 101 (1979)
42. H. Noguchi, Y. Tamaki and T. Yushima, Appl. Ent. Zool. 14, 225 (1979)
43. A.S. Hill and W.L. Roelofs, J. Chem. Ecol. 7, 655 (1981)
44. A.A. Sekul and A.N. Sparks, J. Econ. Ent. 60, 1270 (1967)
45. E.R. Mitchell and R.E. Doolittle, J. Econ. Ent. 69, 324 (1976)
46. W.L. Roelofs, A.S. Hill, R.T. Cardé and T.C. Baker, Life Sci. 14, 1555 (1974)
47. J.A. Klun, J.R. Plimmer, B.A. Bierl-Leonhardt, A.N. Sparks and O.L. Chapman, Science 204, 1328 (1979)
48. W. Roelofs, A. Comeau, A. Hill and G. Milicevic, Science 174, 297 (1971)
49. M. Beroza, B.A. Bierl and H.R. Moffitt, Science 183, 89 (1974)
50. W. Roelofs, J. Kochansky, E. Anthon, R. Rice and R. Cardé, Environ. Ent. 4, 580 (1975)

51. K. Nakamura, K. Nakazawa and K. Norikoshi, Shokubutsu-Boeki 29, 7 (1975)
52. N. Watanabe, Shokubutsu-Boeki 30, 342 (1976)
53. I. Kudo, Shokubutsu-Boeki 35, 285 (1981)
54. F. Tanaka and S. Yabuki, Jap. J. Appl. Ent. Zool. 22, 162 (1978)
55. A.K. Minks and D.J. DeJong, J. Econ. Ent. 68, 729 (1975)
56. S. Shirasaki and M. Yamada, Tohoku Agric. Res. 27 149 (1980)
57. Y. Miyahara, M. Shimazu and T. Wada, Jap. J. Appl. Ent. Zool. 21, 59 (1977)
58. M. Borikiri, S. Fukamachi and H. Kamiwada, Proc. Assoc. Plant Protection Kyushu 24, 117 (1978)
59. K. Nakamura, personal communication
60. T. Sugino, Ann. Rept. Pheromone Experiments, p. 1-6, Japan Plant Protection Association, Tokyo (1975)
61. F. Nakasuji and K. Kiritani, Protection Ecol. 1, 23 (1978)
62. I. Teich, R.M. Waters, M. Jacobson and S. Neumark, J. Environ. Sci. Health, A12, 291 (1977)
63. K. Yanagisawa, Shokubutsu-Boeki 33, 406 (1979)
64. M. Kobayashi, T. Wada and H. Inoue, Proc. 1st Japan/USA Symp. IPM, Tsukuba (Japan), p. 32-40, Research Council, MAFF (1981)
65. T. Negishi, T. Ishiwatari and S. Asano, Appl. Ent. Zool. 12, 178 (1977)
66. T. Negishi, T. Ishiwatari, M. Uchida and S. Asano, Appl. Ent. Zool. 14, 478
67. K. Shimada, Jap. J. Appl. Ent. Zool. 24, 81 (1980)
68. T. Negishi, T. Ishiwatari, S. Asano and H. Fujikawa, Appl. Ent. Zool. 15, 113 (1980)
69. T. Negishi, Proc. 16th Internatl. Congr. Ent., Kyoto, p. 222 (1980)
70. M. Ohtaishi and T. Horikawa, Proc. 1st Japan/USA Symp. IPM, Tsukuba (Japan), p. 41-49, Research Council, MAFF (1981)
71. Y. Tamaki, H. Noguchi, H. Sugie, A. Kariya, S. Arai, M. Ohba, T. Terada, T. Suguro and M. Mori, Jap. J. Appl. Ent. Zool. 24, 221 (1980)
72. K. Nakamura and K. Kawasaki, Appl. Ent. Zool 12, 162 (1977)
73. K. Kawasaki, K. Nakamura, Y. Tamaki and H. Noguchi, unpublished data
74. N. Ohbayashi, Ann. Rept. Pheromone Experiments, p. 67-73, Japan Plant Protection Association, Tokyo (1979)
75. H.H. Shorey, L.K. Gaston and C.A. Saario, J. Econ. Ent. 60, 1541 (1967)
76. T. Yushima, Y. Tamaki, S. Kamano and M. Oyama, Appl. Ent. Zool. 10, 237 (1975)
77. M. Oyama, Y. Noguchi and Y. Tamaki, Proc. Ann. Meeting Jap. Soc. Appl. Ent. Zool. p. 7 (1980)
78. S. Tatsuki and H. Kanno, Management of Insect Pests with Semiochemicals, ed. E.R. Mitchell, p. 313-325, Plenum, New York (1981)
79. P.S. Beevor and D.G. Campion, Chemical Ecology: Odour Communication in Animals, ed. F.J. Ritter, p. 313-325, Elsevier, Amsterdam (1979)
80. Y. Tamaki, Chemical Control of Insect Behavior: Theory and Application, ed. H.H. Shorey and J.J. McKelvey, Jr., p. 253-285, John Wiley & Sons, New York (1977)
81. Y. Tamaki, H. Noguchi, H. Sugie, M. Ohtaishi, T. Horikawa, and M. Ohba, in this issue

NEW APPROACHES TO THE SEARCH FOR BIOACTIVE FUNGAL METABOLITES

Shingo Marumo

Department of Agricultural Chemistry, Nagoya University, Chikusa-ku, Nagoya 464, Japan

Abstract - The bioactivity of natural products may be classified as acting against another species (interspecies), against another individual of their own species (intraspecies) or within the individual itself (strain level). Application of such a classification system to two important classes of microbial products, growth inhibitors and reproduction regulators, led to the categories shown in Table 1.
A search for new types of bioactive natural products in microbiology, based on this approach, led to fruitful investigation. In the category of aversion factors, lunatoic acid A (3) was isolated from Cochliobolus lunata, and was later found to be an asexual chlamydospore-inducing substance - the first chemically identified in nature. A survey was conducted for growth self-inhibitors (or autoantibiotics) among phytopathogenic fungi, and two active substances (5) and (6) were isolated from Diaporthe citri and Pleospora herbarum, respectively. Asexual spore-inducing substances were investigated in several fungi, e.g., a major arthrospore-inducing substance of Sclerotinia fructicola, exhibiting activity at 0.001 µg/ml, was shown to be 7. The arthrospore-inducing substance of Cephalosporium acremonium and the aerial mycelium-inducing substance of Streptoverticillium species were recently isolated and their structures are now under investigation. Interestingly, the former substance enhanced production of cephalosporin C, an antibiotic produced by this fungus.
In a second approach, the production of new secondary metabolites by fungi was examined in relation to light regime during culture, revealing that Botrytis cinerea, a serious phytopathogenic fungus, produced abscisic acid, a plant hormone. The production was considerably influenced by the type of lights, being enhanced by blue light, whereas it was entirely inhibited under irradiation with black light blue lamp (λ_{max} 360 nm).

INTRODUCTION

Numerous organic compounds have been isolated from microorganism sources, some of them merely as metabolic products with no regard to biological activity. However, much effort has been devoted by natural product chemists to the search for biologically active compounds among metabolic products of microorganisms; for example, various toxic compounds affecting the growth of plants (1, 2), insects (2) and animals (3), have been identified chemically from pathogenic fungi and bacteria. Among these, gibberellin, a plant hormone, was originally detected as a fungal metabolite (4). Factors essential for growth of microorganisms have also been investigated; mevalolactone, an important biosynthetic precursor of isoprenoids, was first isolated from Lactobacillus homohiochi (5) and the ethanol fermentation broth (6). New antibiotics have been sought for the last three or four decades on a grand scale, and more than three thousands antibiotics have been isolated up to the present day.

In order to increase the efficiency of a search for bioactive natural products, it is desirable to avoid repeated isolation of known compounds in the isolation process: to this end, scientists have built up their own search systems by devising novel isolation procedure for microorganisms, a variety of culture conditions, and new bioassay methods.

Our own search for new types of bioactive fungal metabolites was organised along two lines. Firstly, the basic classification used for bioactive natural products was applied to microbial products, i.e., allelochemics (interspecies in Table 1), pheromones (intraspecies) and endogenous growth regulators (strain level). Application of these classification to two types of important fungal metabolites, growth-inhibitory substances and reproduction-regulating substances, is summarized in Table 1.

Of these five types of bioactive fungal metabolites, we selected three as subjects for research, i.e., aversion factors, autoantibiotics (or growth self-inhibitors) and asexual spore inducing substances. Later, aerial mycelium-inducing substances were added to our research

Table 1.	Interspecies	Intrapsecies	Strain level
Growth-inhibitory substances	antibiotics	aversion factors	autoantibiotics (growth self-inhibitors)
Reproduction-regulating substances	------	sexual organ-inducing substances	asexual spore-inducing substances

programs.

When different strains of the same fungal species are inoculated on the same nutrient agar medium in a Petri dish and incubated, mutual inhibition of mycelial growth is sometimes observed between the growing colonies of different strains. This phenomenon was named "aversion" by Caylay in 1923 (7), and it should be noted that aversion was reported five years before the discovery of the first antibiotic, penicillin (1928): penicillin was classified as an allelochemics (interspecies) (8). Since then, intensive investigation of antibiotics has continued for more than fifty years, and the immense impact of antibiotics on human welfare has mashed Caylay's finding that a similar antibiotic action was also observed among strains of the same species. We were interested in aversion, since it might be caused by some growth-inhibitory substance(s) produced by either strain or as a result of cosynthesis by both strains, and so we started isolating the active principles responsible for this phenomenon, "aversion factors", from several fungal species. As a result, we have succeeded in isolation and chemical characterization of aversion factors in two fungal species, as is described in the experimental section.

The terms, "autoantibiotics, self-inhibitors or autoinhibitors", were first used by Lingappa and Lingappa (9) in reference to substances accumulated in the culture medium that inhibit or significantly retard the growth and development of the organisms producing them: they actually isolated two autoantibiotics, phenethyl alcohol and tryptophol, from Candida albicans (9). Since no other chemical works on autoantibiotics have not been reported, except those on spore-germination inhibitors (10, 11, 12), we made a survey for autoantibiotics among phytopathogenic fungi, to determine their frequency of occurrence in the fungi. Rather surprisingly, autoantibiotic activity was found in about 30% of all strains of fungi tested (13). Of these, two fungi, Diaporthe citri and Pleospora herbarum, were selected for examination and the autoantibiotics contained in them were shown to be 5 and 6, respectively (14). A direct search for autoantibiotics in a pathogenic fungus which we wish to control can save both the labor and the expence otherwise necessary for wide screening, and should be conducted more often with phytopathogenic or other fungi.

One of the most intriguing types of bioactive natural products in microbiology is the reproduction-regulating substances of fungi. There are two types of reproduction systems, i.e., sexual and asexual processes, in the life cycle of fungi. Much work has been done on the sexual process, and several sexual reproduction-regulating substances such as trisporic acid (15), sirenin (16), antheridiol (17), oogoniol (18) and cyclic AMP (19), have been chemically identified. More recently, the mating pheromones of Saccharomyces (20) and Rhodosporidium (21) species were chemically identified by Japanese workers. On the other hand, asexual reproduction in fungi is principally controlled by the light conditions under which the fungi were grown (22). They can be classified into three groups: (i) the first group of fungi need an irradiation of light for asexual sporulation, (ii) the second group were able to sporulate only under dark conditions, (iii) the other fungi sporulate with no regard to light conditions. We selected fungal species belonging to each of the three types, and looked for any sporulation-stimulating substance contained in the sporulating mycelium. First, Pleospora herbarum (23), as the first type of fungus, produced a heavily spore-bearing mycelium under fluorescent lighting, and this mycelium was extracted with ethyl acetate. Addition of the ethyl acetate extract to the sporeless mycelium grown in the dark, induced a dramatic production of spores in the mycelium. The active substance contained in the extract was partially purified through chromatographic separation, however, instability of the active substance made the final purification difficult (24), and this work is still in progress. As a member of the second group of fungus, Sclerotinia fructicola was cultured on nutrient agar in the dark, when the fungus produced asexual arthrospores abundantly. Three kinds of arthrospore-inducing substances were isolated from the dark-cultured materials. The major substance, which exhibited activity at 0.001 μg/ml, was shown to be a sesquiterpene, named sclerosporin (25), whose structure was finally determined as 7, confirmed by total synthesis of the racemic compound (26). Two minor active substances of S. fructicola were identified as R(-)-glycerol monolinolate (9) (27) and dolichol-23 (10) (28), respectively. Interestingly, the former compound was active only in its R enantiomer, and the latter new metabolite was produced only in submerged culture.

Arthrospore-inducing substance of Cephalosporium acremonium was also investigated in relation to the production of cephalosporin C, an antibiotic produced by this fungus, whose semisynthetic derivatives have been clinically used worldwide as antibacterial agents. Our research was based on Nash and Huber's observation in 1971 (29) that a parallel correlation existed between formation of arthrospores and production of the antibiotic, indicated by the finding that strains producing more cephalosporin C produced more arthrospores. Thus, we started searching for arthrospore-inducing substances contained in the spore-forming mycelium. Once the spore-inducing substance was isolated, it would be expected also to stimulate production of cephalosporin C. As the result of examining the culture broth of arthrospore-producing mycelium, two components were extracted. Interestingly, addition of these two components together was found to be necessary for inducing activity. One of these two was successfully isolated, and the pure substance, at concentrations less than 0.03 μg/ml in the presence of another component, induced arthrospores even under "unsporulatable" culture conditions. Moreover, as expected, the production of cephalosporin C was remarkably enhanced by addition of these substances (30).

The last subject to which our first approach was directed was aerial mycelium-inducing substances. Recently, much attention was focussed on the induction of aerial mycelium from substrate mycelium in Streptomycetes. This induction is one of the most important differentiation in the life cycle of Streptomycetes, and several reports on this subject were published in relation to various phenotype characters such as antibiotic production and nutrient auxotrophy. The involvement of transposable genetic determinants in aerial mycelium induction was also suggested. Some known antibiotics, such as lincomycin and chloramphenicol, were reported to exhibit aerial mycelium-inducing activity (31), and a new antibiotic, pamamycin, was isolated with similar activity (31). We have succeeded in the isolation of an aerial mycelium-inducing substance from *Streptoverticillium* species (32). The active substance was isolated in quite minute amount (ca. 60 μg) from 200 liters of cultured nutrient agar materials, and its very low concentration at 0.0001 μg/disc induced aerial mycelium formation on a spontanous bald mutant isolated from the same strain. Interestingly, the substance exhibited activity only in the presence of inosine (or adenosine); these nucleosides were also isolated from the same cultured materials.

In our second approach to the search for bioactive fungal metabolites, fungi were cultured under irradiation by various colored lights, and their antibiotic as well as phytotoxic activity were compared with those of the dark culture. We expected that the light irradiation might stimulate them to produce new metabolites which had never been detected under dark culture conditions. As a result, *Botrytis cinerea*, a serious phytopathogenic fungus, was shown to produce abscisic acid, a plant hormone, when grown in blue light (33). The yield of abscisic acid, which was also produced in the dark culture, was increased fourfold in the blue light culture. Interestingly, irradiation of the fungus with black light blue (λ_{max} 360 nm) inhibited production of abscisic acid to a trace amount. Since previous studies on secondary metabolites of microorganisms were conducted mostly on those produced in dark culture, irradiation by any specific colored light during the culture might be a promising method for finding new microbial products, and our study is continuing in this direction.

EXPERIMENTAL AND RESULTS

Aversion factors of *Cochliobolus setariae* (34) and *Cochliobolus lunata* (35, 36)

More than ten species of fungi, which had been reported to cause aversion, were collected from the Institute for Fermentation, Osaka (IFO), Japan. Our reinvestigation of aversion with these strains confirmed that two species, *Cochliobolus setariae* and *Cochliobolus lunata* caused aversion, showing a clear inhibitory zone between growing colonies of different strains of the same species. First, our preliminary examination on *C. setariae* revealed that the aversion was due to respective production from each strain of active substances which were extractable with organic solvents and exhibited selective inhibition of mycelial growth in the opposite strain. Two strains, IFO 6635 and IFO 6387, which showed aversion, were separately cultured in a malt-dextrose medium by shaking, and aversion factors were isolated from each cultured filtrate. As a result, an aversion factor of strain 6635 was shown to be the bisacetal (**1**) of prehelminthosporol and prehelminthosporal. **1** was fairly unstable, decomposing to each component, and the structure proposed was finally confirmed as its stable acetyl derivative. The aversion factor of strain 6387 was identified as ophiobolin A (**2**), a known metabolite isolated from several *Cochliobolus* and *Helminthosporium* species. Ophiobolin A (**2**) completely inhibited growth of the opposite strain at 3 μg/ml,

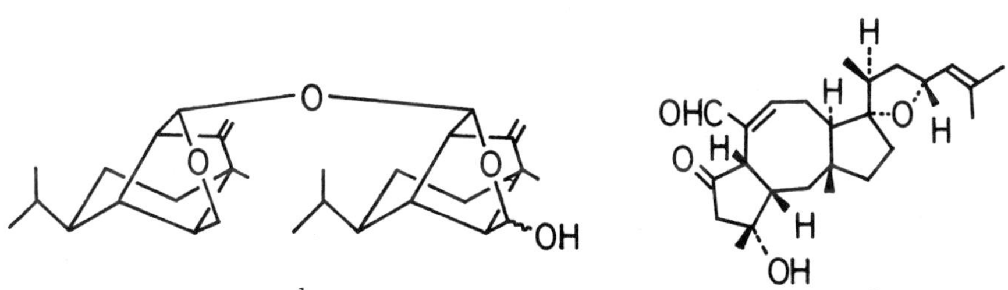

1 **2**

whereas strain 6387 itself was not suppressed even at 500 µg/ml. On the other hand, the bisacetal compound (1) inhibited growth of the opposite 6387 strain at 25 µg/ml, and 100 µg/ml was necessary for complete inhibition of growth of strain 6635 itself. Interestingly, prehelminthosporal, the right hand component of structure 1, was more toxic than the bis-acetal (1) to strain 6635 itself, inhibiting its growth at 25 µg/ml. It was assumed that the fungus converted prehelminthosporal, with high toxicity, into the bisacetal derivative with low toxicity in order to facilitate normal growth of its own mycelium.
In the case of *C. lunata*, half-aversion was observed. When ten IFO strains of the fungus were grown together on a nutrient agar plate, strain 5997 inhibited growth of eight of the other strains, leaving one strain (IFO 6586) unaffected, whereas the growth of strain 5997 was not inhibited by any of the other nine strains tested. Therefore, an aversion factor was isolated from strain 5997, by shake-culturing it in malt-dextrose medium. As a result, the aversion factor,lunatoic acid A, was isolated from the ethyl acetate extract of the cultured filtrate by repeated TLC, but was more easily purified as its methyl ester derivative, which showed still activity. Thus, lunatoic acid A methyl ester was obtained as yellow needles, mp 109°C, $[\alpha]_D$ -208°, $C_{22}H_{26}O_7$. The structure was elucidated as 3, on the basis of UV, IR, ^{1}H and ^{13}C NMR spectra and chemical derivatization. 2,4-Dimethylhexanoic acid was obtained by alkaline hydrolysis of 3, and its absolute configulation was determined as 2S, 4S from its optical rotation, which was compared with those of synthetic compounds. The chirality of the chromophore at the carbon bearing the dimethylhexanoate moiety was determined as R, based on CD of its dihydro-derivative (Pd hydrogenation of the double bond conjugated with a carboxyl group), which agreed well with, and was of opposite sign to, that of the authentic compound (4), whose absolute stereochemistry was already unambiguously established by X-ray analysis. Lunatoic acid A inhibited growth of eight of nine strains of this fungus in concentrations of 3 to 12 µg/ml. On the other hand, the growth of strain 6586, which did not show aversion with strain 5997 itself, was inhibited by 100 µg/ml, and at this concentration strain 5997 itself was also inhibited. At high concentrations (50 - 100 µg/ml) several other fungi, e.g., *Pyricularia oryzae*, *Glomerella cingulata* and *Fulvia fulva*, were also inhibited, but bacterial growth was not affected at all. From these bioassay results, lunatoic acid A may be considered a novel antifungal substance characterized by its selective activity against different strains of the same *Cochliobolus* species. The rather curious antifungal properties of lunatoic acid A prompted us to investigate microscopically its morphological effect on the mycelial growth of each strain of *C. lunata*, and on other fungi. Interestingly, swollen, thick-walled cells were produced by the action of lunatoic acid A on all nine strains of *C. lunata*. Strain 5997 produced the cells abundantly all over the colony, clearly indicating that their production was due to endogenous production of lunatoic acid A. The morphological features of the cells closely resemble those of chlamydospores of *Fusarium solani*. Thus, after careful examination, we concluded that the induced cells should be chlamydospores or chlamydospore-like cells. Similar swollen, thick-walled cells were also induced by lunatoic acid A on the mycelium of *Curvularia trifolii*, and were concluded to be chalydospore-like cells. Lunatoic acid A is the first chlamydospore-inducing substance chemically identified in fungi (36).

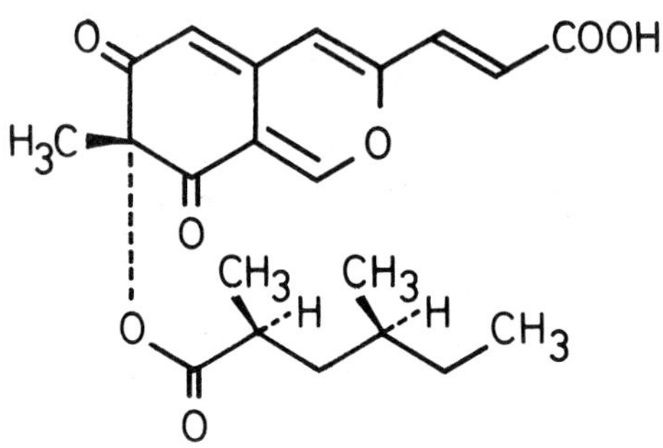

3

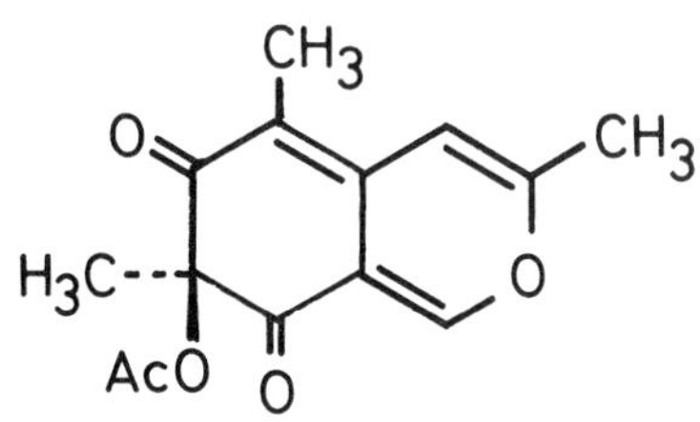

4

Autoantibiotics of *Diaporthe citri* (14) and *Pleospora herbarum* (14)

Autoantibiotics (or growth self-inhibitors) were sought in phytopathogenic fungi, in order to find antifungal agent for use in agriculture by a new method, rather than by the usual screening method of antibiotics. To this end, we modified the screening method as follows: (i) phytopathogenic fungi were widely collected, (ii) they were inoculated on a nutrient agar medium and incubated, and the colonies which grew slowly were selected, (iii) then, they were grown on the agar medium containing active carbon, and the strains growing more rapidly than on the medium without active carbon were finally selected, (iv) these strains were cultured superficially, and (v) autoantibiotics contained in the cultured filtrate were isolated by the usual bioassay technique. We were rather surprized to find, as a result of the screening experiment, that autoantibiotic activity could be found in more than 30% of all phytopathogenic fungi tested (13). Among them, two fungi, *Diaporthe citri* and Pleospora herbarum, were selected for isolation of the autoantibiotics. Thus, an autoantibiotic of D. citri IFO 6443 was obtained as a yellow oil, $C_{12}H_{23}O_3N$, $[\alpha]_D$ +1.5 ± 0.26, CD: $[\theta]_{360\ nm}$ -515. The structure was deduced as 5, on the basis of spectral (UV, IR, ^{1}H and ^{13}C NMR) analysis and chemical reactions, with the stereochemistry undetermined. 5 had an unique α-keto-hydroxamic acid moiety, in which the α-keto group was important for activity, as evidenced by the fact that synthetic hydroxamic acid with a similar carbon chain had no antifungal activity. 5 inhibited growth of D. citri IFO 6443 (which produced 5) at 12.5 µg/ml, Pyricularia oryzae at 3.13 µg/ml and Phytopathora cactorum at 50 µg/ml, but other phytopathogenic fungi tested were inhibited at 100 µg/ml or higher concentrations.

An autoantibiotic of P. herbarum was isolated from the cultured potato-sucrose medium, as colorless needles, mp 91.5°C, $C_{15}H_{24}O_2$. Its characteristic UV: λ_{max} (nm) 225 (ε 8030), 275 (1200), 280 (960), indicated a resorcin type chromophore, on which butyl and pentyl substituents were positioned at 2 and 5, respectively, as ascertained by their specific fragment peaks in the mass spectrum. Thus, 2-butyl-5-pentylresorcin (6) retarded growth of P.herbarum significantly at 6 µg/ml. We can generally recognize the phenomenon of growth self-inhibition occurring widely in nature. We have shown the presence of autoantibiotics in phytopathogenic fungi in the present work. Soil sickness caused by some plants is a serious unresolved problem in agriculture. The isolation and possible role of "overcrowding factors" have been reported in several kinds of insects. We would like to emphasize that such types of bioactive natural products should be further explored in various organisms.

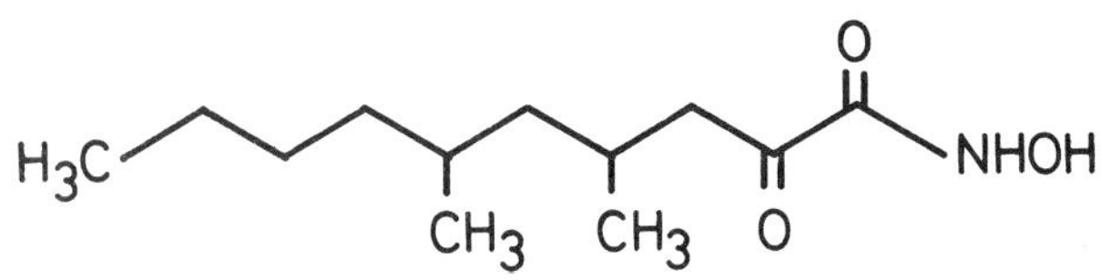

5

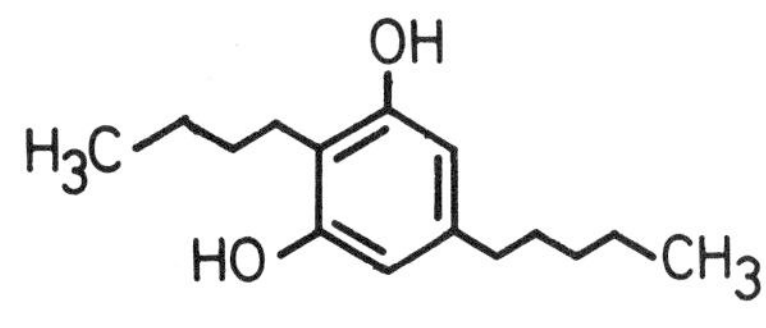

6

Arthrospore-inducing substances of Sclerotinia fructicola (25, 26, 27, 28, 37)

Sclerotinia fructicola was reported in 1933 to produce abundant asexual arthrospores when grown in darkness, but little or none under illumination. Our preliminary investigation revealed that the dark-induced sporulation of this fungus was attributed to spore-induced substances produced only in the dark-cultured mycelium. We have isolated three kinds of sporogenic substances from the dark-cultured matrials and chemically identified their structures as follows. S. fructicola was cultured on potato-sucrose agar medium in the dark, and the cultured materials were extracted with ethyl acetate. The major active substance contained in the extract was purified through repeated TLC on Kiesel Gel 60 and subsequent HPLC on LiChrosorb RP-2 (dioxane-H_2O (6:4)) into a homogenous single peak on chromatograms (yield 182 µg from four liters of the cultured materials), and named sclerosporin (25). Two related metabolites, named sclerosporal (194 µg) and sclerosporene (35 µg), were also isolated (37), although they had no activity. Chemical studies (37) on sclerosporin and sclerosporal were conducted using these quite minute amount of samples, by devising ultramicro-techniques for structure elucidation. For example, 50 µg of sclerosporal was chemically derivatized through successive four steps of reactions: (i) $LiAlH_4$ in Et_2O, (ii) H_2/Pd in EtOH, (iii) TsCl/py, (v) $LiAlH_4$ in Et_2O, into the saturated hydrocarbon, whose mass spectrum was used for identification of the carbon skeleton. First, their structures were considered to have a guaiane skeleton. However, further synthetic work to confirm the proposed structures revealed that the mass spectrum of trans-guaiane was almost indistinguishable from that of trans-cadinane, thus the proposed structures based on the mass spectra should be reinvestigated. In order to obtain enough sample for spectral analysis, the fungus was again cultured repeatedly on the nutrient agar medium, using in all 5050 plates (101 liters) of Petri dishes, and 3.8 mg of pure sclerosporal was isolated. The detailed spectral analysis of sclerosporal with 360 ^{1}H NMR deduced an alternative structure belonging to cis-cadinane (8), thus the newly postulated structures of sclerosporin (7) and sclerosporal (8) were completely confirmed by their successful total synthesis, except for the absolute stereochemistry (26).

The sporogenic activity of sclerosporin was measured on S. fructicola, by adding the sample to unsporulatable mycelium grown under illumination by fluorescent lamps. The bioassay results are shown in Figure 1. Sclerosporin exhibited weak but significant sporogenic activity at 0.001 (4×10^{-9}M) ~ 0.005 µg/ml (2×10^{-8}M), and the activity was enhanced as the amount of the sample increased. At the maxmum concentration (5 µg/ml or 3×10^{-5}M) tested, the 79% production of arthrospores (compared with those in darkness) was observed. Synthetic racemic sclerosporin also produced arthrospores abundantly at 25 µg/ml than those produced in darkness, thus, the structure of sclerosporin was further supported from the biological activity.

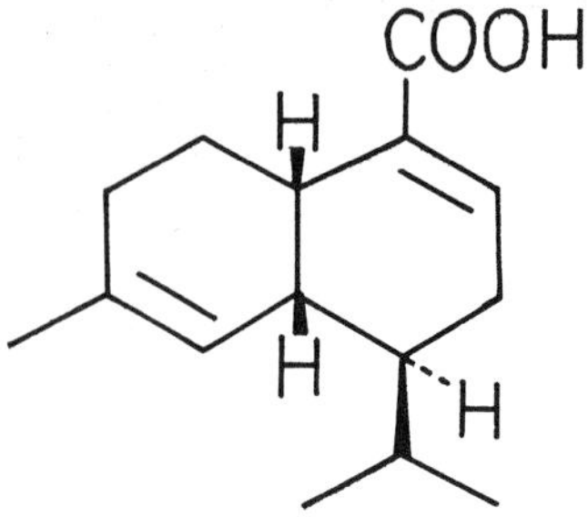

7

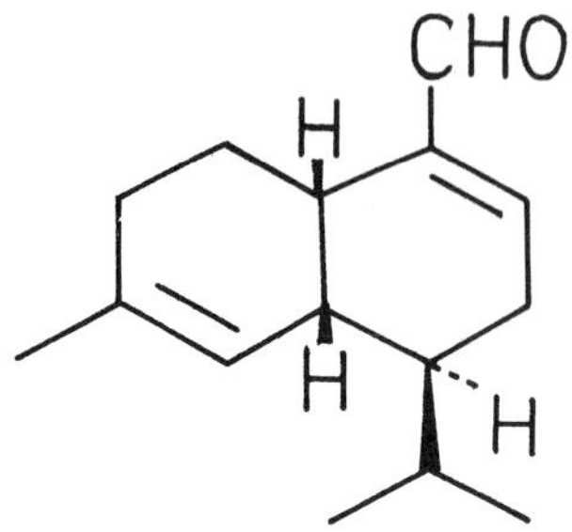

8

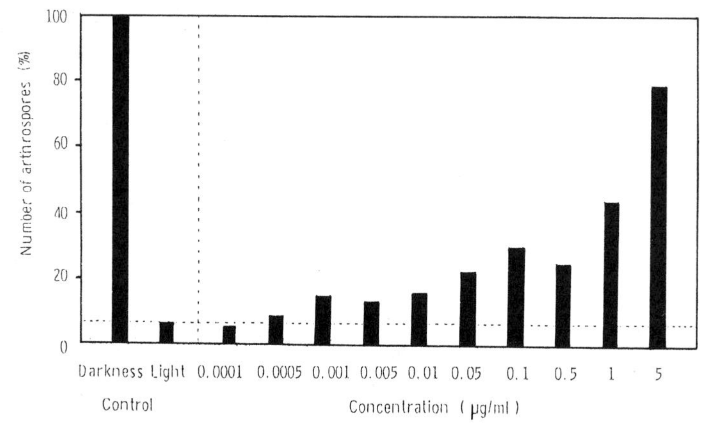

Figure 1. Asexual arthrospore-inducing activity of sclerosporin on the mycelium of S. fructicola grown under fluorescent lighting, in which the fungus does not sporulate.

A minor sporogenic substance was isolated from the same cultured materials, in addition to sclerosporin, and was identified as α -glycerol monolinolate (27). Since it has a chiral center in the molecule, both R and S enantiomers of α -glycerol monolinolate were synthesized from D- and L-mannitol, respectively: interestingly, only the R enantiomer was active. On the other hand, the enantiomeric ratio of the natural substance, measured using its diastereomeric di(+)-MPTA esters, was shown to be a mixture of R(23%)- and S(26%)-glycerol monolinolate and also of its β isomer (42%). Synthetic R(-)-glycerol monolinolate (9) exhibited significant sporogenic activity at 0.05 - 0.1 µg/ml, which was almost one hundredth that of sclerosporin. The 3-phosphate ester of the S(+) enantiomer of 1-monoacyl glycerol has been known to be an obligatory intermediate in biosynthesis of triglycerides and phospholipids. Our present research revealed that the antipode of this important but ubiquitous metabolite was active in inducing asexual arthrospores in S. fructicola. Another minor sporogenic substance was isolated from the shaking culture of the fungus. The active substance was identified as dolichol-23 (10) (28). The cis/trans ratio of double bonds in it was determined as 18:3 from the ^1H NMR, although their precise positions were not clarified. Dolichol-23 exhibited weak but clear activity at 0.02 µg/ml. Maximum sporulation occurred at 0.5 µg/ml, however, even at this concentration the sporulation was not so abundant (ca. 56%) as that in darkness. Moreover, since the sporulation of the fungus occurred actually on the agar plate but not in submerged culture in which 10 was produced, the role of dolichol-23 for the sporulation might be less significant, compared with those of the two sporogenic substances already identified.

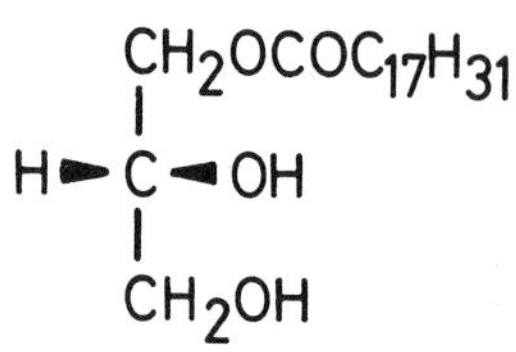

9

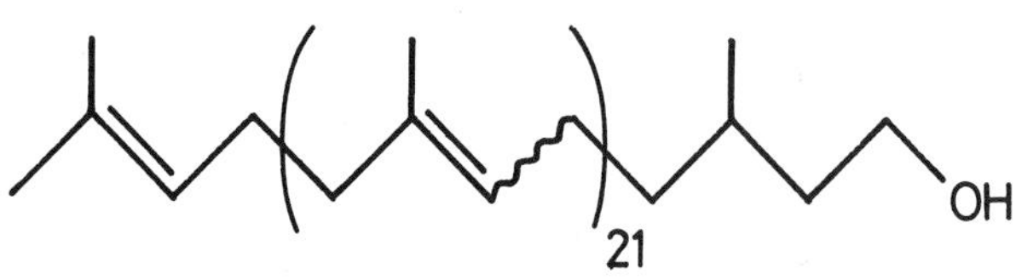

10

Arthrospore-inducing substances of Cephalosporium acremonium (30)

We have an interest in the possible role of asexual reproduction-regulating substances which might be capable of controlling production of important secondary metabolites such as antibiotics. Nash and Huber (29) reported in 1971 that Cephalosporium acremonium showed a parallel correlation between formation of arthrospores and production of cephalosporin C, that is, they observed that the strains bearing more arthrospores tended to produce more antibiotic. Semi-synthetic cephalosporins, derivatized chemically from 7-aminocephalosporanic acid which was obtained from cephalosporin C, have been one of the most important chemotherapeutic agents used in more than 50% consumption of all antibiotics clinically used in the world. We assumed that any arthrospore-inducing substance might be produced when the mycelium was differentiating to arthrospores, and if the active substance were isolated, it could be used for stimulating production of cephalosporin C. C. acremonium ATCC 14553 was cultured by shaking in a sucrose-containing medium in which arthrospores were produced in abundance. Addition of the aqueous acetone extract of the culture broth to non-sporulating mycelium grown in glucose medium induced dramatic arthrospore production. The active substances were purified through successive column chromatography on supports such as active carbon, DEAE-Sephadex A-25 (OH^- and AcO^- form), Sephadex G-10, and HPLC on LiChrosorb RP-18, Nucleosil Phenyl and ODS-5. Two active substances were extracted from the culture broth, and quite interestingly, addition of the two components together was necessary for inducing activity. One of the two was successfully isolated in pure form, in a yield of ca. 200 μg from 200 liters of the culture broth. The active substance exhibited arthrospore-inducing activity at concentrations less than 0.03 μg/ml in the presence of the other component which has not yet been purified. Moreover, the production of cephalosporin C was considerably enhanced by addition of these substances, as we expected. An example of our bioassay results, which were conducted during isolation procedures of the active subsatnce, is shown in Figure 2. Chemical studies on the structure of the active substance are now in progress.

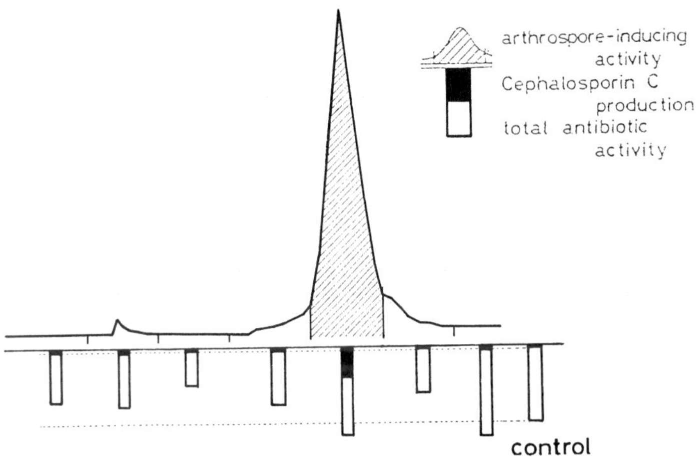

Figure 2. Bioassay results on arthrospore-inducing activity and total antibiotic activity as well as cephalosporin C production-promoting activity of the crude active substance which was purified by Sephadex A-25 (OH^- form) column chromatography. Another active component was added to all tested fractions.

Aerial mycelium-inducing substance of Streptoverticillium species (32)

Streptomycetes have a rather simple asexual life cycle which usually involves three stages: germination of asexual apores to form substrate mycelium, differentiation of the substrate mycelium to aerial mycelium, and asexual spore formation on the aerial mycelium and/or (in some cases) on the substrate mycelium (38). In this life cycle, aerial mycelium formation in particular is an important cellular differentiation, in that it is closely coordinated with various phenotype characteristics such as production of antibiotics, pigments, enzymes, earthy odor, and nutrient auxotrophy (39). Involvement of transposable genetic determinants in these phenomena has also been suggested (40). We were interested in aerial mycelium-inducing substance (AMIS) which might be produced when aerial mycelium was induced from substrate mycelium. In order to examine this possibility, aerial mycelium-negative strains (bald mutants) were isolated from Streptoverticillium species KCC U-0166 - twenty bald mutants were isolated from ca. 5000 colonies of the parent strain. The parent strain produced aerial mycelium heavily when cultured on an inorganic salts-starch agar medium. Extraction of this material with acetone and addition of the aqueous acetone extract to the bald mutants resulted in a dramatic induction of aerial mycelium in two strains. Thus, these two spontaneous bald mutants were used as test organisms for purification of AMIS.

The aqueous acetone extract of the cultured agar materials (200 liters) was, after washing with organic solvents, subjected to successive column chromatography, as illustrated in Figure 3. Finally, 68 μg of active substance was isolated chromatographycally in a single peak by monitoring with UV at 230 nm; the peak was completely superimposable with the histogram of biological activity. Quite interestingly, AMIS exhibited activity only in the presence of inosine (or adenosine); these nucleorosides were also isolated from the same cultured materials. The isolated AMIS induced aerial mycelium in the bald mutant at very low concentrations of 0.0001 - 0.0005 μg/disc by a paper disc diffusion bioassay. The structure elucidation of AMIS, as well as its physiological role in Streptomycetes, are now under investigation.

The cultured materials (200 liters)
↓ extracted with acetone
washed with ethyl acetate
washed with *n*-butanol

Water-soluble residues
↓
Charcoal column
↓ 80% ethanol in water
Octyl Sepharose column
↓ EtOH-H_2O
CM-Sephadex column
↓ 0.1M TEAB-EtOH (1:1)
QAE-Sephadex column
↓ 0.1M TEAB-EtOH (1:1)
Toyopearl HW-40 (super fine) column
↓ 0.1M TEAB-EtOH (1:1)
LiChrosorb RP-18 HPLC
↓ dioxane-H_2O-AcOH (45:55:0.5)
Zorbax NH_2 HPLC
↓ cyclohexane-EtOH (85:15)
Zorbax NH_2 HPLC
↓ cyclohexane-EtOH (85:15)
Zorbax NH_2 HPLC
↓ cyclohexane-EtOH (85:15)
Active substance
yield : 68 μg

Figure 3. The isolation procedure of the aerial mycelium-inducing substance of *Streptoverticillium* species KCC U-0166. TEAB: triethylamine bicarbonate (pH 7.0).

Photocontrolled microbial production of abscisic acid by *Botrytis cinerea* (33)

Botrytis cinerea, a phytopathogenic fungus causing serious gray mold didease on many kinds of cultivated plants, was cultured on a potato-dextrose medium, either in the dark or under continuous blue light irradiation (λ_{max} 450 ± 50 nm, light intensity of 76 μw cm^{-2}). Blue light was already known to have an inhibitory effect on asexual sporulation of *B. cinerea* (41). The cultured mycelium and agar were extracted with acetone, and the aqueous acetone extract was bioassayed on turnip seedlings. As a result, the extract obtained from the dark cultured materials exhibited weak inhibitory activity, whereas, quite interestingly, strong activity was found in the extract obtained from the blue light culture. The active substance contained in the latter extract was purified by TLC on silicic acid, after converting it with diazomethane to the methyl ester derivative. In this way, the methyl ester of the active substance was obtained as a colorless oil in a yield of 5.2 mg/100 ml of the cultured agar materials. The IR($CHCl_3$) and ^1H NMR spectra were identical with those of abscisic acid methyl ester, and its optical rotation, $[\alpha]_D$ +360° (EtOH), indicated it to be natural (+)-abscisic acid. The stereochemistry of the C_2-double bond in the side chain, analyzed by GLC, was shown to be in the ratio *cis* (98%): *trans* (2%). Abscisic acid was also isolated from the dark cultured materials in a yield of 1.4 mg/100 ml of the cultured materials, and the sample was shown by analysis to contain 2.4% of *trans*-abscisic acid. A considerable difference in abscisic acid yield between the dark and the blue light culture prompted us to examine the effect of other colored lights. A black light blue (BLB) lamp (λ_{max} 360 nm, light intensity of 236 μw cm^{-2}) was similarly used for irradiation of the fungus. The production of abscisic acid was in striking contrast to the case of the blue light culture, decreasing to a yield of 0.2 mg/100 ml of the cultured materials, which was less than one twentieth that of the blue light and one seventh that of the dark culture. Green,red, and far red lights were also used for irradiation of the fungus, and all of them had similar promising effects on the production of abscisic acid. B. cinerea had been reported to produce several sesquiterpenoids of the perhydroindane skeleton, by shake-culturing in "the dark" (42). In contrast, abscisic acid, which is also a sesquiterpenoid, was isolated from "the blue light culture" of the same fungus. Our present research suggests that culturing of fungi under irradiation by some colored lights may be a promising method for finding new microbial products, and further studies are continuing in this direction.

AcKnowledgment - We wish to thank Prof. W. D. Crow, The Australian National Univ., for his kind reading of the manuscript.

REFERENCES

1. "Toxins in Plant Disease", Ed. by R. D. Durbin, Academic Press, New York (1981).
2. N. Takahashi, S. Marumo and N. Ohtake, "Biologically Active Natural Products" (in Japanese), 2nd Ed., Tokyo Univ. Press, Tokyo (1981).
3. "Microbial Toxins I - VI", Ed. by S. J. Ajl, A. Ciegler, S. Kadis, T. C. Montie and G. Weinbaum, Academic Press, New York (1971).
4. T. Yabuta and Y. Sumiki, Bull. of Agric. Biol. Chem. Soc. Japan, 14, 1526 (1938).
5. G. Tamura, J. Gen. Appl. Microbiol., 12, 431 (1956).
6. K. Folkers, H. R. Shiggs, L. D. Wright, D. E. Wolf and C. H. Hoffman, J. Am. Chem. Soc. 78, 4499, 5273 (1956): 79, 1486, 2316 (1957).
7. D. M. Caylay, J. Genetics, 13, 353 (1923).
8. R. H. Whittaker and P. P. Feeny, Science, 171, 757 (1971).
9. R. T. Lingappa and Y. Lingappa, Bact. Proc., G-117 (1964).
10. V. Macko, R. C. Staples and J. A. A. Renwick, Science, 170, 539 (1970).
11. V. Macko, P. J. Allen and J. A. A. Renwick, Science, 173, 835 (1971).
12. H. Abe, M. Uchiyama, Y. Tanaka and H. Saito, Tetrahedron Lett., 3807 (1976).
13. K. Kitaori's master thesis presented to Faculty of Agriculture, Nagoya University(1978).
14. Their manuscripts are in preparation for Agric. Biol. Chem.(Japan).
15. L. Caglioti, G. Canelli, B. Camerino, R. Mondelli, A. Prieto, A. Quilico, T. Salvatori and A. Selva, Tetrahedron, Suppl., 7, 175 (1966).
16. L. Machlis, W. H. Nutting, M. W. Williams and H. Rapoport, Biochem., 5, 2147 (1966).
17. T. C. McMorris, A. W. Barksdale, Nature, 215, 320 (1967); G. P. Arsenault, K. Biemann, A. W. Barksdale and T. C. McMorris, J. Am. Chem. Soc., 90, 5635 (1968).
18. T. C. McMorris, R. Seshadri, G. R. Weihe, G. P. Arsenault and A. W. Barksdale, J. Am. Chem. Soc., 97, 2544 (1975).
19. I. Uno and T. Ishikawa, Molec. Gen. Genet., 113, 228 (1971).
20. A. Sakurai, S. Tamura, N. Yanagishima and C. Shimada, Agric. Biol. Chem., 41, 395(1977).
21. Y. Kamiya, A. Sakurai, S. Tamura, K. Abe, E. Tsuchiya and S. Fukui, Agric. Biol. Chem., 41, 1099 (1977).
22. C. M. Leach, "Method in Microbiology", Vol. IV, Ed. by C. Booth, Academic Press, pp 609 - 664, New York (1971).
23. C. M. Leach, Mycologia, 60, 532 (1968).
24. S. Marumo, Shokubutsu Boeki, 33, 421 (1979) (in Japanese).
25. M. Katayama and S. Marumo, Agric. Biol. Chem., 42, 505 (1978).
26. The manuscript was submitted to Tetrahedron Lett.
27. M. Katayama and S. Marumo, Agric. Biol. Chem., 42, 1431 (1978).
28. M. Katayama and S. Marumo, Agric. Biol. Chem., 42, 1967 (1978).
29. C. H. Nash and F. M. Huber, Appl. Microbiol., 22, 6 (1971).
30. The manuscript is in preparation for Nature.
31. P. A. McCann and B. M. Pogell, J. Antibiot., 32, 673 (1979).
32. The manuscript is in preparation for publication.
33. S. Marumo, M. Katayama, E. Komori, Y. Ozaki, M. Natsume and S. Kondo, Agric. Biol.Chem. 46, 1967 (1982).
34. M. Nukina and S. Marumo, Agric. Biol. Chem., 40, 2121 (1976).
35. M. Nukina and S. Marumo, Tetrahedron Lett., 2603 (1977).
36. M. Nukina and S. Marumo, Agric. Biol. Chem., 46, 2339 (1982).
37. M. Katayama and S. Marumo, Tetrahedron Lett., 1773 (1979).
38. S. A. Waksman, "The Actinomycetes", Vol. I, Williams & Wilkins Com. (1959).

39. P. A. Redshaw, P. A. McCann, M. A. Pentella and B. M. Pogell, J. Bacteriol., 137, 891 (1959).
40. M. Okanishi, T. Ohta and H. Umezawa, J. Antibiot., 23, 45 (1970).
41. K. K. Tan, J. Gen. Microbiol., 82, 191 (1974).
42. H. -W. Fehlhaber, R. Geipal, H. -J. Mercker, R. Tshesche and K. Welmer, Chem. Ber., 107, 1720 (1974); A. P. Shaw and J. R. Hanson, J. C. S. Perkin I, 741 (1980).

MILDIOMYCIN, AN EFFECTIVE ERADICANT FOR POWDERY MILDEW

Takashi Iwasa

Central Research Division, Takeda Chemical Industries Ltd., Osaka 532, Japan

Abstract - Mildiomycin is a nucleoside antibiotic produced by an actinomycete, *Streptoverticillium rimofaciens* B-98891. Its antimicrobial activity on agar media is not so strong, but it shows an excellent control effect against various kinds of powdery mildews without phytotoxicity. It also shows systemic property. Since powdery mildew fungus is an obligate parasite, disc-plate method with *Rhodotorula rubra* and high-performance liquid chromatography were used to detect mildiomycin *in vitro*. Mildiomycin contains 5-hydroxymethylcytosine in its molecule. Biosynthetic study showed that 5-hydroxymethylcytosine was formed by the hydrolysis of hydroxymethyl cytidinemonophosphate derived from the hydroxymethylation of cytidinemonophosphate presumably synthesized through the biosynthetic pathway of pyrimidine nucleotide.

INTRODUCTION

Powdery mildew is an important plant disease that causes extensive damage to cereals, vegetables, fruit trees, and garden plants; consequently, an effective eradicant, without side effects, of powdery mildew has been sought. Culture broths of actinomycetes were screened by the brush inoculation method (1) in which anti-mildew activity was evaluated on 7 day-old barley seedling in a test tube (70 x 15 mm). In this effort an actinomycete, *Streptoverticillium rimofaciens* B-98891 (2), was found to secrete an active substance in its culture broth. The active substance was isolated by monitoring the *in vivo* activity, the *in vitro* activity and by high-performance liquid chromatography (HPLC)(3). It was confirmed (4, 5) that the substance was a new nucleoside antibiotic with 5-hydroxymethylcytosine (HMC); it was named mildiomycin (MIL) because of its specific activity against powdery mildew fungi (6).

Mildiomycin ($C_{19}H_{30}N_8O_9$)

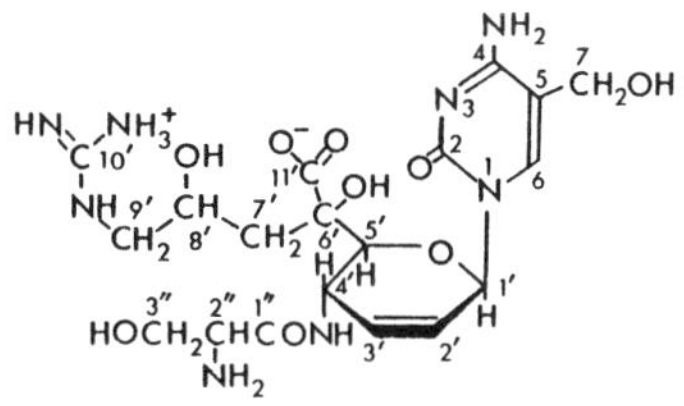

Assay methods of MIL, its biological activities and the biosynthesis of pyrimidine chromophore are reviewed in the following paragraphs.

ASSAY METHODS

Difficulty existed in detecting activity against powdery mildew fungi, which is an obligate parasite, during isolation and purification of MIL. A microbiological assay method and chemical assay method using high-performance liquid chromatography were devised to detect MIL.

Microbiological assay method

In searching for *in vitro* test microorganisms other than powdery mildew fungus, 1,400 strains of yeasts were examined. Of these, 29 strains, including 21 strains of *Rhodotorula*, were selected as highly susceptible to MIL, and finally *R. rubra* IFO 0907 was chosen as the test organism. From the results of experiments for a suitable assay condition, the disc-plate assay for MIL was established (2) as shown in Fig. 1.

High-performance liquid chromatography

MIL and related antibiotics were analyzed by HPLC with a fine reversed phase adsorbent which was well-suited for the best column packing for aminoacyl nucleosides (3). For MIL, the mobile phase of 2.5 % methanol-0.005M citrate buffer (pH 5.8) gave the best correlation between the injection amount and the peak height by UV detection as shown in Fig. 2. From the standard curve the content of MIL in crude or purified samples, in culture filtrates or in solution, could be readily determined.

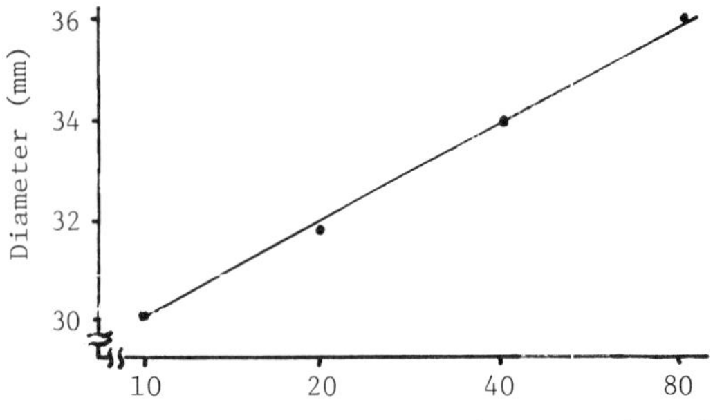

Fig. 1. Relation between diameter of inhibition zone and concentration of mildiomycin

Assay media: Potato dextrose agar (pH 5) for base layer and potato sucrose agar (pH 5) for seed layer.
Inoculum: 2-4 x 10^9 cells/ml. The inoculum size is 5 % of the seed layer medium.
Incubation: 28°C for 18-20 hours.

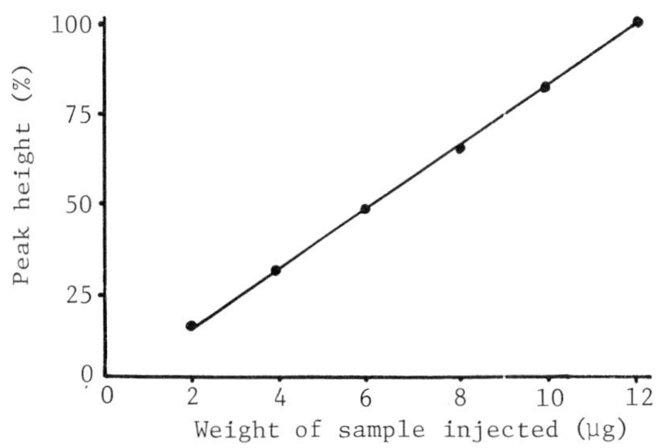

Fig. 2. The standard curve of mildiomycin on HPLC

μ Bondapack C_{18}, 2.5 % methanol-0.005M citrate buffer, flow rate, 1.0 ml/min.
The sample was measured at the UV range, 0.2 , at a sample concentration of 2 mg/ml

ANTIMICROBIAL SPECTRUM OF MILDIOMYCIN

The antimicrobial activity of MIL on agar media (2) examined by the agar dilution method is shown in TABLE 1. MIL showed activity against *Mycobacterium phlei*, *Rhodotorula rubra* and some phytopathogenic fungi such as *Cochliobolus miyabeanus*, *Sclerotinia sclertiorum*, *Botrytis cinerea*, *Guignardia laricina* and *Alternaria kikuchiana*. No growth inhibition by MIL was observed at a concentration of 500 μg/ml in the following microorganisms; *Candida albicans* IFO 0853, *C. tropicalis* IFO 0006, *Saccharomyces cerevisiae* IFO 0209, *Aspergillus niger* IFO 4066, *Penicillium chrysogenum* IFO 4626, *Trichophyton rubrum* IFO 5467, *Pyricularia oryzae* IFO 5279, *Helminthosporium sigmoideum* var. *irregulare* IFO 5273, *Venturia pirina* IFO 6189, *Diaporthe citri* IFO 9170, *Elsinoe fawcetti* IFO 8417, *Pythium aphanidermatum* IFO 7030, *Gibberella zeae* IFO 7160, *Bacillus subtilis* IFO 3513, *B. cereus* IFO 3466, *B. brevis* IFO 3331, *Staphylococcus aureus* IFO 3061, *Sarcina lutea* IFO 3232, *Proteus vulgaris* IFO 3045. The mechanism of action of MIL has been studied using *E. coli* and *R. rubra* (7, 8) and it is suggested that MIL inhibits the protein synthesis.

ACTIVITY AGAINST POWDERY MILDEW

Activity of MIL against powdery mildews on 15 kinds of plants caused by 13 species of powdery mildew fungi of 8 genera was examined (6, 9). The effects were determined by the % area of mildew on the leaves. The % disease control was calculated using the formula;

$$\% \text{ disease control} = 100 \times \left(1 - \frac{\% \text{ area of mildew on treated plants}}{\% \text{ area of mildew on untreated plants}}\right)$$

TABLE 1. Antimicrobial spectrum of mildiomycin

Test organisms	Condition of assay Media a)	Temp. (°C)	Time (hour)	M.I.C. (μg/ml)
Rhodotorula rubra IFO 0870	A	28	40	50
Trichophyton mentagrophytes IFO 5809	D	28	88	500
Cochliobolus miyabeanus IFO 5277	A	28	40	250
Sclerotinia sclerotiorum IFO 9395	A	28	40	500
Botrytis cinerea TKF 12	A	20	88	250
Guignardia laricina IFO 7888	A	28	88	100
Alternaria kikuchiana IFO 8414	A	28	88	250
Escherichia coli IFO 12734	B	37	20	500
Pseudomonas aeruginosa IFO 3449	B	37	20	500
Mycobacterium phlei IFO 3158	C	37	40	50
M. smegmatis ATCC	C	37	40	250

a) A: Modified Pfeffer's agar (10) B: Nutrient agar C: Glycerol-nutrient agar D: 1 % glucose, 0.4 % ammonium phosphate, dibasic, 0.07 % magnecium sulfate 0.1 % potassium phosphate, monobasic, 0.1 % sodium chloride, 0.005 % ferrous sulfate. 1.5 % agar

TABLE 2. Control of powdery mildew by mildiomycin

Host plant (Cultivar)	Pathogen	Chemicals a) & concn. (mg a.i./l)	Disease control (%)	Date Inoculation	Spray	Assessment
Cucumber (Shinko)	*Sphaerotheca fuliginea*	MIL 25	95.5	Nov.14	Nov.16	Nov.29
		MIL 50	99.1		Nov.22	
		DINO 148	82.7			
		QUINO 62.5	100.0			
		W.S. 2500	100.0 b)			
Melon (Ginsen)	*S. fuliginea*	MIL 25	80.4	Feb.12	Feb.14	Feb.29
		MIL 50	92.8			
		DINO 148	94.8			
Rose (Francis)	*S. pannosa*	MIL 25	96.0	-	Mar.11	Apr.1
		MIL 50	97.8		Mar.18	
		DINO 148	63.2			
Strawberry (Hogyoku)	*S. humuli*	MIL 25	96.0	-	Nov.21	Dec.6
		MIL 50	96.3		Nov. 29	
		DINO 148	78.9			
		QUINO 83	50.0			
		POLY 100	80.9			
Tobacco (MC)	*Erysiphe cichoracearum*	MIL 25	92.1	-	Feb.8	Feb.19
		MIL 50	93.0			
		DINO 148	94.0			
Tomato (Fukuju No.2)	*E. cichoracearum*	MIL 25	87.0	Jun.10	Jun.12	Jul.2
		MIL 50	94.8			
		DINO 148	83.3			
Barley (Shiga-hakkoku)	*E. graminis*	MIL 25	90.0	Mar.12	Mar.14	Mar.26
		MIL 50	94.5			
		QUINO 83	90.0			
Garden pea (Usumiendo)	*E. pisi*	MIL 25	87.1	Jun.28	Jul.1	Jul.10
		MIL 50	88.4			
		DINO 148	87.4			
Red clover	*E. polygoni*	MIL 25	85.1	-	Jun.20	Jun.27
		MIL 50	90.3			
		DINO 148	46.1			

a) MIL: Mildiomycin 5.5 % WP, DINO: Dinocap 37 % EC, QUINO: Quinomethionate 25 % WP, TH-M: Thiophanate methyl 70 % WP, POLY: Polyoxin AL 10 % WP, W.S.: Wettable sulfur 75 % WP

b) Chlorosis

TABLE 2. Control of powdery mildew by mildiomycin (Continued)

Host plant (Cultivar)	Pathogen	Chemicals & concn. (mg a.i./1)		Disease control (%)	Date Inoculation	Spray	Assessment
Oxalis	*Microsphaera ruselli*	MIL	25	97.0	Jun.28	Jun.29	Jul.6
		MIL	50	98.7			
		DINO	148	83.5			
Apple (Rall's Janet)	*Podosphaera leucotricha*	MIL	25	87.9	May.22	May.24	May 31
		MIL	50	91.8			
		DINO	148	92.7			
		POLY	160	81.9			
Mulberry (Ichinose)	*Phyllactinia moricola*	MIL	25	81.6	-	Sep.3	Oct.8
		MIL	50	82.5		Sep.10	
		DINO	148	88.9			
Grape (Muscut berry A)	*Uncinula necator*	MIL	25	100.0	-	Jun.26	Aug.7
		MIL	50	100.0		Jul.3	
		TH-M	476	66.7		Jul.10	
						Jul.17	
Green pepper (Ise)	*Leveillula taurica*	MIL	50	86.5	Apr.18	Apr.19	Apr.29
		DINO	148	41.5			
Oak	*Cystotheca wrightii*	MIL	25	50.3	-	Apr.26	May 3
		MIL	50	93.4			
		DINO	148	89.2			
		QUINO	83	55.1			

All powdery mildews tested were controlled by MIL. MIL was also active against the powdery mildew of green pepper caused by an endoparasitic fungus, *Leveillula taurica,* which had been resistant to fungicides on the market. Thus, MIL is regarded to have a broad anti-mildew spectrum. No phytotoxicity has been observed so far.

Insufficient control by benomyl of powdery mildew of cucumber has been encountered owing to the possible occurrence of benomyl-resistant strain. The controlling effect of MIL against powdery mildew fungus from benomyl-treated plot was tested. As a result MIL was effective against inocula from both untreated and benomyl-treated plots (TABLE 3.).

TABLE 3. Effect of mildiomycin against benomyl-resistant strain of *Sphaerotheca fuliginea* on cucumber

Treatment	Concn. (mg/1)	Area mildewed[a] (%) Sources of inoculum: Benomyl plot[b]	Untreated plot
Mildiomycin	50	0	0
Benomyl	250	89.2	59.2
Thiophanate-methyl	250	95.0	48.3
Dinocap	148	0	0
Untreated	-	96.7	88.3

a) Inoculation: May 10 Spray: May 11 Assessment: May 17
b) Inocula from plants sprayed 15 times with benomyl (250 mg/1)

When roots of cucumber seedlings were soaked in a 6 mg/1 solution of MIL, powdery mildew at the cotyledon and leaf were well controlled (TABLE 4.). To examine further the systemic effect, possible translaminar action was tested by spraying the upper surfaces of tobacco leaves with MIL (50 mg/1) 2 days after inoculating the under surface. Although the upper surfaces were exposed daily to infections by conidia, MIL controlled powdery mildew on that surface remarkably well, being slightly superior to quinomethionate (83 mg/1). On the under surface, good control was obtained by MIL and it was superior to quinomethionate (TABLE 5). Similar results were also observed on cucumbers.

The effect of MIL on the germination of conidia was investigated on the epidermis of an onion bulb, floated in an MIL solution. In the control plot, germination took place after 6 hours and the germination rate reached 52 % after 48 hours. In a 6 mg/1 solution of MIL, germination also occurred after 6 hours but the germ tube was abnormal , *e.g.* spherical or

TABLE 4. Effect of mildiomycin against powdery mildew on cucumber seedlings in root soaking

Chemicals	Concn. (mg/1)	Area mildewed a) (%) Cotyledon	Leaf
Mildiomycin	0.06	100.0	100.0
	0.6	72.5	55.5
	6.0	0	0
Dimethirimol	0.01	0	0
Untreated	-	100.0	100.0

a) 14 days after inoculation

TABLE 5. Effect of mildiomycin against powdery mildew of tobacco by spraying the upper surface of the leaves

Chemicals	Concn. (mg/1)	Leaf area mildewed a) (%) Dec. 29		Jan. 5	
		Upper	Under	Upper	Under
Mildiomycin	50	1.3	2.6	0.7	5.0
Quinomethionate	83	1.5	5.2	2.3	16.3
Untreated	-	23.9	12.4	54.7	19.1

a) Inoculation: Dec. 21 Spray: Dec. 23 and 29

TABLE 6. Effect of mildiomycin on the germination of *Sphaerotheca fuliginea* conidia on the epidermis of onion bulb

Time (hour)	Germination rate (%) Mildiomycin (mg/1)			
	0	1.5	6	12
24	41	55	0 (17)a)	0 (0)
48	52	57	0 (52)	1 (1)

a) Germ tubes were spherical or oval-shaped

oval-shaped. In a 12 mg/1 solution of MIL, germination was inhibited almost completely (TABLE 6.). The good control of MIL against powdery mildew may be attributed to its effect on the germination of conidia, that may play an important role in the powdery mildew infection(11).

TOXICITY

LD 50 of MIL for female mice was 599 mg/kg administered intravenously and 5250 mg/kg administered orally. LD 50 of MIL for female rats was 700 mg/kg administered intravenously and 4120 mg/kg administered orally (9). In 30-day feeding trials no significant adverse effects were observed in mice or rats at 200 mg/kg daily. In a 3-month subacute toxicity study in rats the maximum non-effect level was 50 mg/kg daily (9). LC 50 of MIL for fishes were as follows;>40 mg/1 (72 hours) for carp (*Cyprinus carpio*),>40 mg/1 (168 hours) for Japanese killifish (*Oryzias latipes*) (9).

BIOSYNTHESIS OF PYRIMIDINE CHROMOPHORE

MIL has a 5-hydroxymethylcytosine (HMC) in its molecule. HMC has only been found so far in the deoxyribonucleic acid of T-even phage and has been known to be formed by hydroxymethylation at 5-position of deoxycytidine monophosphate (5'-dCMP) (12). Investigation was carried out to confirm how HMC in the MIL molecule was formed by the MIL producer (13). With the crude enzyme prepared from the mycelium of the organism HMC was formed from 5'-CMP and paraformaldehyde or L-serine in the presence of tetrahydroforic acid. This enzymatic reaction was enhanced by 2-mercaptoethanol and ferous ion and inhibited by aminopterin. Cytidine (CR), cytosine (C) and 5'-dCMP were not the substrate of the enzymatic reaction. Experiments of enzymatic degradation of pyrimidine nucleotides and nucleosides revealed that the producing organism had 5'-nucleotidase activity but that it lacked nucleosidase and nucleosidephosphorylase activities. HMCMP, however, was enzymatically hydrolyzed to yield HMC. The biosynthetic pathway of HMC has been proposed (13) as shown in Fig. 3.

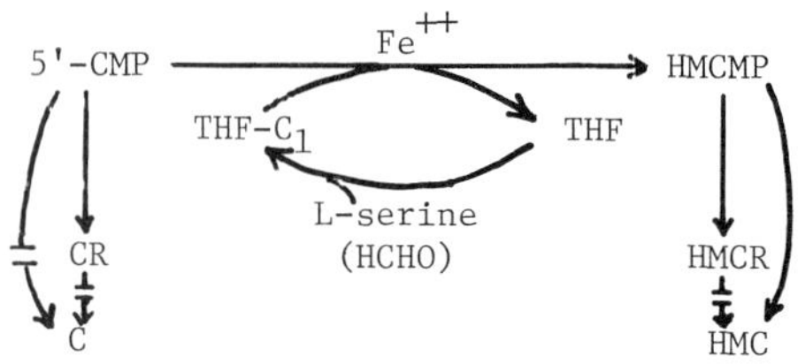

Fig. 3. Proposal pathway of HMC biosynthesis

CONCLUSION

MIL is a unique antibiotic both from microbiological and chemical points of view. The pyrimidine base of MIL is 5-hydroxymethylcytosine which has only been found so far in the DNA of T-even phage, and known to be formed by the hydroxymethylation of 5'-dCMP. In MIL hydroxymethylcytosine is formed in a different way; it is formed by the hydrolysis of hydroxymethylcytidine monophosphate derived from the hydroxymethylation of 5'-CMP.

On agar media MIL shows only weak and narrow activity against most of fungi and bacteria tested, but it shows a broad anti-mildew activity on various plants; MIL was effective against 13 species in 8 genera of powdery mildew fungi. It is noteworthy that MIL is low toxic to mammals and fishes. It also shows no irritation in cornea and skin in rabbits. Any phytotoxicity has not been observed so far. Thus, it may be said that MIL is an excellent fungicide for powdery mildew control.

REFERENCES

1. T. Kusaka, K. Suetomi and T. Iwasa, J. Pesticide Sci. 4, 345-348 (1979)
2. T. Iwasa, K. Suetomi and T. Kusaka, J. Antibiotics 31, 511-518 (1978)
3. S. Harada and T. Kishi, ibid 31, 519-524 (1978)
4. S. Harada, E. Mizuta and T. Kishi, J. Am. Chem. Soc. 100, 4895-4897 (1978)
5. S. Harada, E. Mizuta and T. Kishi, Tetrahedron 37, 1317-1327 (1981)
6. K. Suetomi and T. Kusaka, J. Pesticide Sci. 4, 349-353 (1979)
7. J. Gen, I. Yamaguchi and T. Misato, The 6th Anual Meeting of Pesticide Sci. Soc. Japan (1981)
8. J. Gen, I. Yamaguchi and T. Misato, The 7th Anual Meeting of Pesticide Sci. Soc. Japan (1982)
9. T. Kusaka, K. Suetomi, T. Iwasa and S. Harada, Proc. 1979 British Crop Protection Conf.-Pests and Diseases 589-595
10 T. Iwasa, E. Higashide and M. Shibata, J. Antibiotics 24, 114-118 (1971)
11. K. Suetomi and T. Kusaka, The 3rd Anual Meeting of Pesticide Sci. Soc. Japan (1978)
12. J. G. Flaks and S. S. Cohen, J. Biol.Chem. 234, 1501-1506 (1959)
13. H. Sawada, T. Suzuki, S. Akiyama and Y. Nakao, Anual Meeting of Soc. Fermentation Technology, Japan (1981)

INHIBITORS OF FUNGAL CELL WALL BIOSYNTHESIS FROM MICROBIAL ORIGIN

Kiyoshi Isono, Masakazu Uramoto, and Makoto Ubukata

Antibiotics Laboratory, The Institute of Physical and Chemical Research, Wako-shi, Saitama 351, Japan

Abstract- Two new antifungal antibiotics, neopeptins A and B have been discovered in our screening studies for inhibitors of microbial cell wall biosynthesis at the enzyme level. The antibiotics were isolated from a fermentation broth of *Streptomyces* sp. K-710. They have the molecular formulae corresponding to $C_{53}H_{81}N_{11}O_{19}$ and $C_{54}H_{83}N_{11}O_{19}$ respectively. They inhibited β-1,3-glucan synthetase and proteoheteroglycan synthetase from *Saccharomyces cerevisiae*. They are also inhibitory to a variety of phytopathogenic fungi causing swelling of mycelia. They were also preventive to cucumber powdery mildew disease in pot tests. Structural studies indicated that neopeptins are peptolides consisting of eight amino acids including 2 moles of serine and each 1 mole of aspartic acid, *N*-methylphenylalanine, *threo*-β-hydroxyglutamic acid, *N*-methylaspartic acid, β-methylglutamic acid and an unknown amino acid. Neopeptin A has the side chain fatty acid, 12-methyltridecanoic acid, whereas neopeptin B possesses 12-methyltetradecanoic acid.

INTRODUCTION

Selective toxicity is the important concept and basis for the development of useful antibiotics. As in the case of β-lactam antibiotics in bacterial cell wall biosynthesis, polyoxins (1) have been proved to be a non-toxic potent antifungal antibiotics, whose site of action is the inhibition of cell wall chitin synthetase. Thus, polyoxins have been used as an agricultural fungicide for the recent fifteen years in Japan. For this reason, we have focused our interest on specific inhibitors of fungal cell wall biosynthesis. Our strategy is to utilize enzymes responsible to fungal cell wall biosynthesis. We deviced the assay methods for cell wall-chitin, -β-1,3-glucan and -proteoheteroglycan synthesis employing enzymes from *Pyricularia oryzae* and *Saccharomyces cerevisiae*. Thus, we have discovered neopolyoxins A, B, and C (2) as specific inhibitors of chitin synthetase. The structure study (3) has shown that they are nucleoside peptides analogous to the polyoxins. However, neopolyoxin A has 2-oxo-4-imidazoline-4-carbaldehyde instead of uracil and showed higher activity against a variety of fungi including *Candida albicans* than the polyoxins. Subsequently, lipopeptins A and B (4,5,6) have been discovered as specific inhibitors for proteoheteroglycan synthesis. They are peptolides with a fatty acid side chain having the following structures.

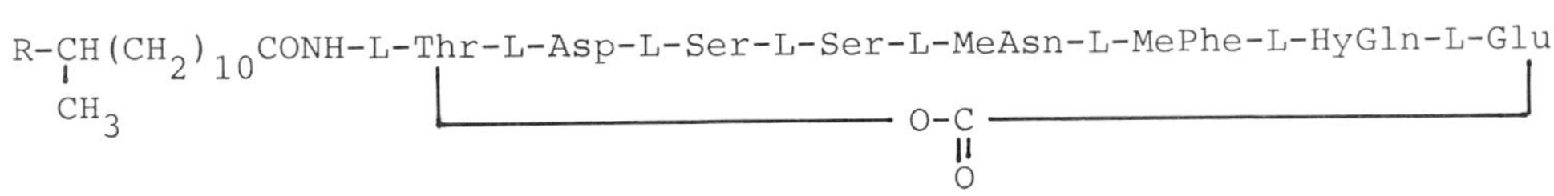

lipopeptin A: R = CH_3CH_2

lipopeptin B: R = CH_3

As an extension of this study, we have been able to isolate two new antifungal antibiotics from a fermentation broth of *Streptomyces* sp. K-710, which resembles *Actinomyces malachiticus*. Because the compounds are considered to be peptolides analogous to lipopeptins, they have been designated

PC 2 - C*

as neopeptins A and B. This paper describes fermentation, isolation, biological activity and structural study of neopeptins.

EXPERIMENTAL

Materials

Saccharomyces cerevisiae GS-1-36 used for enzyme source in this study was kindly provided by Dr. E. Cabib of NIH, Maryland, U.S.A. *Streptomyces* sp. K-710 was newly isolated from a soil sample collected in Aizuwakamatsu-shi, Fukushima-ken, Japan.

Analyses

IR spectra were taken on a Perkin Elmer 521 grating infrared spectrometer. ^{1}H-NMR spectra were taken on a JNM-FX400 spectrometer. GC/MS was run on a Hitachi RMU-6MG with a OV-1 column. High resolution mass spectrum, field desorption (FD) and secondary ion (SI) mass spectra were taken on a Hitachi M-80 spectrometer. Amino acid analysis was performed with a JEOL JLC:6AH amino acid analyzer.

Biological assay

Preparation of β-1,3-glucan synthetase from *S. cerevisiae* and the assay procedure are essentially the same to Cabibs' method (7) with some modification. The assay method of proteoheteroglycan synthetase was already described (6). In the present study, the enzyme preparation from *Saccharomyces cerevisiae* was used. For minimal inhibitory concentration, conventional agar dilution method was employed using potato-sucrose agar. Experimental cucumber powdery mildew disease in pot test was performed in Fungicide Laboratory (Dr. T. Misato) of this institute.

RESULTS

Fermentation

140 ml of a pre-culture (48 hrs) of *Streptomyces* sp. K-710 in 500 ml shaking flasks were used to inoculate to a jar fermenter containing 18 liters of a medium composed of glucose (2%), soluble starch (1%), meat extract(0.1%), dry yeast (0.4%), soybean flour (2.5%), sodium chloride (0.2%) and potassium phosphate, dibasic (0.005%). Fermentation was carried out at 30° for 72 hrs with aeration (18 liters/min) and agitation (400 rpm/min).

Isolation

Outline of the procedure is shown in Scheme I. Fermentation broth (pH 7.6) was filtered with the aid of Celite and the mycelium was extracted with 70% methanol. The filtrate and the mycelium extract were combined and passed through a column of Diaion HP-10. The column was washed with 10% methanol and the antibiotics were eluted with 70% methanol. The eluate was concentrated *in vacuo* to a small volume and extracted with butanol. The extract was was concentrated *in vacuo* to dryness and the residue was purified with

Scheme I. Isolation procedure of neopeptins

Culture broth
→ Broth filtrate | Mycelium
→ (combined) Diaion HP-10
→ Butanol extraction
→ Silicic acid column
→ Sephadex LH-20
→ HPLC (Nucleosil $5C_{18}$)
→ Neopeptin A | Neopeptin B

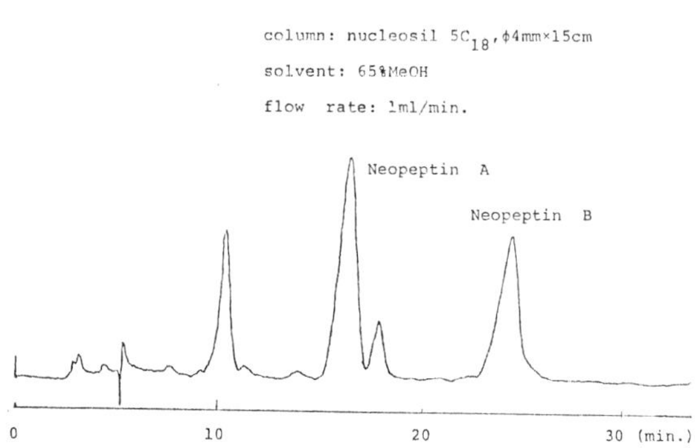

Fig. 1. HPLC pattern of neopeptins.

Column: Nucleosil $5C_{18}$
Solvent: 65% methanol

silicic acid chromatography using the following stepwise solvent systems: chloroform ⟶ chloroform-methanol (9:1 ⟶ 4:1 ⟶ 1:1). Active fractions were combined and concentrated to give a crude powder. Further purification was done by a Sephadex LH-20 column using methanol affording 950 mg of a white powder. The final purification was achieved by HPLC using a Nucleosil $5C_{18}$ column with 65% methanol affording two separated biologically active peaks (Fig. 1). From the first fraction, neopeptin A was obtained as purified white powder. Similarly neopeptin B was obtained from the second peak. The yield ratio of neopeptins A and B was approximately 2:1.

Physico-chemical properties

Neopeptins A and B were obtained as amorphous white powder which decompose gradually over 200°. They are soluble in water and lower alcohols but hardly soluble in acetone, chloroform, ether, and hexane. They showed positive

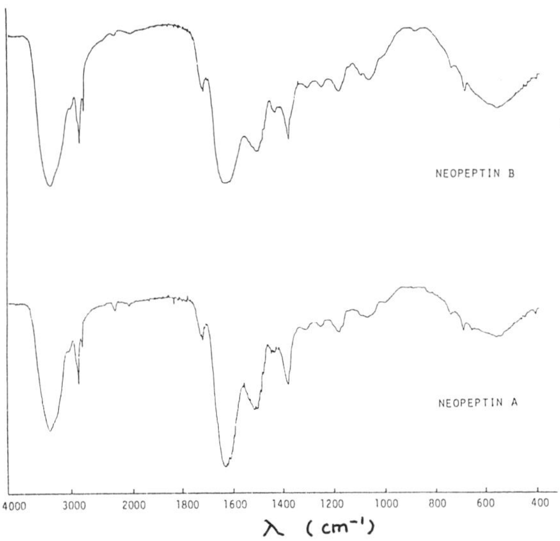

← Fig. 2. IR spectra of neopeptins (in potassium bromide)

↓ Fig. 3. 400MHz ^{1}H-NMR spectrum of neopeptin A in methanol-$\underline{d}_4$

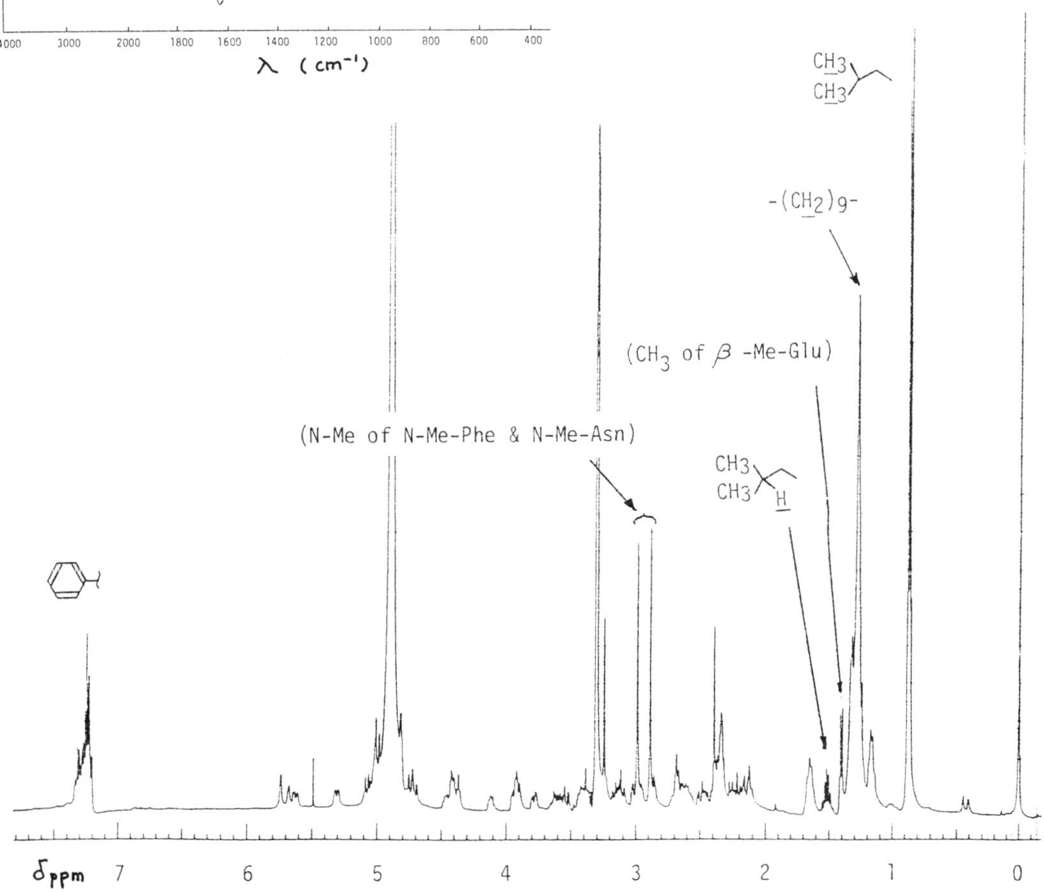

reaction to Rydon-Smith, iodine vapor tests, but negative to ninhydrin and anthrone tests. They are optically active: $[\alpha]_D20$ -9.2° (c 0.48, methanol) for neopeptin A and $[\alpha]_D20$ -28.6° (c 0.124, methanol) for neopeptin B. Paper-electrophoresis showed that they are amphoteric compounds having isoelectric points at acidic pH (~4). Elementary analysis and molecular weight determination by secondary ion mass spectroscopy (SIMS) gave the following molecular formulae.

Neopeptin A. Calcd.for $C_{53}H_{81}N_{11}O_{19}$: C, 54.11; H, 6.94; N, 13.10. Found: C, 53.94; H, 7.19; N, 12.78. SIMS: $(M+1)^+$ 1176, $(M+Na)^+$ 1198, $(M+K)^+$ 1214.

Neopeptin B. Calcd. for $C_{54}H_{83}N_{11}O_{19}$: C, 54.49; H, 7.03; N, 12.95. Found: C, 53.96; H, 7.12; N, 12.24. SIMS: $(M+1)^+$ 1190, $(M+Na)^+$ 1212, $(M+K)^+$ 1228.

They showed end absorption in UV region and IR spectra of neopeptins A and B were nearly identical (Fig.2). The presence of amide (1650, 1530 cm^{-1}) and lactone (1740 cm^{-1}) was suggested. The ^1H-NMR spectrum of neopeptin A with some assignment is shown in Fig. 3.

Structure of fatty acid

After acid hydrolysis of neopeptins A and B (6N hydrochloric acid, 110°, 17 hrs), each hydrolysate was extracted with chloroform and concentrated to dryness. The residue was esterified with diazomethane and analyzed by GC/MS (Fig.4). The fatty acid from neopeptin A was determined to be 12-methyltridecanoic acid. As shown in Fig 4a, molecular ion peak, M^+ 242 of the methyl ester indicated that it is a C_{14} fatty acid and the intense $(M-C_3H_7)^+$ 199 ion indicated the *iso*-structure. The spectrum was superimposable with the authentic methyl 12-methyltridecanoate. The fatty acid from neopeptin B was determined to be 12-methyltetradecanoic acid. As shown in Fig.4b, the spectrum of the methyl ester indicated the peaks M^+ 256, $(M-C_4H_9)^+$ 199, $(M-C_2H_5)^+$ 227 and $(M-OCH_3)^+$ 225. Enhanced abundance of ion 199 suggested branching at C-12. The *anteiso* structure is further reflected by the unusual ion abundance ratio $(M-C_2H_5)^+ > (M-OCH_3)^+$ in contrast to normal chain esters (8). Authentic methyl 12-methyltetradecanoate gave an essentially identical spectrum.

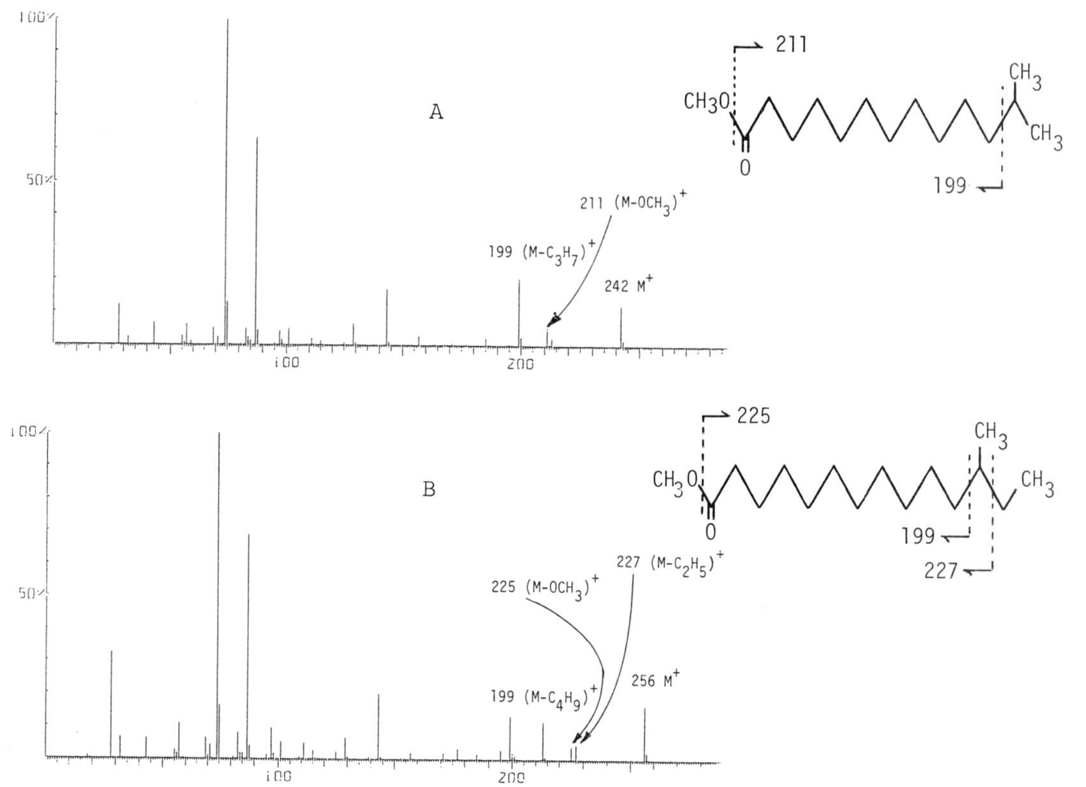

Fig. 4. GC/MS spectra of the fatty acids. A: Methyl ester of the fatty acid from neopeptin A. B: Methyl ester of the fatty acid from neopeptin B. Column, OV-1.

Amino acid composition

Amino acid analysis of the acid hydrolysate revealed the presence of serine and aspartic acid in 2:1 ratio. In addition, several other unusual amino acids were indicated. The hydrolysate was trimethylsilylated with BSA and subjected to GC/MS analysis. The results correspond to the following amino acid derivatives: N-methylphenylalanine(2TMS), $(M-CH_3)$ 308; aspartic acid (3TMS), M^+ 349, $(M-CH_3)^+$ 334; β-hydroxyglutamic acid(4TMS), $(M-CH_3)^+$ 436, N-methylaspartic acid(3TMS), M^+ 363, $(M-CH_3)^+$ 348; β-methylglutamic acid (3TMS), M^+ 377, $(M-CH_3)^+$ 362; serine(3TMS), M^+ 321, $(M-CH_3)^+$ 306. Isolation of each amino acid was done by combination of Dowex 50W (5% pyridine), Avicel chromatography (n-propanol-1N ammonium hydroxide, 7:3) and preparative TLC (75% phenol). ^{1}H-NMR analysis of the isolated amino acids supported the structures of N-methylphenylalanine, threo-β-hydroxyglutamic acid and N-methylaspartic acid. The structure of the new amino acid, β-methylglutamic acid was deduced from the spectrum analysis. Analytical data with assignment is shown below. The assignment was supported by spin decoupling experiment.

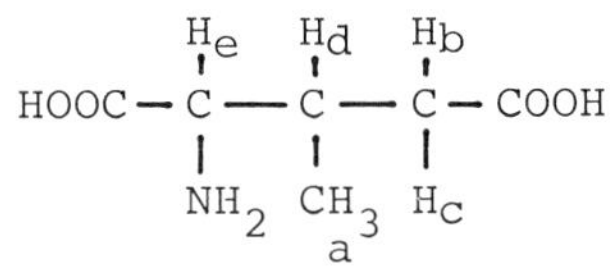

δ in ppm (D_2O): 0.94 (3H(a), d, $J_{a,d}$ = 7Hz), 2.29 (1H(b), dd, $J_{b,c}$ = 14 Hz, $J_{b,d}$ = 9 Hz), 2.47 (1H(c), dd, $J_{c,b}$ = 14 Hz, $J_{c,d}$ = 6.4 Hz), 2.50 (1H(d), dddd, $J_{d,a}$ = 7 Hz, $J_{d,b}$ = 9 Hz, $J_{d,c}$ = 6.4 Hz, $J_{d,e}$ = 3.2 Hz), 3.70 (1H(e), d, $J_{e,d}$ = 3.2 Hz).

Sum-up of the seven amino acids and one fatty acid indicated the presence of one more unusual amino acid, which is now under investigation.

Open-chain neopeptin A

The presence of lactone group was proved by obtaining an open chain lipopeptide, $(M+H)^+$ 1194 (SIMS) by treatment of neopeptin A with 0.035 M sodium hydroxide at 37°for 12 hrs. Treatment with carboxypeptidase (9) liberated β-methylglutamic acid and the residual lipopeptide, $(M+1)^+$ 1052, $(M+Na)^+$ 1074 (SIMS) was obtained. Therefore, the C-terminal amino acid which participate in lactone formation is possibly β-methylglutamic acid.

BIOLOGICAL PROPERTIES

As shown in Fig. 5 and 6, neopeptins A and B inhibited β-1,3-glucan synthetase and proteoheteroglycan synthetase from *Saccharomyces cerevisiae* and *Pyricularia oryzae*. ID_{50} of neopeptins A and B for both enzyme were calculated to be 300 - 350 mcg/ml. Chitin synthetase was not inhibited by 1 mg/ml of neopeptins. The antibiotics inhibited growth of a various plant pathogenic fungi. Minimum inhibitory concentration is shown in Table 1. The inhibition

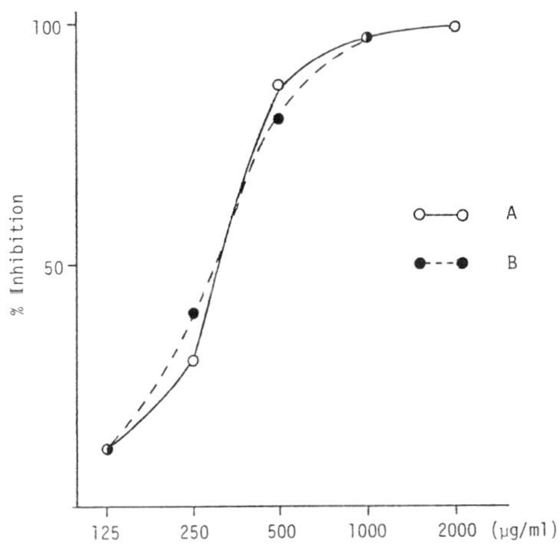

Fig.5. Inhibition of β-1,3-glucan synthetase by neopeptins

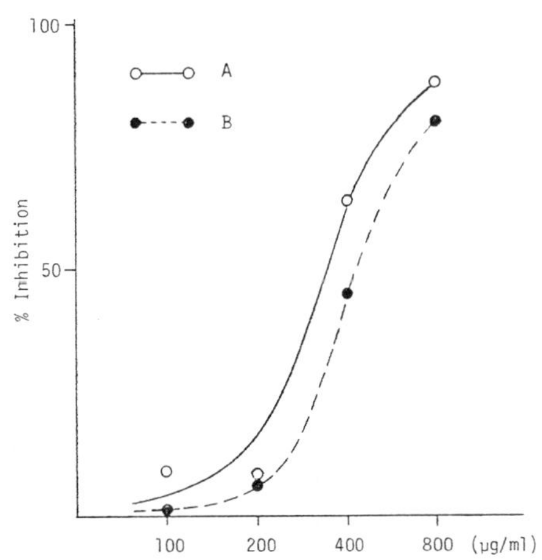

Fig.6. Inhibition of proteoheteroglycan synthetase by neopeptins (For neopeptin B, an enzyme from *P. oryzae* was used.)

was accompanied by swelling of mycelia. Neopeptins (~30 ppm) were shown to be preventive to experimental powdery mildew disease caused by Sphaerotheca fuliginea in pot test without any phytotoxicity (data not shown). The antibiotics were of low toxicity to mice. Mice torelated intravenous injection of 200 mg/Kg of a mixture of neopolyoxins (A:B, approximately 2:1).

Table 1. Antifungal activity of neopeptins

Test organism	Minimal inhibitory concentration (mcg/ml)	
	Neopeptin A	Neopeptin B
Cochliobolus miyabeanus IFO 5277	62.5	125
Colletotricum lagenarium IFO 7513	4.0	250
Pyricularia oryzae IFO 5994	500	150
Glomerella cingulata IFO 9767	250	250
Botrytis cinerea IFO 5365	250	>500
Alternaria mali IFO 8984	250	>500
Rhizoctonia solani IFO 6258	>500	>500
Aspergillus oryzae	>500	>500
Penicillium chrysogenum	>500	>500

DISCUSSION

The new antibiotics, neopeptins A and B were isolated from the culture broth of Streptomyces sp. K-710 which resembles Actinomyces malachiticus. The structural studies indicated that neopeptins A and B are peptolides with the fatty acid side chain, 12-methyltridecanoate and 12-methyltetradecanoate respectively. The constituent amino acids of neopeptin A has been shown to be serine (2), aspartic acid, N-methylphenylalanine, threo-β-hydroxyglutamic acid, N-methylaspartic acid and a new amino acid, β-methylglutamic acid which participates in lactone formation. The presence of one more unknown amino acid is presumed. From the biosynthetic standpoint , it is interesting if β-methylglutamic acid originates from glutamic acid or isoleucine. The structural feature so far elucidated shows resemblance with lipopeptins in many respects, which were reported previously from our laboratory (5), except the presence of β-methylglutamic acid and the absence of glutamic acid and threonine. Remarkable difference was observed in thier biological activities. Whereas neopeptins inhibit β-1,3-glucan synthetase from S. cerevisiae, lipopeptins (1000 mcg/ml) were not inhibitory to the same enzyme. In contrast, both antibiotics were equally inhibitory to proteoheteroglycan synthetase. Inhibition of β-1,3-glucan and proteoheteroglycan syntheses as well as swelling formation of mycelium may explain that the site of action of neopeptins is related to fungal cell wall biosynthesis. Low toxicity of the antibiotics to mice and plants here again may verify our strategy.

Acknowledgements - We are grateful to Drs. T. Misato and K. Ko of this institute for pot-tests and Drs. K. Izaki and T. Nakajima of Tohoku University for their helpful discussions. We thank Dr. H. Kambara of Hitahi Co. Ltd. for secondary ion mass spectroscopy.

REFERENCES

1. K. Isono and S. Suzuki, Heterocycles, 13, 333 (1979) and references cited therein.
2. K. Kobinata, M. Uramoto, M. Nishii, H. Kusakabe, G. Nakamura and K. Isono, Agric. Biol. Chem., 44, 1709 (1980)
3. M. Uramoto, K. Kobinata, K. Isono, T. Higashijima, T. Miyazawa, E.E. Jenkins and J.A. McCloskey, Tetrahedron, 38, 1599 (1982)
4. K. Tsuda, T. Kihara, M. Nishii, G. Nakamura, K. Isono and S. Suzuki, J. Antibiotics, 33, 247 (1980)
5. M. Nishii, T. Kihara, K. Isono, T. Higashijima, T. Miyazawa, S.K. Sethi and J.A. McCloskey, Tetrahedron Lett., 21, 4627 (1980)
6. M. Nishii, K. Isono and K. Izaki, Agric. Biol. Chem., 45, 895 (1981).
7. E.M. Shematek, J.A. Braatz and E. Cabib, J. Biol. Chem., 255, 888 (1980)
8. R. Ryhage and E. Stenhagen, Arkiv. Kemi., 15, 291 (1960)
9. Y. Narahashi and K. Yoda, J. Biochem., 86, 683 (1979)

PHYTOTOXINS PRODUCED BY PLANT PATHOGENIC MICROORGANISMS

Akitami Ichihara and Sadao Sakamura

Department of Agricultural Chemistry, Hokkaido University, Sapporo 060, Japan

Abstract - The chemistry and biochemistry of several phytotoxins recently isolated from plant pathogenic bacterium and fungus are described in this paper. In *Pseudomonas* phytopathogens, several phytotoxins have been structurally confirmed. One of them, coronatine is an extracellular toxin produced by *Pseudomonas syringae* pv. *atropurpurea*, the incitant of the chocolate spot disease on Italian ryegrass. Coronatine induces necrosis with the chlorotic halo symptom of the disease in host leaves as well as in nonhosts and is thus nonspecific. Coronatine also induces marked hypertrophy on potato tuber tissues. From the culture fluid of the bacterium, coronatine was isolated. The structure and stereochemistry of coronatine were determined from spectroscopic data, x-ray analysis and synthesis of coronamic acid, the amino acid portion of coronatine. Since coronafacic acid, the acidic portion of coronatine, has been synthesized by intermolecular and intramolecular Diels-Alder reaction, a formal total synthesis of coronatine has been achieved. Stereoisomers and analogs of coronatine were synthesized by replacing the coronamic acid moiety with other amino compounds, and the hypertrophic response of potato tubers was examined. Stereospecific cleavage of 1-aminocyclopropanecarboxylic acid in the formation of ethylene in fruit ripening was elucidated by the conversion of (+)-allocoronamic acid to 1-butene. Pyrenocine A and pyrenochaetic acid A are phytotoxins isolated from culture filtrates of *Pyrenochaeta terrestris*, a phytopathogenic fungus of pink root disease of onion. Synthesis of pyrenocine A and pyrenochaetic acid A from the same starting material, 5-acetyl-4-methoxy-6-methyl-2-pyrone has been effected.

INTRODUCTION

Characterization of many toxins chould now proceed rapidly because of widespread availability of modern instruments of analysis (1). Information about the structure of many more toxins and synthetic analogs should also lead to further insight into structure-toxicity relationships, and allow us to utilize in a useful way. In this paper we describe the chemistry of several phytotoxins, one of which is isolated from a bacterium, *Ps. syringae* pv. *atropurpurea*, and the others from a fungus, *Pyrenochaeta terrestris*.

CORONATINE

Pseudomonas syringae pv. *atropurpurea* causes chocolate spot disease on Italian ryegrass (2). During the study of bacterial physiology, it was found that the virulent isolates of the bacterium caused outgrowths on potato tuber tissues. The same activity was also found in the filtrates of the culture fluids. These facts suggest that the activity may be one of the essential requirements for the pathogenicity of the bacterium and used as a bioassay in isolation. In 1975 the substance responsible for the activity was isolated and named 'coronatine'. Coronatine is a vivotoxin, since it was present in the leaves of Italian ryegrass infected by the bacterium.

Isolation

Coronatine was isolated from the culture fluid of a virulent isolates of *Ps. syringae* pv. *atropurpurea*. This bacterium was incubated at 23°C for 3 days in glucose-potassium nitrate medium under aeration. The cultured cells were removed by centrifugation and the supernatant was processed as shown in Fig. 1. The supernatant and 2% active carbon-celite (1 : 1 w/w)was mixed well and the adsorbent was packed in a column, which was washed with water and eluted with acetone. The eluate was concentrated to small volume *in vacuo*, adjusted to pH 2.5, and extracted with ethyl acetate. The extracts were concentrated, and the concentrate was chromatographed on a column containing silicic acid and Hyflo Supercel (10 : 1 w/w). The column was first eluted with benzene, then stepwise with benzene-ethyl acetate and finally with methanol. Fractions from the column were tested for hypertrophy-inducing activity on potato tuber discs. The fractions showing physiological activity were combined and further chromatographed on a silicic acid column which was eluted successively with isopropyl ether-acetic acid (95 : 5 v/v), acetone, and methyl alcohol. Coronafacic acids were obtained from the isopropyl ether-acetic acid eluate. The acetone eluates were separated twice on silicic acid columns using ether and benzene-acetone (1 : 1 v/v) as eluent. Finally the active fraction was purified by preparative TLC developing with benzene-acetone (1 : 1 v/v). Recrystallization from ethyl acetate yielded pure coronatine as needles, m.p. 151–153°C.

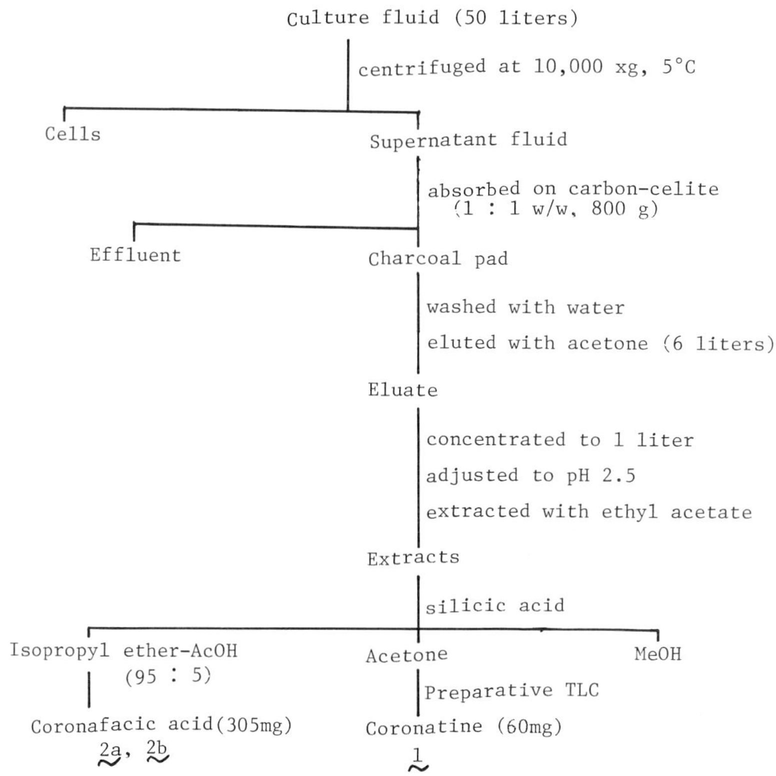

Fig. 1 Isolation procedures of coronatine (1) and coronafacic acid (2a, 2b)

Phytotoxic effects of coronatine

Coronatine produced lesions on leaves of Italian ryegrass on the injection (1 μl) of an aqueous acetone solution at 3.2 to 3.200 ng/l. The necrosis with chlorotic halo produced by coronatine was similar to the symptom on the leaves inoculated with the pathogenic bacterium. In addition, a substance isolated from infected plants had some properties identical with those of coronatine, while such substance was isolated neither from healthy plants nor from the bacterial cells (3). From the results of the phytotoxicity tests, coronatine was suggested to be a chlorosis-inducing toxin in the pathogenesis. In order to determine host-specificity, tests were carried out on many plant species, and coronatine was toxic to 21 species of plant in 17 genera in 4 families out of 25 species in 20 genera in 6 families tested. Evidently, coronatine is not a host-specific toxin.

Structure of coronatine

Coronatine 1, needles, mp 151–153°C, was fomulated as $C_{18}H_{25}O_4N$ by elemental analysis and high resolution mass spectrometry (m/z M^+ 319.1753, calcd, 319.1731) (4). The UV, IR and NMR spectra of coronatine indicate the presence of following moiety, UV λ_{max}^{EtOH} 208nm, (ε 8378) (O=C-C=C-), IR ν_{max}^{KBr} 1740 (five membered ring C=O), 1620 (C=C), 3270, 1645, 1525 cm^{-1} (-CONH-), NMR $\delta_{TMS}^{d\text{-}acetone}$ 0.94 (6H, t, J=7Hz, CH_2CH_3 x 2), 3.15 (1H, br.q -CHCO-), 6.50 (1H, s, =CH). The high resolution mass spectrum of 1 indicates that coronatine consists of two fragments, $C_{12}H_{15}O_2$ (m/z 191.1075) and $C_6H_{10}O_2N$ (m/z 128.0682), which are bonded to each other by an amide linkage. Other ion peaks below m/z 191 are quite similar to those of coronafacic acids 2a and 2b, which were isolated directly from the culture broth. In fact, hydrolysis of coronatine gave an acid, whose Rf value on TLC is identical with that of 2a, and an α-amino acid, later identified as coronamic acid (4a) (Fig. 2).

Treatment of coronatine with acetic anhydride-pyridine afforded anhydrocoronatine 3, m/z 301 (M^+), whose IR spectrum exhibited characteristic peaks at 1800, 1640, 1605 cm^{-1} assignable to an azlactone moiety. Since the NMR spectrum of 3 (and 1 also) shows the presence of two ethyl groups, one of which is known to be from coronafacic acid moiety, the amino acid must be depicted as 4, considering the degree of unsaturation. The structure including relative configuration (NH_2/CH_2CH_3 trans) was also confirmed by the synthesis of (±)-coronamic acid (4)(5).

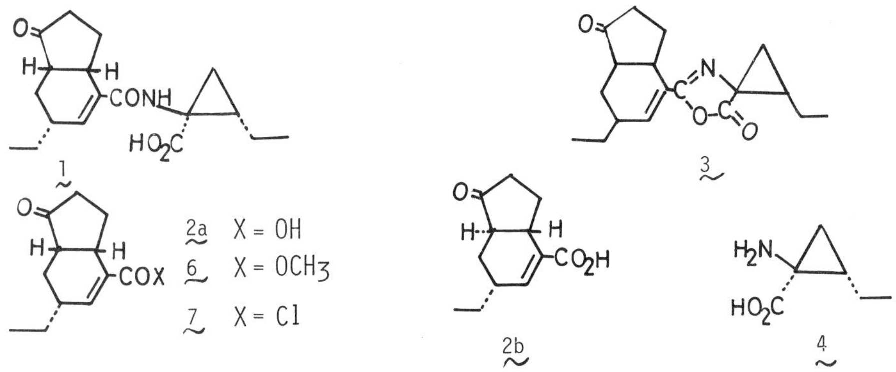

Fig. 2 Structure of coronatine and its derivatives

Coronafacic acids exist as two stereoisomers, 2a and 2b depending on the conditions of recrystallization. The isomer 2b is easily convertible through enolisation to 2a. Esterification of each of 2a and 2b by methanolic HCl afforded the same methyl ester 6. The UV spectrum ($\lambda_{max}^{CH_3OH}$ 217nm, ε 8558) of 2b is compatible with α,β-unsaturated acid, whose double bond is located in a six-membered ring. The IR spectra (1740 cm^{-1} in $CHCl_3$, five-membered ring ketone) of 2a and 2b, D_2O treatment of 2b (m/z M^+ 211), the NMR spectrum of 2a (3.15, quintet, J=10Hz, 7Hz, 6Hz, CO•CH•(CH)•CH_2), and the mass spectrum of 2a (m/z 55, =-C≡O) suggest a 1-hydrindanone structure (2a) for coronafacic acid. The structure of coronafacic acid has been definitely established as 2a and 2b by X-ray analysis, and the plane structure of coronatine was confirmed.

Stereochemistry of coronatine

The relative configurations of coronafacic acid (2a) and coronamic acid (4) were already confirmed by X-ray analysis and synthesis respectively. The absolute configuration of coronatine (1) has now been established by the partial synthesis of coronatine (1) from natural coronafacic acid (2a) and optically active, synthetic coronamic acid (4a) whose absolute configurations were determined separately (5,6).

Stereochemistry of coronafacic acid (2a). The absolute configuration of 2a has been confirmed by ORD and CD measurements, which exhibited positive Cotton effect, ($[\alpha]_{290}$ + 2912°, $[\alpha]_{276}$ + 2641) and ($[\theta]_{285}$ + 333, $[\theta]_{225}$ + 1333). Since the octant projection of 2a indicates that all the carbon atoms, C-5, C-6, C-7, C-9 and C-10 lie in the positive octant in the most plausible conformation, the absolute configuration must be as depicted in 2a (5).

Stereochemistry of coronamic acid (4a). Possible four steroisomers (4a, 4b, 5a, 5b) of coronamic acid are synthesized as shown in Fig. 3. Synthetic (±)-coronamic acid (4) was identical with the natural sample in behavior on paper chromatography and retention time on the amino acid analyzer. Optical resolution of (±)-coronamic acid (4) was carried out using the quinine salts of N-formyl coronamic acid and after several fractional recrystallizations, the two crystalline materials obtained were separately hydrolysed to yield optically active 4a, $[\alpha]_D^{20}$ + 14.7 and 4b, $[\alpha]_D^{23}$ - 14.2 respectively. Enzymatic resolution of (±)-N-acetyl-coronamic acid using L-acylase also gave directly 4a, and the recovered 4b acetate was hydrolysed to 4b. In the same way (±)-allocoronamic acid (7) was stereoselectively synthesized as shown in Fig. 3 and resolved through the quinine salt to give (+)-allocoronamic acid (5a) $[\alpha]_D^{25}$ + 65.0 and (-)-allocoronamic acid, 5b, $[\alpha]_D^{21}$ - 68.4. It was expected that if (+)-coronamic acid has the stereochemistry 4a and is cleaved at a by hydrogenolysis, D-isoleucine and L-alloisoleucine would be produced (6) (Fig. 4). In fact, hydrogenolysis of 4a over 10% Pd-C under pressure of 14 kg/cm at 80°C occurred at all three bonds (a,b and c) of the cyclopropane ring and afforded four amino acids, isoleucine, alloisoleucine, norleucine, and 2-amino-2-methyl valeric acid, whose structures were identified by the NMR spectra and amino acid analyzer. When the reaction products were treated with L-amino acid oxidase, only the peak ascribed to alloisoleucine was decreased in the amino acid analyzer. On the other hand, treatment of the reaction products with D-amino acid oxidase resulted to decrease isoleucine. These observations indicate that the alloisoleucine and isoleucine have L- and D-configuration respectively, and the stereochemistry of their precursor, (+)-coronamic acid, should be represented as (+)-(1S,2S)-1-amino-2-ethylcyclopropane-1-carboxylic acid (4a). The same treatment of (-)-coronamic acid (4b) and (+)-allocoronamic acid (5a) confirmed that these have (1R, 2R) and (1R, 2S) configuration respectively. The absolute configuration of 4b was further confirmed by X-ray analysis of its N-acetate. Condensation of the acid chloride 7 with 4a afforded synthetic coronatine (1) which is identical with natural sample in spectral data and biological activity. From these results, the absolute configuration of coronatine should be depicted as 1.

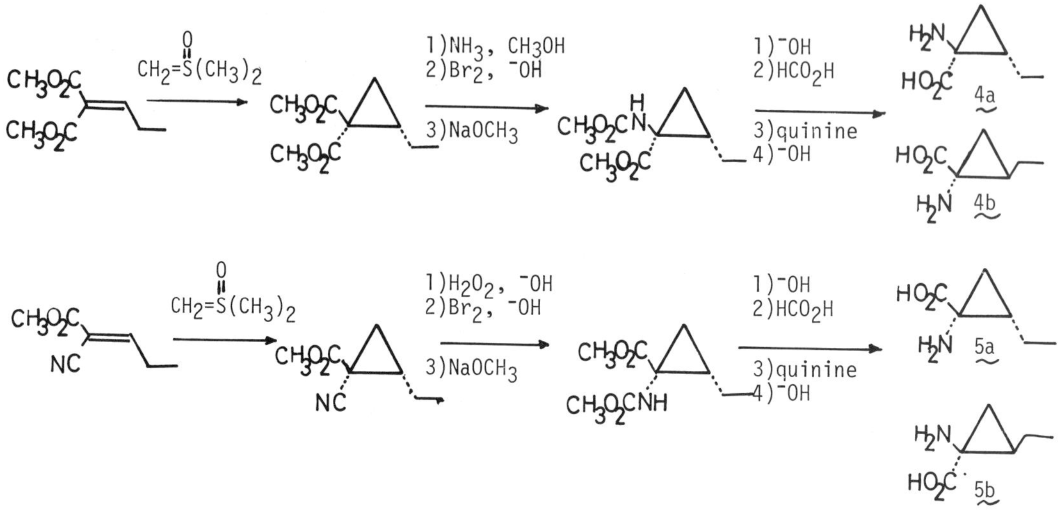

Fig. 3 Synthesis of stereoisomers of coronamic acid

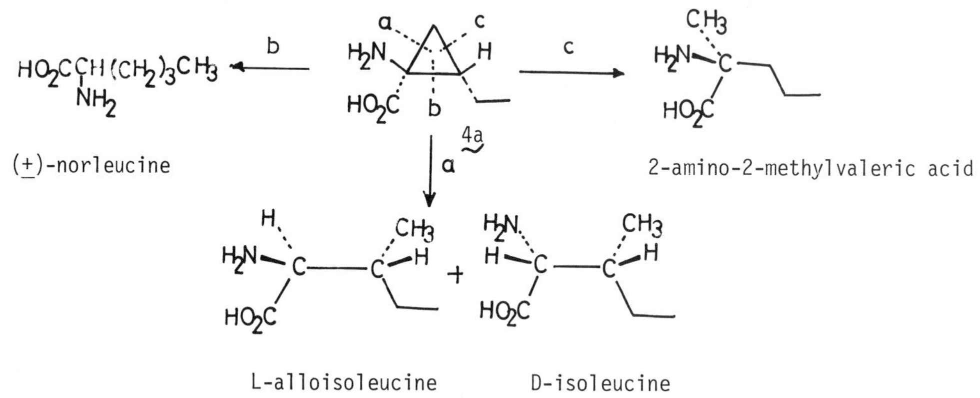

Fig. 4 Hydrogenolysis products of (+)-coronamic acid

Synthesis of coronatine : synthesis of (+)-coronafacic acid (2a)
Since partial synthesis of coronatine (1) from natural coronafacic acid and optically active coronamic acid has been completed, the synthesis of (±)-coronafacic acid means the total synthesis of 1 in a formal sense. Synthesis of 2a has been carried out by two routes, one through intermolecular (8) and the other through intramolecular Diels-Alder reaction (9). Here only the latter route is described (Fig. 5). Condensation of the enamine from butanal and dimethylamine with diethyl maleate, quaternization with p-TsOMe, and subsequent elimination yielded the known diester 8. The stereochemistry of the diester 8 was confirmed as be trans which is a necessary requirement for formation of E,E-diene through conrotatory ring opening at a later stage. Reduction of 8, oxidation and ketalization afforded an acetal, which was futher oxidized to an aldehyde 9. A methyl ketone 10 was prepared from dimethylfulvene and methyl vinyl ketone. Aldol condensation of the methyl ketone 10 with the aldehyde 9 yielded a ketol 11, which was treated with mesyl chloride and then diazabicycloundecene to give an α,β-unsaturated ketone. Selective reduction of the conjugated double bond was accomplished using sodium dihydrobis (2-methoxyethoxy) aluminate to give a saturated ketone 12. Thermal reaction of 12 involved three successive reaction, 1) conratatory opening of the cyclobutene ring, 2) retro-Diels-Alder reaction, and 3) intramolecular Diels-Alder reaction, affording 92% yield of a single products 13. Jones oxidation of 13, accompanied by deacetalization, isomerization, and oxidation, produced (±)-coronafacic acid (2a), whose spectral data are identical with those of a natural sample.

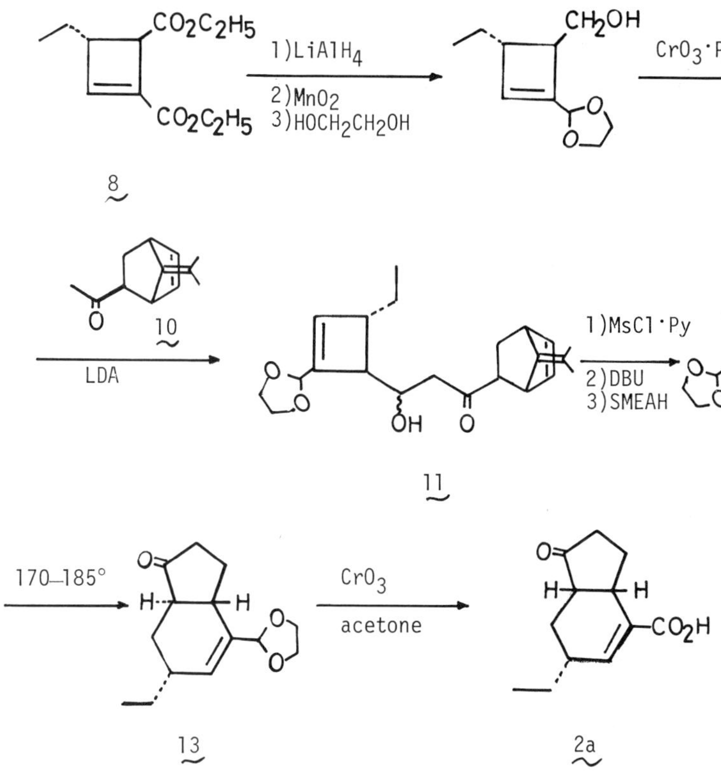

Fig. 5 Synthesis of coronafacic acid

Structure-activity relationships

The stereoisomers and analogs of coronatine were synthesized by replacing the coronamic acid moiety with other amino compounds. The hypertrophic response of potato tubers was used for bioassay of the analogs (10). A carboxyl group in coronamic acid was essential for induction of the activity. Moreover, the configuration at the α-carbon atom in the amino acid was closely related to increase in activity. Bulkiness of the alkyl groups in the amino acid moiety was associated with the activity.

Utilization of coronamic acids

1-Aminocyclopropane-1-carboxylic acid (ACC) is a key intermediate in the biosynthesis of ethylene, a fruit ripening hormone in plants, and consequently there has been interest in the biotransformation to and from ACC. Two metabolic pathways from ACC were investigated, one to ethylene (11) and the other to α-ketobutyrate (12). However, in these transformations, stereospecificity cannot be recognized due to the symmetrical nature of the cleavage in ACC. In order to determine whether ACC conversion to ethylene by plant tissues proceeds in a stereospecific fashion, the four stereoisomers of coronamic acid were administered to post-climacteric apple, excised preclimacteric cantaloupe, and etiolated mungbean hypocotyls (11). In each case, (+)-allocomonamic acid was the prefered substrate yielding 1-butene. This observation leads to the suggestion that the enzyme interacts with amino, carboxyl,and pro-(S) methylene groups. Another example was found in the deamination of ACC to α-ketobutyrate by ACC deaminase (12). Since (+)-coronamic acid was preferably deaminated by the same enzyme to produce α-keto-n-caproic acid, it was deduced that C_1-pro-(S) carbon would be cleaved stereospecifically in the deamination.

PYRENOCINE A AND PYRENOCHAETIC ACID A

Pyrenocine A (14) and pyrenochaetic acid A (15) were isolated from the culture filtrate of the phytopathogenic fungus (*Pyrenochaeta terrestris*) of pink disease in onion (13). The very similar substitution patterns of these metabolites suggest that they are closely related to each other in their biosynthesis. For the purpose of biosynthetic studies, these two compounds have been synthesized (14, 15).

Synthesis of pyrenocine A (14) and pyrenochaetic acid (15)
Condensation of acetylacetone and malonyl chloride afforded 5-acetyl-4-hydroxy-6-methyl-α-pyrone (16). Methylation of 16 with methyl iodide in the presence of silver oxide gave a single product 17, which was treated with trimethylsilyl chloride to yield silyl enol ether 18. Aldol condensation of 18 with acetaldehyde afforded pyrenocine B, which was converted to pyrenocine A (14) by acetylation (Fig. 6). The Diels-Alder reaction of the

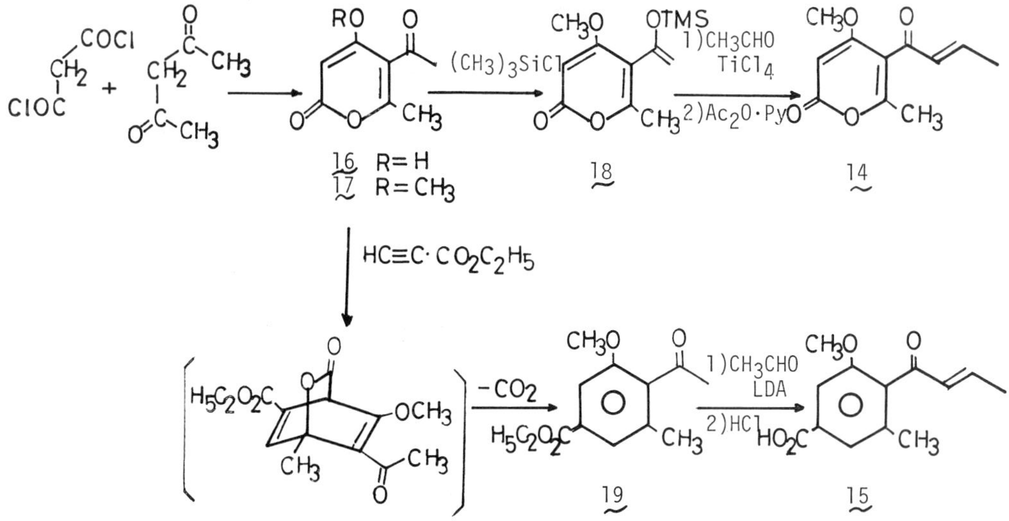

Fig. 6 Synthesis of pyrenocine A and pyrenochaetic acid A

α-pyrone 17 with ethyl propiolate afforded a benzoic acid derivatives 19. Aldol condensation of 19 with acetaldehyde and then hydrolysis yielded pyrenochaetic acid (15).

Acknowledgements - We would like to express our thanks to our coworkers, whose names are given in the references, for their contributions to the work described above.

REFERENCES

1. R. D. Durbin, ed. Toxins in Plant Disease, Academic Press, New York (1981)
2. K. Nishiyama, R. Sakai, A. Ezuka, A. Ichihara, K. Shiraishi, M. Ogasawara, H. Sato and S. Sakamura, Ann. Phytopathol. Soc. Japan, 42, 613 (1976)
3. K. Nishiyama, R. Sakai, A. Ezuka, A. Ichihara, K. Shiraishi and S. Sakamura, Ann. Phytopathol. Soc. Japan, 43, 219 (1977)
4. A. Ichihara, K. Shiraishi, H. Sato, S. Sakamura, K. Nishiyama, R. Sakai, A. Furusaki, T. Matsumoto, J. Am. Chem. Soc., 99, 636 (1977)
5. A. Ichihara, K. Shiraishi, S. Sakamura, K. Nishiyama, R. Sakai, Tetrahedron Lett., 269 (1977)
6. A. Ichihara, K. Shiraishi, S. Sakamura, A. Furusaki, N. Hashiba and T. Matsumoto, Tetrahedron Lett., 365 (1979)
7. K. Shiraishi, A. Ichihara and S. Sakamura, Agric. Biol. Chem., 41, 2497 (1977)
8. A. Ichihara, R. Kimura, K. Moriyasu and S. Sakamura, Tetrahedron Lett., 4331 (1977)
9. A. Ichihara, R. Kimura, S. Yamada and S. Sakamura, J. Am. Chem. Soc., 102, 6353 (1980)
10. K. Shiraishi, K. Konoma, H. Sato, A. Ichihara and S. Sakamura, Agric. Biol. Chem., 43, 1753 (1979)
11. N. E. Hoffman, S. F. Yang, A. Ichihara and S. Sakamura, Plant. Physiol. in press.
12. H. Honma, T. Shimomura, K. Shiraishi, A. Ichihara and S. Sakamura, Agric. Biol. Chem., 43, 1677 (1979)
13. H. Sato, K. Konoma and S. Sakamura, Agric. Biol. Chem., 43, 2409 (1979), H. Sato, K. Konoma, S. Sakamura, A. Furusaki, T. Matsumoto and T. Matsuzaki, Agric. Biol. Chem., 45, 795 (1981), H. Sato, K. Konoma and S. Sakamura, Agric. Biol. Chem., 45, 1675 (1981)
14. A. Ichihara, K. Murakami and S. Sakamura, Tetrahedron Lett., 22, 4005 (1981)
15. A. Ichihara, K. Murakami and S. Sakamura, in preparation.

CHEMICAL BASIS OF HOST RECOGNITION BY *ALTERNARIA* SPECIES (see Note a)

T. Ueno, T. Nakashima and H. Fukami

Pesticide Research Institute, College of Agriculture, Kyoto University, Kyoto 606, Japan

Abstract - Alternaria mali and A. kikuchiana, the causal fungi of Alternaria leaf spot disease of apples and black spot disease of Japanese pears, produce host-specific toxins, named AM-toxin I, II and III and AK-toxin I and II, as the primary determinants of these diseases. These toxins were isolated as crystals and their structures were elucidated to be 1, 2 and 3 in Fig. 1 and 9 and 10 in Fig. 3. The AM- and AK-toxins not only showed extremely potent toxic activity, but solutions of these toxins also induced the same necrotic symptoms only on the leaves of the host plants as those observed on inoculation with the spores of the causal fungi and caused almost instantaneous electrolyte loss from leaf tissues of susceptible cultivars. An early ultrastructural change in cells treated with the toxins appeared to be alternation of the plasma membrane. This indicates that AM- and AK-toxins play an important role in host recognition of A. mali and A. kikuchiana during the early stage of infection. The results of NMR conformation analyses of AM-toxins including synthesized analogs, 4, 6, 7 and 8 in Fig. 1, indicate that the ring conformation of the molecules is strongly related to expression of the toxic activity.

INTRODUCTION

At present, "host-specificity" of plant pathogens is the most intriguing problem in plant pathology. It is assumed that many complex biochemical mechanisms are involved in host-specificity, but in some cases the causal fungi recognize their host plants and invade their tissues by exuding highly potent chemicals, namely "host-specific toxins", which display specific toxicity only to the host plants at an initial stage of the infection process (Ref. 1). It is well known that such toxic substances participate in establishing disease in the several diseases caused by Alternaria, Helminthosporium and other species (Ref. 2), and structures of some host-specific toxins have been elucidated in these several years (Ref. 3 - 12). Alternaria mali and A. kikuchiana cause leaf spot disease of apples and black spot disease of Japanese pears respectively, and produce necrotic blotches especially on the leaves, shoots and fruits of susceptible cultivars. However, great differences in tolerances to these diseases are observed among apple and Japanese pear cultivars (see Table 1). As the results of a series of plant pathological experiments on these diseases, Sawamura and Tanaka observed that the culture filtrates of these fungi induced the same necrotic symptoms as did the spore inoculations (see Table 1) and suggested the presence of host-specific toxins in the culture filtrates (Ref. 14 & 15). In this paper, we describe isolation, structure elucidation and biological significance of the host specific toxins produced by A. mali and A. kikuchiana, named AM-toxin I, II and III and AK-toxin I and II after the name of the causal fungi.

Table 1. Pathogenicity of A. mali and A. kikuchiana and host-specific toxicity of AM- and AK-toxins

pathogenic fungi	apple cultivars			Japanese pear cultivar	
	Indo	Fuji	Jonathan	Nijisseiki	Chojuro
A. mali (strain No. I-716)					
spore inoculation	+++	++	+	++	-
culture filtrate	+++	++	+	++	-
AM-toxin I, II and III	+++	++	+	++	-
A. kikuchiana (strain No. AS-1223)					
spore inoculation	-	-	-	+++	-
culture filtrate	-	-	-	+++	-
AK-toxin I and II	-	-	-	+++	-

Note a. Preceding paper in series: T. Ueno, T. Nakashima and H. Fukami, The Physiological and Biochemical Basis of Plant Infection, Y. Asada et at. (eds). Japan Sci. Soc. Press, Tokyo (1982) in press.

AM-TOXINS, HOSTSPECIFIC TOXINS PRODUCED BY A. MALI

A. mali produces host-specific AM-toxin I (alternariolide) (1), II (2) and III (3). Chemistry of them has been extensively developed by two groups in Japan. Both of them proposed the same structure for 1 almost at the same time and one of them reported the isolation and structure elucidation of 2 and 3 (Ref. 3 - 6).

Chemical studies on AM-toxins

The isolated AM-toxins (1 - 3) have the following physicochemical properties; 1: mp 204 - 208°C, $[\alpha]_D$ -79°(c=1.0 in chloroform, at 19°C), $C_{23}H_{31}N_3O_6$, 2: mp 212 - 214°C, $[\alpha]_D$ -1.9(c=0.55 in dimethyl sulfoxide, at 27°C), $C_{22}H_{29}N_3O_5$ and 3: mp 228°C, $C_{22}H_{29}N_3O_6$. Their IR, PMR and MS spectra suggested that they were analogous depsipeptides. Presence of a lactone linkage in 1 was also confirmed by the results of methanolysis of 1 which gave a methyl ester of a linear peptide (1'), mp 143°C, $C_{24}H_{35}N_3O_7$. Acid hydrolysis of 1 and 1'gave each equimolar amount of L-alanine (L-Ala), L-α-amino-δ-(p-methoxyphenyl)-valeric acid (L-Amv), L-α-hydroxy-isovaleric acid (L-Hyv), pyruvic acid and ammonia. Catalytic hydrogenation of 1' gave a mixture of two diastereomers (1''), $C_{24}H_{37}N_3O_7$,by uptake of one molar hydrogen which produced another one molar alanine instead of pyruvic acid and ammonia by acid hydrolysis. These experimental results indicate that 1 and 1' contain one molar dehydroalanine(Dha) as a structural component in addition to L-Ala, L-Amv and L-Hyv. The sequence of these four components in 1' was unequivocally decided from mass spectral investigation of 1' and 1'' (Ref. 5). As the results, 1 was concluded to be a cyclic tetradepsipeptide composed of L-Hyv, L-Amv, Dha and L-Ala shown in Fig. 1 (Ref. 5). The structures of 2 and 3 were also determined on the basis of NMR and mass spectral correlation to those of 1 and 1' (see Fig. 1) (Ref. 5 - 7). These proposed structures were also confirmed by total synthesis (Ref. 16 - 18). Further details of isolation and structure elucidation of AM-toxins should be referred in Note a and Ref. 5, 6 and 7.

	X	R	n
1	CH_2=	CH_3O-	3
2	CH_2=	H-	3
3	CH_2=	HO-	3
4	CH_3 , H	CH_3O-	3
5	CH_3 , H	CH_3O-	3
6	CH_2=	CH_3O-	1
7	CH_2 , H	CH_3O-	1
8	CH_3 , H	CH_3O-	1

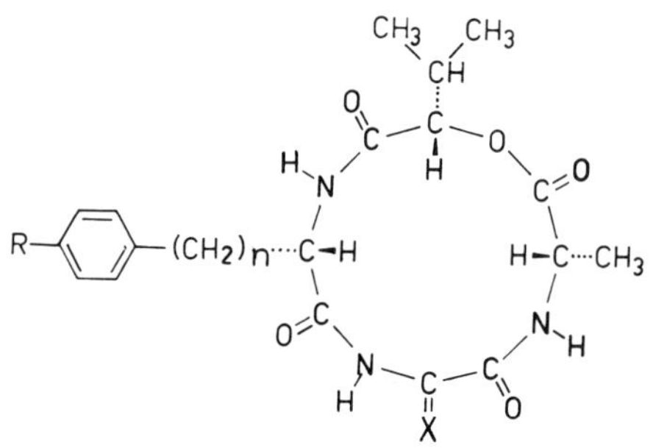

Fig. 1 Structures of AM-toxin I (1), II (2), III (3) and synthesized analogs (4 - 8)

Biological activity of AM-toxins

The AM-toxins (1, 2 and 3) not only showed extremely potent biological activity, but solutions of them also induced the same necrotic symptoms on apple leaves as those observed on inoculation of the causal fungus. When the cuttings of shoots were soaked in the solutions, the threshold concentrations of the toxins inducing necrosis of apple cultivars after 12hr were found to be 10^{-5}- 10^{-3}μg/ml for the extremely susceptible group (e.g. Indo), 10^{-3}- 10^{-1}μg/ml for the moderately susceptible group (e.g. Fuji) and 10^{-1}- 10μg/ml for the resistant group (e.g. Jonathan). These host-specifc activity of the toxins show good correspondence with the results obtained by spore inoculation of the causal fungi and with empirical observations in orchards. A mali has a wide potential host range, for instance, some cultivars of Japanese pear (e.g. Nijisseiki), in addition to apple cultivars and AM-toxins were shown to induce veinal necrosis on all of the leaves of the host plants (see Table 1). On inoculation of an avirurent mutant of A. mali (nonpathogenic) with a droplet of the dilute toxin solution, the nonpathogenic mutant can invade the host tissue with the aid of the toxin just as the pathogenic strains do. This fact indicates that AM-toxins play an important role in the host recognition during the early stage of infection. Several of the cellular responces of the host plants occur very quickly after exposure to the toxin. The mechanism of these effects is not clear yet. Electron microscope pictures have shown that AM-toxins cause changes in plasma membrane and chloroplast of the host cell within 1hr after treatment. Quite similar alternations of the host cell are observed in infected tissue of the host leaves upon inoculation of spores of A. mali (Ref. 19). Such morphological responces to the toxin are in accord with the results of physiological experiments. 1 is capable of inducing destruction of the microstructure of chloroplasts and electrolyte leakage from the host tissue almost immediately after treatment (Ref. 20). The relatioship between the toxin concentration and electrolyte leakage in susceptible and resistant tissue is sigmoidal in form. However, a resistant cultivar, Jonathan, tolerates the toxin at approximately 100,000 times higher concentration than a susceptible cultivr, Indo. These physiological and morphological observations suggest that the primary attack of the toxin may involve destruction of the membrane system.

The structure-toxicity relationship of AM-toxins

From the results of biological assay using synthesized analogs (4 - 8 in Fig. 1), 5 and 6 indicate fairly high activity against susceptible cultivar Indo. This fact suggests that the double bond of Dha and the length of methylene group of L-Amv moiety in the molecule do not play substantial roles for expression of activity of AM-toxins. Although the structural difference between 4 and 5 depends on the absolute configuration of Ala which was introduced in stead of Dha, the biological activity was not observed in 4. PMR spectra of 1, 2, 3, 5 and 6 showed that their ring protons appeared as well-resolved and quite similar patterns with almost the same chemical shifts in the measured organic solvent. On the other hand, PMR spectrum of 4 in the same solvent showed different complex patterns. These observations suggest that main portion of 4 has different conformations from that of 1, 2, 3, 5 and 6 (Ref. 21). This finding implies the ring conformation of the molecules is strongly related to expression of their biological activity. From the results of conformation analyses using NMR saturation transfer and line shape analyses, it was concluded that the major conformation of 1 and 2 corresponds with that of 5 which is shown in Fig. 2 (Ref. 22). If these investigations are also applicable to the active site in the host plant tissue, it is concluded that the ring conformation of the toxin molecule play the most important role to express the toxic activity.

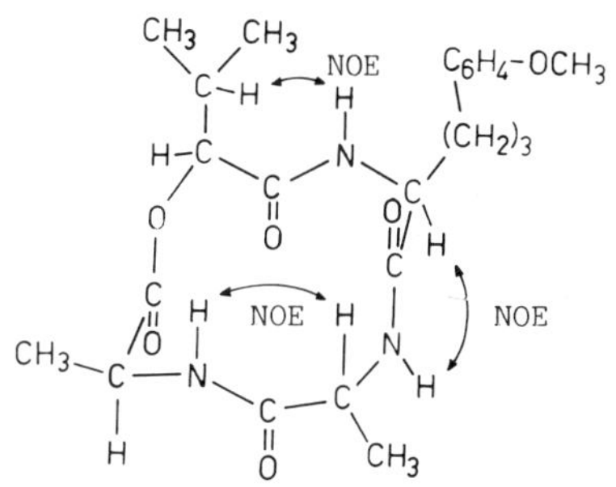

Fig. 2 Conformation of [D-Ala]²-AM-toxin I (5)

AK-TOXINS, HOST-SPECIFIC TOXINS PRODUCED BY A. KIKUCHIANA

As a necrosis inducing factor, Sugiyama et al. reported the isolation, structure elucidation and synthesis of altenin produced by A. kikuchiana, but its host-specificity was not reported (Ref. 23 - 25). Based on the strict plant pathological experiments, we reported the isolation and structure elucidation of the two host-specific toxins (9) and (10) from the culture broth of the causal fungi (Ref. 10).

Isolation of AK-toxins

The isolation procedures of AK-toxins are summarized in Table 2. Every step of the isolation procedures was monitored by the bioassay on young leaves of the susceptible cultivar (Nijisseiki). The active priciple was extracted from the culture broth of A. kikuchiana (strain No. AS-1223) which was cultured in a jar fermenter at 28°C for 3 days in the modified Richards' medium (sucrose 25g, KNO_3 5g, KH_2PO_4 2.5g and $MgSO_4 \cdot 7H_2O$ 1.25g/litter). Repeated chromatographic purification using Amberlite XAD-2, silica gel, droplet counter-current and Sephadex LH-20, and recrystallization from methanol gave two acidic compounds, named AK-toxin I [mp. 168°C(decomp.),$[\alpha]_D$ 164°(c=0.128 in methanol at 25°C)] and II [mp. 168°C(decomp.), $[\alpha]_D$ 125° (c=0.132 in methanol at 23°C)].

Structure elucidation of AK-toxins

The high resolution of mass spectrum (In-Beam EI) of AK-toxin I ($M^{+\cdot}$ at m/z 413.1827) suggestd the molecular formula $C_{23}H_{27}NO_6$ (calcd. 413.1836) which was consistent with the result of elemental analysis (found: C; 67.26, H; 6.70 and N; 3.27%, calcd. for $C_{23}H_{27}NO_6$: C; 66.81, H; 6.58 and N; 3.39%) and CMR data shown in Table 3. Three carbonyl groups (see Table 3) were infired from the IR spectrum (in KBr) to be an ester ($\nu_{C=O}$ 1750cm^{-1}), an amide ($\nu_{C=O}$ 1680 and 1550cm^{-1}) and a conjugated acid ($\nu_{C=O}$ 1690cm^{-1}).
The presence of N-acetyl-β-methyl-phenylalanyl moiety in AK-toxin I was deduced from the PMR spectrum (see Table 4) where acetyl methyl protons (3H, s, δ 1.84), phenyl protons (5H, broad s, δ 7.23), methyl protons (3H, d, δ 1.30, J=7.1Hz) coupling with a methine proton (double q, δ 3.22, J=7.1 and 8.3Hz), the latter coupling with another methine proton (d, δ 4.73, J=8.8Hz) were observed and also from the spectrum obtained in DMSO-d_6 where a doublet signal of the amide proton (δ 8.29, J=6.5Hz) appeared and coupled with the methine proton (double d, δ 4.86, J=6.1 and 6.5Hz) that was observed as a doublet signal at δ 4.73 in the spectrum in CD_3OD. This conclusion was also confirmed from the following characteristic ions observed in the high resolution mass spectrum of AK-toxin I (In-Beam EI 70eV); methyl tropyrium cation at m/z 105.0672 (100%, calcd. for C_8H_9 105.0703), Ph-CH(CH_3)-CH=$\overset{+}{N}H_2$ at 134.0974 (52%, calcd. for

Table 2. Isolation procedures of AK-toxin I and II

culture filtrate (600ℓ)
- absorbed on Amberlite XAD-2 at pH 3.0
- eluted with acetone

aceton eluate
- concentrated
- extracted with ethyl acetate

extract
- extracted with sat. $NaHCO_3$ solution

→ ethyl acetate phase

→ $NaHCO_3$-phase
- reextracted with ethyl acetate at pH 3.0

ethyl acetate (acidic) phase
- evaporated

resisue (30g)

column chromatography (Kieselgel 60, 70-230 mesh ASTM, E. Merck, 200g)
- eluted with $CHCl_3$-ethanol mixture (98.5:1.5 - 97:3 v/v)

active fractions
- evaporated

residue (8g)

droplet counter-current chromatography (descending method)
- developed with CCl_4-$CHCl_3$-benzene-methanol-water mixture (3:3:6:8:2 v/v)

active fractions
- evaporated

residue (3g)

column chromatography (Kieselgel 60, 70-230 mesh ASTM, E. Merck, 90g)
- eluted with $CHCl_3$-ethanol mixture (98.5:1.5 - 97:3 v/v)

active fractions
- evaporated

residue (1.6g)

column chromatography (Kieselgel 60, 70-230 mesh ASTM, E. Merck, 30g)
- eluted with benzene-ethyl acetate-ethanol mixture (50:50:2 - 25:75:2 v/v)

active fractions

→ crystal (4.5mg)
- recrystallized from methanol

AK-toxin II

→ mother liquor
- evaporated

column chromatography (LH-20, 1M-phosphate buffer at pH 5.5)
- eluted with benzene-n-butanol mixture (99.5:0.5 v/v)

crystal (4.5mg)
- recrystallized from methanol

AK-toxin I

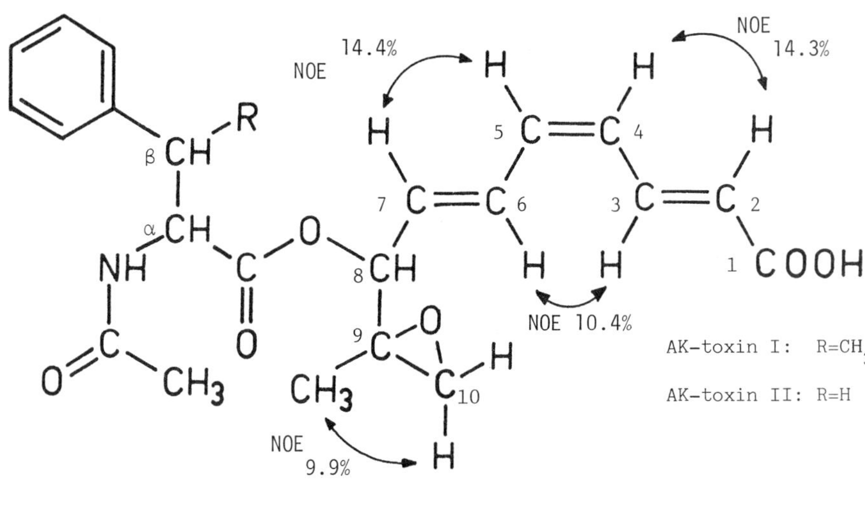

AK-toxin I: $R=CH_3$

AK-toxin II: R=H

Fig. 3 Structures of AK-toxins

Table 3. CMR spectrum of AK-toxin I (50MHz in CD_3OD)

No.	Chemical shift(δ ppm)	Remarks*	No.	Chemical shift(δ ppm)	Remarks*
1	17.75	$-CH_3$	12	129.43	-CH=
2	18.99	$-CH_3$	13	129.55	-CH= x 2
3	22.18	$-CH_3$	14	130.64	-CH=
4	42.98	>CH-	15	132.23	-CH=
5	52.83	$-CH_2-$	16	136.48	-CH=
6	57.77	>C<	17	140.06	-CH=
7	59.40	>CH-	18	143.37	>C=
8	77.57	>CH-	19	170.22	-CO-
9	124.20	-CH=	20	171.70	-CO-
10	128.04	-CH=	21	173.04	-CO-
11	128.80	-CH= x 2			

* Assigned by off-resonance decoupling and peak height

Table 4. PMR spectra of AK-toxin I and II (200MHz in CD_3OD)

AK-toxin I			AK-toxin II		
Chemical shift (δ ppm)	No. of protons	Remarks	Chemical shift (δ ppm)	No. of protons	Remarks
1.30	3	d *J*=7.1Hz			
1.31	3	s	1.29	3	s
1.84	3	s	1.93	3	s
2.61	1	d *J*=4.8Hz	2.61	1	d *J*=4.6Hz
2.76	1	d *J*=4.8Hz	2.75	1	d *J*=4.6Hz
3.22	1	dq *J*=8.8, 7.1Hz	2.97 - 3.16	2	m
4.73	1	d *J*=8.8Hz	4.66	1	t
5.35	1	d *J*=7.1Hz	5.22	1	d *J*=7.0Hz
5.87	1	dd *J*=15.2, 7.1Hz	5.70	1	dd *J*=15.2, 7.0Hz
5.95	1	d *J*=15.1Hz	5.94	1	d *J*=15.1Hz
6.24	1	dd *J*=11.2, 11.1Hz	6.21	1	dd *J*=10.7, 10.7Hz
6.39	1	dd *J*=11.1, 11.0Hz	6.27	1	dd *J*=10.7, 10.7Hz
6.95	1	dd *J*=15.2, 11.0Hz	6.81	1	dd *J*=15.2, 10.7Hz
7.23	5	bs	7.25	5	bs
7.77	1	dd *J*=15.1, 11.2Hz	7.73	1	dd *J*=15.1, 10.7Hz

$C_9H_{12}N$ 134.0968), $Ph-CH(CH_3)-CH=\overset{+}{N}H-CO-CH_3$ at m/z 176.1100 (43%, calcd. for $C_{11}H_{14}NO$ 176.1075) and $Ph-CH(CH_3)-CH(C\equiv\overset{+}{O})-NH-CH_3$ at m/z 204.1011 (22%, calcd. for $C_{12}H_{14}NO_2$ 204.1023). Another structural moiety of AK-toxin I was concluded to be 9,10-epoxy-8-hydroxy-9-methyl-2*E*, 4*Z*,6*E*-decatrienoic acid from the following experimental results. AK-toxin I gave a monomethyl ester ($M^{+\cdot}$ m/z 427.2024, In-Beam EI, calcd. for $C_{24}H_{29}NO_6$ 427.1993) by treatment with diazomethan in methanol and a hexahydro derivative $(M+1)^+$ m/z 420, FD-MS; $M^{+\cdot}$ m/z 419.2034, In-Beam EI, calcd. for $C_{23}H_{33}NO_6$ 419.2306 by catalytic hydrogenation on PtO_2 in methanol. Taking account of rather lower value of chemical shift of an olefinic proton (δ 7.77), the presence of C=O streching band of conjugated acid at $1690cm^{-1}$ in the IR spectrum and UV_{max} (ε=27,600 in methanol), all of the six olefinic protons and a methine proton in PMR spectrum of AK-toxin I were reasonably assigned to H on C-2 (δ 5.95), H on C-3 (δ 7.77), H on C-4 (δ 6.24, H on C-5 (δ 6.39), H on C-6 (δ 6.95), H on C-7 (δ 5.87) and H on C-8 (δ 5.35) (see Table 4) of 8-oxy-2*E*,4*Z*,6*E*-trienoic acid. The fact that large paramagnetic shifts were observed on H on C-2 and H on C-3 by addition of $Pr(NO_3)_3$ shift reagent in D_2O indicated that the two protons should locate on α and β position from the terminal carboxyl group. Informations about their geometrical arrangements of the conjugated olefinic protons were obtained from their coupling constants and enhancement of proton signals on NOE experiments. The values of the coupling constants, J(between H on C-2 and H on C-3)=15.1(trans), J(between H on C-3 and H on C-4)=11.2(vicinal), J(between H on C-4 and H on C-5)=11.1(cis), J(between H on C-5 and H on C-6)=11.0(vicinal), J(between H on C-6 and H on C-7)=15.2(trans) and J(between H on C-7 and H on C-8)=7.1Hz(vicinal), suggested the arrangement of trans, cis, trans trienoic structure, which was confirmed by observation of NOE enhancement between H on C-2 and H on C-4, H on C-3 and H on C-6, and H on C-5 and H on C-7 as shown in Fig. 1. Remaining one methyl (s, δ 1.31) and one methylen signals with AB type (1H, d, δ 2.61 and 1H, d, δ 2.76, J=4.8Hz) should be assigned to methyl-ethyleneoxide group attached to C-8 of the oxy-trienoic acid by the fact that NOE enhancement was also observed between the methyl protons and one of the methylene protons (δ 2.61) on C-10. This investigation was also supported from the chemical shifts of a singlet carbon (δ 57.77) and a triplet carbon signal (δ 52.83) in the CMR spectrum of AK-toxin I (see Table 3). On the basis of these experimental results, the structure of AK-toxin I was determined to be 8-(α-acetylamino-β-methyl-β-phenyl-propionyloxy)-9,10-epoxy-9-methyl-2E,4Z,6E-decatrienoic acid as shown in Fig. 3.

The molecular formula of AK-toxin II was determined to be $C_{22}H_{25}NO_6$ ($M^{+\cdot}$ m/z 399.1676, calcd. 399.1679) by high resolution mass spectrometry (In-Beam EI 70eV). The PMR spectra of AK-toxin I and II (see Table 4) indicated that their difference was in the substitution on the β-position of N-acetyl-phenylalanyl moiety with or without a methyl group. In the PMR spectrum of AK-toxin II, a multiplet methylene (2H on C-β) and a triplet methine signal (1H on C-α) with an ABX system were observed at δ2.97 - 3.16 and 4.66 instead of the doublet methyl (CH_3 on C-β, δ 1.30), the double quartet methine (1H on C-β, δ 3.22) and the doublet methine signal (1H on C-α, δ 4.73) of AK-toxin I, and other all of the proton signals showed quite similar patterns with almost the same chemical shifts as those of AK-toxin I. The high resolution mass spectrum of AK-toxin II (In-Beam EI 70eV) gave every 14 mass unit decreased peaks, compared with the characteristic ions for N-acetyl-β-methyl-phenylalanyl moiety of AK-toxin I; tropyrium cation at m/z 91.0566 (50%, calcd. for $C_7H_7$91.0547), $Ph\text{-}CH_2\text{-}CH{=}\overset{+}{N}H_2$ at m/z 120.0823 (100%, calcd. for $C_8H_{10}N$, 120.0813), $Ph\text{-}CH_2\text{-}CH{=}\overset{+}{N}H\text{-}CO\text{-}CH_3$ at m/z 162.0912 (62%, calcd. for $C_{10}H_{12}NO$ 162.0917) and $Ph\text{-}CH_2\text{-}CH(C{\equiv}\overset{+}{O})\text{-}NH\text{-}CO\text{-}CH_3$ at m/z 190.0863 (42%, calcd. for $C_{11}H_{12}NO_2$ 190.0867). These data clearly demonstrated that AK-toxin II contained N-acetyl-phenylalanine as the structural moiety, and consequently AK-toxin II was the β-demethyl derivative of AK-toxin I as shown in Fig. 3 (10).

Biological activity of AK-toxins

The results of biological assay showed the crstalline AK-toxin I and II had a host-specific phytotoxic property resemble to that of the causal fungus when they were applied to young fresh leaves of Japanese pear cultivars. the threshold concentrations of these toxins inducing necrosis observed after 16hr at room temperature were 0.065μg/ml respectively when droplets of the toxin solution were placed on leaves of a susceptible cultivar, Nijisseiki. But in the case of a resistant cultivar, Chojuro, even 6.5μg/ml solutions of the toxins did not induce any necrosis on the leaves. These results show apparently that AK-toxin I and II have a host-specific phytotoxic activity for japanese pear cultivars which are susceptible to *A. kikuchiana*.

REFERENCES

1. P.B.Pringle and R.P.Scheffer, Ann. Rev. Phytopathology, 2, 133 (1964)
2. R.P.Scheffer and O.C.Yoder, Phytotoxins in Plant Diseases (R.K.S.Wood et al.,eds) Academic Press, London, New York, 251 (1972)
3. T.Okuno, Y.Ishita, K.Sawai and T.Matsumoto, Chem. lett., 1974, 635
4. T.Okuno, Y.Ishita, A.Sugawara, A.Mori, K.Sawai and T.Matsumoto, Tetrahedron Lett.,1975,335
5. T.Ueno, T.Nakashima, Y.Hayashi and H.Fukami, Agr. Biol. Chem., 39, 1115 (1975)
6. T.Ueno, T.Nakashima, Y.Hayashi and H.Fukami, Agr. Biol. Chem., 39, 2081 (1975)
7. T.Ueno, T.Nakashima, M.Uemoto, H.Fukami, S.Lee and N.Izumiya, Biomedical Mass Spectrometry, 4, 134 (1977)
8. A.T.Bottini and D.G.Gilchrist, Terahedron Lett., 1981, 2719
9. A.T.Bottini, J.R.Bowen and D.G.Gilchrist, Terahedron Lett., 1981, 2723
10. T.Nakashima, T.Ueno and H.Fukami, Terahedron Lett., 1982, submitted for publication.
11. Y.Kono and J.M.Daly, Bioorganic Chem., 8, 391 (1979)
12. Y.Kono, S.Takeuchi,A.Kawarada,J.M.Daly and H.W.Knoche, Tetrahedron Lett., 1980, 1537
13. J.M.Liesch, C.C.Sweeley,G.D.Staffeld, M.S.Anderson, D.J.Webber and R.P.Scheffer, Tetrahedron, 38, 45 (1982)
14. K.Sawamura, Bull. Hort. Res. Stn. Japan, C4, 43 (1966)
15. S.Tanaka, Mem. Coll. Agr. Kyoto Imp. Univ., 28, 1 (1933)
16. S.Lee, H.Aoyagi, Y.Shimohigashi, N.Izumiya, T.Ueno and H.Fukami, Terahedron Lett.,1976,843
17. Y.Shimohigashi, S.Lee, T.Kato, N.Izumiya, T.Ueno and H. Fukami, Chemistry Lett.,1977,1141
18. T.Kammera, H.Aoyagi, M.Waki, T.Kato, N.Izumiya, K.Noda and T.Ueno, Tetraheron Lett.,1981, 1785
19. P.Park, M.Tsuda, Y.Hayashi and T.Ueno, Can. J. Bot., 55, 2383 (1977) (1976)
20. K.Kohmoto, I.D.Kahn. Y.Renbutsu, T.Taniguchi and S.Nishimura, Physiol. Pl. Path.,8,141
21. Y.Shimohigashi, S.Lee, T.Kato, N.Izumiya, T.Ueno and H.Fukami,Agr.Biol.Chem.,41,1533(1977)
22. T.Higashijima, T.Inubushi, T.Ueno and T.Miyazawa, FEBS Lett., 105, 337 (1979) (1966)
23. N.Sugiyama, C.Kashima, M.Yamamoto, T.Sugaya and R.Mohri, Bull. Chem. Soc. Japan, 39,1573
24. N.Sugiyama, C.Kashima, Y.Hosoi, T.Ikeda and R.Mohri, Bull. Chem. Soc. Japan, 39,2470(1966)
25. N.Sugiyama, C.Kashima, M.Yamamoto and R.Mohri, Bull. Chem. Soc. Japan, 40, 345 (1967)

GIBBERELLIN BIOSYNTHESIS IN *ZEA MAYS*: THE 3-HYDROXYLATION STEP GA_{20} TO GA_1

Bernard O. Phinney and Clive Spray

Department of Biology, University of California, Los Angeles, USA

Abstract - Elongation growth in *Zea mays* (maize) is dependent on the presence of the gibberellin, GA_1, which originates biosynthetically via an early-13-hydroxylation pathway. GA_1 is apparently the only biologically active gibberellin, per se, in this pathway. Other gibberellins in the pathway are active through their metabolism to GA_1. The four gibberellin mutants of maize, d_5, d_3, d_2 and d_1 control specific and different steps in the pathway. The d_5 gene blocks an early step, CPP to *ent*-kaurene, the d_3 and d_2 genes control intermediate oxidation steps and the d_1 gene controls the terminal step, GA_{20} to GA_1. The data presented here show that 3-chloro-substitution of GA_{20} resulted in the loss of activity when assayed on the d_5 mutant. At low levels no bioactivity was observed. At high levels (greater than 0.1 µg per plant) the bioactivity was 10% that of GA_1. The bioassay data for 3-chloro-GA_{20} support the position that hydroxylation at carbon-3 is necessary for the bioactivity of GA_{20}.

INTRODUCTION

Gibberellins (GAs) are tetracyclic diterpene acids (Fig. 1) that were originally identified by the Japanese as secondary metabolites from the fungus, *Gibberella fujikuroi*. They were subsequently shown to be present in higher plants and found to control a wide variety of responses associated with the growth and differentiation of flowering plants. They are now accepted as a class of plant hormones. The subject has been covered in a number of books and reviews (1-8) and considerable information has been accumulated on the biosynthetic origin of the GAs, especially in the fungus (2). Information is only now appearing on the biosynthesis of GAs in higher plants.

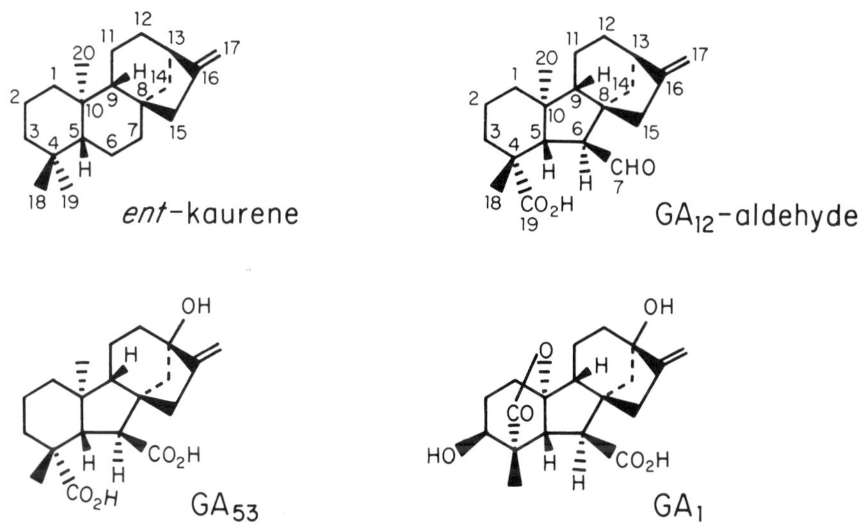

Fig. 1. Numbering system for the gibberellin precursors, *ent*-kaurene and GA_{12}-aldehyde, and the structures for GA_{53} (a C_{20} gibberellin) and GA_1 (a C_{19} gibberellin).

GA biosynthesis originates via a diterpene pathway which begins with mevalonic acid (MVA) and leads to GA_{12}-aldehyde, the common precursor for all of the known GAs (Fig. 2). The details are probably the same for the fungus and higher plants. Subsequent to GA_{12}-aldehyde, branches occur, each of which leads to a series of C_{20} and C_{19} GAs. These branches differ from each other in the presence or absence of hydroxylation and in the pattern and timing of hydroxylation. There are at least three different pathways subsequent to GA_{12}-aldehyde: a non-hydroxylation pathway leading to GA_9, an early-3-hydroxylation pathway leading to GA_1 and GA_3 and an early-13-hydroxylation pathway leading to GA_1 only. There is also evidence for the presence of a fourth pathway, a 1β-hydroxylation pathway in Triticum aestivum [wheat] (9, 10). While the details of the pathways in the fungus Gibberella fujikuroi are well known, similar information for higher plants is only slowly accumulating in the literature (9-12). The current evidence suggests that the pathway(s) present in a higher plant depends on the species being studied; it may also depend on the particular organ under study and stage of development of that organ. The control of GA-dependent growth in higher plants cannot be understood until the details of these pathways are known.

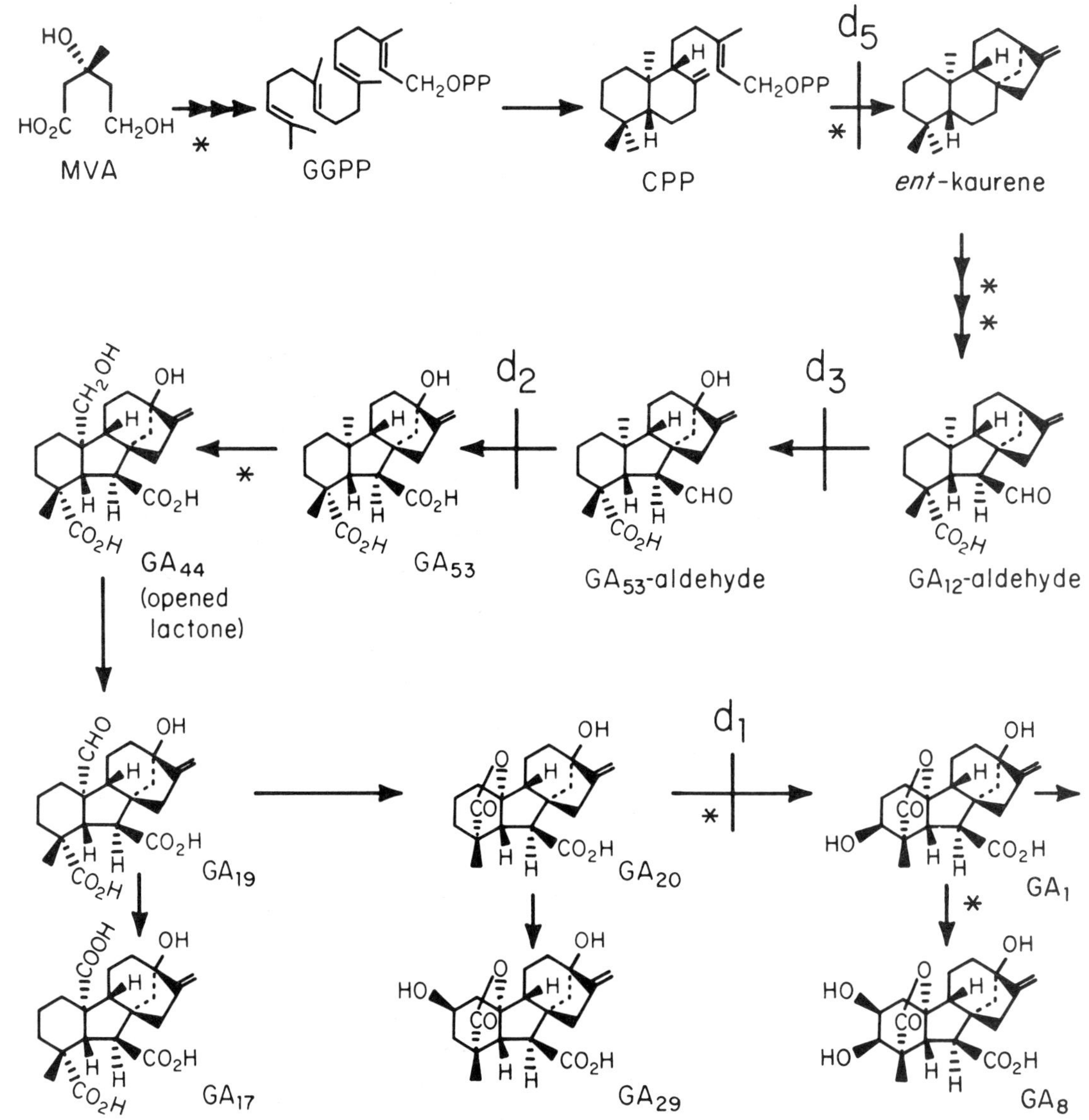

Fig. 2. A hypothetical GA biosynthetic pathway for Zea mays L. (maize). The first part of the pathway, MVA to GA_{12}-aldehyde, is the same for the fungus, Gibberella fujikuroi, and for higher plants. The second part, an early-13-hydroxylation pathway, originates from GA_{12}-aldehyde and terminates with GA_1. It is unique to higher plants. Specific steps documented by radio-feeds are indicated by an asterisk (*). Since GA_8 and GA_{29} are biologically inactive, they are shown as branches from the main pathway. GA_{17} is also shown as a branch because radio-feeds to other plant systems show it to be unmetabolized. The positions of the genetic blocks for the GA-mutants of maize are also given.

ENDOGENOUS GIBBERELLINS AND THE BIOSYNTHETIC PATHWAY

Seven GAs have been identified by GC-MS or by GC-SICM from young tassels of normal maize (11). On the basis of their structures these GAs are presumptive members of an early-13-hydroxylation pathway (Fig. 2). There is also evidence for the presence of this pathway in other species of higher plants (12-16). The pathway does not occur in the fungus, Gibberella fujikuroi (2,6). In maize at least three of the steps in the early-13-hydroxylation pathway have been defined by radio-feeds; e.g. the label from [^{14}C]GA_{53} has been recovered in GA_{44} (16). Also [^{3}H]GA_{20} and [^{3}H]GA_1 have been fed to maize and the label found in GA_1 (17) and GA_8 (18) respectively. There is also evidence in maize for specific steps in the pathway from MVA to GA_{12}-aldehyde. The label from [^{14}C]CPP has been found in ent-kaurene (19) and the label from [^{14}C]ent-kaurenol and ent-kaurenal has been recovered in ent-kaurenal and ent-kaurenoic acid, respectively (20). GA_{17} is shown in Fig. 2 as a branch from the main pathway based on studies with Cucurbita maxima (21). In this material a cell-free system was shown to metabolize radiolabelled GA_{19} to GA_{20} with no evidence for the metabolism of radiolabelled GA_{17} to either GA_{20} or its presumptive metabolites. GA_8 and GA_{29} are shown as branches from the main pathway since 2β-hydroxylation results in loss of bioactivity. Apparently GA_1 is the terminal gibberellin in this early-13-hydroxylation pathway. It is the only GA in the pathway that is biologically active per se (22, and see below). This presumptive pathway provides a basis for determining the specific steps controlled by the GA (dwarf) mutants in maize.

THE GIBBERELLIN MUTANTS

The four dwarf mutants, d_5, d_3, d_2 and d_1, are simple recessives and non-allelic to each other (23). They have internodes and leaves (stem units) that are shorter than normals; they are GA mutants in that they respond by normal growth to exogenous GA and to no other growth factor (Figs. 3-5). The implication of the genetic information is that these mutants may be controlling specific and different steps in a pathway leading to a native GA responsible for elongation growth in maize. This interpretation also requires that only the terminal GA in the pathway be biologically active, per se. GAs earlier in the pathway would be biologically active only as a consequence of their metabolism to the terminal GA. The genetic information can also be used to resolve whether there is more than one biosynthetic pathway controlling elongation growth in maize. Growth response data have now been obtained relating bioactivity of the maize GAs and their precursors for each of the four mutants (22). The information suggests that each mutant gene controls a specific and different step in the early-13-hydroxylation pathway of maize as follows (Fig. 2): (1) dwarf-5, the cyclization step, CPP to ent-kaurene, (2) dwarf-3, the 13-hydroxylation step, GA_{12}-aldehyde to GA_{53}-aldehyde, (3) dwarf-2, the carbon-7 oxidation step, GA_{53}-aldehyde to GA_{53} and (4), dwarf-1, the 3-hydroxylation step, GA_{20} to GA_1. (GA_{53}-aldehyde is only a tentative substrate in the pathway, since it is not known at what step carbon-7 is oxidized from the aldehyde to the acid. It is possible that GA_{12}-aldehyde is metabolized to GA_{12} and then to GA_{53}. This would reverse the order of the d_2 and d_3 genes in the pathway.)

In this report additional evidence will be presented to support the position that 3-hydroxylation of GA_{20} (i.e. metabolism of GA_{20} to GA_1) is necessary for the observed bioactivity of GA_{20}.

MATERIALS AND METHODS

The mutants used in these studies came from genetic stocks that were segregating in the ratio of 3 normal to 1 dwarf. Seed were presoaked for 24 hr, planted in vermiculite and grown to the early seedling stage in the greenhouse. Individual plants were then removed and transferred to liquid culture for seedling bioassays, or to soil for repeated treatments. Treatments were made as described by Phinney and Spray (22). The gibberellins, GA_1 and GA_3, were supplied by Grenetta Harris, Abbott Laboratories, North Chicago, Ill. GA_{20} was a gift from Jake MacMillan, University of Bristol, U.K.; 3-chloro-GA_{20} was synthesized from GA_3 as follows. Methyl-3-keto-GA_3-13-acetate was prepared as described by Beale et al. (24). This compound was reduced to the 3α-alcohol of GA_1 by the addition of two equivalents of "L-Selectride" (Aldrich trade mark) dissolved in tetrahydrofuran at -60°C in the presence of a trace of ethanol. After 15 minutes the solution was allowed to reach room temperature. The resulting product, methyl-3-epi-GA_1-13-acetate, was extracted with ethyl acetate and purified by column chromatography on silica gel, eluting with ethyl acetate-petroleum ether. This compound was 3β-chlorinated after the methods of Beale et al. (24). The product, methyl-3β-chloro-GA_1-13-acetate was deacetylated with 0.5M sodium methoxide, demethylated using the method of Bartlett and Johnson (25) and recrystallized to give 3-chloro-GA_{20}. GLC showed the purity of the three GAs and 3-chloro-GA_{20} to be greater than 99%.

RESULTS AND DISCUSSION

The responses of d_5 and d_1 mutants to multiple treatments of GA_1 and GA_{20} are shown in Figs.

3 and 4. In these treatments, dosages were set at levels that would give a normal-type growth response to GA_1 for the mutants of each set. The cumulative dosage was 200 µg per plant. The single treatment responses of d_5 seedlings to GA_1 and GA_{20} are shown in Fig. 6. For the d_5 mutant both GA_1 and GA_{20} were highly active. In contrast GA_{20} was biologically inactive in multiple treatments to d_1 plants while the activity of GA_1 was high and indistinguishable from the activity on d_5 plants. This absence of activity of GA_{20} on d_1 plants has been attributed to the inability of the d_1 mutant to hydroxylate carbon-3 of GA_{20} (22).

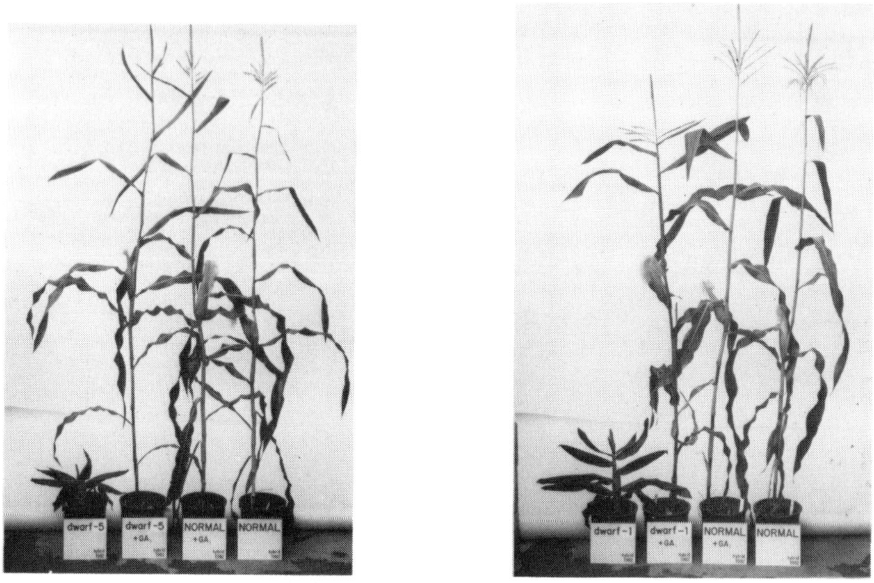

Fig. 3. Response of the d_5 mutant (left) and the d_1 mutant (right) to multiple treatments of GA_1. Plants read from left to right: dwarf, no treatment; dwarf + GA_1; normal + GA_1; normal, no treatment. Both the amounts and timing of treatments were chosen to give a normal-type growth response for the treated dwarfs. Dosages for all treated plants were identical.

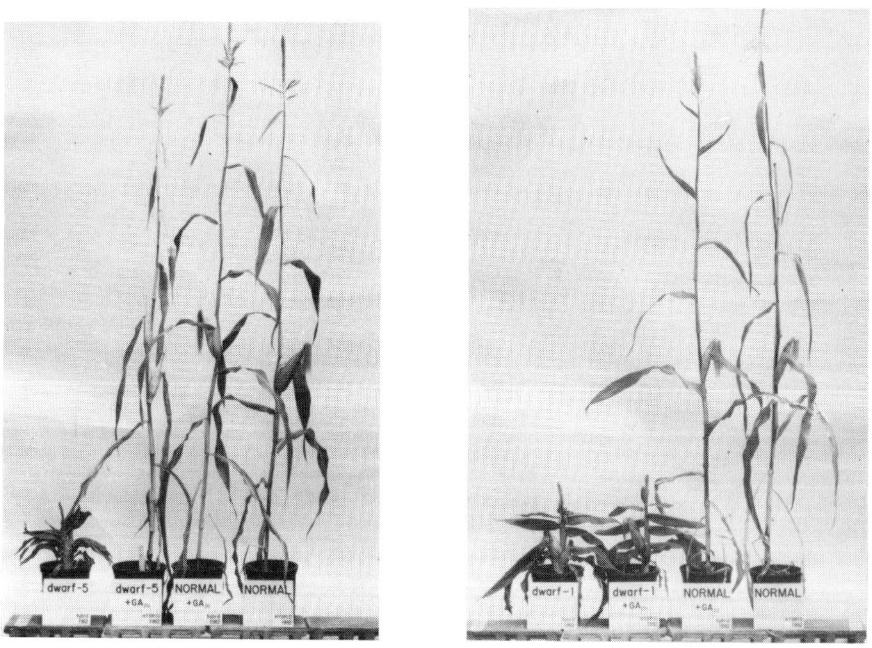

Fig. 4. Response of the d_5 mutant (left) and the d_1 mutant (right) to multiple treatments of GA_{20}. Plants read from left to right: dwarf, no treatment; dwarf + GA_{20}; normal + GA_{20}; normal, no treatment. Both the amounts and timing of treatments were chosen to give a normal-type growth response for the treated dwarfs. Dosages for all treated plants were identical.

This interpretation must mean that the activity of GA_{20} on d_5 plants is a result of its metabolism to GA_1. In other words, GA_{20} is itself inactive. If this interpretation is true, chemical substitution at carbon-3 of GA_{20} should effectively block enzymatic hydroxylation at that position and result in loss of bioactivity. In order to test this interpretation, 3-chloro-GA_{20} was synthesized and tested in single and multiple treatments to d_5 plants. Multiple treatments were set at levels identical to those used for GA_1 and GA_{20}. The results are shown in Figs. 5 and 6; 3-chloro-GA_{20} was inactive in multiple treatments to d_5 plants and 10% as active as GA_{20} in the single treatments in the d_5 seedling bioassay. In these single treatments, 3-chloro-GA_{20} was inactive at dosages below 0.1 μg per plant. The low (10%) bioactivity of 3-chloro-GA_{20} at higher dosages could be due to configurational similarities between the hydroxyl group and the chlorine atom.

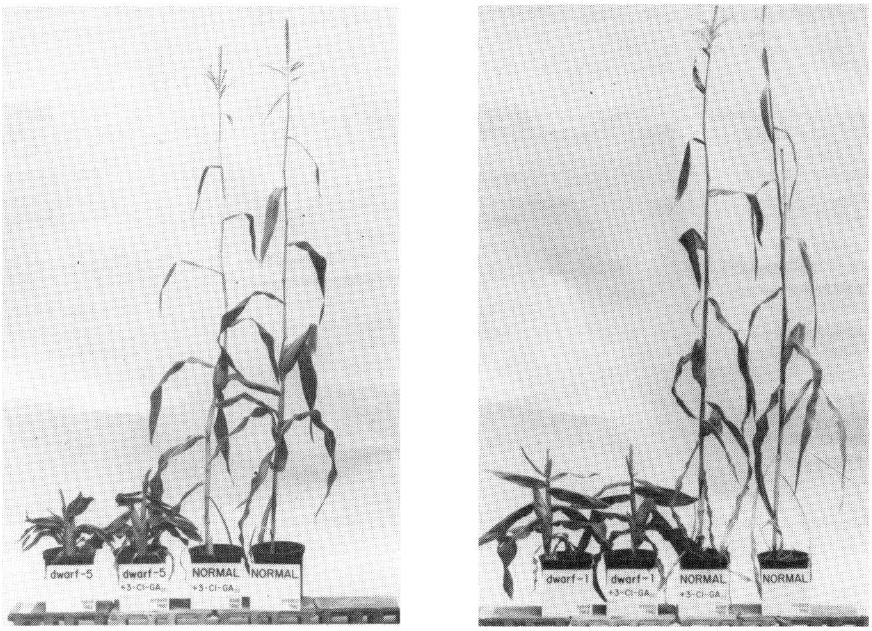

Fig. 5. Response of the d_5 mutant (left) and the d_1 mutant (right) to multiple treatments of 3-chloro-GA_{20}. Plants read from left to right: dwarf, no treatment; dwarf + 3-chloro-GA_{20}; normal + 3-chloro-GA_{20}; normal, no treatment. Both the amounts and timing of treatments were identical to those used for GA_1 and GA_{20} (see Figs. 3 and 4).

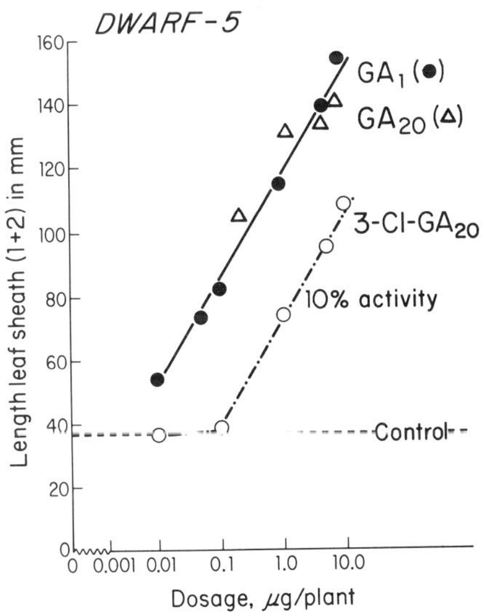

Fig. 6. Dosage response data in the seedling d_5 bioassay (single treatments) for GA_1, GA_{20} and 3-chloro-GA_{20}. Plants were treated at the time of unfolding of the first seedling leaf from the coleoptile; 0.1 ml of an acetone-water (1:1) solution was added into the axil of the leaf. Plants were then grown for one week at 30°C in continuous light after which the lengths of the first and second leaf sheaths were measured, summed and averages of these sums determined (sample size = 10).

It is concluded that the loss of bioactivity from the 3-chlorination of GA_{20} is due to the chemical blockage of hydroxylation at that position.

Acknowledgements - This work was supported by a grant from the National Science Foundation (PMC 80 21588). We wish to thank Peter Lorenz for his assistance in the bioassays reported here. We also thank Jake MacMillan for encouraging the use of Ockham's razor in our studies.

REFERENCES

1. A. Crozier, The Biochemistry and Physiology of Gibberellins, 1 and 2 (in press) (Ed. A. Crozier). Praeger Press (1983).
2. P. Hedden, J. MacMillan and B. O. Phinney, Ann. Rev. Plant Physiol. 29, 149 (1978).
3. P. Hedden, ACS Symposium Series 111, 19 (1979).
4. J. E. Graebe and J. Ropers, In: Phytohormones and Related Compounds: a Comprehensive Treatise (Eds. D.S. Letham, P.B. Goodwin and T.J.V. Higgins) 1, 107, Elsevier/North Holland (1978).
5. J. MacMillan, Hormonal Regulation of Development I. Molecular Aspects of Plant Hormones. Encyclopedia Plant Physiology N.S. (Ed. J. MacMillan) 9, 1, Springer-Verlag (1980).
6. B.O. Phinney, ACS Symposium Series III, 57 (1979).
7. N. Takahashi, Chemical Regulation of Plants (in Japanese) 7, 1 (1972).
8. N. Takahashi, Chemical Regulation of Plants (in Japanese) 16, 65 (1981).
9. P. Gaskin, P.S. Kirkwood, J.R. Lenton, J. MacMillan and M.E. Radley, Agric. Biol. Chem. 44, 1589 (1980).
10. P.S. Kirkwood and J. MacMillan, J.C.S. Perkin I, 689 (1982).
11. P. Hedden, B.O. Phinney, R. Heupel, D. Fujii, H. Cohen, P. Gaskin, J. MacMillan and J.E. Graebe, Phytochemistry 21, 391 (1982).
12. Y. Kamiya and J.E. Graebe, Phytochemistry 21, (in press) (1982).
13. P. Hedden and J.E. Graebe, J. Plant Growth Regul. 1 (in press) (1982).
14. J.D. Metzger and J.A.D. Zeevaart, Plant Physiol. 65, 623 (1980).
15. J.A.D. Zeevaart, T. Gianfagna and W. Lusk, Plant Physiol. 70 (in press) (1982).
16. R.C. Heupel, Ph.D. Dissertation, University of California, Los Angeles (1982).
17. S.B. Rood, Ph.D. Dissertation, University of Calgary, Alberta (1981).
18. L. Rappaport, L. Davies, S. Lavee, R. Nadeau, R. Patterson and C.F. Stolp, In: Plant Growth Substances IX (1973). Tokyo, Hirokawa, 314 (1974).
19. P. Hedden and B.O. Phinney, Phytochemistry 18, 1475 (1979).
20. E.S. Wurtele, P. Hedden and B.O. Phinney, J. Plant Growth Regul. 1, 15 (1982).
21. J.E. Graebe, P. Hedden and W. Rademacher, In: Gibberellins-Chemistry, Physiology and Use (Ed. J.R. Lenton) Monograph 5, British Plant Growth Regulator Group, 31 (1980).
22. B.O. Phinney and C.R. Spray, Plant Growth Substances XI (1982) (in press) Academic Press (1982).
23. E.H. Coe and M.G. Neuffer, In: Corn and Corn Improvement (Ed. G. Sprague) Agron. 18, 111 (1977).
24. M.H. Beale, P. Gaskin, P.S. Kirkwood and J. MacMillan, J.C.S. Perkin I, 885 (1980).
25. P.A. Bartlett and W.S. Johnson, Tetrahedron Lett. 4459 (1970).

METABOLITES OF ABSCISIC ACID IN HIGHER PLANTS

K. Koshimizu and N. Hirai

Department of Food Science and Technology, Faculty of Agriculture, Kyoto University, Kyoto 606, Japan

Abstract - Abscisic acid levels in plants are known to be controlled by biosynthesis or degradation depending on the physiological state of a plant. A systematic survey for abscisic acid metabolites was made to gain a better understanding of this metabolic pathway. Among the fruits investigated, avocado contained a new conjugated metabolite that released dihydrophaseic acid on alkaline hydrolysis. The isolation procedure was guided by HPLC analysis of dihydrophaseic acid released on hydrolysis to afford a dihydrophaseic acid conjugate. The structure of the metabolite was shown by spectral and chemical evidence to be dihydrophaseic acid-4'-O-β-glucoside.

INTRODUCTION

Abscisic acid (ABA) is metabolized to phaseic acid (PA) via hydroxyabscisic acid (HOABA), then to dihydrophaseic acid (DPA) and its epimer (*epi*-DPA) (1-3). ABA is present in its conjugated forms. The presence of three ABA conjugates, 1'-O-α- and 1'-O-β-glucoside and maltosyl ester were reported, after the isolation of ABA glucosyl ester (4-6). ABA metabolites also are converted to conjugates (7,8) that may act in the regulation of ABA metabolism in plant tissues. Only three conjugates, however, β-hydroxy-β-methylglutaryl-hydroxyabscisic acid (HMG-HOABA), PA-1'-O-β-glucoside and PA glucosyl ester are known (4,9, 10). We report the screening of alkali-hydrolyzable conjugates in fruits and the isolation of a new conjugate of DPA from avocado fruit.

RESULTS AND DISCUSSION

Screening of conjugates of ABA metabolites in fruits

Qualitative and quantitative analyses of ABA metabolites were carried out by HPLC which did not require such preliminary derivatization of samples as methylation or trimethylsilylation. Of the two HPLC columns examined, a μ-Bondapak C_{18} column was useful for qualitative and quantitative evaluations of ABA metabolites. ABA, *t*-ABA, PA, DPA and *epi*-DPA were separated on a μ-Bondapak C_{18} column using 35 % (v/v) methanol in 0.1 % (v/v) acetic acid at a flow rate of 0.6 ml/min (Fig. 1). ABA, *t*-ABA and PA were separated on a μ-Porasil column with a solution of 15 % (v/v) acetonitrile in chloroform acidified with 0.1 % (v/v) acetic acid at a flow rate of 30 ml/min, but DPA and *epi*-DPA were not eluted within 30 min because of their higher polarity.

Avocado (*Persia americana*) fruit was chosen for the examination of the hydrolysis conditions and extraction method, because alkaline hydrolysis of the extract of avocado fruit has been shown to release ABA (11). The acidic aqueous solution from the acetone extract was washed with ethyl acetate four times to remove free metabolites. The resulting aqueous layer then was divided by volume into two equal portions. One portion was hydrolyzed at pH 12 and 60° for 1 hr to give an ethyl acetate-soluble acidic fraction (HE-fraction). Because free metabolites of ABA (especially DPA and *epi*-DPA) were not completely removed from the aqueous solution by ethyl acetate extraction, it was possible to overestimate the net amount of metabolites released by hydrolysis. Thus, the other portion of the unhydrolyzed aqueous solution was extracted with ethyl acetate. The ethyl acetate-soluble acidic fraction (CE-fraction) obtained was used as the control for the HE-fraction. The free forms of metabolites in the HE- and CE-fraction of avocado fruit were analyzed by the HPLC procedure.

A peak corresponding to DPA was detected in both the HE- and CE-fraction. A compound from this peak was collected by preparative HPLC and converted to its methyl ester, which was identified as methyl dihydrophaseate (MeDPA) by GC-MS. The levels of DPA were 130 μg/100 g fruit in the HE-fraction and 29 μg/100 g fruit in the CE-fraction. This indicates the presence in avocado fruit of a conjugate(s) that releases DPA on alkaline hydrolysis. ABA was not detected in either fraction.

PC 2 - D

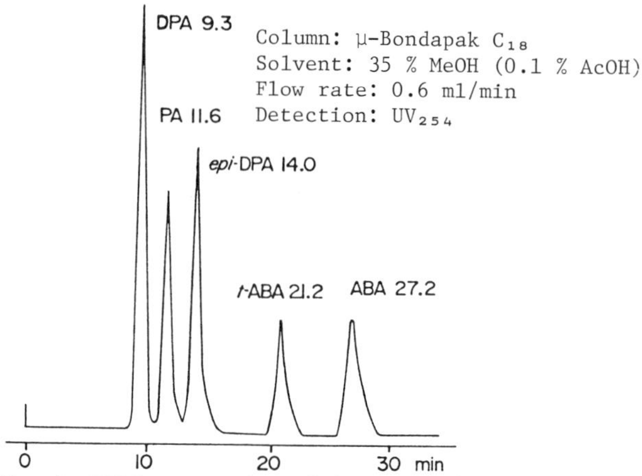

Fig. 1. HPLC separation of ABA metabolites

The conjugates of ABA metabolites in 11 kinds of fruits were examined with this screening method. The results summarized in Table 1 show that fruits of the cherry, tomato, peach, prince melon and orange contain alkali-hydrolyzable conjugates of ABA metabolites. The extracts of apple, kiwi, papaya, citron, longan and papaw did not release detectable amounts of ABA metabolites on alkaline hydrolysis. These results do not prove that there were no conjugates of ABA metabolites in these fruits: conjugated forms that are not hydrolyzed by alkali might be present.

Table 1. ABA metabolites released by alkaline hydrolysis of fruit extracts (μg/100 g fruit)

	Avocado		Tomato		Peach		Prince melon		Orange		Cherry	
	CE[a)]	HE[b)]	CE	HE	CE	HE	CE	HE	CE	HE	CE	HE
ABA[c)]	ND[d)]	ND	ND	ND	5	31	ND	ND	ND	77	ND	ND
PA	ND	ND	ND	ND	4	8	ND	8	ND	ND	ND	100
DPA	29	130	ND	ND	10	73	ND	16	ND	ND	ND	ND
epi-DPA	ND	ND	3	45	ND	ND	ND	14	ND	ND	ND	ND

a) Ethyl acetate-soluble acidic part of control
b) Ethyl acetate-soluble acidic part of hydrolysate
c) ABA + *t*-ABA
d) Not detected

Isolation and structure of a new conjugate of the dihydrophaseic acid from avocado fruit

Because avocado fruit contained a higher concentration of the DPA conjugate than the other fruits tested, we attempted the isolation of the conjugate by monitoring DPA with alkaline hydrolysis.

The aqueous concentrate obtained from the acetone extract of mature avocado fruit (24 kg) was washed successively with *n*-hexane and ethyl acetate at pH 4. After neutralization, the aqueous solution was chromatographed on charcoal and a sample of each eluate was hydrolyzed. HPLC analysis showed that DPA was released from the 10 and 20 % acetone eluate by hydrolysis. A small portion of the combined eluate was analyzed by HPLC on a μ-Bondapak C_{18} column (Fig. 2). The compound with a peak at R_t 14.0 min was a DPA conjugate. The combined 10 and 20 % acetone eluate then was chromatographed successively on silica gel and Sephadex LH-20. The final purification by preparative HPLC gave 42 mg of a DPA conjugate (CDPA).

CDPA, $[\alpha]_D^{27}$ -20° (EtOH; *c* 0.209), had a UV absorption maximum at 257 nm (ε 15600) and IR absorption bands at 3400, 2920, 1690, 1630 and 1600 cm^{-1}. The ^1H NMR spectrum of CDPA showed that it consisted of one mole each of DPA and β-glucose. The doublet ascribable to the β-anomeric proton was observed at δ 4.35 (1H, *J*=7 Hz). CDPA was hydrolyzed more easily with acid than with alkali to release glucose. CDPA also was hydrolyzed by β-glucosidase to yield DPA and glucose. Treatment of CDPA with diazomethane gave a monomethyl ester (MeCDPA) whose ^1H NMR spectrum showed a singlest assignable to a carbomethoxyl at δ 3.07 (3 H). These chemical properties indicate that CDPA is a β-glucoside of DPA, not a β-glucosyl ester.

Acetylation of MeCDPA with pyridine and acetic anhydride introduced four acetyl groups, when the glucose moiety was attached to the oxygen at the C-4' of DPA. But, glucosidic linkage to the C-1' oxygen should form the pentaacetate in the same treatment. MeCDPA gave an acetyl derivative, whose ^1H NMR spectrum (Fig. 3) exhibited a broad singlet (12 H) at δ 2.07 due to four acetoxyls. This indicates that CDPA is dihydrophaseic acid-4'-O-β-glucoside (DPA-4'-β-GS). This structure was validated by results of CIMS using isobutane. CIMS of the tetraacetate showed a quasi-molecular ion peak at m/z 627 due to the protonated tetraacetyl-β-glucoside of MeDPA. An oxonium-type sugar (tetraacetylglucose) ion and an aglycon (MeDPA) ion, produced by cleavage of the glucosidic linkage, were found at m/z 331 and 279, respectively. The structure was finally confirmed by comparing the spectral data for the tetraacetate with those of a sample synthesized from MeDPA and α-acetobromoglucose.

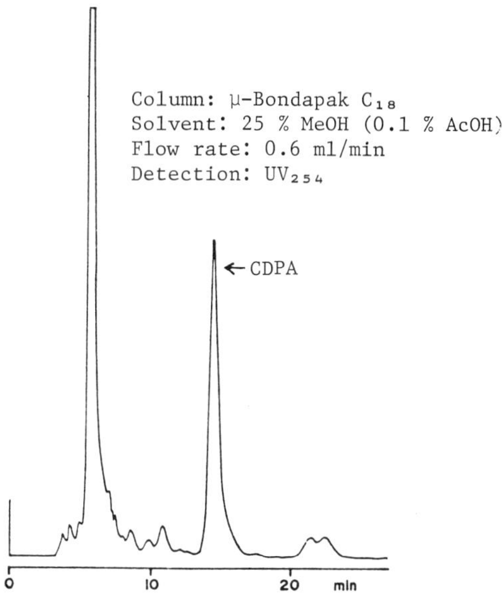

Fig. 2. HPLC trace of 10 and 20 % acetone eluates of a charcoal column

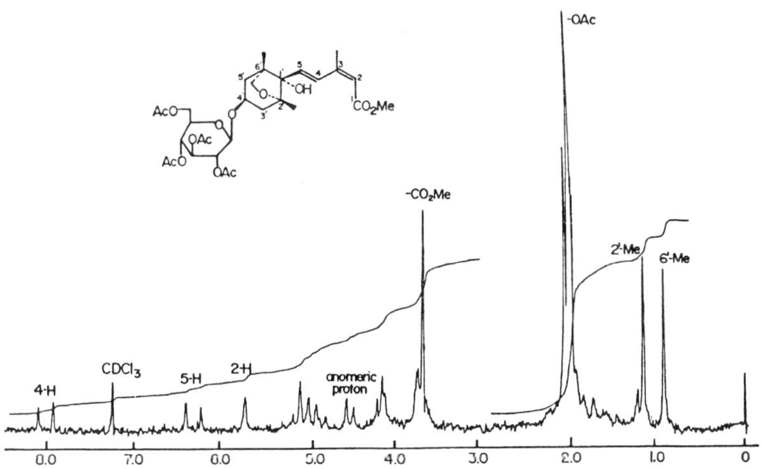

Fig. 3. ^1H NMR spectrum of tetraacetyl methyl ester of CDPA (90 MHz, $CDCl_3$)

ABA metabolites hitherto characterized are summarized in Fig. 4. On the further screening, DPA-4'-β-GS also was found in the fruit of grape (*Vitis vinifera*) analyzed by HPLC and ECD-GC. Neither DPA-4'-β-GS nor DPA inhibited the growth of rice seedlings at a concentration of 100 ppm.

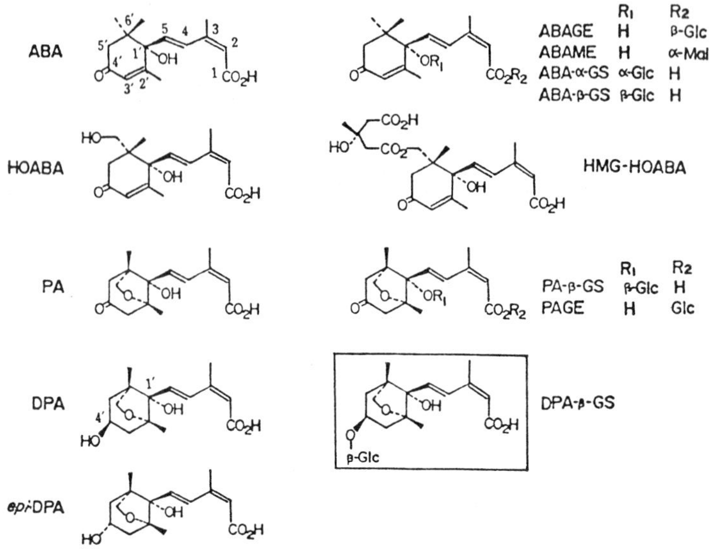

Fig. 4. Characterized ABA metabolites

Acknowledgments - This work was supported in part by a grant from the Ministry of Science and Culture Education, Japan. We thank Drs. M. Suzuki, K. Hara and N. Takeda of Meijo University for the CIMS measurements.

REFERENCES

1. B.V. Milborrow, *Chem. Commun.*, 966 (1969)
2. D.C. Walton and E. Sondheimer, *Plant Physiol.*, 49, 285 (1972)
3. E.T. Tinelli, E. Sondheimer, D.C. Walton, P. Gaskin and J. MacMillan, *Tetrahedron Lett.*, 139 (1973)
4. B.V. Milborrow, *"Plant Growth Substances 1979"*, ed. F. Skoog, Springer-Verlag, Berlin, 1980, p. 262
5. G. Sembdner, W. Dathe, V.I. Keferi and M. Ktacek, *ibid.*, p. 254
6. K. Koshimizu, M. Inui, H. Fukui and T. Mitsui, *Agric. Biol. Chem.*, 32, 789 (1968)
7. B.V. Milborrow, *Phytochemistry*, 14, 123 (1975)
8. J.A.D. Zeevaart and B.V. Milborrow, *Phytochemistry*, 15, 493 (1976)
9. N. Hirai, H. Fukui and K. Koshimizu, *Phytochemistry*, 17, 1825 (1978)
10. N. Hirai and K. Koshimizu, *Phytochemistry*, 20, 1867 (1981)
11. B.V. Milborrow, *Ann. Rev. Plant Physiol.*, 25, 259 (1974)

2,3-DIOXABICYCLO[4.4.0]DECANES AS PLANT GROWTH REGULATORS

M. L. Bolte*, W. D. Crow*, T. Osawa**, D. M. Paton* and S. Yoshida***

Faculty of Science, Australian National University, Canberra, Australia
***Department of Food Science & Technology, Nagoya University, Nagoya, Japan*
****Department of Agricultural Chemistry, University of Tokyo, Tokyo, Japan*

Abstract - Naturally occurring derivatives of 2,3-dioxabicyclo[4.4.0]decane from *Eucalyptus grandis* exercise control over a range of physiological functions in plants. These include root strike in cuttings, water uptake, membrane permeability, frost resistance and inhibition of electron transport in photosynthesis. The synthesis and breakdown of these compounds *in vivo* and *in vitro* are discussed. Synthetic approaches to the naturally occurring compounds and related structures are presented in some detail, and some preliminary structure-activity relationships for synthetic analogues are discussed.

Over the last decade there has been increasing attention brought to bear on the rate of use of material resources, particularly those associated with the production of energy. It is both natural and appropriate that we should therefore direct our research efforts more towards those materials that we can produce economically from plant sources. The green plants represent a photosynthetic factory that must be maintained anyway, since they are responsible for maintenance of the earth's atmospheric balance as well as the recycling of essential mineral elements: we should therefore seek to make the maximum use of their presence. In effect, this means not only seeking new uses of plant materials, but also optimising the use of those that we already exploit with some success. The chemical basis for the control of plant growth processes thus emerges as an area of growing importance for the future.

Trees of the genus *Eucalyptus* (family Myrtaceae) are essentially confined to Australia, although they have been distributed to many other parts of the world, where the inhabitants are now firmly convinced that the trees are part of the native flora. Over 500 species occur in Australia, ranging from small shrubs to large trees. The genus has successfully adapted itself to the wide range of environmental conditions that occur in the continent and representatives are found from sea level to the snow line and from arid sandy deserts to rich, wet rainforest gullies. For this reason it is usually possible to select a species suitable for planting in most areas of the world where a fast-growing hardwood timber species is required: thus there is considerable interest in the genus *Eucalyptus* outside Australia. When grown outside Australia, there is an additional advantage in that the insect pests of its new habitat are usually not equipped to deal with its particular chemistry. Thus it is not unusual to find that a given species will grow much better in areas outside Australia than it does in its native habitat.

There is a strong tendency for different species of *Eucalyptus* to hybridise and a number of the so-called species described by systematists may well be such hybrids: for this reason, classification and identification within the genus is not easy. For the commercial user of *Eucalyptus*, however, this ease of hybridisation has far more serious implications, in that it presents problems in maintaining a pure plantation of a selected strain: regrowth seedlings will not necessarily have the desirable characteristics of their (presumed) parents. There are, for example, wild strains of *E. macrorrhyncha* that are suited to commercial extraction of rutin (Ref.1) and of *E. dives* that give high yields of oil: seedling progeny from such parents may, however, prove quite useless in a commercial plantation intended for production of these materials. The main use of the genus is in timber production for a variety of purposes, where the rate and form of growth is of primary importance, together with such factors as resistance to frost and to insect attack.

While it is possible to select out strains with desirable characteristics, even to deliberately hybridise and breed for such characteristics, it is essential that subsequent propagation be by vegetative means. Root strike in cuttings has been examined in some detail (Ref.2), showing that, in nearly all cases, it occurs only with great difficulty. In *E. grandis* it was established that rooting will occur in seedling material, taken from below the 12th node, but that above this the characteristics of the mature plant take over and root strike does not occur. It was proposed that this was due to endogenous inhibitors and later chemical examination resulted in isolation (Ref.3) of the G-regulators 1, shown to be capable of inhibiting root strike at concentrations of 10-100 μM (3-30 ppm) - well below the amount present in adult leaves. There was ample evidence that other species contained materials with similar physiological action, although of different structure. Ability to propagate *Eucalyptus* species by vegetative means is thus seen to depend upon an understanding of the action of such compounds - the *raison d'etre* for the work described here.

BIOSYNTHESIS AND PHYSIOLOGY OF THE G-REGULATORS

Biosynthetic studies employing ^{14}C, ^{13}C and ^{18}O established (Ref.4) the probable pathway shown in Scheme 1, progressing from the acetate/methionine derived syncarpic acid 2 to the 2-alkylidene-1,3-diones 3 by condensation with an aldehyde or aldehyde equivalent, followed by uptake of oxygen to generate the G-regulator structures 1. There are several points about the scheme that are worthy of comment. The initial observation (Ref.3) of both R- and S-chirality in the G-regulators at positions 1 and 4, coupled with the presence of the peroxyhemiketal structure, had caused us some uneasiness: there is ample precedence for oxidation during silica chromatography (Ref.5) and the possibility existed that the true natural product was in fact the compound 3. This was strongly reinforced when synthetic studies, described below, showed that 3 was indeed readily converted to 1 on silica gel. Re-isolation of the G-regulators in an atmosphere of $^{18}O_2$, however, showed no incorporation of the isotope. It is evident that the uptake of oxygen during biosynthesis is not sterically controlled, i.e., not enzyme-mediated, in the case of the G-regulators. The existence of a photo-oxygenation pathway has been shown in the case of conversion of ergosterol into its peroxide by *Penicillium rubrum* and *Gibberella fujikuroi* (Ref.6).

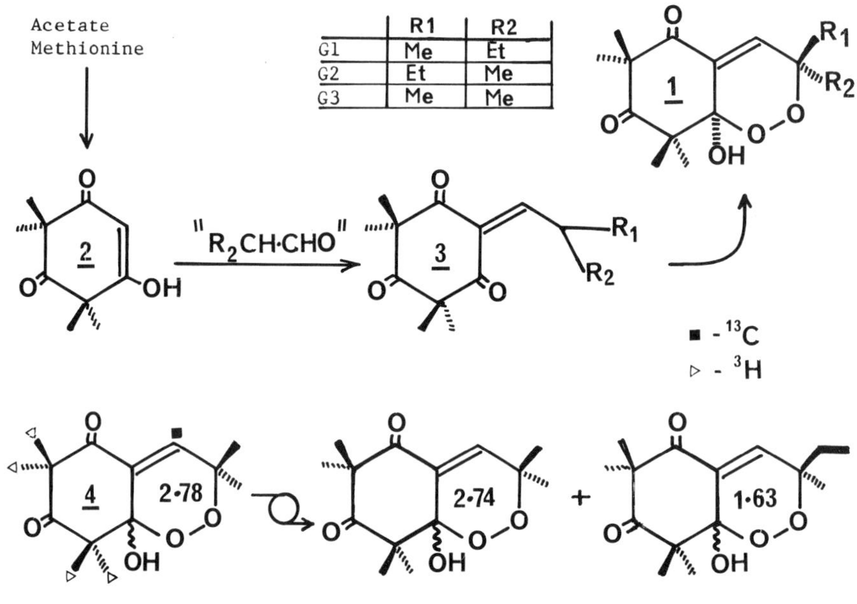

Scheme 1: Biosynthesis of G-regulators.

The matter of the aldehyde equivalent, involved in condensation with syncarpic acid, remains in doubt at the present time. The use of labelled valine and isoleucine indicated that these compounds were incorporated into the structures of G3 and G1/2 respectively. Rather surprisingly, there was some evidence for incorporation of valine into G1/2 and of isoleucine into G3. Subsequent work established that the G-regulators are capable of interconversion within the plant, although the exact mechanism is by no means clear at this stage. Doubly labelled G3, with a tritium/carbon ratio of 2.78 (4) was fed to an isolated twig of *E. grandis*, from which the three inhibitors G1-3 were subsequently isolated, with the tritium/carbon ratios shown. It is evident that the interconversion mechanism is more complex than we had anticipated and further work is in progress in an attempt to unravel the problem.

Chemical assays have established that the G-regulator content of an *E. grandis* seedling rises progressively from node 1 upwards, as shown in Figure 1, while the Mung bean bioassay response for rooting shows an exactly inverse relationship to node number. It is a matter of some interest that the concentration observed in adult leaves of *E. grandis* (2 mM) exceeds the solubility of the compound in water, leading to the suggestion that much of the compound is actually bound as some loose conjugate and is not necessarily physiologically active within the cell. Bioassay responses at concentrations lower than 10^{-5}M, rather surprisingly, show substantial *promotion* of root strike, i.e. the G-regulators show a concentration-dependant response typical of such growth regulators as auxin and ABA.

Diurnal variation of G-content has been studied over all seasons of the year and the results are shown in Fig. 2. Winter-grown material shows high G-content during the period of exposure to frost hazard in the hours before dawn, then the content falls - evidently in response to light. Other frost-hardy *Eucalyptus* species contain high amounts of non-G substances with a similar inhibitory nature: Paton (Ref.7) proposes the hypothesis that frost resistance in the genus can be ascribed to this rapid hardening - dehardening cycle. This role of the G-regulators is possibly associated with reduced stomatal conductance and CO_2-assimilation, probably by inhibition of electron transport in Photosystem II (8).

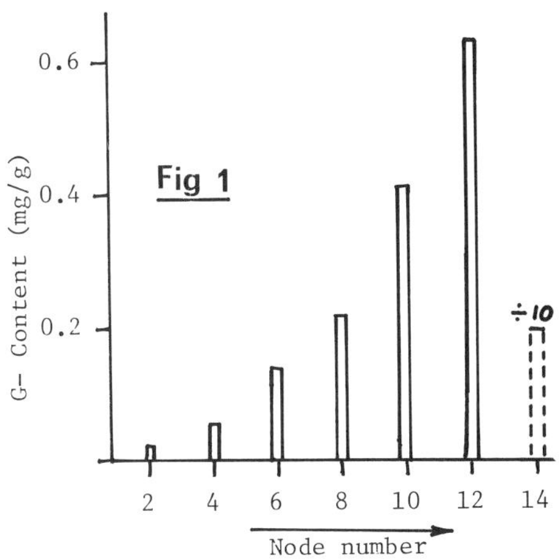

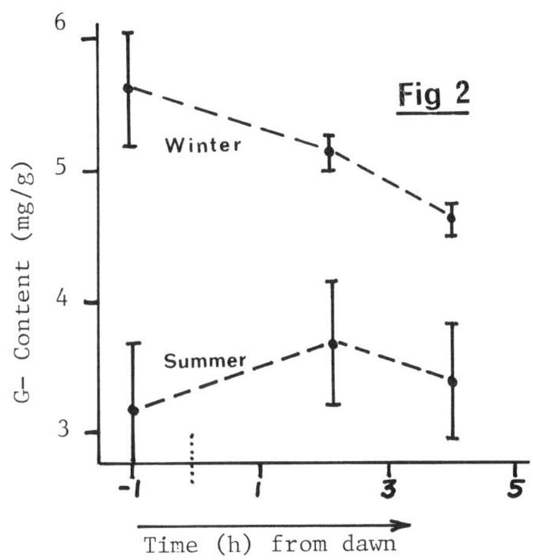

SYNTHETIC APPROACHES TO G-REGULATOR STRUCTURES

The first synthesis of the G-regulators was effected through the standard Knoevenagel reaction (Ref.9), but this proved to be unsuited to more extensive synthetic work.

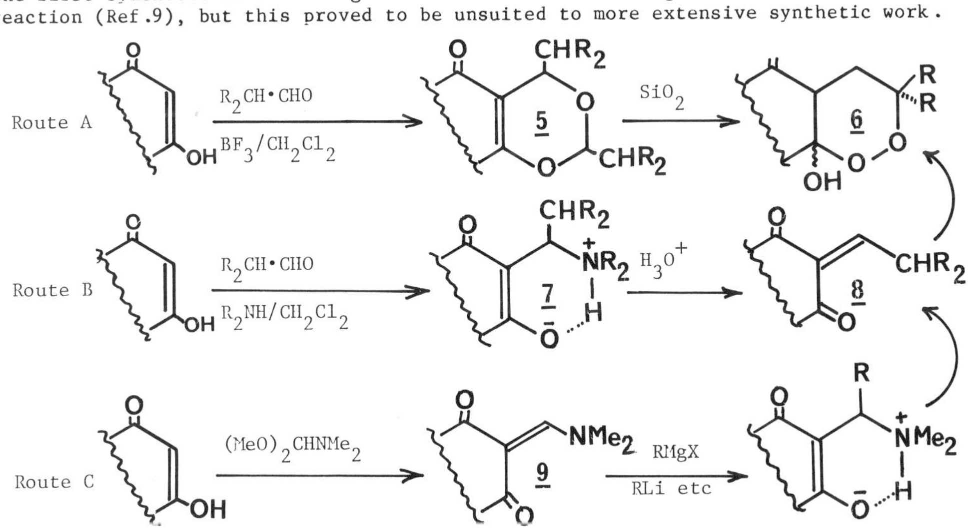

Three routes, A, B and C have been elaborated for synthesis of structures of this type (Refs.10,11,12). Route A was specifically designed to avoid base catalysis or acid catalysis in a nucleophilic solvent and is based on the Prins Reaction of alkenes. A range of Lewis acids were effective, with yields of the 4H-1,3-dioxins 5 usually lying in the range 80-95%. The reaction was not, however, without its limitations as far as choice of 1,3-diketones was concerned. Although N,N-dimethylbarbituric acid reacted in 95% yield, the product obtained was the 2-alkylidene-1,3-diketone 8 rather than the expected product 5. Similar deviations were observed with indan-1,3-dione (20%) and pentan-2,4-dione (45%), while syncarpic acid itself proved quite unsuitable as a substrate. Product variation in the Prins Reaction is not unusual, and the compounds 8 were considered equally acceptable for further elaboration.

Conversion of the 4H-1,3-dioxins 5 to the G-regulator structures 6 was found to occur during chromatography over silica gel (attempted separation of the stereoisomers of 5, presumably through hydrolysis to 8 and attack of oxygen adsorbed on the silica or dissolved in the solvent. Indeed, use of rigorously degassed solvents and silica that had been deoxygenated resulted in formation of the keto-enol pair 10 - 11, observed by n.m.r. Observation of these compounds in the presence of oxygen led to the conclusion that enolisation precedes uptake of oxygen, although the mechanism of this last step is still under examination.

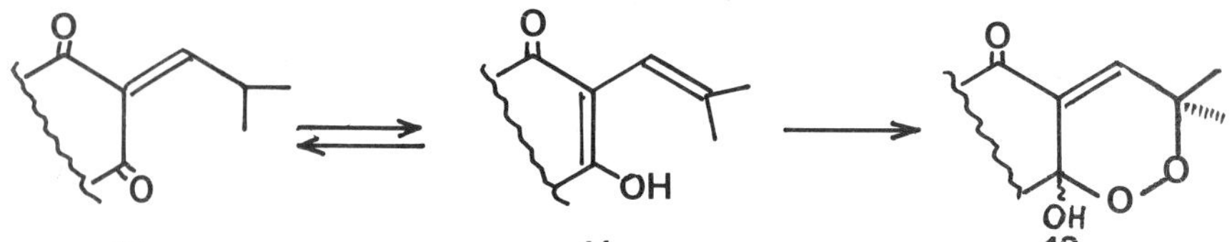

10 11 12

Route B arose from a recognition of the role of the hydroxylic solvent in the normal Knoevenagel condensation, and essentially halts the reaction at the Mannich base stage. Spectroscopic studies show that these compounds exist as internal salts (Ref.12) with a strong intramolecular H-bond when in aprotic media. This essentially prevents the amino-group from taking up a conformation suitable for E2 elimination to 8, thus preserving the substrate from further attack by another molecule of 1,3-diketone... the basic reason for failure in the Knoevenagel condensation. When subjected to hydroxylic solvents, however, protonation and solvation remove the need to retain the particular conformation, and elimination proceeds readily to give 8, with subsequent uptake of oxygen occurring as before. Examination of models suggested that this reaction could be induced to fail if either (a) the base was too sterically demanding or (b) the aldehyde component did not provide sufficient steric inhibition to movement within the Mannich bases. Experiments with a range of larger bases indeed caused failure; use of aldehydes without a substituent on the α-carbon similarly led to failure.

Route C was elaborated to meet the need for sidechains with protected functions, where the use of organometallic reagents offered advantages. The enamino-diketones 9 were readily available from syncarpic acid and related cyclohexan-1,3-diones such as dimedone. In the case of syncarpic acid, little trouble was experienced with a range of Grignard reagents or alkyl lithiums, either of which could be used to generate the Mannich bases. With dimedone, however, the reaction failed, presumably due to formation of an enolate ion; even with two moles of reagent, only starting material was recovered.

PROTEIN BINDING STUDIES AND REACTIONS WITH AMINES

Observations that the concentration of the G-regulators in leaf tissue was greater than their solubility in water led inevitably to the conclusion that these compounds are probably bound in some form for storage, a conclusion that is reinforced by the rapid diurnal variation observed. Early experiments on isolation of low molecular weight protein fractions from *E. grandis* leaves showed that G-regulators could be isolated from this fraction by pH change and extraction with solvents. These experiments were followed up by examining the action of amines on the G-regulators: the expected Michael addition occurred readily to give a series of compounds 13, rather analogous to the Mannich bases 7 and similarly existing as zwitterions (Ref.13).

Treatment of these compounds with aqueous acid revealed two modes of decomposition, one leading to reformation of the G-regulator, the other to decomposition into acetone and the enamino-diketone analogous to 9. The balance between these two pathways was seen to depend upon the steric needs of the attacking base: axial attack by the amine would lead to the initial structure 14a, where the advantages of delocalisation would naturally result in the zwitterionic structurs 14b. The freedom of rotation now permits the molecule to minimise its steric interactions, perhaps by taking up the conformation 15, where the hydroperoxyalkyl group is placed for elimination. While this explanation serves admirably for the experimental situation *in vitro*, the situation in the plant cell is no doubt more complicated: the balance between the pathways observed in the laboratory cannot be used to predict what might happen in the cell.

In summary, there is evidence for some form of binding within the cell, for some form of storage/release mechanism that permits rapid fluctuation, and for a reversible reaction with amines. When these data are taken in conjunction, they form the basis of a plausible hypothesis for the action of the G-regulators in the cell. There is clearly a need for further probing of this hypothesis and experiments to this end are in progress. In the meantime, it forms the basis for our preliminary attempts to synthesise analogues of the G-regulators in a search for the structural features that are responsible for their activity.

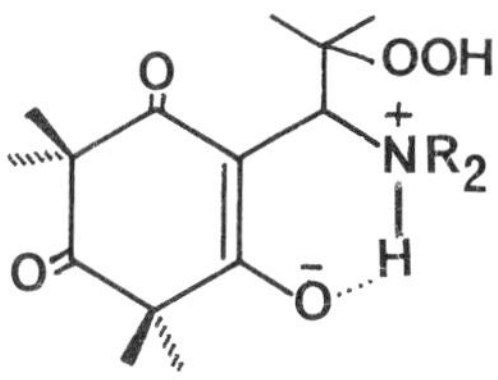

13

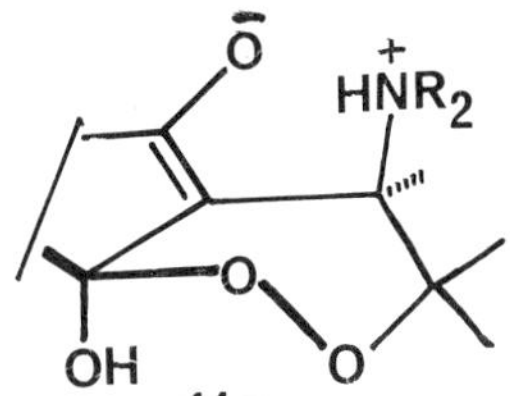

14a

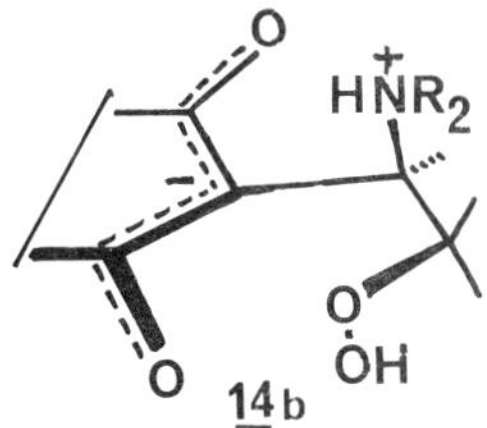

14b

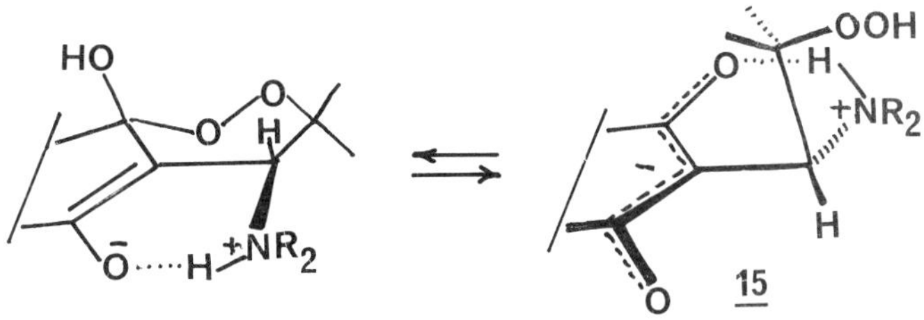

15

STRUCTURE - ACTIVITY RELATIONSHIPS IN G-ANALOGUES.

At this stage only a limited range of bioassay techniques have been used, concentrating on the observed inhibition of root strike in cuttings and on the promotory effects that are seen at lower concentration. For these purposes we have employed the Mung bean hypocotyl rooting assay as well as root growth in germinating rice seed: the qualitative nature of the tests necessarily introduce some uncertainty in the results and only major effects are noted.

The first group of compounds tested were direct analogues of the G-regulators 1, possessing the basic structural feature 16: variations to the A-ring and to the B-ring substituents are

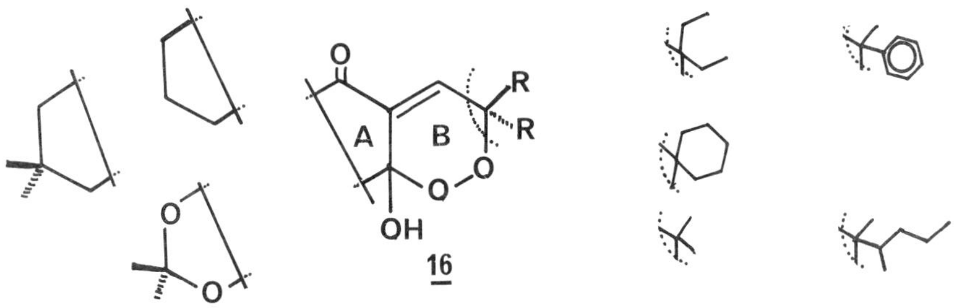

16

shown beside the formula. All showed inhibitory effects at 10^{-4} - 10^{-5} M, with some indication that alkyl substitution on the A-ring was desirable, but that too heavy alkyl substituents on the B-ring reduced the effect. The most active members of the group were comparable to the G-regulators themselves, and some also showed promotory effects at lower concentrations.

Working backwards along the presumed biosynthetic pathway, the next group tested were the 2-alkylidene-1,3-diones, with the basic structure 17 and variations as shown. All these derivatives had no available site for addition of oxygen (where such a site exists, oxygen is added spontaneously during synthesis) and showed reduced inhibitory action. Examination of further representatives would, however, be needed before any particular significance could be assigned to this result.

The closest derivatives obtainable to the 2-alkylidene-1,3-diones that *do* possess a site for oxygen addition are the Mannich bases 7, and a variety of these, with the basic structure and variations 18 were tested for activity. In general, they were slightly more active than the corresponding peroxides 1 (to which they were expected to convert in the cell) and there was no suggestion that the degree of alkyl substitution was important, or that the organic base had any effect. A comparison between a Mannich base 7, the derived peroxide structure 1 and the perhydroxy-Mannich base derived from it (13), showed some interesting points. While the last two were practically identical in bioassay results, the Mannich bases 7 tended to show promotory effects at low concentration to a greater degree than the others. There was, however, considerable variation within each group.

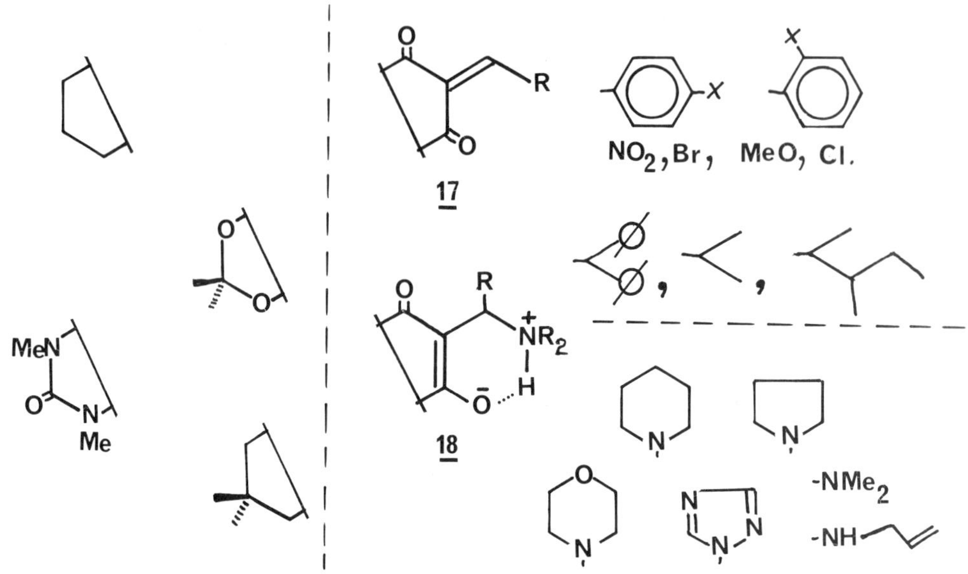

Perhaps the most encouraging aspect of the preliminary bioassay results is the fact that very few of the compounds tested failed to show any activity at all, suggesting that the basic model chosen is at least close to reality. It is, of course, too early to be able to offer explanations for the variations observed: penetration to the action site, degree of ionisation and other factors are yet to be examined. The Mannich bases 7, for example, are eminently water-soluble, as befits a small zwitterion, yet show much the same activity as the peroxides 1 ... almost insoluble in water. Further work to examine these points is in progress.

REFERENCES

1. F. R. Humphreys, Econ. Botany, 18, 195-253 (1964).
2. D. M. Paton, R. R. Willing, W. Nicholls and L. D. Pryor, Aust. J. Bot., 18, 175-180 (1970).
3. W. D. Crow, W. Nicholls and M. Sterns, Tetrahedron Lett., 1353-1356 (1971).
4. W. D. Crow and T. Osawa - unpublished data.
5. R. Caputo, L. Mangini, L. Previtera and R. Iaccarino, Tetrahedron Lett., 3731-3734 (1971).
6. M. L. Bates, W. W. Reid and J. D. White, J. Chem. Soc. Chem. Commun., 44-45 (1976).
7. D. M. Paton, U.S. - Japan Seminar on Frost Resistance, Academic Press, New York, 1982 - in press.
8. T. D. Sharkey, G. F. Stevenson and D. M. Paton, Plant Physiol., 69 (1982) - in press.
9. W. D. Crow, T. Osawa, K. M. Platz and D. S. Sutherland, Aust. J. Chem., 29 2525-2531 (1976).
10. W. D. Crow, M. L. Bolte and S. Yoshida, Aust. J. Chem., 35 (1982) - in press.
11. W. D. Crow, M. L. Bolte and S. Yoshida, Aust. J. Chem., 35 (1982) - in press.
12. M. L. Bolte and W. D. Crow - unpublished data.
13. W. D. Crow, M. L. Bolte and S. Yoshida, Aust. J. Chem., 35 (1982) - in press.

ACKNOWLEDGMENTS

The work described here is part of a continuing project supported by the Australian Research Grants Committee, whose financial assistance is gratefully acknowledged. The work also forms part of a collaborative programme between Australian and Japanese scientists under the auspices of the Science and Technology Exchange Agreement between the two governments.

NEUROHORMONES IN SILKWORM, *Bombyx mori*

Akinori Suzuki, Hiromichi Nagasawa, Shogo Matsumoto, Hiroshi Kataoka, Akira Isogai, Saburo Tamura, Hironori Ishizaki*, Syo Sakurai**, Hajime Fugo***, Haruyuki Sonobe† and Nobuo Ogura‡

Department of Agricultural Chemistry, The University of Tokyo, Tokyo 113, Japan
**Faculty of Science, Nagoya University, Nagoya 464, Japan*
***Faculty of Science, Kanazawa University, Kanazawa 920, Japan*
****Faculty of Agriculture, Tokyo University of Agriculture and Technology, Tokyo 183, Japan*
†Department of Biology, Konan University, Kobe 658, Japan
‡Department of Medical Zoology, Dokkyo University School of Medicine, Tochigi 321-02, Japan

Abstract-Prothoracicotropic (PTTH) and eclosion (EH) hormones were extracted from adult heads of *Bombyx mori* and PTTH was isolated by extensive chromatographic purification. A hormone (melanization and reddish coloration hormone, MRCH) inducing cuticular melanization and epidermal reddish coloration in the armyworm larvae of *Leucania separata* was also extracted from *Bombyx* adult heads. The chemical and biological properties of these hormones were investigated.

INTRODUCTION

In insect endocrinology, the silkworm *Bombyx mori* has historically played important roles (1) and in the life cycle of this insect has also been reported the involvement of neurohormones, such as prothoracicotropic hormone (PTTH)(2,3), diapause hormone (DH)(4,5) and eclosion hormone (EH)(6). Interestingly, it has been found that the neurosecretory organs of *B. mori* contain the hormone termed melanization and reddish coloration hormone (MRCH), which induces cuticular melanization and epidermal reddish coloration in the armyworm larvae (7), although the role of MRCH is still obscure in *B. mori*. In contrast to extensive biological studies, however, little is known of the chemical nature of these neurohormones due to the difficulty of obtaining pure hormones; the major problem in isolating these hormones in a pure form is that only minute amounts of the hormones are present in each insect. In the case of silkworm *B. mori*, the adult heads are suitable as starting materials for large scale purification because millions of male silkworm moths are available from commercial silkworm eggs producers. With a view to clarifying the chemical and biological properties of silkworm neurohormones as a whole, we have already confirmed the presence of these neurohormones in the extracts of *Bombyx* adult heads, collected more than ten millions of the adult heads as starting materials for extraction and have recently succeeded in isolating one of the PTTH and clarifying some chemical and biological properties (8). Some details of our studies on PTTH, EH and MRCH are disclosed in the following sections.

NEUROHORMONES EXTRACTED FROM *Bombyx* ADULT HEADS

The heads of silkworm moths *B. mori* were separated with a razor blade, stored at -20°C until use and extracted as outlined in Fig. 1. The acetone powder of heads was homogenized with 80% ethanol and the resulting mixture was filtered. From the filtrate, ethanol was removed *in vacuo* and the residual aqueous solution was heated on a boiling water bath for 10 min. After cooling, the aqueous solution was mixed with cold acetone and the precipitates yielded with 50% acetone were removed. Acetone solution was concentrated *in vacuo* and the residual

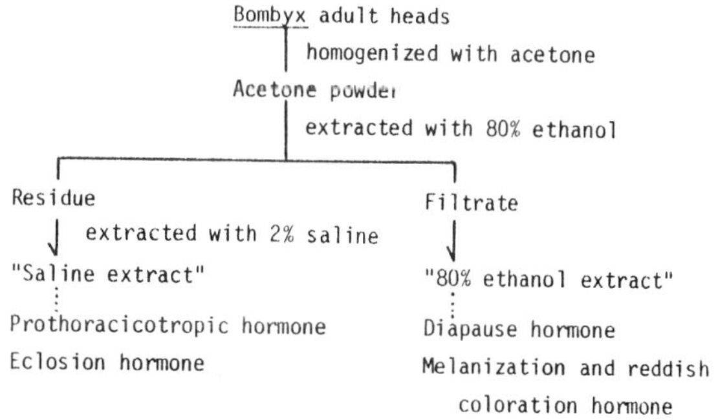

Fig. 1. Neurohormones extracted from *Bombyx* adult heads

aqueous solution was lyophilized to afford the crude extract termed '80% ethanol extract,' which was subjected to bioassay. The residual powder of 80% ethanol extraction was suspended in 2% saline and the mixture was filtered. The residue was re-extracted twice with 2% saline and the combined filtrate was heated on a boiling water bath for 5 min and, after removal of precipitates and lyophilization, the extract termed 'saline extract' was bioassayed.

The 'saline extract' derived from 0.1 heads exhibited PTTH activity (9) to a brainless *Bombyx* pupa and also to a debrained pupa of *Samia cynthia ricini*. The PTTH activity to debrained *Samia* was precipitated with 50-75% acetone, and that to brainless *Bombyx* with 25-50% acetone. The 'saline extract' corresponding to 5 heads also stimulated precocious eclosion behavior in a pharate adult of *B. mori* (6), suggesting the presence of EH. Marked activities of DH and MRCH were not observed in 'saline extract.'

When injected to a female *Bombyx* pupa, '80% ethanol extract' derived from 20 heads remarkably increase the content of 3-hydroxykynurenine in the ovary (10), indicating the presence of DH in the extract. Cuticular melanization in an isolated abdomen of *L. separata* was induced by injection with '80% ethanol extract' derived from 20 *Bombyx* heads (11). Thus DH and MRCH activities were confirmed in '80% ethanol extract,' whereas PTTH and EH activities were absent

In conclusion, the adult heads of *B. mori* were usable as starting materials for extraction of PTTH (12-14), DH (10, 15), EH and MRCH.

PROTHORACICOTROPIC HORMONE

Introduction

PTTH is possibly produced in the brain neurosecretory cells, released from corpora allata at specific times in the insect's life cycle and stimulates the prothoracic glands to produce ecdysone. In 1958 Kobayashi and Kirimura first succeeded in the preparation of extract possessing hormonal activity to brainless *Bombyx* pupae from the pupal brains of *B. mori* (2). Subsequently Ichikawa and Ishizaki found that an aqueous extract of *Bombyx* brains stimulated the adult development of debrained *Samia* pupae (3) and concluded that the active principle must be a protein (16). Since these pioneering works were published, several attempts have been made to purify PTTH, establishing the proteinaceous or peptidal nature of PTTH (17-20). For these several years, we have been carrying out the purification of PTTH extracted from the adult heads of *B. mori* and have recently succeeded in isolating PTTH which induces the adult development of a brainless *Samia* pupa at a dose of 0.1 ng (8). Some chemical and biological properties have also been clarified.

Bioassay for purification of PTTH

The bioassay was performed using debrained pupae of the Eri-silkworm *Samia cynthia ricini*, according to Ishizaki's method (9). Titers of PTTH activity were determined by *Samia* unit; one *Samia* unit was defined as the minimum amount necessary to cause adult development in more than 50% of assay pupae.

Isolation of PTTH[+]

The procedure for isolating PTTH is illustrated in Fig. 2. The 'highly purified PTTH' was routinely obtained through the 12-step procedure from the adult heads of *B. mori* and one run dealt with 192,000-264,000 heads (21-23). Several batches of the 'highly purified PTTH' were pooled and the resulting solution derived from 648,000 heads was applied on DEAE-Sepharose column. The elution was made with the linear gradient of aqueous sodium chloride from 0.1 M to 0.5 M containing 0.05 M Tris-HCl buffer (pH 7.8) and the fractions eluted with ca. 0.3 M

Bombyx adult heads
↓
Step 1. Acetone powder
↓
2. Washing with 80% ethanol
↓
3. Extraction with 2% NaCl
↓
4. Heat treatment on boiling water
↓
5. Precipitation with 80% saturation of ammonium sulfate
↓
6. Precipitation with 50-75% acetone
↓
7. Precipitation with 90% saturation of picric acid
↓
8. Precipitation with 80% acetone
("crude PTTH")
↓
9. Chromatography on Sephadex G-50 (fine)
↓
10. Chromatography on DEAE-Sepharose CL-6B
↓
11. Chromatography on SP-Sephadex C-25
↓
12. Chromatography on Sephadex G-50 (superfine)
("highly purified PTTH")
↓
13. Chromatography on DEAE-Sepharose CL-6B (gradient elution)
↓
14. Chromatography on Sephadex G-50 (superfine)
↓
15. High performance liquid chromatography
(PTTH)

Fig. 2. Purification procedure for PTTH

[+]This work was done in part with the collaboration of Prof. F. Guo and his colleagues, Institute of Zoology, Academia Sinica, Peking, China.

and ca. 0.4 M sodium chloride possessing PTTH activity. After lyophilization, a part (1296×10^3 Samia units) of the former fraction (fraction A) was chromatographed on Sephadex G-50 column using 0.2 M ammonium acetate containing 2% butanol as a solvent. The fraction with PTTH activity was lyophilized and dissolved in a small volume of 10 mM ammonium acetate. The solution was applied onto high performance liquid chromatography (HPLC): Partisil 10 ODS 3 (whatman), 4.6 x 250 mm column, linear gradient with acetonitrile from 10% to 40% in 10 mM ammonium acetate. Only the fraction eluted with ca. 25% acetonitrile revealed PTTH activity, affording pure PTTH (the purity was assessed as described in the following section). As summarized in Table 1, 50 µg of PTTH was isolatee from 648,000 heads and ca. 2×10^6-fold purification was finally attained in a recovery of ca. 8% from the saline extract.

Table. 1. Purification of PTTH from 648,000 *Bombyx* heads

	Purification step	Weight (mg)	Total activity (*Samia* unit)	Specific activity (ng/*Samia* unit)
3	Saline extract	$1,108 \times 10^3$	6480×10^3	171,000
8	Crude PTTH	19,440	6480	3,000
12	Highly purified PTTH	37.6	6480	5.8
13	DEAE-Sepharose			
	fraction A	11.5	2268	5.1
	fraction B	6.8	1620	4.2
14	Sephadex G-50	3.6	1037	3.5
15	HPLC	0.05	518	0.1

Chemical properties of the isolated PTTH

By N-terminal analysis using dansyl (DNS) method, the isolated PTTH afforded only DNS-glycine and O-DNS-tyrosine, suggesting that the isolated PTTH is a single chain peptide whose N-terminal is glycine.
To determine the amino acid composition, the isolated PTTH was hydrolyzed with constant boiling HCl (Pierce Chemical) at 110°C for 20 or 72 hr.
For determination of tryptophane, hydrolysis was done with constant boiling HCl containing thioglycolic acid at 110°C for 20 hr. Each hydrolyzate was analyzed with an amino acid analyzer and the results indicated reasonable integral amino acid ratios: Asx(4), Thr(3), Ser(1), Glx(4), Pro(1), Gly(4), Ala(3), 1/2Cys$_2$(4), Val(4-5), Leu(5-6), Tyr (1-2), Phe(2), His(1) and Arg(3). The molecular weight of the isolated PTTH was calculated as 4330-4740 daltons on the basis of amino acid composition, which coincides with that previously estimated (4400±400 daltons) by gel-filtration on Sephadex G-50 (22).
The results obtained by N-terminal determination and amino acid analyses indicated that the isolated PTTH was sufficiently pure to permit an attempt to determine its structure.

Biological properties of the isolated PTTH

The minimum amount of isolated PTTH necessary to cause adult development in a brainless *Samia* pupa was 0.1 ng (ca. 0.02 pmol).
The changes in titers of ecdysteroids in the hemolymph of debrained *Samia* pupae (male; weight, 1.7-2.0 g) after injection of the isolated PTTH (0.5 ng, 5 *Samia* units /pupa) was measured. Ecdysteroids titers were determined by radioimmunoassay (RIA) according to the method reported by Bollenbacher et al (24). In the debrained pupae injected with the isolated PTTH, no increase of ecdysteroids was observed on Day-1 (one day after injection), but during the following two days, the ecdysteroids level rose gradually. After wing apolysis occurred (Day-3 or -4), the ecdysteroids level greatly increased and reached a maximum (ca. 1.1 µg/ml hemolymph) on Day-6.
In the normal intact pupae also, ecdysteroids titers greatly increased after wing apolysis and reached a maximum (ca. 2.4 µg/ml hemolymph) 2-3 days after the apolysis, although the initial titers of ecdysteroids in the normal intact pupae (ca. 0.047 µg/ml hemolymph) was much higher than that in the brainless pupae (ca. 0.01 µg/ml hemolymph).

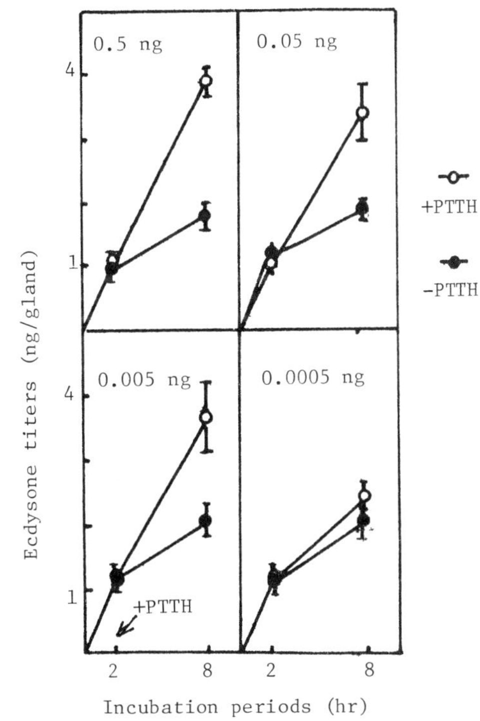

Fig. 3. Ecdysone titers released from the prothoracic gland of *Samia* pupa cultured *in vitro* with PTTH

Almost all the debrained pupae injected with 0.5 ng PTTH eclosed on Day-17~22, and the normal intact pupae eclosed 14-15 days after pupation. These results suggest that the isolated

PTTH injected into the brainless Samia pupae could cause the pupal-adult development through increasing ecdysone titers in the hemolymph.
In order to know whether the isolated PTTH directly stimulates the prothoracic gland (PG) of Samia to release ecdysone or not, PGs of the pupae just after pupation were cultured with the isolated PTTH. PGs were dissected from male Samia pupae within 8 hr after pupation, when PGs had not yet been exposed to endogenous PTTH. A pair of PGs from one pupa was individually preincubated in 100 µl of Grace's medium for 2 hr at 25°C. Then they were transferred to 100 µl of fresh Grace's medium with or without PTTH, respectively, and incubated for another 6 hr. Aliquots were taken from the cultured medium at 2 hr and 8 hr after incubation, and subjected to RIA for ecdysone. As shown in Fig. 3, the results clearly indicated that more than 10^{-11}M of the isolated PTTH stimulated PG to release ecdysone in vitro.

ECLOSION HORMONE

Introduction

Since very early ages, the adult eclosion of certain insects has been well known to occur only at a specific times of the day.
Truman and Riddiford demonstrated by interchanging the brains between Hyalophora cecropia and Anthraea pernyi that the biological clock of the eclosion behavior exists in the brain and successfully showed that a series of the adult eclosion behavior can be induced by a neurotropic hormone termed eclosion hormone (EH) in the brain homogenates (25). Their subsequent studies clarified that EH in Manduca sexta is an acidic peptide with molecular weight of 8500 daltons (26) and is involved throughout the process of ecdysis (27).
Morohoshi and Fugo succeeded in preparing extract possessing EH activty from the male adult heads and pupal heads of B. mori (6). Following their work, we have attempted to purify EH from Bombyx adult heads.

Bioassay for purification of EH

The pupae of B. mori used for bioassay were hybrids of J. 106 x Daizo. Pupal periods for adult eclosion were 10±1 days under the photoperiod of 16-hr light (16L-8D) at 25°C. Under these conditions the moths emerge within only 2 hr after light-on. Samples at each purification step were lyophilized, dissolved in 0.01 M Tris-HCl (pH 7.8) and injected into the pharate adults at the beginning of the last period before emergence. After injection the pupae were maintained under continuous light to observe the result of bioassay.
When the sample possessed EH activity, adult eclosion occurred 1-3 hr after injection and the control pupae emerged 6-9 hr after injection. One EH unit was designated as the minimum amount to induce eclosion in more than 50% of the assayed pupae.

Purification of EH

In the purification of EH, EH activity was not separated from PTTH activity in steps 1 through 9 in the purification procedure of PTTH (Fig. 2). At step 10, EH activity was not adsorbed to DEAE-Sepharose column with 0.2 M ammonium acetate, whereas PTTH activity was completely retained on the column. The fraction possessing EH activity (derived from 264,000 heads) was adjusted to pH 4.2, applied onto SP-Sephadex column and eluted with 0.1 M ammonium acetate buffer (pH 4.2, 4.7, 7.0 and 9.0). The active fraction recovered with the buffer of pH 7.0 was diluted twice (0.05 M) and applied to QAE-Sephadex column. Solid ammonium acetate was added to the break through solution containing EH to give 2 M solution, which was then applied to Octyl-Sepharose column.
The EH activity was eluted with both 0.5 M and 0.1 M ammonium acetate. After lyophilization, the active fraction dissolved in a small volume of 0.01 M Tris-HCl buffer (pH 7.8) was applied onto Sephadex G-50 column using 0.2 M ammonium acetate containing 2% butanol as a solvent and the active fraction showed EH activity at a dose of 1.8 µg/pupa. The results of purification are summarized in Table 2.

Table 2. Purification of EH from 264,000 Bombyx heads

	Purification step	Weight (mg)	Total activity (EH units)	Specific activity (µg/EH unit)
3	Saline extract	45,200	53,000	8,560
10	DEAE-Sepharose	3,850	19,250	200
11	SP-Sephadex	2,800	14,740	190
12	QAE-Sephadex	1,375	8,590	160
13	Octyl-Sepharose	104	8,670	12
14	Sephadex G-50	21	11,700	1.8

The pharate adult head possesses 5-10 times as much activity as the adult head used in this experiment. Purification of EH from the pharate adult heads has also been performed by the same method. Since chromatographic behavior of EH from pharate adult heads was very similar to that of EH from adult heads, both EHs seem to be the same molecule.

Chemical properties of EH

The molecular weight of EH was estimated to be ca. 7000 daltons by gel-filtration on Sephadex G-50. Pronase, trypsin and α-chymotrypsin inactivated EH, whereas glycosidases did not, suggesting that EH is peptidal. These properties of Bombyx EH are quite similar to those of Manduca EH (26).

MELANIZATION AND REDDISH COLORATION HORMONE

Introduction

B. mori hibernates at the embryonic stage and the entrance into diapause of the embryo is determined beforehand by the secretion of DH from the suboesophageal ganglion (SG) at the pupal stage of the mother moth (4,5). DH is extractable with 80% ethanol from pupal SG and adult brain-SG complex. From the adult heads of B. mori, DH was quantitatively recovered in '80% ethanol extract.' The purification of DH has been extensively done by two independent Japanese groups (10,24).

Interestingly, it was found that '80% ethanol extract' also possesses MRCH activity, which is responsible for cuticular melanization in the armyworm larvae, L. separata (11). Some armyworm larvae are known to show polymorphism depending on their population density, i.e. so-called phase variation, and the larval color change is the most conspicuous aspects of phase variation (28). In the larva of L. separata, crowded conditions more or less induce cuticular melanization , which is controlled by MRCH (29). In B. mori, however, larval coloration has been suggested to be associated mainly with juvenile hormone (30). Concerning the role of MRCH in B. mori, Ogura proposed that DH and MRCH may be the same hormone, based on transplantation experiments of cephalic organs of B. mori and L. separata (7,31).

Bioassay for purification of MRCH

The bioassay of MRCH was performed using the penultimate instar larvae of L. separata according to the method already reported (32). One unit of MRCH is defined to be the minimal dose of MRCH required to induce marked melanization in 50% of test insects.

Bombyx adult heads
↓
Step 1. Acetone powder
↓
2. Extraction with 80% ethanol
↓
3. Heat treatment
↓
4. Removal of 50% acetone precipitate (Crude extract)
↓
5. Chromatography on SP-Sephadex C-25
↓
6. Chromatography on QAE-Sephadex A-25 (stepwise)
↓
7. Chromatography on QAE-Sephadex A-25 (gradient)
↓
8. Chromatography on Sephadex G-50
↓
9. Chromatography on DEAE-Sepharose CL-6B
↓
10. High performance liquid chromatography (HPLC), Reverse phase (1st)
↓
11. HPLC, Reverse phase (2nd)
↓
12. HPLC, Reverse phase (3rd)

Fig. 4. Purification procedure for MRCH

Purification of MRCH

The purification procedure starting from 450,000 Bombyx adult heads is shown in Fig 4 and the results are summarized in Table 3. Up to step 5, the purification process was as previously reported (32). In step 7, gradient elution of aqueous sodium chloride in 0.02 M Tris-HCl (pH 8.1) on QAE-Sephadex column resulted in the separation of MRCH activity into two fractions and the active fraction eluted with ca. 0.25 M sodium chloride was used in the following step. In step 8 and 10, gel-filtration on Sephadex G-50 column was done with 0.05 M ammonium acetate and 0.05 M sodium chloride, respectively. In reverse phase HPLC (Develosil ODS-3) with linear gradient elution using acetonitrile and 10 mM ammonium acetate as solvent systems, MRCH activity was found in three separate fractions, indicating heterogeneity of MRCH. Two components of MRCH were nearly purified and the specific activities were 13 and 20 ng/unit, respectively.

Table 3. Purification of MRCH from 450,000 Bombyx heads

	Purification step	Weight (mg)	Total activity (units)	Specific activity (μg/unit)
2	80% Ethanol extract	99,000	22,500	4,400
5	SP-Sephadex	36,000	22,500	1,600
7	QAE-Sephadex*	84	5,625	15
10	Sephadex G-50	6.1	2,250	2.7
11	1st HPLC fraction A	0.053	560	0.098
	B	0.047	560	0.086
	C	0.051	280	0.18
13	3rd HPLC fraction A	0.0036	280	0.013
	C	0.0028	140	0.020

* In this step, MRCH was separated into two fractions. Purification was conducted by using the fraction with more MRCH units.

Chemical properties of MRCH

The distribution coefficient (ca. 0.43) on Sephadex G-50 indicated that the molecular weights of MRCH were ca. 6400-8000 daltons. Inactiviation experiments have been reported previously (11,32); MRCH is a peptide, whose N- and C-terminals may be blocked.

Biological properties of MRCH

MRCH seems to control all the larval color changes in the armyworm species, because the partially purified MRCH caused blackening of the cuticle of L. separata, L. loreyi, Spodoptera litura and Mamestra brassicae (32) and also of S. exempta (S. Yagi, personal communication). Furthermore, MRCH induced reddish pigmentation in the epidermis with cuticular melanization in the isolated abdomen of yellow solitary larva of L. separata.

Recently we confirmed that DH and MRCH are different hormones (32). MRCH also differs from the tanning hormone, bursicon, because the partially purified MRCH had no effect on the cuticular tanning in the wing of adult *M. sexta* at the time of eclosion (L. M. Riddiford, personal communication).

Acknowledgment-These works were suported in part by Grants-in-Aid for Scientific Research from the Ministry of Education, Science and Culture of Japan.

REFERENCES

1. M. Kobayashi,'The Silkworm, an important laboratory tool,' ed. by Y. Tazima, Kodansha, Tokyo, 1978, pp159.
2. M. Kobayashi and J. Kirimura, *Nature*, 181, 1217 (1958).
3. M. Ichikawa and H. Ishizaki, *ibid.*, 191, 933 (1961).
4. K. Hasegawa, Proc. *Japan Acad.*, 27, 667 (1951).
5. S. Fukuda, Proc. *ibid.*, 27, 672 (1951).
6. S. Morohoshi and H. Fugo, *ibid.*, 53, 75 (1977).
7. N. Ogura, *Appl. Ent. Zool.*, 10, 216 (1975).
8. A. Suzuki, H. Nagasawa, H. Kataoka, Y. Hori, A. Isogai, S. Tamura, F. Guo, X.-C. Zhong, H. Ishizaki, M. Fujishita and A. Mizobuchi, *Agric. Biol. Chem.*, 46, 1107 (1982).
9. H. Ishizaki and A. Suzuki,'Neurohormonal Techniques in Insects,' ed. by T. A. Miller, Springer-Verlag, New York, 1980, pp244.
10. H. Sonobe and E. Ohnishi, *Science*, 174, 835 (1971).
11. A. Suzuki, S. Matsumoto, N. Ogura, A. Isogai and S. Tamura, *Agric. Biol. Chem.*, 40, 2307, (1976).
12. M. Kobayashi and M. Yamazaki, *Appl. Ent. Zool.*, 13, 129 (1978).
13. H. Ishizaki, *Develop. Growth Different.*, 11, 1 (1969).
14. J. Nishiitsutsuji-Uwo and M. S. Nishimura, *Experientia*, 31, 1105 (1975).
15. M. Isobe and T. Goto,'Neurohormonal Techniques in Insects,' ed. by T. A. Miller, Springer-Verlag, New York, 1980, pp216.
16. M. Ichikawa and H. Ishizaki, *Nature*, 198, 308 (1963).
17. H. Ishizaki and M. Ichikawa, *Biol. Bull.*, 133, 355 (1967).
18. M. Yamazaki and M. Kobayashi, *J. Insect Physiol.*, 15, 1981 (1969).
19. J. Nishiitsutsuji-Uwo, *Botyu-Kagaku*, 37, 93 (1972).
20. H. Ishizaki, A. Suzuki, A. Isogai, H. Nagasawa and S. Tamura, *J. Insect Physiol.*, 23, 1219 (1977).
21. A. Suzuki, A. Isogai, T. Horii, H. Ishizaki and S. Tamura, *Agric. Biol. Chem.*, 39, 2157 (1975).
22. H. Nagasawa, A. Isogai, A. Suzuki, S. Tamura and H. Ishizaki, *Develop. Growth Different.*, 21, 29 (1979).
23. H. Nagasawa, F. Guo, X.-C. Zhong, B.-Y. Xia, Z.-S. Wang, X.-J. Qui, D.-Y. Wei, E.-Y. Chen, J.-Z. Wang, A. Suzuki, A. Isogai, Y. Hori, S. Tamura and H. Ishizaki, *Scientia Sinica*, 23, 1053 (1980).
24. W. E. Bollenbacher, N. Agui, N. A. Granger and L. I. Gilbert, *Proc. Natl. Acad. Sci.* USA, 76, 5148 (1979).
25. J. W. Truman and L. M. Riddiford, *Science*, 167, 1624 (1970).
26. S. E. Reynolds and J. W. Truman,'Neurohormonal Techniques in Insects,' ed. by T. A. Miller, Springer-Verlag, New York, 1980, pp137.
27. J. W. Truman, P. H. Taghert, P. F. Copenhaver, N. J. Tulbitz and L. M. Schwartz, *Nature*, 291, 70 (1981).
28. S. Iwao, *Colloques. int. Cent. natn. Rech. scient.*, 173, 185 (1968).
29. N. Ogura, *J. Insect Physiol.*, 21, 559 (1975).
30. K. Kiguchi, *J. Seri. Sci.* Tokyo, 42, 293 (1973).
31. N. Ogura and T. Saito, *Appl. Ent. Zool.*, 8, 46 (1973).
32. S. Matsumoto, A. Isogai, A. Suzuki, N. Ogura and H. Sonobe, *Insect Biochem.*, 11, 185 (1981).

SIMULTANEOUS DISRUPTION OF PHEROMONAL COMMUNICATION OF THE TWO TORTRICID MOTHS IN THE TEA PLANTATION

Y. Tamaki*, H. Noguchi*, H. Sugie*, M. Ohtaishi**, T. Horikawa*** and M. Ohba***

*National Institute of Agricultural Sciences, Tsukuba, Ibaraki 305, Japan
**National Research Institute of Tea, Kanaya, Shizuoka 428, Japan
***Shizuoka Tea Experiment Station, Kikugawa, Shizuoka 439, Japan

Abstract - The tea tortrix moth, Homona magnanima, and the smaller tea tortrix moth, Adoxophyes sp., the key pests of the tea plant, occur together 4 to 5 times a year. Female sex pheromones of these species are a four-component system for Adoxophyes (Z9-14Ac, Z11-14Ac, E11-14Ac, 10Me-12Ac) and a three-component system for Homona (Z11-14Ac, Z9-12Ac, 11-12Ac). Field screening of the 6 pheromonal components and their geometrical isomers under in-trap and out-of-trap conditions indicated several potential disruptants for the two species. Mating inhibition tests in small field cages were also conducted to confirm the disruption effect. Of these compounds, Z11-14Ac, the common pheromonal component of the two species, was selected as the most effective common disruptant. A trial on the simultaneous disruption of pheromonal communication of the two species by Z11-14Ac brought about an effective disruption of orientation, apparent suppression of mating of feral females, and appreciable reduction in larval densities in the field. Systematic screenings based on inhibitory effects in trapping by in-trap and out-of-trap evaporation of potential disruptants and those based on mating suppression in small field cages will increase the efficiency in evaluating candidate disruptants for these and other insect species.

INTRODUCTION

The tea tortrix, Homona magnanima, and the smaller tea tortrix, Adoxophyes sp., are key pests of the tea plant. Both species occur 4 to 5 times a year and their occurrence frequently overlaps (1). Although highly toxic organophosphorus insecticides have been routinely used for the control of these tortricid species, control efficacy by these insecticides is not necessarily efficient and this has caused outbreaks of other pests by destruction of natural enemies in the tea plantation (2). Development of an alternative control method is, therefore, highly desirable from the viewpoint of integrated pest management in the tea plantation. The sex pheromone of Homona has been identified as a three-component mixure comprised of (Z)-11-tetradecenyl acetate (Z11-14Ac), (Z)-9-dodecenyl acetate (Z9-12Ac) and 11-dodecenyl acetate (11-12Ac) at a ratio of 30/3/1 (3). The pheromone of Adoxophyes sp. is a four-component system comprising Z9-14Ac, Z11-14Ac, E11-14Ac and 10-methyldodecyl acetate (10Me-12Ac) at a ratio of 63/31/4/2 (4,5). This paper deals with experiments to develop a common disruptant of pheromonal communication in the two tortricid species.

MATERIALS AND METHODS

The pheromonal chemicals were systhesized by NIAS or provided by Takeda Chemical Ind., Otsuka Pharmaceutical Co., and Shin-etsu Chemical Co. Dispensers for the trapping experiments were a plastic capsule (8 x 17.8 mm) for electron-microscopic use (YK-1, Yasumoto Kasei) or a rubber septum (9 x 15 mm) (septum b, Takeda Chemical Ind.). Pheromonal chemicals were dissolved in hexane and loaded on the dispensers. Chemicals were also loaded on sheet-type dispensers of various size by Nitto Electric Ind. for the field-cage disruption experiments. For field experiments on communication disruption, plastic tubes (0.8 mm ID x 200 mm) filled with pheromonal chemicals were prepared by Sin-etsu Chemical Co.; the chemicals evaporate through the wall of the tube.

Traps were of the sticky type (Takeda Chemical Co.). The size of the sticky board is 25 x 30 cm. Traps were placed on the upper surface of tea plants and locations in the field were systematically changed each day. Dispensers of test chemicals were placed at various distance from the trap to evaluate the influence of test chemicals on the attractancy of the pheromone source in the trap. In "in-trap" treatments, one dispenser of test chemicals were placed in the trap with the pheromone source. In "out-of-trap" treatments, the dispenser of test chemical was placed at 0.3, 1.0, or 5.0 m one direction from the trap or at 0.3 m four directions from the trap.

Small screen cages (1 x 1 x 1 m) placed on a lawn ground were used to evaluate the efficiency of mating suppression of each chemical. A laboratory-reared virgin female was tethered with a fine thread on a rod about 30 cm above the ground. Twenty 2- to 3-day-old males were released for 10 tethered females of the same age in each screen cage. The test chemical was evaporated from a sheet-type dispenser attached on each of the four screen walls. Mating of tethered females was assessed on the basis of spermatophores found in the females.

A field trial on communication disruption was conducted in a farmer's tea field (2,250 m^2) at Haibara, Shizuoka Prefecture in the first flight season of the tortricid moths. Tube-type dispensers were attached just below the plucking surface of the tea plant at the rate of 4,000 tubes per ha before the initiation of moth flight. Results of the disruption trial were evaluated by comparing trap catches in monitoring traps, percentages of mating of feral females collected in the fields, and larval densities between the treated field and the control field.

RESULTS

Pheromonal interaction between Homona and Adoxophyes

Because of simultaneous occurrence of *Homona* and *Adoxophyes* in the tea field, pheromonal interaction between the two species is possible. Trapping of male moths is apparently influenced by the pheromone of the other species evaporated in the vicinity of the trap (Table 1). Male catches of *Homona* by the *Homona* pheromone were decreased by the *Adoxophyes* pheromone evaporated at 0 and 0.3 m from the trap. However, male catches of *Adoxophyes* by the *Adoxophyes* pheromone, while decreased by the *Homona* pheromone evaporated at 0.3 m to 1.0 m from the trap, were unaltered by the in-trap evaporation of the *Homona* pheromone. These results suggest at least two points of interest. Firstly, a common lure for the two tortricid moths will be impossible, because *Homona* trapping is adversly affected by the *Adoxophyes* pheromone, even though *Adoxophyes* trapping is not affected by the *Homona* pheromone in the same trap, and secondly, the pheromonal communication in one species will be adversely affected by the pheromone of the other species released near (0.3 m to 1 m) the female.

TABLE 1. Effect on male trapping by pheromone of another species placed at different distances from the trap

distance from trap	No. male/trap/night	
	Adoxophyes	*Homona*
0 m	8.7^{ab}	2.3^{b}
0.3	3.5^{c}	2.9^{b}
1.0	7.0^{b}	7.3^{a}
5.0	10.2^{a}	6.4^{a}

Adoxophyes pheromone: Z9-14Ac/Z11-14Ac/E11-14Ac/10Me-12Ac = 0.63/0.32/0.04/2.0 mg in plastic capsule. *Homona* pheromone: Z11-14Ac/Z9-12Ac/11-12Ac = 1.5/0.15/0.05 mg in rubber septum. Values with the same letter are not significantly different from each other at 5% level in each column of this Table.

TABLE 2. Effect on *Adoxophyes* tapping by pheromonal components of *Homona* evaporated by in-trap and out-of-trap conditions

Pheromone components	No. male *Adoxophyes*/trap/night	
	in-trap	out-of-trap
None	13.1^{a}	35.1^{a}
Z11-14Ac	8.8^{a}	5.2^{b}
Z9-12Ac	2.2^{b}	6.3^{b}
11-12Ac	11.3^{a}	28.7^{a}

Composition of the lure for *Adoxophyes* is the same in Table 1. Loaded amount of pheromone component is 1 mg for Z9- and 11-12Ac and 2 mg for Z11-14Ac per rubber septum. Out-of-trap: 0.3 m four directions. The values with the same letter are not significantly different from each other at 5% level in each column of this Table.

Examination of individual components of the *Homona* pheromone in in-trap conditions revealed that only Z9-12Ac caused a reduction of trap catch for *Adoxophyes*. In out-of-trap conditions (0.3 m from the trap), both Z11-14Ac and Z9-12Ac have inhibitory effects on trap catches of Adoxophyes. These facts indicate that the active ingredient in the Homona pheromone, responsible for the adverse effect on Adoxophyes trapping at 0.3 m, is Z11-14Ac, the major component of the Homona pheromone (Table 2). In a similar examination of pheromonal components of Adoxophyes, no particular component was found showing apparent inhibitory effects for Homona trapping under in-trap conditions (Table 3). This suggests that the inhibitory effect of the Adoxophyes pheromone for Homona trapping under in-trap conditions would be a combined effect of the multiple components. The factor responsible for the adverse effect of the Adoxophyes pheromone at a 0.3 m distance from the trap for Homona was found to be Z9-14Ac and Z11-14Ac (Table 3). Z11-14Ac showed a greater effect than Z9-14Ac under these conditions.

TABLE 3. Effect on Homona trapping by pheromonal components of Adoxophyes evaporated by in-trap and out-of-trap conditions

Pheromone components	No. male Homona/trap/night	
	in-trap	out-of-trap
None	8.8[a]	2.0[a]
Z9-14Ac	5.7[a]	0.8[b]
Z11-14Ac	7.6[a]	0.5[b]
E11-14Ac	6.7[a]	1.9[a]
10Me-12Ac	13.0[a]	1.3[a]

Composition of the lure for Homona is the same in Table 1. Loaded amount of pheromone component is 1 mg per rubber septum. Out-of-trap: 0.3 m four directions. The values with the same letter are not significantly different from each other at 5% level in each column of this Table.

These facts suggest the existence of pheromonal interaction between Adoxophyes and Homona. Particular pheromonal components of the two species seemed to be responsible for the interaction, an inhibitory effect on the attraction of males of the other species. Therefore, more detailed examinations of pheromone components of the two species and related compounds seemed to be valuable for development of a disruptant of pheromonal communication commonly effective for the both species.

In-trap and out-of-trap screening of pheromonal compounds

Effects of pheromonal components and several related chemicals on male catches of the both species were compared under in-trap (0 m) and out-of-trap (0.3 m) conditions. Results on Adoxophyes trapping are summarized in Fig. 1. All the chemicals except for 11-12Ac showed

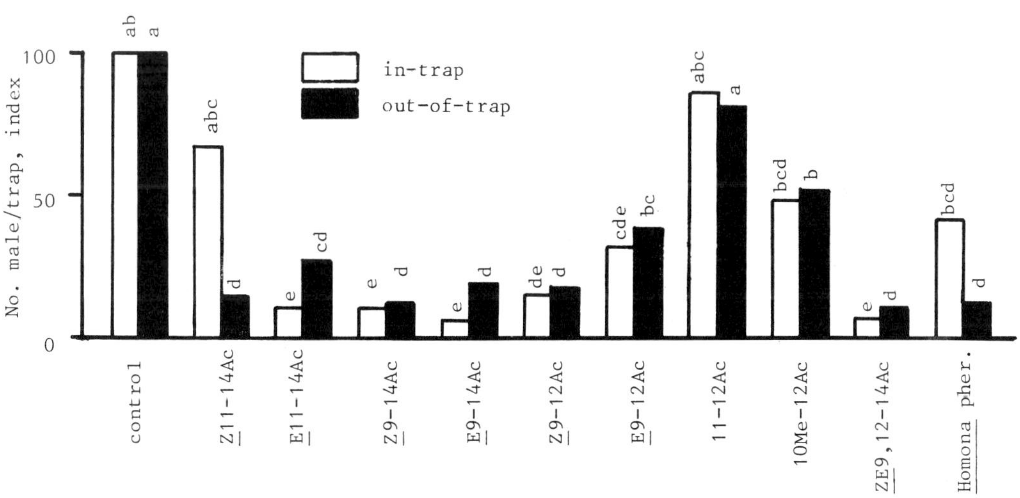

Fig. 1. The influence on Adoxophyes trapping of pheromonal components and related compounds under the conditions of in-trap and out-of-trap evaporation. The composition of Adoxophyes pheromone is the same in Table 1. Columns with the same letter are not significantly different from each other at 5% level in each evaporation condition.

an influence on male catches. Of these, Z11-14Ac is unique. Although no influence was evident in in-trap evaporation of this compound, it caused a remarkable decrease of male catch in out-of-trap evaporation. The inhibitory effects of E11-14Ac and E9-14Ac were greater by in-trap evaporation than by out-of-trap evaporation. Other compounds showed no difference between the two evaporation conditions.

The influence of these compounds on Homona trapping were also examined under the conditions of out-of-trap evaporation. The results indicated that Z11-14Ac, Z9-14Ac, and Z9-12Ac as well as the Adoxophyes pheromone, apparently inhibited the male catches of Homona (Fig. 2). From these results a possible disruptant of pheromonal communication which will be commonly effective to both Adoxophyes and Homona, was considered to be Z11-14Ac, Z9-14Ac, Z9-12Ac, or combinations of these compounds.

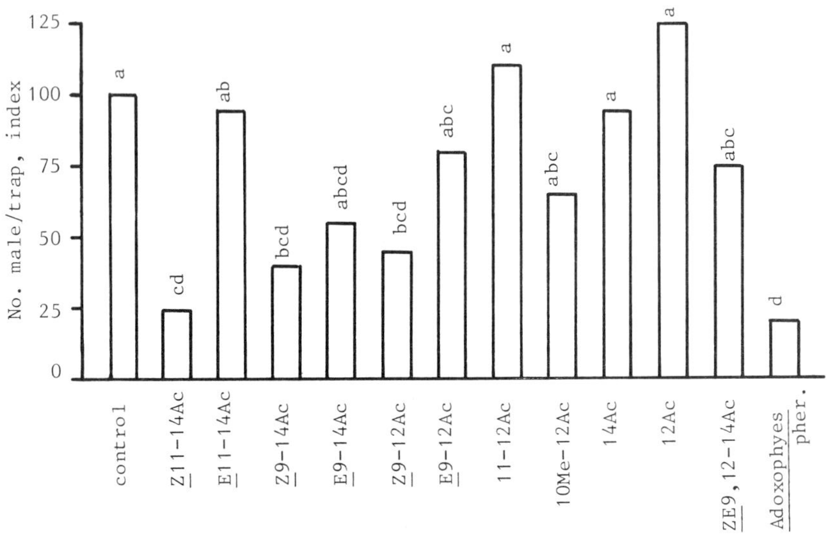

Fig. 2. Influence on Homona trapping of pheromone components and related compounds under the conditions of out-of-trap evaporation. Composition of Homona pheromone is the same in Table 1. The columns with the same letter are not significantly different from each other at 5% level.

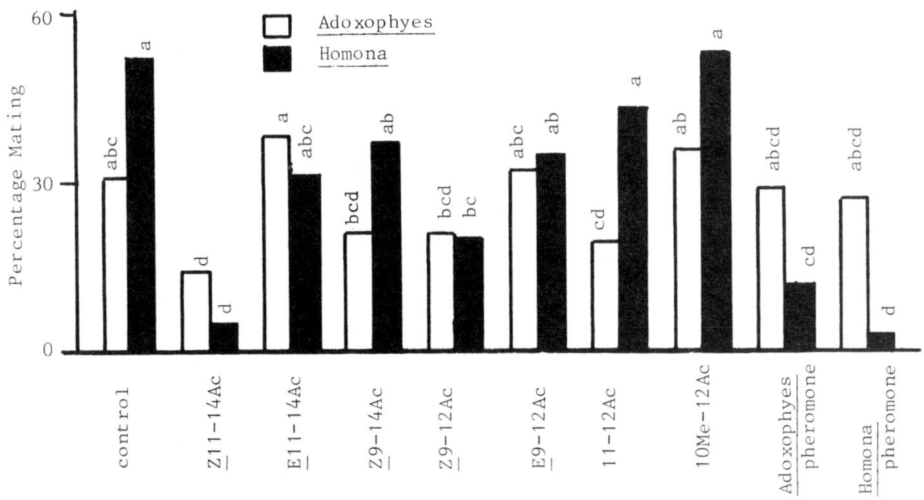

Fig. 3. Mating suppression of Adoxophyes and Homona by pheromonal components. All the compounds were evaporated from the sheet-type dispensers; the evaporation rate is 1 mg/day/dispenser. Adoxophyes pheromone: Z9-14Ac/Z11-14Ac/E11-14Ac/10Me-12Ac = 70/30/5/20. Homona pheromone: Z11-14Ac/Z9-12Ac/11-12Ac = 60/3/1.

Inhibition of mating of Adoxophyes and Homona by pheromonal components

Relative effectiveness of pheromonal components as mating inhibitors was evaluated in 1 x 1 m screen cage placed on a lawn ground. Results for the two tortricid species are shown in Fig. 3. Z11-14Ac showed apparent effectiveness on the mating suppression of both Adoxophyes and Homona. The sex pheromones of both Adoxophyes and Homona were also effective for the mating suppression of Homona, but these pheromones are not effective for Adoxophyes sp. under these conditions. Results on Homona were comparable with the data from trapping experiment under out-of-trap evaporation presented in Fig. 2. These results suggest that Z11-14Ac could be used as a common disruptant for the two tortricid species, though the disruption effect of Z11-14Ac may be smaller for Adoxophyes than for Homona.

Control trial of Adoxophyes and Homona by simultaneous disruption of the pheromonal communication

Simultaneous disruption of pheromonal communication of Adoxophyes and Homona by Z11-14Ac was compared under field conditions with the normal disruption by their respective pheromones (Table 4). Evaporation rates were 125 mg to 140 mg/hr/ha. Percentage disorientation evaluated by monitoring traps was very high for treatment with Z11-14Ac and the respective pheromones. Percentages of mating were surveyed on wild females collected from each field. The effect of mating suppression was low in Adoxophyes; 70.5% and 92.2% of females were mated in the fields treated by pheromone and Z11-14Ac, respectively. In Homona the corresponding values showed 31.7% and 48.8% for pheromone and Z11-14Ac, indicating the disruption to be much more effective than in the case of Adoxophyes. Larval densities apparently decreased with the disruption treatments by the respective pheromones or by a common disruptant, Z11-14Ac. A higher effect was noticed on Homona than on Adoxophyes. Although the effectiveness of the common disruptant, Z11-14Ac, was smaller than respective pheromones, the difference seemed minimal.

TABLE 4. A trial of simultaneous disruption of Adoxophyes and Homona in a tea field at Haibara-cho, Shizuoka Prefecture. First flight season of 1981, 2,250 m^2 field.

Compound used for treatment	No. males caught by monitoring trap	Percentage disorientation	Percentage mating of wild female	Index of larval density after treatment
		Adoxophyes		
pheromone	36.5	98.8	70.5	29
Z11-14Ac alone	16.0	99.5	92.2	39
control	3,024.5	-	100.0	100
		Homona		
pheromone	8.0	99.4	31.7	1
Z11-14Ac alone	3.0	99.8	48.8	13
control	1,303.0	-	98.0	100

Composition of pheromone for Adoxophyes is Z9-14Ac/Z11-14Ac/E11-14Ac/10Me-12Ac of 51/27/4/16 ratio and that for Homona is Z11-14Ac/Z9-12Ac/11-12Ac of 84/8/2 ratio. Evaporation rates of Z11-14Ac, Adoxophyes pheromone and Homona pheromone are 125, 140 and 128 mg/hr/ha, respectively.
Index (I) was calculated on larval densities of control (C) and treatment (T) before (C_b,T_b) and after (C_a,T_a) the treatment by the equation, $I = 100T_aC_b/T_bC_a$.

DISCUSSION

Z11-14Ac, a common disruptant develped here, is the common pheromonal component of both Adoxophyes and Homona. This compound is unique in its activity, because the inhibitory effect is particularly large when it was evaporated around the trap. In the case of Adoxophyes trapping, evaporation of Z11-14Ac at a distance of 0.3 to 1.0 m from the trap remarkably suppressed the attractancy of pheromone trap, but no adverse effect occurred when it was evaporated from the inside of trap. Although the mechanism is not known, this particular activity of Z11-14Ac is a useful characteristics as a disruptant of pheromonal communication.

It has been often indicated that a potent inhibitor of male attraction under the conditions of in-trap evaporation is not necessarily a good disruptant when it was evaporated around the trap (6-14). Z11-14Ac for Adoxophyes and Homona is an example of a reversed case; it is a weak inhibitor by in-trap evaporation but a strong disruptant by out-of-trap conditions.

The first step in developing a communication disruption method for a particular pest insect or a complex of insects is the selection of an effective disruptant. In general, the respective pheromone blend for each species is used as a disruptant (15). This is based on the suggestion of maximal disruption effect by the natural blend of the pheromonal component (16). However, multiple application of respective pheromonal blends for each pest species of a particular crop is impractical. A common disruptant for multiple pests on the crop is highly desirable, and this was indicated to be possible in the case of Adoxophyes and Homona. Although the effectiveness of Z11-14Ac seemed to be smaller than those of the respective pheromones, further improvement will be possible. The techniques such as in-trap and out-of-trap evaporation, small screen cage test for mating inhibition, and small plot field trials for feral insects will be efficient for the selection of the effective disruptant for the pest complex on a particular crop.

Acknowledgements - We are indebted to Takeda Chemical Ind., Otsuka Pharmaceutical Co., Shin-etsu Chemical Co., and Nitto Electric Ind. for their supply of synthetic pheromonal chemicals and formulations, and to Drs. N. Takahashi and W.S. Bowers for their reading the draft.

REFERENCES

1. J. Minamikawa and M. Osakabe, Insect Pests of Tea Plant, Japan Plant Protection Assoc., Tokyo, pp. 322 (1979).
2. M. Ohtaishi and T. Horikawa, Proc. 1st Japan/USA Symp. on IPM, Research Council, MAFF, Japan, p. 41-49 (1981).
3. H. Noguchi, Y. Tamaki and T. Yushima, Appl. Ent. Zool. 14, 225 (1979).
4. Y. Tamaki, H. Noguchi, T. Yushima and C. Hirano, Appl. Ent. Zool. 6, 139 (1971).
5. Y. Tamaki, H. Noguchi, H. Sugie, R. Sato and A. Kariya, Appl. Ent. Zool. 14, 101 (1979).
6. J.R. McLaughlin, E.R. Mitchell, D.L. Chambers and J.H. Tumlinson, Environ. Ent. 3, 677 (1974).
7. R.J. Marks, Bull. Ent. Res. 66, 243 (1976).
8. E.R. Mitchell, W.W. Copeland, A.N. Sparks and A.A. Sekul, Environ. Ent. 3, 778 (1974).
9. E.R. Mitchell, Environ. Ent. 5, 770 (1976).
10. J.R. McLaughlin, L.K. Gaston, H.H. Shorey, H.E. Hummel and F.D. Stewart, J. Econ. Ent. 65, 1592 (1972).
11. G.E. Daterman, G.D. Davis, Jr. and R.G. Smith, Environ. Ent. 4, 944 (1975).
12. R.S. Kaae, H.H. Shorey, L.K. Gaston and H.H. Hummel. Environ. Ent. 3, 87 (1974).
13. R.T. Cardé, C.C. Doane, J. Granett and W.L. Roelofs, Environ. Ent. 4, 793 (1975).
14. G.H.L. Rothschild, Ent. Exp. Appl. 17, 294 (1974).
15. W.L. Roelofs, Establishing Efficasy of Sex Attractants and Disruptants for Insect Control, Ent. Soc. Amer. pp. 97 (1979).
16. W.L. Roelofs, Proc. Symp. Insect Pheromones and Their Application, Japan Plant Protection Assoc., Tokyo, p. 123-134 (1976).

SEX PHEROMONE OF THE CARIBBEAN FRUIT FLY: CHEMISTRY AND FIELD ECOLOGY

James L. Nation

Department of Entomology and Nematology, University of Florida, Gainesville, Florida 32611, USA

Abstract - Male Caribbean fruit flies, *Anastrepha suspensa* (Loew) produce and release 4 chemical compounds as a sex pheromone to attract sexually mature females. Active extracts prepared from the entire body of 9-day-old male flies were purified by column chromatography, and 2 alcohols and 2 lactones were isolated. The 2 alcohols have been identified as Z-3-nonen-1-ol and Z,Z-3,6-nonadien-1-ol, and these were synthesized and shown to have behavioral activity when bioassayed in the laboratory with 10-day-old female flies. Extracts of male *A. suspensa* attracted female *A. ludens*, the Mexican fruit fly, and extracts of male *A. ludens* attracted female *A. suspensa*. Analyses of *A. ludens* showed the presence of the same 4 compounds found in *A. suspensa* pheromone extracts, but in different relative proportions. It seems probable that the two species utilize the same 4 compounds as a sex pheromone.

INTRODUCTION

Male Caribbean fruit flies, *Anastrepha suspensa* (Loew), produce and release 4 chemical compounds as a sex attractant for females (1, 2). The male pheromone also acts as an aggregation pheromone for both sexes in the field (3). In an earlier report, 2 of the compounds were shown to be 9 carbon alcohols from NMR, IR, mass spectral, and GLC data. Alcohol I had 1 double bond (MW 142) and alcohol II had 2 double bonds (MW 140) (2).

Identification of these 2 alcohols as Z-3-nonen-1-ol and Z,Z-3,6-nonadien-1-ol, respectively, and their synthesis and bioassay are reported in this paper.

MATERIALS AND METHODS

Laboratory reared flies for pheromone extraction and for bioassay were supplied by Dr. R.M. Baranowski, University of Florida, AREC, Homestead, FL. The laboratory bioassay routinely used was the same as that published earlier (2). A field bioassay has also been published (3, 4).

All analytical gas-liquid chromatography (GLC) was performed on a Packard 7831 gas chromatograph equipped with hydrogen flame ionization detectors. Silicic acid and silicic acid with 20% silver nitrate for column chromatography were obtained from Applied Sciences Laboratory, State College, PA.

RESULTS

Positions of Double Bonds in the 2 Alcohols

Alcohol I. Microozonolysis (5) and GLC analysis of products were used to locate the positions of double bonds. About 10 μg of Alcohol I was subjected to ozonolysis in cold pentyl acetate, and the ozonide was reduced with 1 mg triphenyl-phosphine. After warming to room temperature, GLC showed hexanal (4.30 min, 12% DEGS, 80°C, N_2 flow 56 ml/min and 4.53 min., 3% OV-1, room temperature, N_2 flow 26 ml/min.) as a product. Known hexanal gave identical retention times. The data indicated a double bond at position 3, and Alcohol I was identified as 3-nonen-1-ol.

Alcohol II. Ozonolysis of about 10 μg Alcohol II yielded propionaldehyde (2.85 min, 12% DEGS, room temperature, N_2 flow 48 ml/min). A synthetic sample of E-6-nonen-1-ol (courtesy of Dr. Martin Jacobson, USDA, Beltsville, MD) was used as a reference compound, and it also yielded propionaldehyde upon ozonolysis. The data indicated that 1 double bond in Alcohol II was located at position 6. The second double bond was located by ozonolysis of the acetate derivative of Alcohol II, which yielded acetoxy propionaldehyde (8.61 min., 12% DEGS, 111°C, N_2 flow 56 ml/min). As a reference compound the acetate of E-3-hepten-1-ol (Chemical Samples Co., Ohio) was prepared, and upon ozonolysis it also produced acetoxy propionaldehyde. These data indicated a double bond at position 3 in a 9 carbon alcohol, and thus Alcohol II was identified as 3,6-nonadien-1-ol.

Synthesis of 3-nonen-1-ol. The Z and E isomers of 3-nonen-1-ol were synthesized from nonyne-1-ol (obtained from Chemical Samples Company, Columbus, OH). The Z isomer was made by hydrogenation of 1 g nonyne-1-ol in pyridine in a low pressure Parr hydrogenator with 0.1 g of 5% Pd on charcoal as a catalyst. The reaction consumed 99% of the theoretical calculation for hydrogen over a 3 hour period. The product was filtered, acidified with 3N HCl, extracted into ether, and the ether layer was washed with $NaHCO_3$ solution to remove excess HCl. The product, Z-3-nonen-1-ol, had an identical retention time (12.8 min.) with natural alcohol I on a 12% DEGS column, 105°C, N_2 flow, 77 ml/min.

The E isomer was made by addition of 1 g nonyne-1-ol to liquid NH_3 in a dry ice-alcohol bath followed by addition of 3 equivalents of Na metal. The mixture was stirred for 5 hours, and then the NH_3 was allowed to evaporate as the bath warmed to room temperature. The product was extracted into ether and washed with water. It was further purified by column chromatography over 20 g Hi-Flosil-Ag^R (silicic acid impregnated with 20% silver nitrate) and eluted with 200 ml 4% ether in petroleum ether, 100 ml 10% ether in petroleum ether, and 100 ml 15% ether in petroleum ether. The presence of E-3-nonen-1-ol in 10 ml fractions was monitored by GC and fractions 10-25 were combined and concentrated on a rotary evaporator. The E-3-nonen-1-ol had a shorter retention time (13 min.) than the Z isomer and natural alcohol I (14.8 min.) on a 5% carbowax 20M col., 105°C, N_2 flow 38 ml/min).

Synthesis of 3,6-nonadien-1-ol. The Farchan Division of Storey Chemical Company supplied a custom synthesis of 3,6-nonadiyne-1-ol. One g of the 3,6-nonadiyne-1-ol in 4 ml pyridine was hydrogenated overnight with 0.15 g 5% Pd on charcoal as catalyst. The reaction mixture was neutralized with 3N HCl, shaken with hexane, and the hexane layer was washed with $NaHCO_3$ to remove residual HCl. The product, Z,Z-3,6-nonadien-1-ol, was further purified by column chromatography on 5 g Hi-Flosil-Ag^R (silicic acid with 20% silver nitrate). The column was washed with successive 12 ml portions of a mixture of 50% ether in petroleum ether until impurities (monitored by GC) were eluted, and then 100% ether was used to elute the Z,Z-3,6-nonadien-1-ol. Comparison of the Z,Z-3,6-nonadien-1-ol and natural alcohol II by GC showed identical retention times (16.7 min., 5% carbowax 20M, 120°C, N_2 flow 22 ml/min; 16.5 min, 12% DEGS, 120°C, N_2 flow 50 ml/min).

Laboratory Bioassay. Laboratory bioassays were conducted in the apparatus and by the procedure previously published (2). When tested alone, 50 μg of Z-3-nonen-1-ol attracted a mean of 16±5.5 (SD) females while the control (solvent only) attracted 9±5.8 females. When 1 μg was tested in combination with the other 3 components of the pheromone mixture, Z-3-nonen-1-ol did not increase the attractiveness of the mixture. Similar results were obtained in some tests reported with the natural Z-3-nonen-1-ol isolated from male flies (2). Combination tests with amounts greater than 1 μg of Z-3-nonen-1-ol are continuing, but the function of this alcohol may be to mediate some close range behaviors rather than attraction.

Synthetic Z,Z-3,6-nonadien-1-ol (1 μg) does increase the attractiveness of mixtures by about 2 fold. In combination with the other 3 components of the pheromone, 1 μg of Z,Z-3,6-nonadien-1-ol, gives an activity ratio (2) of 2.58 when compared against the attractiveness of the 3 other components without Z,Z-3,6-nonadien-1-ol.

Lactone Components of the Pheromone. Earlier published data (2) was interpreted to indicate a molecular weight of 196 and an empirical formula of $C_{11}H_{16}O_3$ for the two lactone esters, but more recent data indicate a molecular weight of 194 with a formula consistent with $C_{12}H_{18}O_2$. These two components are gamma lactones, and are diasteriomers. Partial synthesis has been effected, but assignment of isomerism in the molecules has not been completed. These data will be reported elsewhere.

DISCUSSION

Two 9 carbon alcohols, Z-3-nonen-1-ol and Z,Z-3,6-nonadien-1-ol, have been identified in extracts of male Caribbean fruit flies. Synthesis of these alcohols and laboratory bioassays confirm them as behaviorally active components of the sex pheromone of male flies. An isomer of them, E-6-nonen-1-ol, was identified as 1 component among several others in the sex pheromone of Mediterranean fruit fly males. Preliminary evidence indicates that Z-3-nonen-1-ol and Z,Z-3,6-nonadien-1-ol, as well as the 2 lactone esters from Caribbean fruit flies, are present in extracts of male Mexican fruit flies, *Anastrepha ludens* (6), and females of each species are attracted in laboratory bioassays to the heterospecific extract. These 2 species, however, are not known at present to be sympatric, and no behavioral interactions between the 2 species have been reported. There are many additional species of *Anastrepha* (7), and it will be of interest to determine if the *A. suspensa* compounds attract any other species.

TABLE 1 -- Proportions of alcohols and lactones in extracts of male flies.

Compound	μg/male *A. suspensa*	μg/male *A. ludens*
Z-3-nonen-1-ol (I)	0.012	0.030
Z,Z-3,6-nonadien-1-ol (II)	0.016	0.018
lactone III	0.120	0.039
lactone IV	0.410	0.150

Acknowledgement - I thank Ms. Kathy Dennis for technical assistance, Dr. R.M. Baranowski and Dr. A. Burditt for providing flies, and Dr. R. Ramer for assistance with the synthesis of 3-nonen-1-ol. This research was supported, in part, by a grant from Florida Citrus Commission.

REFERENCES

1. J.L. Nation, Ann. Entomol. Soc. Amer. 65, 1364-1367 (1972).
2. J.L. Nation, Environ. Entomol. 4, 27-30 (1975).
3. A.J. Perdomo, J.L. Nation and R.M. Baranowski, Environ. Entomol. 5, 1208-1210 (1976).
4. A.J. Perdomo, R.M. Baranowski and J.L. Nation, Fla. Entomol. 58, 291-295 (1975).
5. M. Beroza and B.A. Bierl, Anal. Chem. 39, 1131-1135 (1967).
6. J.L. Nation, Proc. Int. Soc. Citriculture 2, 481-485 (1977).
7. A. Stone, USDA Misc. Publ. 439, 1-112 (1942).

ALARM AND AGGREGATION PHEROMONES OF MITES

Yasumasa Kuwahara

Institute of Applied Biochemistry, University of Tsukuba, Sakura, Niihari, Ibaraki 305, Japan

Abstract - The mold mite Tyrophagus putrescentiae (Schrank) was used as an assaying mite in order to investigate the structural requisites of neryl formate for inducing alarm pheromone activity. There was found to be no need to preserve the acyclic monoterpenoid structure for the development of biological activity, and the basic requisite for the activity was the presence of a (Z)-allylic primary alcohol formate within an n-octane or n-nonane carbon skeleton.

The composition of the citral when emitted by the citral producing mites is neral; however, during the solvent extraction process, a part of neral is isomerized to geranial. This reaction was catalyzed by the mites' bodies, and part of the citral was further reduced to geraniol and nerol. Several carbonyl compounds were also reduced to the corresponding alcohols.

Strong attraction and aggregation behavior of test mites to the extracts of Lardoglyphus konoi was noted during bioassay of the alarm pheromone. The active principle isolated as the aggregation pheromone was active not only con-species but also with other related mites. The structure of the pheromone was identified as 1,3,5,7-tetramethyldecyl formate by physico-chemical measurements and chemical degradation. The synthesized diastere-omeric mixture of racemates had one-tenth the activity of the natural pheromone. The absolute configuration of C_1 was found to be R. The pheromone has been assigned the trivial name lardolure.

INTRODUCTION

Much effort has been made to elucidate chemical structures and to investigate their feasibility in pest control in the field of pheromone research on Arthropoda noxious to human being. Most of this effort has been limited to Insecta. Little work has been done on Arachnoidea, another important class, except on sex pheromones of ticks(1) and mites(2), and on the biological studies of the aggregation pheromones of ticks(3).

It has been found during the maintenance of a culture of the mold mite, Tyrophagus putrescentiae (Schrank)(TP), a cosmopolitan species capable of infesting many types of foods and stored products, that TP contained an alarm pheromone which it excreted on being disturbed. The pheromone has been isolated and identified as neryl formate, 3,7-dimethyl-(Z)-2,6-octadienyl formate(I)(4,5). In order to investigate the species-specificity of the mite's alarm pheromone, the following four species of mites were collected along with TP: Aleuroglyphus ovatus(AO), Lardoglyphus konoi(LK), Carpoglyphus lactis(CL) and Dermatophagoides farinae(DF). TP and AO belong to the same subfamily, acarinae; LK belongs to the same family, acaridae, as TP and AO; CL belongs to another family, carpoglyphidae, of the same super-family, acaroidea, and DF belongs to epidermoptidae and differs at the coholt level from the other four species. Citral(a mixture of neral and geranial, (Z)- and (E)-3,7-dimethyl-2,6-octadienal) has been isolated from four species of mites(AO, CL, LK and DF)(6), and its function has been assigned(7) as an alarm pheromone for LK and CL, and possibly as a defence substance because of its anti-fungal properties(8) for DF and AO. Citral has also been isolated as a minor component of the alarm pheromone in TP(10). Significant differences have been noted during studies on the function of citral not only in the quantity of citral emitted but also in the composition of the citral, between mites on being disturbed and when at rest(7). The initial composition of citral when discharged from the glands consists of more than 90% neral in the three species CL, AO and DF; LK consists of 75% neral(7). During the study, aggregation behavior of mites upon filter paper impregnated with hemolymph or crude extracts of LK has been observed, especially after the alarm pheromone activity faded out, and the presence of an aggregation pheromone has been suggested. Three new developments based on the above-mentioned results on mite pheromones are presented in this paper.

STRUCTURAL REQUISITES FOR THE MOLD MITE ALARM PHEROMONE

A survey of the alarm pheromone activity of all available monoterpenoids and related compounds has shown that nerol and its derivatives, such as the formate(pheromone, I), acetate and neral, showed activity, and formate(I) was the most active(1-10 ppm). Nerol and its acetate showed activity at 100-1,000 ppm, and neral at 10-100 ppm. All of the corresponding geraniol and citronellol derivatives except geranial(100-1,000 ppm) are inactive. Therefore, the presence of primary allyl alcohol moiety with (Z)-geometry in the terpenoid molecule has been supposed indispensable for the activity. In fact, the synthetic monoterpenoid, (Z)-3,7-dimethyl-2-octenol and its formate(II) showed activity equal to nerol and its formate (I), respectively(10). None of the cyclic monoterpenoids or their related compounds show any activity. In order to test the structural need for an acyclic monoterpenoid carbon skeleton, three groups of non-terpenoid pheromone analogues (a total of 16 compounds)(Fig. 1), were synthesized, and their biological activity was determined(11).

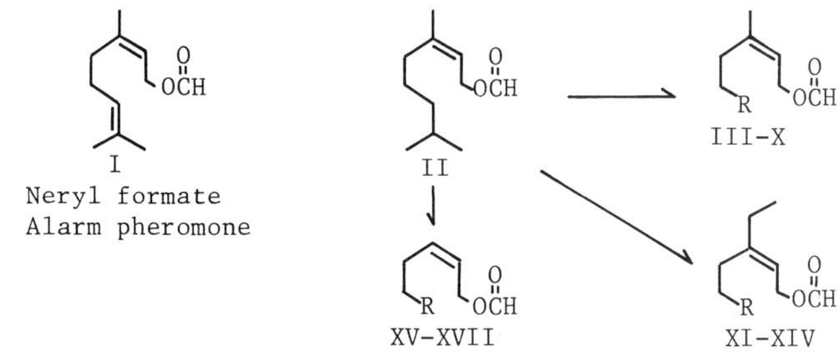

Fig. 1. Structure of neryl formate(I) and summary of structural modification processes from (Z)-3,7-dimethyl-2-octenyl formate(II).

Materials and methods

TP was reared and bioassayed as reported(5). Each compound was dissolved in hexane in a successive ten-fold dilution series starting from 10,000 ppm. Pheromone activity was designated by the lowest concentration(ppm) at which mites showed a positive response to the filter paper being tested. All C_3-methyl(III-X) and C_3-ethyl compounds(XI-XIV) were prepared by way of a Wittig reaction of an appropriate 2- or 3-alkanone with ethoxycarbonylmethylene triphenylphosphorane, separation of (Z)- and (E)-2-alkenoate, reduction of the (Z)-2-alkenoate with $LiAlH_3(OEt)$, and subsequent formylation. C_3-Non-substituted compounds(XV-XVII) were prepared by way of an appropriate alkylation of propargyl alcohol derivatives, selective reduction to (Z)-2-alkenols and subsequent esterification(11).

Results and discussion

The synthetic compounds, their purities, GLC-t_R and pheromone activities are summarized in Table 1. All of the corresponding (E)-analogues of the compounds listed in Table 1 were inactive. Alarm pheromone activity was demonstrated in almost all the compounds(14 out of 17), the exceptions being those with overly long alkyl chain analogues(IX, X and XIV). A relationship between GLC-t_R(OV-1) and biological activity was demonstrated, and the optimum

Table 1. List of synthetic compounds, purities, GLC-t_R, and pheromone activities

(Z)-2-Alkenyl formate	purity (%)	Log t_R OV-1, 90°C	Pheromone activity (ppm)
3-Methyl, heptenyl(III)	91.8	0.041	1,000-10,000
Octenyl(XV)	91.8	0.114	1,000-10,000
3,6-Dimethyl, heptenyl(IV)	81.8	0.322	100-1,000
7-Methyl, octenyl(XVI)	100	0.322	100-1,000
Nonenyl(XVII)	100	0.398	1,000-10,000
3-Methyl, octenyl(V)	91.1	0.398	10-100
3,7-Dimethyl, octenyl(II)	92.8	0.602	1-10
3-Ethyl, octenyl(XI)	94.0	0.612	10-100
Neryl(pheromone)(I)	100	0.653	1-10
3-Methyl, nonenyl(VI)	94.4	0.698	10-100
3-Ethyl-7-methyl, octenyl(XII)	80.8	0.785	10-100
3,8-Dimethyl, nonenyl(VII)	93.3	0.806	100-1,000
3-Ethyl, nonenyl(XIII)	80.9	0.919	100-1,000
3-Methyl, decenyl(VIII)	94.5	0.954	100-1,000
3-Ethyl, decenyl(XIV)	93.8	1.187	Inactive
3-Methyl, undecenyl(IX)	94.8	1.204	Inactive
3-Methyl, dodecenyl(X)	86.0	1.462	Inactive

range of vapor pressure for the activity was determined. Substitution of a methyl residue at C_3(II, V. VI) enhanced the activity of the corresponding (Z)-2-alkenyl formate(XV, XVI, XVII). Substitution of an ethyl residue at C_3(XI, XII, XIII) also improved the activity, as did methyl substitution at C_7 on the (Z)-2-octenyl formate skeleton(II, XII, XVI).

In the present study, no compound showed higher activity than I and II(1-10 ppm); however, it was concluded that there was no need to preserve the monoterpenoid structure for the development of biological activity. Therefore, the (Z)-allylic primary alcohol formate moiety, with a suitable chain length and within the optimum range of vapor pressure was elucidated as the basic requisite for developing alarm pheromone activity.

EFFECT OF MITES' BODIES ON THE CHANGE OF CITRAL COMPOSITION

As previously reported(7), citral is emitted from CL and AO into the environment and the quantity of this discharge is 10 to 50 times larger when mites are disturbed than when at rest. Furthermore the composition of citral differs significantly in the disturbed state (neral 74-86%) and when at rest(neral 54-66%). A similar compositional change is thought to occur during solvent extraction process. This compositional change of citral seems to be characteristic of these acarid mites, and is thought to be a mechanism to nullify the information formerly obtained as the alarm pheromone. This process was quantitatively investigated, mainly using CL.

Materials and methods

Pure neral and geranial were prepared from the corresponding alcohols by active MnO_2 oxidation. Prior to use, the mites' bodies were washed in the following manner, if not otherwise noted: mites(ca. 3 ml) separated from the culture medium by the flotation method(12) using saturated saline were dipped into hexane(20 ml) and suspended for 10 min. After removing the solvent by decantation, new hexane was added and the same procedure was repeated two times. The mites' bodies were then placed on filter paper and kept for 30 min at room temperature to evaporate the remaining hexane. The mites thus prepared were subsequently used for experiments. For the qualitative and quantitative determinations of citral, GLC was employed, using a Yanaco GLC model G-180F on a glass column packed with 10% PEG-20M on Chromosorb W at 110°C and 25 ml/min N_2 flow rate, or a FFAP G-SCOT column(0.25 mm id x 20 m) at 130°C and the split ratio(100:1). The amount of citral was determined using nonyl acetate(50 or 500 ppm) as the internal standard. The following incubation method was used, unless otherwise noted: the mites(0.5 g) were placed in a test tube, and a mixture of substrate(neral, geranial or citral, 100 or 1,000 ppm in hexane, 1 ml) with an internal standard was added and kept at room temperature with occasional stirring. A one μl portion of the supernatant layer was subsequently injected into the GLC at appropriate intervals.

Results and discussion

A preliminary experiment had indicated that part of the intrinsic neral from the secretory gland was changed to geranial by the presence of mites' bodies and that, without the mites' bodies, the citral composition remained unchanged. Therefore the compositional change of citral were investigated using known amounts of citral and mites' bodies. In Table 2, the results of the incubations of neral and geranial are summarized. Within an average 26.7 min for neral and 26.0 min for geranial, 50% of the substrate was consumed. It took 90 min for neral and an average of 60 min for geranial to equilibrate as a mixture of 40% neral and 60% geranial. Three hours after incubation initiated, the concentration of citral was almost unchanged, 38 ppm from neral and 31 ppm from geranial. Therefore, 62%(from neral) and 69% (from geranial) of the citral was lost during incubation for causes other than the cis-trans isomerization reaction. However, in the chromatogram(GLC), two new peaks appeared in the process of time, which were identified as nerol and geraniol. Even though all four components were put together, the total response of the components still indicated a gradual decrease(ca. 5 ppm/hr) and the presence of some other mechanism was considered.

In Table 3, the effects of the incubation solvent and the treatment of mites on the compositional change of citral were summarized. More than 81% of the citral was recovered under

Table 2. Cis-trans isomerization of citral by CL bodies.

Substrate (100 ppm)	Exp. No.	Time for consuming 50% of substrate	Final concentration* of Neral	Geranial	Citral	Time to equilibrate as Neral 40% & geranial 60%
	1	25 min	17 ppm	26 ppm	43 ppm	90 min
Neral	2	27	14	21	35	90
	3	28	15	21	36	90
	1	22	13	20	33	60
Geranial	2	36	11	15	26	80
	3	20	13	20	33	40

* Final observation at 180 min after start of incubation.

Table 3. Effects of incubation solvents and treatment of mites on the compositional change of citral starting from neral(100 ppm).

Condition		Substrate consumption 25%	Substrate consumption 50%	Final concentration of Neral	Final concentration of Geranial	Final concentration of Citral
Solvent	EtOH	190 min		76 ppm	24 ppm	100 ppm
	Acetone	106		61	43	94
	Benzene	30	77 min	33	48	81
	Hexane	8	20	12	17	29
	Ether	5	16	20	32	52
Treatment of mites	3% Formalin	140		69	22	91
	10% TCA*	170		66	20	86
	Water	18		40	59	99

* Trichloroacetic acid

all conditions except in the cases of hexane and ether. The yield of citral was the lowest with hexane. The speed of the isomerization from neral to geranial was inhibited more than 14-fold in EtOH, acetone, 3% formalin and 10% trichloroacetic acid. In the case of water, the isomerization reaction was not affected; however, reduction to alcohol was completely blocked. As a result, it was concluded that the cis-trans isomerization was at least partly dependent upon the nature of the mite's protein and that the reduction to alcohol was an enzymic reaction.

Using citral as the substrate, the yields of alcohols were compared to give the following correlative results: at 100 ppm 43% yield; at 1,000 ppm, 16%; and at 10,000 ppm, 11%. As a substrate for reduction, n-nonanal, n-decanal and 2-octanone were incubated with the mites' bodies to yield the corresponding alcohols in detectable amounts. In the case of 2-octanone , S(+)-1-methyl-heptanol(50% e.e) was obtained.

In Table 4, the results of neral(1,000 ppm) incubation with CL and three other species(TP, AO and LK) are presented. Neral was isomerized to geranial and the presence of the corresponding alcohols was detected with all species. The order of the speed consuming neral was as follows: CL > AO > TP > LK. In CL and LK, citral functions as an alarm pheromone, and in AO, its role is considered that of a defence substance(7). No correlation between the isomerization reaction and the function of citral is known at present.

Table 4. Results of neral(1,000 ppm) incubation with four species of mites

Species of mite	Substrate consumption 25%	Substrate consumption 50%	Final concentration of Neral	Final concentration of Geranial	Final concentration of Nerol	Final concentration of Geraniol
C. lactis	3 min	17 min	210ppm	290ppm	83ppm	80ppm
A. ovatus	15	35	180	192	21	40
T. putrescentiae	22	59	240	240	57	68
L. konoi	39	130	449	348	42	12

IDENTIFICATION AND SYNTHESIS OF THE AGGREGATION PHEROMONE OF LK

The presence of an aggregation pheromone in LK which attracts and arrest not only conspecies, but also the other three species of mites(CL, AO and TP), has been demonstrated and a trial isolation has been attempted(13). The present paper deals with the isolation, identification, and synthesis of the pheromone(14).

Isolation

Based on the observation that the aggregation pheromone accumulated in the culture medium(13) , the mites and the culture medium were dipped into hexane to extract the pheromone. Two methods were used to isolate the pheromone from the hexane extract by monitoring the activity of all the resulting fraction, using CL as the test mite. One method involved extraction of MeOH-soluble parts from the hexane-extracted oil(from 1 l of mites and medium) and repeated column chromatographies(SiO_2 and Sephadex LH-20) to give the pure pheromone(6.3 mg, active at 0.1 ppm). The other method used hydrolysis of the oil, extraction of the alcohol(s) and a subsequent formylation instead of extraction of the MeOH-soluble parts. The pure aggregation pheromone(13.6 mg) was isolated from 1.23 l of materials. The resultant pheromones were combined and used for structure elucidation.

Structure elucidation

A PMR spectrum(100 MHz) of the pheromone(in $CDCl_3$, with TMS as an internal standard)gave the following chemical shifts: at δ8.052(1H, s) and at ca. δ5.3(1H, m), which was coupled with a

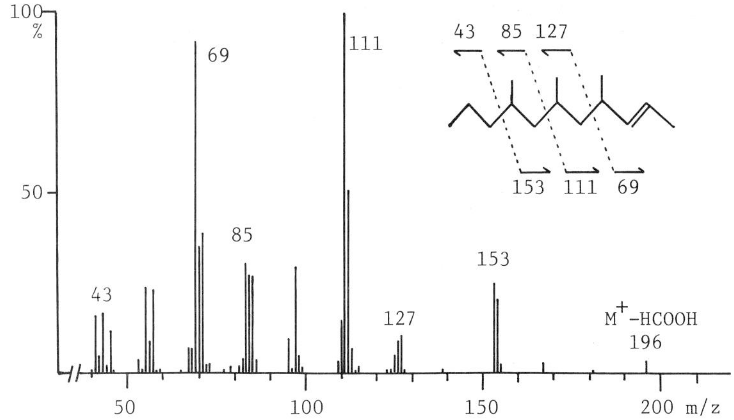

Fig. 2. EI-mass spectrum(20 eV) of the aggregation pheromone.

methyl doublet at δ 1.264(J=6.3Hz), and also with many protons at the methyl-methylene region, which indicated the presence of an α-methyl substituted alkyl formate. The presence of a formate moiety had been suggested by preliminary experiments of hydrolysis and subsequent formylation. Oxidation of the alcohol by the Jones or Cornforth reagent gave a ketone as the sole product. The ketone was found to be a methyl ketone by haloform oxidation. The EI-mass spectrum of the pheromone(Fig. 2) gave the highest mass fragment at m/z 196(4%), and the following characteristic ions: 153, 127, 111(base ion peak), 85, 69 and 43. CI-mass spectrum(methane) also supported these results, and gave $M^+ + 1$ ion at m/z 197(81.7%). Its molecular ion was suggested as m/z 196, and taking the formate into consideration, the molecular formula was tentatively assigned as $C_{11}H_{20}O_2$.

The PMR spectrum, however, suggested no evidence of olefinic protons, nor did the CMR spectrum indicate any sp^2 carbons. The presence of a formate carbon at 190.8 ppm and an alkoxy-substituted carbon at 69.043 ppm was also observed from CMR spectrum. A full decoupled CMR spectrum indicated at least 13 lines of chemical shifts, and more than 13 carbons were suggested in the alkyl moiety, even if the presence of some higher alkyl formate as an impurity was taken into consideration. Therefore the highest ion of the pheromone was reconsidered and reassigned as M^+ - HCOOH, and consequently, the molecular weight of the pheromone was concluded to be m/z 242($C_{15}H_{30}O_2$).

The pheromone was changed to a ketone by hydrolysis and oxidation as stated above. The Wolf-Kischner reduction of this ketone gave the following mass spectrum shown in Fig. 3. Although M^+ was not observed, the following diagnostic ions were observed: m/z 169, 155, 127,

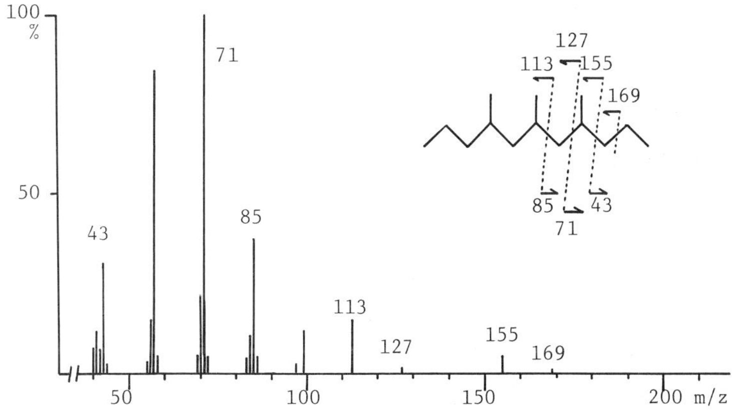

Fig. 3. EI-mass spectrum of the hydrocarbon derived from the aggregation pheromone by way of hydrolysis, oxidation and Wolf-Kischner reduction, at 20 eV.

113, 99, 85, 71(base ion peak) 57 and 43. All the fragment ions except those at 99 and 57 were explainable as indicated in Fig. 3. Therefore, the structure of the pheromone-hydrocarbon was unambiguously identified as 4,6,8-trimethylundecane, and consequently, the structure of the aggregation pheromone was concluded to be 1,3,5,7-tetramethyldecyl formate, for which the trivial name lardolure was proposed.

Synthesis

A sample of a mixture of lardolure and its stereoisomer was synthesized for structure confirmation and biological testing. The synthetic route and the yield of each step is summarized in Fig. 4. The synthesized lardolure theoretically consisted of 8 sets of diastereomers, and was partially separated by GLC using G-SCOT column systems(6 peaks by OV-101, 4 peaks by

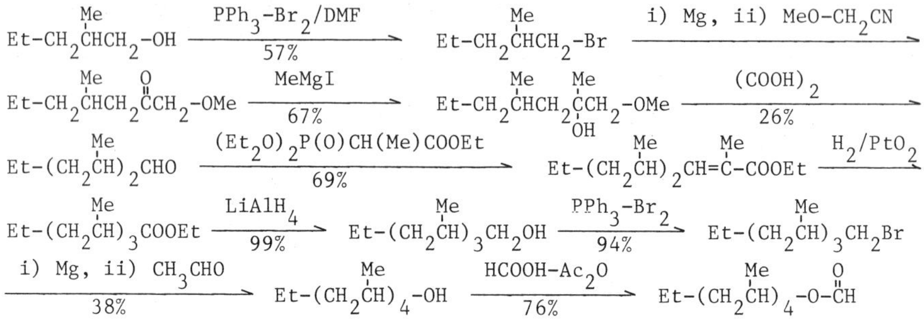

Fig. 4. Summary of the synthesis of a mixture of lardolure and its stereoisomers.

FFAP and 6 peaks by SS-4). All peaks appearing in those chromatograms gave identical mass spectra, and the t_R of the natural lardolure was identical to that of the shortest t_R-peak in all column systems. The synthetic lardolure showed aggregation pheromone activity at 1 ppm with CL; however, with the other mites(TP, LK and AO) it showed no activity. Therefore some stereoisomer may act to inhibit the pheromone activity, as was observed in other optically active pheromones.

Stereo chemistry of C_1 of the lardolure

The natural lardolure showed a plain + cotton curve by ORD; $[\alpha]^{25}_{205}$ -515°, $[\alpha]^{25}_{217}$ 0° and $[\alpha]^{25}_{235}$ 400°, and $[\alpha]^{25}_{D}$ + (data not readable at C = 0.1 in hexane). (S)-1-Methylheptyl formate is known to give $[\alpha]^{20}_{D}$ -3.80°(purity 91%). By PMR study using a chiral shift reagent[Eu(TFC)3], the chemical shift of the methyl residue of (S)-1-methylheptyl formate was observed as a doublet at the higher magnetic field, when spiked by a racemic formate. A similar pair of methyl doublet was confirmed by the synthetic lardolure, and under the same conditions, the natural lardolure gave a doublet at lower magnetic field when spiked by the synthetic lardolure. Therefore the natural lardolure was concluded to be optically pure at least at C_1, and the absolute configuration of C_1 was assigned as R. The absolute structure of the other three asymmetric carbons are presently unknown, although from the t_R data of the G-SCOT column systems, their configurations seemed to be regular.

Acknowledgement - The author wishes to thank Prof. Emeritus S. Ishii and Prof. H. Fukami of Kyoto University, Assoc. Prof. K. Matsumoto and Dr. Y. Wada of Tokyo Women's Medical College, Dr. L.T. My-Yen, Dr. Y. Tominaga, Miss L. Sakuma and Mr. H. Suzuki of this university for their encouragement, collaboration and technical assistance.

REFERENCES

1. R.S. Berger, Science 177, 704-705 (1972), W.F. Wood, M.G. Leahy, R. Galun, G.D. Prestwich J. Meinwald, R.E.Purnell, R.C. Payne, J. Chem. Ecol. 1, 501-509 (1975), D.E. Sonnenshine, R.M. Silverstein, E. Plummer, J.R. West, T. McCullough, J. Chem. Ecol. 2, 201-209 (1976).
2. S. Regev, W.W. Cone, Environ. Entomol. 4,307-311 (1975), ibid, 5,133-138 (1976).
3. M.G.Leahy, Recent Advances in Acarology 2, p.297-308, Academic Press, New York (1979).
4. Y. Kuwahara, S. Ishii, H. Fukami, Experientia 31, 1115-1116(1975).
5. Y. Kuwahara, H. Fukami, S. Ishii, K. Matsumoto, Y. Wada, Jap. J. Sanit. Zool. 30, 309-314 (1979).
6. Y. Kuwahara, S. Ishii, H. Fukami, K. Matsumoto, Y. Wada, ibid, 31, 49-52 (1980).
7. Y. Kuwahara, S. Ishii, H. Fukami, K. Matsumoto, Y. Wada, ibid, 31, 73-80 (1980).
8. L. Cole, M. Blum, R. Roncadori, Mycologia, 67, 701-708 (1975), M. Okamoto, K. Matsumoto, Y. Wada, H. Nakano, Jap. J. Sanit. Zool. 29, 255-260 (1978).
9. L.T. My-Yen, K. Matsumoto, Y. Wada, Y. Kuwahara, Appl. Ent. Zool. 15, 474-477 (1980).
10. Y. Kuwahara, Appl. Ent. Zool. 17, 127-132 (1982).
11. Y. Kuwahara, L. Sakuma, Appl. Ent. Zool. (1982), Agr. Biol. Chem. (1982), in press.
12. K. Matsumoto, Jap. J. Sanit. Zool. 21, 213-219 (1970).
13. L.T. My-Yen, Y. Wada, K. Matsumoto, Y. Kuwahara, Jap. J. Sanit. Zool. 31, 249-254 (1980)
14. Y. Kuwahara, L.T. My-Yen, Y. Tominaga, K. Matsumoto, Y. Wada, Agr. Biol. Chem. (1982), in press.

COMPOUNDS DERIVED FROM THE APHID ALARM PHEROMONE OF POTENTIAL USE IN CONTROLLING COLONISATION AND VIRUS TRANSMISSION BY APHIDS

Geoffrey G. Briggs, Glenn W. Dawson, Richard W. Gibson, David C. Griffiths, John A. Pickett, Adrian D. Rice, Mary F. Stribley and Christine M. Woodcock

Rothamsted Experimental Station, Harpenden, Hertfordshire, AL5 2JQ, UK

Abstract. New 1,4-cycloaddition products of the aphid alarm pheromone (E)-β-farnesene are synthesised and tested for activity against colonisation and virus transmission by aphids. The most active compound, the adduct of (E)-β-farnesene with diundecyl acetylenedicarboxylate, persists for 7 days on the plant but neither structural modification nor use of antioxidants extend the period of activity. The sodium salt of the diacid from the adduct with maleic anhydride is systemically active, but only against aphid settling.

INTRODUCTION

The damage to crops by aphids, either by feeding or by transmitting virus disease can be prevented to some extent by insecticides, but aphids are developing increased resistance, particularly to systemic organophosphates (Ref. 1). Also, such insecticides do not prevent damage to crops by non-persistent viruses, such as potato virus Y, since these are rapidly acquired and transmitted by aphids. The fast-acting pyrethroids may control infection with non-persistent viruses but are less effective with the more resistant biotypes of Myzus persicae (Ref. 2), so alternative novel approaches appear desirable.

Of the chemicals that influence aphid behaviour, the most active is the alarm pheromone which, for most important pest species, is the sesquiterpene hydrocarbon, (E)-β-farnesene (1) (Refs. 3,4,5 & 6). Synthetic (E)-β-farnesene (1) substantially increases the effectiveness of contact pesticides such as permethrin against aphids in the laboratory (Ref. 7) and this approach is being investigated in field crops (Ref. 8). Because (E)-β-farnesene (1) is highly volatile and readily oxidised in air, it cannot be used directly for long term protection of plants. So, more stable and less volatile compounds derived from (E)-β-farnesene (1) by 1,4-cycloaddition (Diels-Alder) reactions were examined. These inhibit colonisation of plants and acquisition of plant virus by aphids (Refs. 8 & 9).

(1) 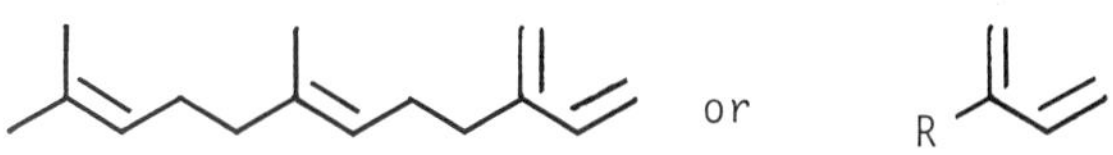

The structures of some of these earlier compounds and their relative biological activities are given in Table 1. The sulpholene (2) readily gave (E)-β-farnesene (1) by the retro-Diels-Alder reaction but compounds (3) to (5) which released (1) either in very small amounts or not at all showed equal or greater activity (Fig. 1).

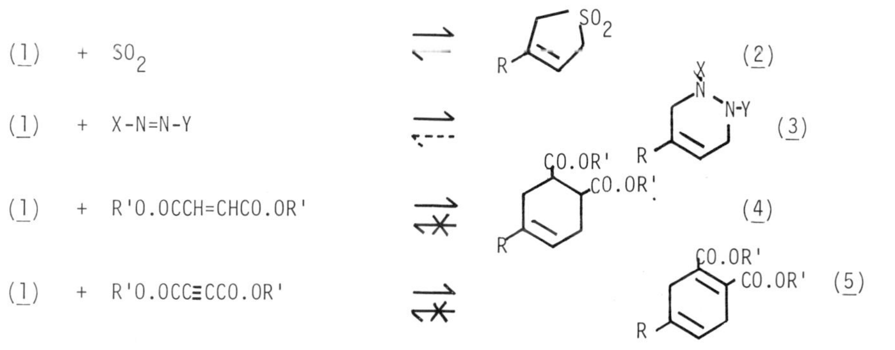

Fig. 1. Reversible and irreversible 1,4-cycloaddition reactions of (E)-β-farnesene (1).

The purpose of the present study, following these promising results, was to examine new biological and chemical aspects of the effect, in order to identify structure/activity relationships, to increase persistence and to investigate the possibililty of designing compounds with systemic activity.

TABLE 1. (E)-β-farnesene derivatives and relative biological activity

Compound		Interference with:- Aphid settling	Potato virus Y acquisition
(2)		*	*
(3a)	X=Y=$CO.OCH_2CH_3$	*	*
(3b)	X=$CO.OCH_2CH_3$ Y=H	**	*
(3c)	X=Y=CH_3	**	*
(4a)	R'=CH_2CH_3	**	*
(4b)	R'=$(CH_2)_9CH_3$	**	*
(5a)	R'=CH_2CH_3	*	*
(5b)	R'=$(CH_2)_9CH_3$	***	***

EXPERIMENTAL

Chemicals

1,4-Cycloaddition products (5) from (E)-β-farnesene (1) were obtained by the general methods described previously (Ref. 9). The high molecular weight compounds were purified by elution from Florisil with increasing ether in hexane. Alcohols used in preparation of the dienophiles were obtained either from commercial sources or by standard methods. Compounds (5) were characterised by nuclear magnetic resonance (NMR) spectroscopy and all had spectra consistent with those for the compounds reported previously. Each 1,4-cycloaddition product contained ca. 60% of the (E)-isomer, ca. 30% of the corresponding (Z)- isomer and other isomers containing terminal methylenes arising from the isomeric composition of the (E)-β-farnesene sample.

The compounds derived from (E)-β-farnesene and the other test compounds (obtained commercially or prepared by standard methods) were prepared as aqueous emulsions using Ethylan BV at 10% of active ingredient (w/w) as emulsifying agent and applied to leaves at 0.01 ml/cm^2. Concentrations w/v for emulsions of (E)-β-farnesene derivatives (5) were calculated from weights of the complete isomeric mixtures. Antioxidants, 2,6-ditertbutyl-4-methylphenol, N-phenyl-N'-octyl-1,4-phenylenediamine and 1,4-dihydroxybenzene were added at 10%, of active ingredient w/w.

Sodium salt of 1,2-dicarboxy-4-(4,8-dimethyl-3,7-nonadienyl)cyclohex-4-ene(8). The 1,4-cycloaddition product (9) from (E)-β-farnesene (1) and maleic anyhydride (Ref. 9) (300 mg, 1 mmole) was stirred overnight with sodium hydroxide (80mg, 2 mmole) in water (45 ml) to give a clear solution of compound (8) containing 1% a.i. ready for dilution and testing.

Decomposition of compound (5b)

Compound (5b) (100mg) on glass (4 cm^2) was exposed to natural light for 20 hr. After extraction with hexane (10 ml) a portion (0.4 μl) was analysed by gas chromatography (Flexsil, 25m x 0.2mm, OV 101, 50° 10 min, 4°/min, 280^oC)-coupled mass spectrometry (V.G. M.M. 70-70F, 200^oC, 70eV) (GC-MS) and results compared with those from samples of undecomposed (5b) and authentic decan-1-ol.

Bioassay

Non-systemic tests These tests have been described previously (Ref. 2,9 & 10). Briefly the settling test involves confining aphids, *Myzus persicae*, for 24 hrs on upper surfaces of Chinese cabbage (*Brassicae pekinensis*) leaves, allowing choice between the halves treated with test chemical and formulation control.

The potato virus Y (PVY) and beet yellows virus (BYV) tests involve placing *Myzus persicae* on infected plants treated with test chemicals or formulation control and then transferring them to healthy plants, recording those that become diseased.

Active compounds (significantly different from controls at $P<0.05$) were retested at successively lower doses until activity ceased.

Systemic tests For the systemic settling test Chinese cabbage leaves were severed from the plant under water, to prevent air from entering the stems, and transferred to the test solution 3 hrs before the start of the test (preliminary studies using a dye solution having indicated that this would allow enough time for an even distribution of solution throughout the leaf). The control leaves (of similar age) were placed in distilled water. The leaves were then cut from the tip to *ca.* 25 mm down the midrib. This allowed half a test leaf to be placed alongside half a control leaf (Fig. 2). (The dye test indicated that this split did not influence distribution through the leaf.)The two halves of the leaves were joined with a strip of Blu-tack (Bostik). A petri-dish containing 20 apterous *Myzus persicae* was placed in the centre of the joined leaves, offering the aphids equal areas of treated and untreated surface. Each test had 10 replicates and results were recorded at 24 hrs.

A similar technique of overlapping leaves was used to investigate uptake of systemic compounds through the roots, and their transfer from one leaf to another.

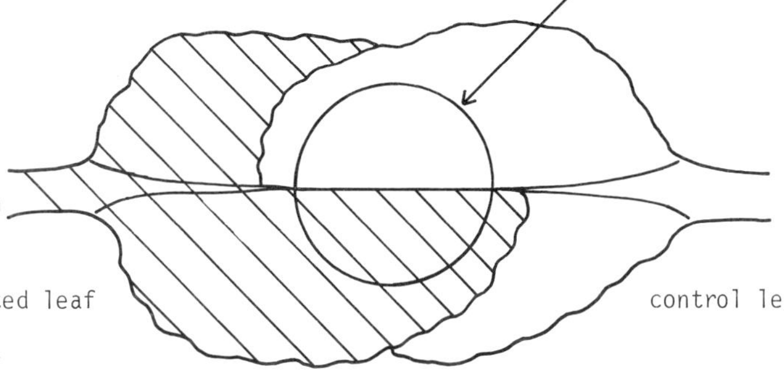

Fig. 2 Diagram of overlapping leaves for testing the effect of systemic action on settling

For investigating interference with PVY acquisition by systemic action, petioles of infector plant leaves were placed in test solutions or water 24 hrs before aphids were allowed access.

RESULTS AND DISCUSSION

Structure/activity relationships

Because compound (5b) was the most active (Ref. 9), influence of varying R' in structure 5 on activity was investigated using the settling test; results are given in Table 2. The most active compound (5e), prepared from diundecyl (C_{11}) acetylenedicarboxylate, differs from (5b) only in having an extra methylene in each n-alkyl group of the diester part of the molecule. The C_{18} or stearyl homologue (5h), the only solid in the series (m.p.38°C), enhanced colonisation and the branched chain alkyl derivative (5i), prepared using catalytically hydrogenated farnesol to give the dienophile hexahydrofarnesyl acetylenedicarboxylate, was inactive. Compound (5j), similar to the most active compound (5e) but prepared using undecan-2-ol in place of undecan-1-ol, had poor activity. Because the unsaturated C_{18} (or oleyl) homologue (5k) was slightly active, the unsaturated C_{11} compounds (5l) and (5m) were prepared but proved to be inactive at the concentrations used in the test.

Although not all compounds in Table 2 have been tested against PVY acquisition, preliminary results suggest that the pattern of activity is similar to that for aphid settling. Thus

TABLE 2. Variation of R' in structure (5) and results of settling tests

No.	R'	Conc. %	Mean no. of aphids settled on leaves: control	treated	significance of difference, P
(5c)	$(CH_2)_7CH_3$	0.5	10.9	5.2	<0.01
		0.1	8.7	7.9	N.S.
(5d)	$(CH_2)_8CH_3$	0.5	13.2	5.1	<0.01
		0.1	11.3	6.0	<0.05
(5b)	$(CH_2)_9CH_3$	0.5	13.4	3.8	<0.001
		0.1	13.0	6.0	<0.001
		0.05	9.4	8.3	N.S.
(5e)	$(CH_2)_{10}CH_3$	0.5	16.8	2.0	<0.001
		0.1	14.4	3.0	<0.001
		0.05	12.0	6.6	<0.05
		0.01	7.0	10.5	N.S.
(5f)	$(CH_2)_{11}CH_3$	0.5	10.7	8.3	N.S.
(5g)	$(CH_2)_{13}CH_3$	0.5	12.6	5.7	<0.01
(5h)	$(CH_2)_{17}CH_3$	0.5	6.6	11.0	<0.05
		0.1	7.3	10.7	N.S.
(5i)	$[(CH_2)_2CH(CH_3)CH_2]_3H$	0.5	10.5	7.7	N.S.
(5j)	$CH(CH_3)(CH_2)_8CH_3$	0.5	11.1	7.3	<0.05
		0.1	9.8	10.3	N.S.
(5k)	$(CH_2)_8\overset{H}{C}=\overset{H}{C}(CH_2)_8H$	0.5	13.0	5.0	<0.01
		0.1	8.2	9.1	N.S.
(5l)	$(CH_2)_9CH=CH_2$	0.5	10.6	6.8	N.S.
(5m)	$(CH_2)_5\overset{H}{C}=\overset{H}{C}(CH_2)_3CH_3$	0.5	10.0	8.4	N.S.

the percentage reduction in numbers of plants infected by aphids given the opportunity to acquire PVY from infected plants (treated with test compound at 0.1%) against control plants was: 78% (P <0.01) for (5b), 80% (P <0.01) for (5e), and the result with the C_{11} compound (5j), was not significant. However, for BYV acquisition the pattern of activity is less similar to that for settling. Most compounds highly active against settling and PVY transmission are inactive at 1% against BYV acquisition except for the C_{14} compound (5g) which is active (69%, P < 0.01).

The sulpholene (2) is highly phytotoxic perhaps because it releases SO_2 and some of the nitrogen containing derivatives also damage plants. However, compounds with structure (5) do not damage leaves even at relatively high rates.

Long-chain carboxylic acids are known to influence aphid settling (Ref. 11 & 12). The carboxylic acids are structurally and physically very different from compounds with structure (5) but the patterns of activity shown on varying the carbon numbers of the carboxylic acids and of the alkyl substituents in the diester part of compounds with structure (5) are surprisingly similar. For example both of the C_{10} compounds, (5b) and decanoic acid, interfere with aphid settling and activity falls as the homologous series is ascended. The C_{18} compounds, (5h) and stearic acid, enhance settling. The unsaturated C_{18} compounds, (5k) and oleic acid, both interfere with aphid settling. However, the carboxylic acid most active in preventing settling, dodecanoic acid (C_{12}), enhanced acquisition of PVY (Ref. 10) whereas the pattern of activities of compounds with structure (5) is generally similar for settling and PVY acquisition. The activities of the corresponding simple alcohols which might be formed by hydrolysis of compounds (5) are given in Table 3. Although decan-1-ol is active and oleyl slightly active, the effects are insufficient to account directly for the activity of the related pheromone derivatives. Furthermore the most active against settling, decan-1-ol, does not interfere with acquisition of PVY.

TABLE 3. Effect of long chain alcohols on aphid settling

	Conc. %	Mean no. of aphids settled on leaves Control	Treated	significance of difference, P
$CH_3(CH_2)_9OH$ (decan-1-ol)	0.5	12.6	5.6	<0.05
	0.1	12.9	6.7	<0.01
$CH_3(CH_2)_{13}OH$(tetradecan-1-ol)	0.5	9.6	8.1	N.S.
$CH_3(CH_2)_{17}OH$(stearyl alcohol)	0.5	7.9	9.3	N.S.
$CH_3(CH_2)_7CHOHCH_3$ (decan-2-ol)	0.5	11.8	5.4	<0.05
$CH_3(CH_2)_7C{=}C(CH_2)_8OH$ (oleyl alcohol)	0.5	12.7	3.4	<0.01
	0.1	11.5	6.6	N.S.
$CH_2{=}CH(CH_2)_8OH$(9-decen-1-ol)	0.5	7.6	8.3	N.S.

Other structures not containing the (E)-β-farnesene moeity were also investigated. Didecyl maleate (6), which is compound (5b) without the (E)-β-farnesene structure, decreases aphid

(6) 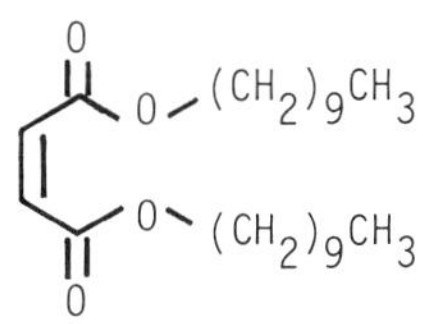

settling at 0.5%. Also the compound obtained from (5b) by catalytic hydrogenation (4 moles of H_2 absorbed, confirmed by NMR) and which thereby contains a substantially modified pheromone moeity also interferes with settling. However, these compounds are substantially less active than (5b) and (5e) which incorporate the pheromone structure.

The most active compound prepared so far, (5e), is active at 0.05% corresponding to a field rate of ca 250 g/ha. The pheromone (E)-β-farnesene(1) causes increased mobility in aphids when applied at levels equivalent to 300 mg/ha. Therefore, if activity of the derivatives is related to pheromonal activity, there is potential for designing compounds with much greater potency than the ones so far described.

Persistence

Compound (5b) applied to leaves at 1% is highly active against PVY acquisition after 7 days (Ref. 9). Compound (5e) on leaves at 0.5% is active against aphid settling after 7 days but not after 14 days. Calculated vapour pressures for these two compounds indicate that evaporative loss would be unimportant. The decomposition thus indicated for compounds with structure (5) on leaf surfaces could be by hydrolysis of the ester linkage and by aerial oxidation of the double bonds and allylic methylenes. Analysis (GC-MS) of products from compound (5b) after contact with air under natural light for 20 hrs gave (5b), (83% recovery) R_t 88 and 95 min for (Z)- and (E)-isomers, and decan-1-ol, (30% theoretical) Rt 30 min, the hydrolysis product. An expected product of oxidation, the aromatic compound (7), was not detected.

(7) 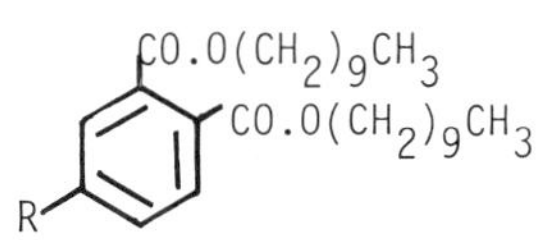

Hydrolysis of compounds (5) would proceed more slowly if the secondary alcohol replaced the primary but the structural modification (5e)→(5j) (R'=undec-1-yl → -2-yl) led to a lower level of biological activity. Various antioxidants were employed but did not improve persistence on plants.

Systemic activity

Known systemically active compounds are all moderately polar with log K_{ow} values in the range -0.5 to 3.5 (Ref. 13) but the compounds with structure (5) are highly lipophilic; the calculated log K_{ow} even for (5a) is >6. Consistent with this, compound (5b) is inactive systemically. Compound (8), obtained by hydrolysis of the maleic anhydride adduct (9) investigated earlier, with a log K_{ow} of -1 (calc. for di-anion), 2 (calc. for mono-anion) and -1 (observed, pH 10.5) should therefore be systemic. Against aphid settling,

(9)

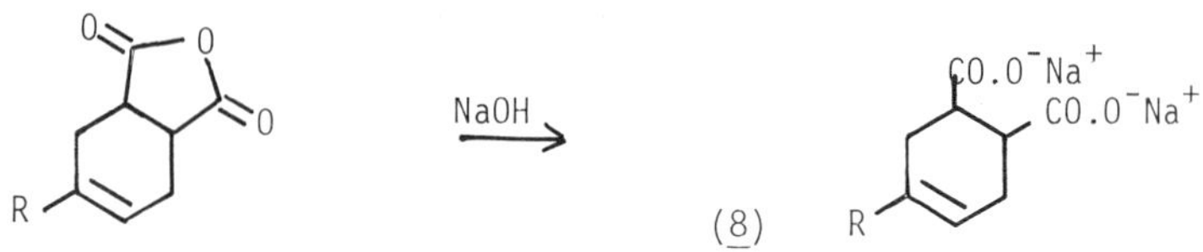

(8)

(8) is active at 0.05% via the cut leaf petiole, at 0.1% through the washed root and via the soil but is inactive by translocation from one leaf to another at 0.5%, higher levels being prohibited by phytotoxic effects. However, at 0.05% via the cut petiole compound (8) is inactive against PVY acquisition.

The activities reported here against aphid settling, and against acquisition of PVY and of BYV show that structure-activity relationships are not always parallel in the different tests, and in some instances differ substantially. This must relate partially to the different time scales (and therefore degree of leaf penetration) in which the two types of test operate: aphids take up to 2 hrs to settle, and BYV is acquired over several hours, yet PVY is acquired in under 2 mins. The cause of the differences in trends in the settling and BYV tests is not yet clear; for instance, initial probing by aphids on leaves appears to be unaffected by treatment with the pheromone derivatives (Ref. 14). Elucidation of the precise mechanisms by which the new compounds interfere with settling and virus acquisition requires further study.

REFERENCES

1. R.M. Sawicki, A.L. Devonshire, A.D. Rice, G.D. Moores, S.M. Petzing and A. Cameron, Pest. Sci. 9, 189-201 (1978).
2. R.W. Gibson, A.D. Rice and R.M. Sawicki, Ann. Appl. Biol., 100, 49-54 (1982).
3. W.S. Bowers, L.R. Nault, R.E. Webb and S.R. Dutky, Science 177, 1121-1122 (1972).
4. L.J. Edwards, J.B. Siddall, L.L. Dunham, P. Uden and C.J. Kislow, Nature (Lond.) 241, 126-127 (1973).
5. W.H. Wientjens, A.C. Lakwijk and T. Van Der Marel, Exp. 29, 658-660 (1973).
6. J.A. Pickett and D.C. Griffiths, J. Chem. Ecol. 6, 349-360 (1980).
7. D.C. Griffiths and J.A. Pickett, Ent. Exp. Appl. 27, 199-201 (1980).
8. J.A. Pickett, G.W. Dawson, R.W. Gibson, D.C. Griffiths, A.D. Rice, R.M. Sawicki, M.C. Smith and C.M. Woodcock, Les Colloques de l'I.N.R.A. 7, 243-252 (1982.
9. G.W. Dawson, R.W. Gibson, D.C. Griffiths, J.A. Pickett, A.D. Rice and C.M. Woodcock, J. Chem. Ecol. (in press).
10. R.W. Gibson, A.D. Rice, J.A. Pickett, M.C. Smith and R.M. Sawicki, Ann. Appl. Biol. 100, 55-59 (1982).
11. A.R. Greenway, D.C. Griffiths and S.L. Lloyd, Ent. exp. appl. 24, 369-374 (1978).
12. M.H. Sherwood, A.R. Greenway and D.C. Griffiths, Bull. Ent. Res. 71, 133-136 (1981)
13. G.G. Briggs, R.H. Bromilow, R. Edmondson and M. Johnston, in Herbicides and Fungicides - Factors affecting their activity. (Chem. Soc. Spec. Pub. No. 29) 129-134 (1977).
14. D.C. Griffiths, J.A. Pickett and C.M. Woodcock, Bull. Ent. Res. (in press).

2-TRIDECANONE: A NATURAL TOXICANT IN A WILD TOMATO RESPONSIBLE FOR INSECT RESISTANCE

George G. Kennedy and Michael B. Dimock

Department of Entomology, North Carolina State University, Raleigh, North Carolina 27650, USA

Abstract - Larvae of the insect pest species *Manduca sexta, Heliothis zea* and *Leptinotarsa decemlineata* are unable to survive on the wild tomato species *Lycopersicon hirsutum f. glabratum*. The resistance of this plant to *M. sexta* and very probably *L. decemlineata* is due to the presence of 2-tridecanone in the tips of the glandular trichomes which abound on the foliage. Although 2-tridecanone is also toxic to *H. zea*, most larvae are not exposed to a lethal dose. Other factors appear to account for most of the resistance to *H. zea*. The level of 2-tridecanone present in the trichomes of resistant foliage is significantly greater when the plants are grown under long than under short daylengths. The toxicity of methyl keytones to *H. zea* is influenced by chain length and is related to the compounds lipophilicity. Position of the carbonyl carbon in the tridecanone molecule does not affect its toxicity.

INTRODUCTION

Certain accessions of the wild tomato species *Lycopersicon hirsutum f. glabratum* C. H. Mull are resistant to attack by a number of important insect pests of the cultivated tomato (Ref. 1). That resistance offers promise for use in a breeding program to develop insect resistant tomato cultivars for use in commercial tomato production. First instar larvae of at least three important insect pest species, the tomato fruitworm (*Heliothis zea*), the tobacco hornworm (*Manduca sexta*) and the Colorado potato beetle (*Leptinotarsa decemlineata*) die, often without feeding, when placed on the foliage of the resistant accession PI 134417 of *L. hirsutum f. glabratum*. Under field conditions PI 134417 is virtually immune to attack by these species.

TRICHOME AND 2-TRIDECANONE INVOLVEMENT

Resistant plants are covered by a dense vesture of a variety of types of glandular trichomes. These trichomes have been implicated in the resistance to several arthropod species (Ref. 2) and at least one type plays a major role in the resistance to *H. zea, M. sexta* and *L. decemlineata*. The removal of trichome exudate by washing the foliage with 70% ethanol and rinsing it with distilled water eliminated the resistance to all 3 species (Table 1). Mortality on the insect-susceptible, cultivated tomato *Lycopersicon esculentum* was 18, 18 and 17% for *H. zea, M. sexta* and *L. decemlineata* respectively.

TABLE 1. Effect of trichome-exudate removal on expression of resistance of *L. hirsutum f. glabratum*.

	% Mortality of		
	H. zea	*M. sexta*	*L. decemlineata*
Exudate present	84 a	93 a	97 a
Exudate removed	26 b	29 b	15 b

Mean separation vertical at $P \leq 0.001$.

Since larvae of all three species became convulsive and subsequently inmobilized shortly after their placement on resistant foliage, it was clear that they were being poisoned rather than becoming entangled in the trichome exudate. Chromatographic separation of chloroform washes of resistant foliage, which contained the trichome exudate, combined with bioassay of each fraction for acute toxicity to *M. sexta* and *H. zea* indicated the acute toxicity of the exudate was due to a single compound. This was identified as the methyl keytone 2-tridecanone (Ref. 3).

Bioassay of 2-tridecanone for toxicity to all 3 insect species by placing first instar larvae on filter paper discs treated with various rates of 2-tridecanone produced the following LC_{50} values: *M. sexta* 17.05 μg/cm^2, *H. zea* 17.1 μg/cm^2 and *L. decemlineata* 26.9 μg/cm^2 treated surface. For *H. zea*, comparable LC_{50} values for the commercial insecticides malathion and methomyl were 4.08 and 2.01 μg/cm^2 treated surface.

Gas chromatographic analysis of surface extracts of resistant and susceptible foliage on numerous occasions over a period of 2 years indicated the amount of 2-tridecanone in the resistant foliage was far greater than that in the susceptible foliage (Table 2). The levels associated with the resistant foliage are well in excess of the LC_{50} values for all three species as determined using treated filter paper discs.

TABLE 2. 2-Tridecanone levels of resistant and susceptible tomato foliage.

Foliage	μg 2-Tridecanone/cm^2 of leaflet	
	Mean	Range
Resistant (*L. hirsutum f. glabratum*)	44.6	5.9 - 148
Susceptible (*L. esculentum*)	0.1	0.0 - 0.2

Direct gas chromatographic analysis of trichome tip exudate collected with a microcapillary indicated a mean of 6.3 ng 2-tridecanone per trichome tip with a range of 0.7 to 10.7 ng/tip. Analysis of chloroform surface extracts of resistant foliage obtained by steeping foliage in chloroform for one hour and subsequent analysis of chloroform extracts of homogenates from these surface extracted leaflets (Ref. 4) indicated that virutally all of the 2-tridecanone present occurs on the leaflet surfaces (99.5%) in association with the glandular trichomes.

TOXICITY OF STRUCTURAL ANALOGS OF 2-TRIDECANONE

The toxicity of 2-tridecanone to several different insect species from at least three different orders (Ref. 3) and its seemingly apparent role in the resistance of *L. hirsutum f. glabratum* to *H. zea, M. sexta* and *L. decemlineata* prompted an investigation of the relationship between structure and activity of 2-tridecanone and congeners varying in chain length and carbonyl position (Ref. 5). In all of these tests, toxicities to *H. zea* were determined by placing newly-eclosed first instar larvae on treated filter paper discs for six hours and then transferring them to artificial diet. After 18 hours on diet, mortality was recorded.

Chain length and toxicity

Methyl-2-keytones varying in chain lengths from 5 to 19 carbons were evaluated for toxicity. The most toxic compounds had chain lengths ranging from 9 to 15 carbons. The LC_{50} values ranged from 17.05 μg/cm^2 for 2-tridecanone to 578.75 for 2-pentadecanone (Table 3).

TABLE 3. LC_{50} values of methyl-2-keytones varying in chain length: *Heliothis zea*.

Compound	LC_{50} ($\mu g/cm^2$)	95% CI
2-Nonanone	245.18	236 - 255
2-Decanone	99.33	93.4 - 106
2-Undecanone	64.19	63.3 - 65.1
2-Dodecanone	25.36	24.5 - 26.3
2-Tridecanone	17.05	15.9 - 18.3
2-Tetradecanone	26.41	18.7 - 37.3
2-Pentadecanone	578.75	552 - 607

These data show a marked relationship between chain length and toxicity to *H. zea* larvae suggesting that activity is contingent upon lipophilicity. Following the example of Hansch (6) and Martin (7), the logarithm of the octanol-water partition coefficient (log P), a measure of lipophilicity, was plotted against the logarithm of toxicity (log $1/LC_{50}$). The resulting plot (Fig. 1) resembles a parabola and an equation was fit to the data using curvilinear regression. For chain lengths of 9-14 carbons, this regression explains 97% of the variation in toxicity among congeners as a function of the octanol-water partition coefficient. Inclusion of 2-pentadecanone in the model lowers the R^2 value from 0.97 to 0.78. A parabolic relationship of this type has been explained by assuming that the toxicity of a congener depends upon the probability that the molecule will reach the site of action. This probability depends at least in part on the ability of the congener to pass through lipid barriers such as the cuticle and the cell membranes. This ability is determined by the lipophilicity of the compound as measured by P. The probability of a compound reaching the active site depends heavily upon this value (Refs. 7 & 8). The peculiarity exhibited by 2-pentadecanone may result from steric effects due to size, although no data relating to this point are available.

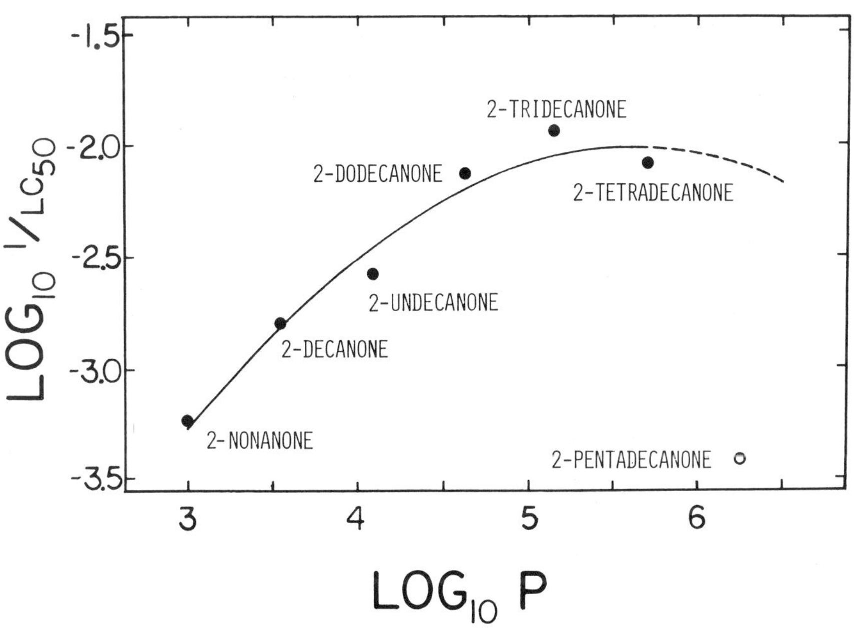

Fig. 1 Relationship between toxicity (=$1/LC_{50}$ in $nmol/cm^2$) and lipophilicity (as indicated by partition coefficient, P) of methyl-2-keytones.

Carbonyl position and toxicity

The preceeding model predicts that the position of the carbonyl carbon in the tridecanone molecule will not affect toxicity since it does not alter P. In fact, 2-, 3-, 5-, and 7-tridecanone do not differ significantly in toxicity (Table 4).

TABLE 4. LC_{50} values for tridecanones varying in position of the carbonyl carbon: *Heliothis zea*

Compound	LC_{50} $\mu g/cm^2$	95% CI
2-Tridecanone	17.05	15.9 - 18.3
3-Tridecanone	16.31	15.3 - 17.4
5-Tridecanone	19.15	18.3 - 20.0
7-Tridecanone	17.16	17.6 - 21.3

Foliage of *L. hirsutum f. glabratum* is known to contain 2-heptanone, 2-undecanone and 2-dodecanone in addition to 2-tridecanone. However, in the insect resistant accession PI 134417, 2-tridecanone is the major component of the essential oil (Ref. 9). It is undoubtedly of evolutionary significance that the most abundant of several toxic keytones present in the essential oil is the one most toxic to insects. The model in Fig. 1 predicts that 2-tetradecanone should be as toxic as 2-tridecanone, although the former is absent from the essential oil. Presumably, a defense based upon 2-tetradecanone would involve a greater commitment of plant resources than one based upon the equally toxic 2-tridecanone.

RELATIONSHIP OF 2-TRIDECANONE AND INSECT RESISTANCE

The preceeding studies showing that 2-tridecanone is involved in the resistance of *L. hirsutum f. glabratum* to *H. zea*, *M. sexta* and *L. decemlineata* represent a classical approach to the isolation and identification of a biologically active substance. They demonstrate that the resistance factor(s) is associated with the glandular trichomes and that the trichome tips contain only a single acutely toxic compound, 2-tridecanone, which is present in apparently sufficient quantities to account for the observed resistance to all three species. This is seemingly clear evidence that 2-tridecanone is the chemical responsible for the resistance of PI 134417. If this hypothesis is valid, then the level of resistance to all three species should reflect the levels of 2-tridecanone on the foliage of plants in populations segregating for 2-tridecanone abundance, or on plants grown under conditions which enhance or diminish the levels of 2-tridecanone present.

Influence of daylength on expression of resistance

Kennedy et al. (Ref. 4) demonstrated that the levels of 2-tridecanone and *M. sexta* resistance in PI 134417 are affected by the light regime under which the plant is grown. In a series of experiments to test the hypothesis that resistance to all three species varies in response to 2-tridecanone levels, PI 134417 plants were raised under light regimes varying in daylength. All plants were raised under nine hours of photosynthetically active radiation. Long days were achieved by interrupting the dark period with two hours of low intensity photomorphogenically active radiation. This avoided the confounding effects of different levels of photosynthesis under long and short days.

The light regime under which the plants were raised had no effect on the susceptibility of *L. esculentum*, the cultivated tomato, as indicated by larval survival. On PI 134417, however, mortality of *M. sexta* and *L. decemlineata* was significantly greater when the plants were grown under a long day regime than when grown under a short day regime. Mortality of *H. zea* did not show a similar, statistically significant response (Table 5).

The mortality of *M. sexta* and *L. decemlineata* reflected the amount of 2-tridecanone per cm^2 leaflet surface, but this was not so for *H. zea* (Table 6). 2-Tridecanone was more abundant in foliage of plants grown under long days. The density of glandular trichomes was also influenced by the daylength under which the PI 134417 plants were raised and it is really the effect of light on trichome density which accounts for its effects on 2-tridecanone level. The amount of 2-tridecanone per trichome tip did not differ significantly between daylengths (Table 6).

TABLE 5. Effect of daylength on insect resistance of *L. hirsutum f. glabratum* - PI 134417

	Mean Percent Mortality		
Daylength	*M. sexta*	*L. decemlineata*	*H. zea*
Long	54	58	78
Short	35*	23*	67 (NS)

* Means for a given species significantly different at $P \leq 0.01$.

TABLE 6. Effect of daylength on 2-tridecanone abundance and glandular trichome density

	Amount of 2-tridecanone		Number of
Daylength	$\mu g/cm^2$	ng/trichome tip	Trichomes/mm^2
Long	16.7	3.2	29.3
Short	7.3*	2.6 (NS)	13.9*

* Means within a column significantly different $P \leq 0.01$.

Involvement of other factors in *H. zea* resistance

The fact that mortality of *M. sexta* and *L. decemlineata* on foliage from plants grown under different daylengths reflected the levels of 2-tridecanone associated with the foliage of these plants provides additional evidence for the role of 2-tridecanone in the resistance of PI 134417 to those species. The absence of a relationship between abundance of 2-tridecanone and mortality of *H. zea* is surprising given its toxicity to *H. zea* and the large quantities that are present. Clearly, other factors are involved in the resistance to *H. zea*.

One possible explanation for the apparent absence of 2-tridecanone involvement is that the larvae are not actually exposed to a lethal dose of 2-tridecanone, although potentially lethal quantities are present in the trichome tips. To obtain an estimate of the relative dosage of 2-tridecanone *H. zea* larvae received on resistant foliage, newly-eclosed larvae were placed on resistant foliage and observed continuously to monitor their behavior and record the number of trichomes disrupted. These observations revealed many of the larvae became incapacitated and convulsive even though they did not disrupt any trichome tips. There was no easily discernible relationship between larval incapacitation and the dosage of 2-tridecanone received, as measured by the number of trichome tips discharged.

2-Tridecanone is toxic to *H. zea* by fumigant action (Ref. 10). Gas chromatographic analysis of samples of air surrounding PI 134417 foliage indicated the presence of 2-tridecanone vapors. These vapors likely account for the incapacitation of larvae which did not disrupt any trichome tips.

Recovery of incapacitated larvae

Continued observation of *H. zea* larvae on resistant foliage over a period of several hours indicated that many of the initially incapacitated larvae recovered (Fig. 2). Recovery of this type suggests the involvement of an inducible detoxification mechanism. This possibility is presently under investigation.

CONCLUSIONS

Data presented clearly indicate that 2-tridecanone, which is acutely toxic to all three insect species, is the principal factor responsible for the resistance to *M. sexta* and, very probably, for the resistance to *L. decemlineata*, but is not the principal factor responsible for resistance to *H. zea*. The results point out the limitations of relying solely on chemical isolation and bioassay data using uniform plant material when attempting to identify a chemical or group of chemicals causing insect resistance in a plant. Where possible, the insect's response and the level of the proposed resistance factor should be measured for a number of plants differing in their level of insect resistance. Such plants can be obtained from populations segregating for resistance or by growing them under a variety of conditions which alter the expression of resistance.

In the present study the method used for bioassaying the toxic factor, while effective for isolating the toxic chemical, did not realistically simulate the way in which insect larvae are exposed to 2-tridecanone on the resistant foliage. Although the procedure worked well for *M. sexta*, it gave misleading results for *H. zea*. With the latter, confinement on treated filter paper apparently resulted in exposure to unrealistically high dosages of 2-tridecanone and overwhelmed ability to recover. When attempting to assign a causal function to a biologically active chemical, it is extremely important that the bioassays used accurately mimic the insect's natural exposure to the chemical under investigation. An in-depth understanding of the insect's response to the plants under study greatly facilitates the design of meaningful bioassays and the interpretation of experimental results.

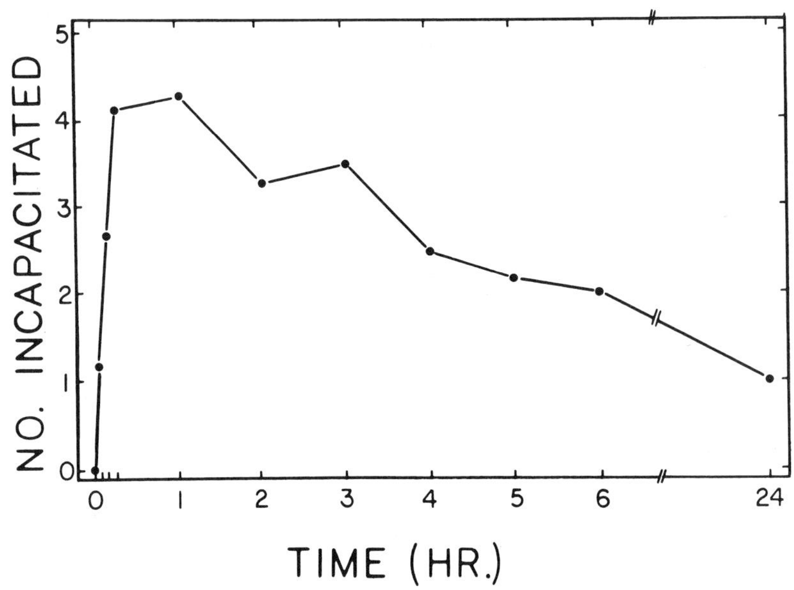

Fig. 2 Incapacitation and recovery of first instar *H. zea* larvae on foliage of PI 134417

Acknowledgement - This material is based upon work supported in part by the U.S. Department of Agriculture under Agreement No. 58-7B30-1-281.

REFERENCES

1. G. G. Kennedy and W. R. Henderson. J. Amer. Soc. Hort. Sci. 103:334-336 (1978).
2. G. G. Kennedy and R. T. Yamamoto. Ent. exp. & appl. 26:121-126 (1979).
3. W. G. Williams, G. G. Kennedy, R. T. Yamamoto, J. D. Thacker and J. Bordner. Science 207:888-889 (1980).
4. G. G. Kennedy, R. T. Yamamoto, M. B. Dimock, W. G. Williams and J. Bordner. J. Chem. Ecol. 7:707-716.
5. M. B. Dimock, G. G. Kennedy and W. G. Williams. J. Chem. Ecol. 8:(in press) (1982).
6. C. Hansch. Acc. Chem. Res. 2:232-239 (1969).
7. Y. C. Martin. Quantitative Drug Design: A Critical Introduction. Marcel Dekker, Inc., New York (1978).
8. J. W. McFarland. J. Med. Chem. 13:1192-1196 (1970).
9. R. K. Soost, R. W. Scora and J. J. Sims. Proc. Amer. Soc. Hort. Sci. 92:568-571 (1968).
10. M. B. Dimock and G. G. Kennedy. Ent. exp. & appl. 29 (in review) (1982).

MILBEMYCIN: A FAMILY OF MACROLIDE ANTIBIOTICS WITH INSECTICIDAL ACTIVITY

Hiroshi Mishima

Fermentation Research Laboratories, Sankyo Co. Ltd., Hiromachi, Shinagawa-ku, Tokyo, Japan

Abstract - The milbemycins, which exhibit a broad spectrum of agricultural pesticidal activity, were isolated from the culture broth of *Streptomyces hygroscopicus* subsp. *aureolacrimosus* subsp. nov. The milbemycins were identified as a series of closely related macrocyclic lactone derivatives, which lacked significant antibacterial or antifungal activity.

INTRODUCTION

Recently, attention has been focused on the utilization of antibiotics for controlling pests, and several reports dealing with the pesticidal activity of antibiotics have appeared.

Aoki, in the course of a screening program in 1973 directed toward the discovery of new pesticidal antibiotics using the two-spotted spider mite as a test insect, found that the metabolite produced by Streptomycete, strain B-41-146, exhibited an extraordinary potency against pests of various orders. The antibiotic, designated as milbemycin, consisted of a mixture of naturally occurring derivatives of a novel 16-membered macrocyclic lactone (Ref. 1 & 2).

Subsequently, the oleandosyl oleandosyloxy compounds(avermectin) of milbemycin were isolated from the mycelium of *Streptomyces avermitilis* by a Merk Sharp & Dohme research group(Ref. 4).

STUDIES ON MILBEMYCIN

The taxonomic and fermentation studies, isolation, structure determination, stereochemistry, biosynthesis, and insecticidal activity of milbemycins are outlined.

Taxonomic studies

The morphological and cultural characteristics of strain B-41-146 were determined by use of the media and methods described by Shirling and Gottlieb. The strain was identified as a new species of *Streptomyces hygroscopicus* and designated as *S. hygroscopicus* subsp. *aureolacrimosus* subsp. nov.

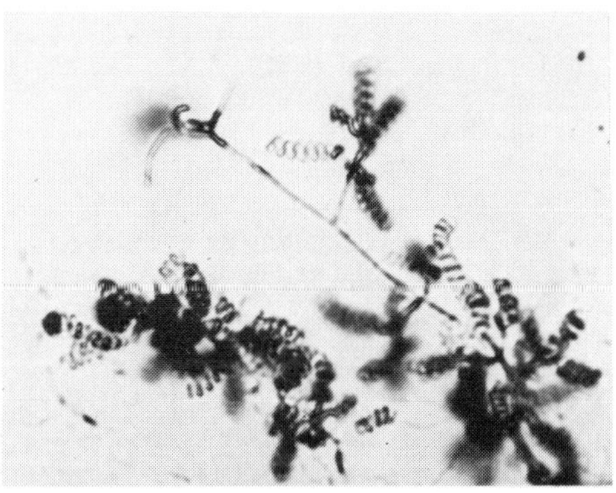

Fig. 1. Scanning electron micrograph of strain B-41-146.

Fermentation studies

The medium used for the production of milbemycin contained the following ingredients(in g/1,000 *ml* water): glucose 40, starch 5, soybean meal 10, corn-steep liquor 2, and NaCl 3. The pH of the medium was adjusted to 6.8 before sterilization. One *l* of the seed culture, grown in 2-liter Erlenmeyer flasks on a rotary shaker(220 rpm, 7 cm) at 28°C for 2 days, was transferred to a 30-liter jar-fermentor with 20 *l* of the medium and fermentation was conducted at 28°C for 10 days, with aeration of 10 *l*/min, agitation of 150 rpm and inner pressure of 0.5 kg/cm^2.

The packed cell volume in the culture broth increased in the first 3 days and remained constant thereafter. The antibiotics were first detected in the broth after 3 days cultivation and increased at a linear rate for the next 6 days. The yield was a maximum at 9 days.

To determine the amount of milbemycins produced, a concentrated extract of the whole culture broth was applied to a silica-gel 60-F_{254} plate and developed with a solvent system composed of CCl_4 and dioxane(82:18). For quantitative assay, the plate was scanned at 240 nm with a dual-wavelength TLC scanner.

Isolation

The cake, obtained by filtration of fermentation broth(120 *l*) containing milbemycin, was extracted twice with methanol(50 *l*). After adding water(50 *l*), the resulting aqueous MeOH was extracted twice with n-hexane(100 *l*). The n-hexane was evaporated under reduced pressure and the residue was dissolved in 2 *l* of MeOH. The resulting solution was allowed to stand overnight at -20°C and the precipitate was removed by filtration. The filtrate was concentrated to obtain 90 g of a brown oily substance. A practical scheme for the isolation of all of the components of milbemycin complex are shown in Fig. 2.

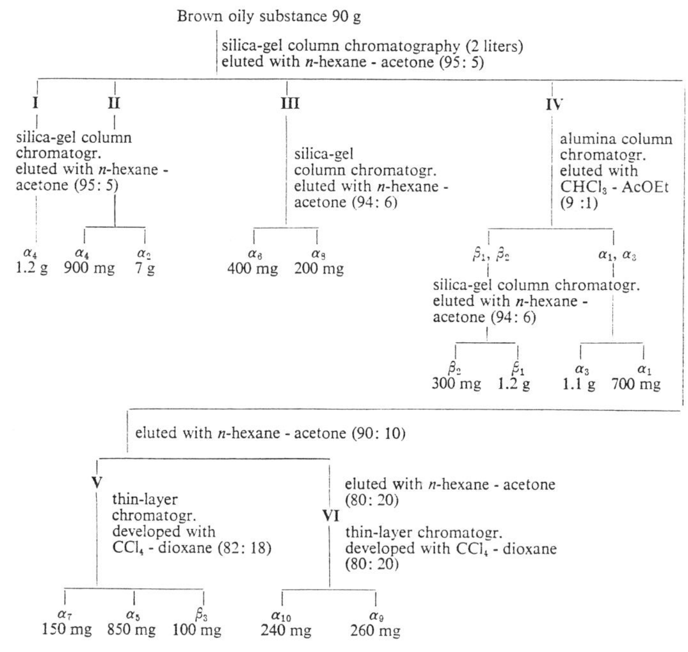

Fig. 2. Separation of milbemycins.

According to the fermentation development, including medium modification and strain improvement, qualitative and quantitative changes in milbemycin components were observed, including disappearance of some components and production of new related compounds.

Structure determination

For the sake of convenience, all components were classified into two groups, α and β series. The degree of unsaturation of the components(α_1 through α_4) was one more than those of β_1 or β_2. The structures of two samples (α_3 and β_1) selected from each series were determined by X-ray diffraction.

On treatment with p-bromophenylisocyanate, α_3 and β_1 gave rise to crystalline α_3 and β_1 p-bromophenylurethane, respectively. The former substance was recrystallized from methanol and the space group belongs to $P2_12_12_1$. A total of 1829 reflections were collected with a 2θ range of 50° using Mo Kα radiation. Structure determination was done by a heavy atom method and all heavy atoms were refined by the block diagonal least-squares method. Difference synthesis could not reveal the hydrogen atoms, since all atoms had rather large temperature factors.

The space group of the latter substance belonged to $P4_1$ and 1884 independent reflections were collected. The structure was solved by the usual heavy atom technique and was currently refined by a block-diagonal least squares method. As can be seen in Fig.6, although the substances of α series have a tetrahydrofuran ring in the molecule, the components belonging to β series lack this feature.

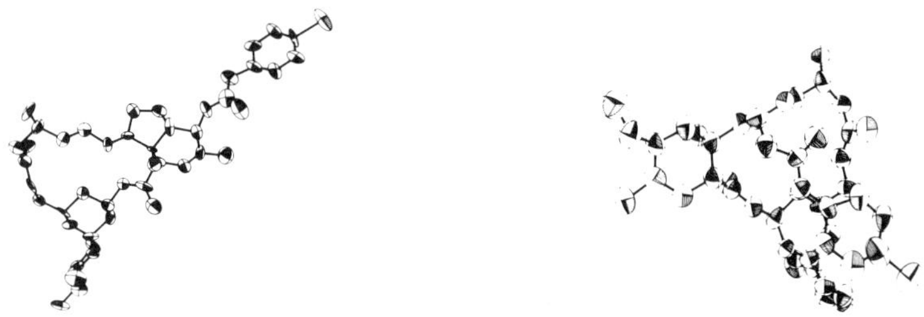

Fig. 3. A computer-generated drawing of milbemycin α_3(left) and β_1(right) with hydrogens omitted for clarity.

The UV spectra of the congeners of the α-series showed a characteristic maximum at 244-247 nm, having two shoulders in the region of 238-254 nm due to a diene chromophore, and those of the compounds(α_9, α_{10}, and F) with the pyrrole ring exhibited an additional maximum at 266 nm. In contrast, the UV spectra of the congeners of the β-series, excluding β_3, showed a single maximum at 245-247 nm. In all IR spectra of milbemycins except for β_3, absorption bands due to hydroxy and the 16-membered lactone groups were observed at 3330-3600 cm^{-1} and 1707-1710 cm^{-1} , respectively. In addition to these absorption bands, the IR spectra of α_5 through α_8 showed on absorption band at 1721-1722 cm^{-1} due to ester group.

Comparison of the mass spectra, with the aid of other spectra including IR, UV, and ^{1}H and ^{13}C NMR was especially useful in the structure determination of other congeners.

The mass spectrum of milbemycin showed relatively few prominent fragment ions in addition to an intense molecular ion. On the basis of the structure elucidated by X-ray analysis, the mass fragmentation pattern could be rationalised in terms of typical fragmentation such as retro Diels-Alder, ester elimination, allyl fission and cleavage α- to an oxygen atom; the structures of diagnostic fragment ions are represented as shown in Fig. 4. The correctness of ionic structures was supported by careful inspection of the corresponding ^{13}C enriched metabolites obtained by biosynthetic studies(*vide infra*).

Comparison of the mass spectrum of α_3($C_{32}H_{46}O_7$, M^+ 542) and α_1($C_{31}H_{44}O_7$, M^+ 528) showed that m/z values of a, b, and c ions of α_1 were 14 mass units less than those of α_3. This indicates clearly that in the structure of α_1 a methyl group(3H, d, 1.13 ppm) is attached at C-25 instead of the ethyl group. In the case of β_1 and β_2, m/z values of a, b, and c ions of β_2 were 14 mass units more than those of β_1. This again indicates that in the structure of β_2 an ethyl group(3H, t, 0.82 ppm) is attached at C-25 instead of the methyl group.

The mass spectra of α_2($C_{32}H_{46}O_7$, M^+ 542) and α_4($C_{31}H_{48}O_7$, M^+ 556) coincided completely with those of α_1 and α_3, respectively, except for their molecular ions, indicating that the methyl group is part of a fragment eliminated from the molecular ion by retro Diels-Alder and moreover must exist as a methoxy group(3H, s, 3.48, 58.77 ppm). Further confirmation was found in the fact that the same dimethoxy derivative was prepared from α_1 and α_3 by treatment with MeI and Ag_2O.

Chemical transformation by $NaBH_4$ reduction served to relate milbemycin J and K to α_1 and α_3 respectively.

In a similar manner, the structure of the other constituents was deduced from careful comparison of the pattern of mass fragmentation and NMR spectroscopic data. NMR assignments are based on general chemical shift considerations, decoupling experiments(^{1}H NMR), and the pattern observed in proton coupled and selective proton decoupled experiments (^{13}C NMR). It became clear that the main variation of the structures exists in the substituents at C-4 and 5 or the cyclohexane and spiroketal moiety.

Stereochemistry

In order to deduce the absolute configuration of the cyclic secondary alcohol at C-5, Mills' rule was employed together with the benzoate sector rule, independently of X-ray crystallography.

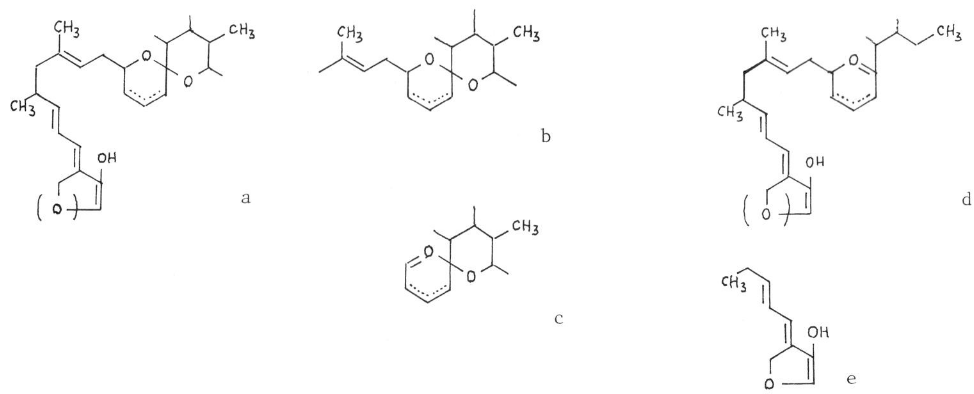

Fig. 4. Diagnostic ion structures of mass spectrum

An α,β-unsaturated ketone obtained by oxidation of milbemycin D with Sarett reagent was reduced by $NaBH_4$ to generate, stereoselectively, the starting material D, probably due to the steric hindrance of the tetrahydrofuran ring and/or the participation of the tertiary hydroxyl group at C-7. For preparation of the C-5 epimer of D, the allylic mesylate was subjected to S_N2 displacement with tetraethylammonium formate followed by hydrolysis with $NaHCO_3$, giving the epimeric alcohol.

The specific rotation of D($[\alpha]_D$ -105°) and its acetate(-92°) were more laevorotatory than the epimer($[\alpha]_D$ -132°) and its acetate(-119°), respectively, showing that the stereochemistry of C-5 is the R configuration. The same conclusion was also supported by CD measurement of the p-dimethylaminobenzoates prepared from the epimeric pair. Each CD of p-dimethylaminobenzoates exhibited an opposite Cotton effect and the benzoate of natural D gave rise to a positive Cotton effect at 295 nm.

The relative as well as the absolute configuration of all centers of 13-deoxyavermectin are shown to be identical with those of milbemycin(Ref. 4).

Biosynthesis

The origin of the carbon skeleton of the macrocyclic lactone ring of milbemycins was studied in shake cultures of the producing organism by feeding the cultures with ^{13}C labelled precursors followed by ^{13}C NMR analysis of the product.

On the basis of time course studies of milbemycin formation in these cultures, the ^{13}C enriched precursors, acetate-1-^{13}C, propionate-1-^{13}C and -3-^{13}C, and DL-valine-2-^{13}C, were added independently to the cultures in the production medium at about 72 hrs after inoculation, and incubation was continued for an additional 48 hrs. Milbemycins α_2, α_4, and D could be isolated from the culture broth in total yields of about 400 mg/*l* by extraction with methanol and purification by column chromatography using Rober Si-60 and PR-8.

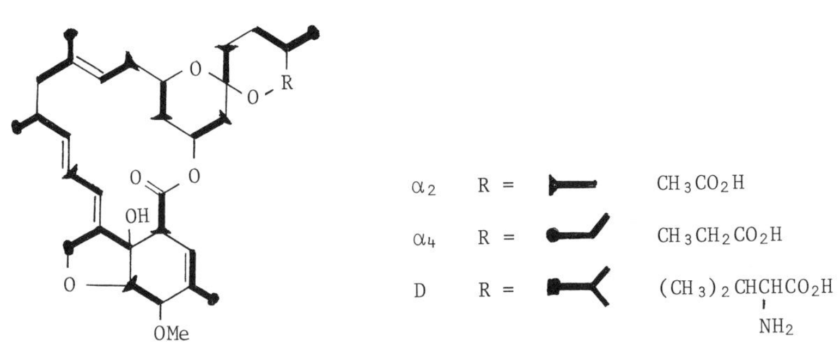

Fig. 5. Biogenesis of milbemycin α_2, α_4, and D.

The 400 MHz ^{13}C NMR spectra of α_2, α_4, and D constituents of milbemycin was well-resolved and showed that the carbons of its carbon skeleton are derived from 7 acetates and 5 propionates, as one would assume *a priori*. It was also shown that the methyl, ethyl, and isopropyl substituents at C-25 and its side chain are derived from

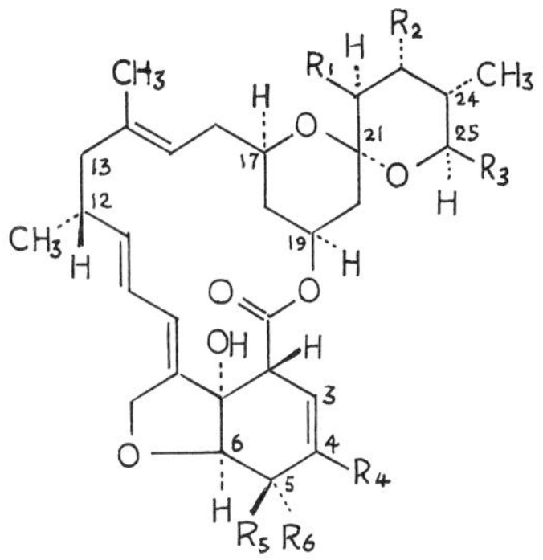

α series of milbemycin

	R_1	R_2	R_3	R_4	R_5	R_6
α_1	H	H	CH_3	CH_3	OH	H
α_2	H	H	CH_3	CH_3	OCH_3	H
α_3	H	H	C_2H_5	CH_3	OH	H
α_4	H	H	C_2H_5	CH_3	OCH_3	H
α_5	OH	$OCOCH(CH_3)C_4H_9$	CH_3	CH_3	OH	H
α_6	OH	$OCOCH(CH_3)C_4H_9$	CH_3	CH_3	OCH_3	H
α_7	OH	$OCOCH(CH_3)C_4H_9$	C_2H_5	CH_3	OH	H
α_8	OH	$OCOCH(CH_3)C_4H_9$	C_2H_5	CH_3	OCH_3	H
α_9	H	H	CH_3	CH_2OCO-(NH)	OH	H
α_{10}	H	H	C_2H_5	CH_2OCO-(NH)	OH	H
D	H	H	$CH(CH_3)_2$	CH_3	OH	H
F	H	H	$CH(CH_3)_2$	CH_2OCO-(NH)	OH	H
G	H	H	$CH(CH_3)_2$	CH_3	OCH_3	H
J	H	H	CH_3	CH_3	=O	
K	H	H	C_2H_5	CH_3	=O	

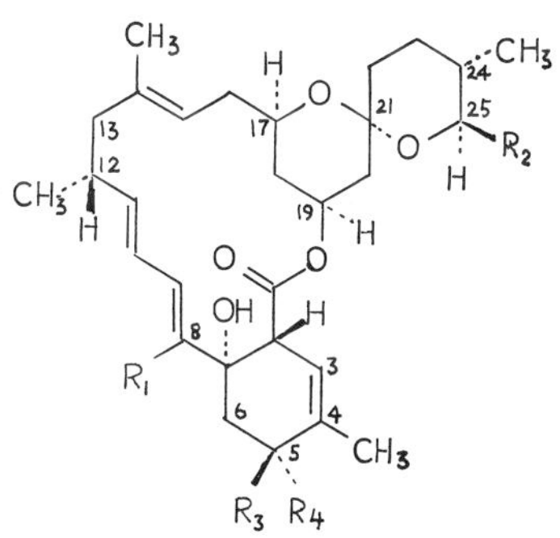

β series of milbemycin

	R_1	R_2	R_3	R_4
β_1	CH_2OH	CH_3	OCH_3	H
β_2	CH_2OH	C_2H_5	OCH_3	H
E	CH_2OH	$CH(CH_3)_2$	OCH_3	H
H	CH_3	$CH(CH_3)_2$	=O	

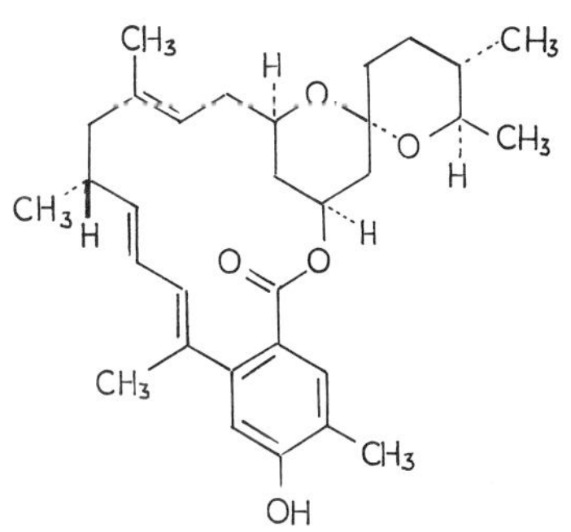

β_3

Fig. 6.

acetate, propionate, and DL-valine, respectively, and that the methyl carbon of the methoxy group at C-5 was enriched by incorporation of L-methionine-methyl-^{13}C.

It is also noteworthy that the incorporation ratio of ^{13}C enriched precursor is conspicuously high at the probable primer unit of C-25 compared with other carbons.

In the mass spectrum of D enriched by incorporation of DL-valine-2-^{13}C, a remarkable increase(about 40%) of abundance at m/z 557, 429, 411, 210, and 182 was observed. Since this indicates retention of the isopropyl group at C-25 in M^+ and fragment ions a, b, and c, conclusive evidence was provided for the interpretation of the mass fragment pattern of milbemycin.

Insecticidal activity

The name milbemycin originated from its high potency against mites of various orders. Most of the twenty components of these natural product exhibited a broad spectrum of activity against agricultural pests such as aphids, mites, tent caterpillars, intestinal worms, and other parasites that prey on crops and livestock. They are promising as agricultural pesticide, because of their potent activity without toxicity to plants and animals at effective dosages. For example, milbemycin D was highly effective against all stages in the life cycle of the two-spotted spider mite and the motile stage of the citrus red mite. When applied in solution directly onto adult and nymphal populations on foliage, D showed and LD_{50} of 0.3 ppm for the former and an LD_{50} of 0.03 ppm for the latter.

Although eggs of the mites were much less sensitive to milbemycin, the antibiotic in petroleum oil showed a remarkable degree of synergistic activity. This formulation was remarkably effective in controlling field populations of the citrus red mite when sprayed on mandarin orange orchards(Ref. 3).

Addendum

A recent article informed that the total synthesis of milbemycin β_3 was accomplished by two research groups(Ref. 5).

Acknowledgement - The above research into milbemycin was carried out in cooperation with the staff of the research laboratories of Sankyo Co. Ltd., for whose help the author is very grateful. He is grateful to Dr. A. Aoki, Hokkai Sankyo Co. Ltd., who found Streptomycete, strain B-41-146 and the biological activities of the metabolite, and also thanks to Prof. S. Okuda, Institute of Applied Microbiology of Tokyo University, for the discussion with respect to the biosynthetic studies.

REFERENCES

1. H. Mishima, M. Kurabayashi, C. Tamura, S. Sato, H. Kuwano, and A. Saito, Tetrahedron Letters, 711(1975)
2. Y. Takiguchi, H. Mishima, M. Okuda, M. Terao, A. Aoki, and R. Fukuda, J. Antibiotics, 33, 1120(1980)
3. S. Yamanoto, A. Nishida, A. Aoki, Jap. J. appl. Ent. Zool., 25, 183(1981)
   S. Yamamoto, A. Nishida, ibid., 25, 286(1981)
   S. Yamamoto, K. Ishikawa, A. Nishida, ibid., 26, 29(1982)
4. G. Albers-Schonberg, B. H. Arison, J. C. Chabala, A. W. Douglas, P. Eskola, M. H. Fisher, A. Lusi, H. Mrozik, J. L. Smith, and R. L. Tolman, J. Am. Chem. Soc., 103 4216(1981)
   J. P. Springer, B. H. Arison, H. H. Hirchfield, and K. Hoogsteen, ibid., 103, 4221 (1981)
   H. Mrozik, P. Eskola, B. H. Arison, G. Albers-Schonberg, and M. H. Fisher, J. Org. Chem., 47, 489(1982) and references cited therein.
5. C&EN News, 40, April 19(1982)

REGULATORY SUBSTANCES IN SEXUAL REPRODUCTION OF FUNGI

Akira Sakurai and Yuji Kamiya

The Institute of Physical and Chemical Research, Wako-shi, Saitama-ken 351, Japan

Abstract - Substances regulating sexual reproduction in yeasts have been investigated chemically. From cells of mating type α each of two species of *Saccharomyces*, peptides were isolated which induce sexual agglutinability in cells of the opposite mating type *a*. The peptides were found to differ in their amino-acid sequences but showed cross interaction between the two species of yeasts. In *Rhodosporidium*, a novel lipopeptide, rhodotorucine *A*, was found, produced by cells of mating type *A* to induce mating tube formation in the opposite mating type *a* cells. Rhodotorucine *A* was also shown to be metabolized specifically by *a* cells into two inactive peptide fragments.

INTRODUCTION

Many kinds of fungi have a sexual reproduction stage in their life cycles. This sexual process involves special regulation systems for sexual differentiation of cells and recognition and exchange of information between mating partner cells, indicative of the presence of regulatory substances. Chemical studies of the regulation systems are of considerable interest, since they may lead to discovery of new types of bio-active substances regulating the life cycles of organisms. Recently, terpenes and steroids were isolated as regulatory substances in the sexual reproduction of fungi belong *Phycomycetes* group, such as sirenin from *Allomyces*; antheridiol and oogoniols from *Achlya* and trisporic acids from *Mucor* (1). We have been studying the regulating substances involved in the mating reaction of Ascomyceteous and Heterobasidiomyceteous yeasts, and three kinds of peptide were isolated as the active principles. These substances are tentatively called mating pheromones, since they are secreted from a mating type cell to act on the mating partner. The peptides isolated as mating pheromones were found to have a common biological function in regulation of cell differentiation and DNA synthesis in the cell.

MATING PHEROMONES OF SACCHAROMYCES YEASTS

One of the most representative yeast; *Saccharomyces*, used commonly in alcoholic fermentation, belongs to *Ascomycetes* and has a sexual reproduction stage in which two haploid cells designated as *a* and α mating types are formed from ascospores of the heterothallic strains. Conjugation takes place between these two mating type cells to form diploid cells through the process of sexual agglutination, cell fusion and karyogamy as shown in Fig. 1: during this process, it has been suggested (2) that secretion of substances from each mating type of cell takes place.

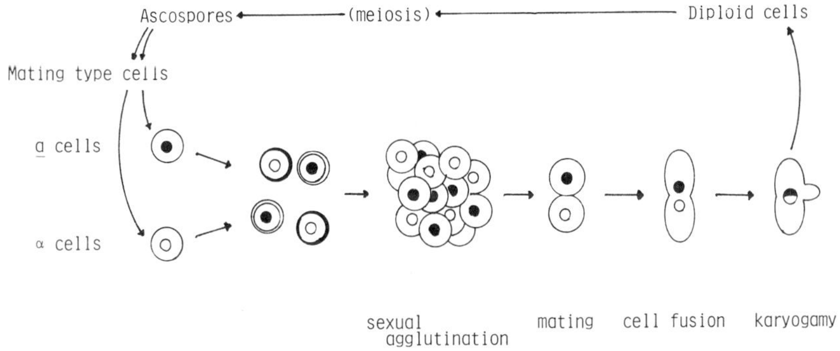

Fig. 1 Mating process in *Saccharomyces*

α Substance-I (α factor) of *Saccharomyces cerevisiae*

Duntze and his co-workers (3) confirmed that the mating type α cells of *S. cerevisiae* secrete some factor which causes morphological changes and inhibition of cell division in the opposite mating type *a* cells. They named it as α factor and isolated four peptides as the active principles. On the other hand, Yanagishima and his co-worker (4) discovered the presence of a regulatory substance in the sexual agglutination reaction of the mating process. They found that a strain of *a* cells did not immediately cause sexual agglutination when mixed with α cells, but that its ability do so was induced by a substance secreted by α cells. We tried to isolate the active principle, named α substance-I, from cultures of α cells of *S. cerevisiae*.

The biological activity of α substance-I was determined by the procedure shown in Fig. 2. *a* Cells were cultured for 2 hr in a medium containing the test sample to induce sexual agglutinability and then mixed with α cells. Before mixing, both cells were killed by heating at 100 °C for 5 min or by adding 10 ppm of cycloheximide to prevent the further induction of agglutinability. If the test sample had biological activity, cell agglutination reaction was observed within 30 min.

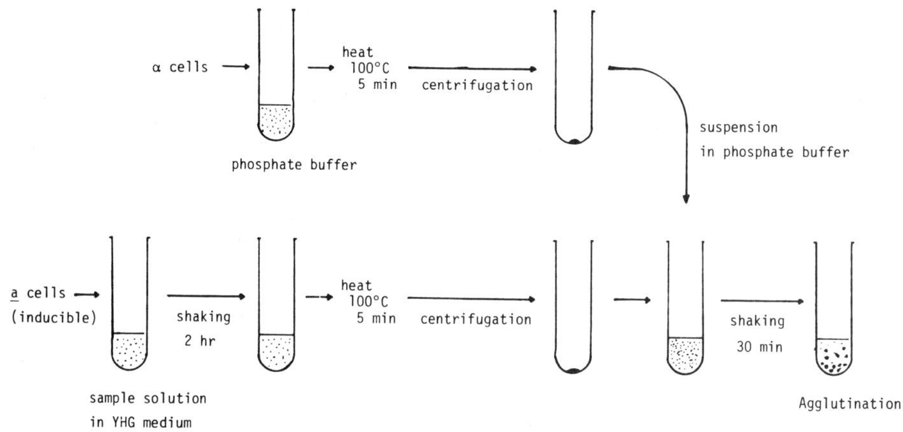

Fig. 2 Bioassay procedure for detection of ability to induce sexual agglutinability in *a* cells of *Saccharomyces*.

We succeeded in isolating 1.1 mg of a peptide as the main active principle from a 300 liter culture of α cells of *S. cerevisiae*. The peptide showed the activity in induction of sexual agglutinability in *a* cells at a concentration of 0.8 ng/ml and is designated as α substance-IA: the amino acid sequence was determined in 1976 as shown below (5).

H-His-Trp-Leu-Gln-Leu-Lys-Pro-Gly-Gln-Pro-Met-Tyr-OH

α Substance-IA

The amino acid sequence of α substance-IA was found to be identical with that of α2 of the α factors isolated by Duntze and his co-workers (6). Thus, in the mating process in *S. cerevisiae*, the mating pheromone secreted by α cells is shown to play several roles; induction of sexual agglutinability, morphological change and inhibition of cell division by arresting DNA synthesis in the opposite mating type *a* cells.

αk Substance of *Saccharomyces kluyveri*

Further investigation of other heterothallic *Saccharomyces* led to the finding that haploid type cell of *S. kluyveri* produces a substance inducing sexual agglutinability in *a* cells of *S. cerevisiae*. This haploid cell, thus denoted as mating type α of *S. kluyveri*, does not form a hybrid with any cells of *S. cerevisiae*. The above evidence suggests the existence of cross interaction of mating pheromones between *S. cerevisiae* and *kluyveri*. We undertook the isolation of the active principle, named αk substance, from the culture of α cells of *S. kluyveri*. Biological activity was determined in the same way shown in Fig. 2.

Isolation. The culture filtrate of α cells (*S. kluyveri* IFO 1894) was treated with Amberlite CG-50 column. The active fraction, eluted with acidic ethanol, was purified as shown in Fig. 3. Finally, 0.75 mg of pure active αk substance was obtained from 70 liter of the culture filtrate and was found by chromatographic analyses (7) to be a peptide different to that from *S. cerevisiae*, α substance-IA.

Culture filtrate (70 liters)
↓
Adsorbed on Amberlite CG-50
↓ washed with H_2O and EtOH-H_2O (1:1)
eluted with EtOH-H_2O-HCl (80:20:0.1)
Countercurrent distribution (10 transfers)
↓ with n-BuOH-AcOH-H_2O (4:1:5)
Sephadex LH-20 chromatography with MeOH-AcOH (98:2)
↓
Partition chromatography on Sehadex G-25
↓ with n-BuOH-n-PrOH-0.5M AcOH
Sephadex G-25 chromatography with 10% AcOH-n-BuOH (9:1)
↓
Fractogel PGM 2000 Chromatography with MeOH-1M AcOH (1:1)
↓
Fractogel PGM 2000 Chromatography with MeOH-1M AcOH (2:8)
↓
α_k Substance (0.75 mg)

Isolation procedure for α_k substance

Fig. 3 Isolation procedure for αk substance

Structural analysis. From the amino acid analysis of the acid hydrolyzate, αk substance was considered to be a peptide composed of Ser 2, Glu 1, Pro 1, Gly 1, Met 1, Leu 1, Tyr 1, Phe 1, Lys 1, His 1 and Trp 1. Micro-scale Edman-dansyl degradation was applied to sequence analyses of αk substance and its trypsin digest, and an amino acid sequence shown below was revealed.

(His)-Trp-Leu-Ser-Phe-Ser-Lys-Gly-Glu-Pro-Met(O)-Tyr-OH

Table 1. FD mass spectra of αk substance and its enzymatic digests

	$[M+H]^+$ observed, m/z	Calculated
α_k Substance	1696	198+1497[His-Trp-Leu-Ser-Phe-Ser-Lys-Gly-Glu-Pro-Met(O)-Tyr]+H
Tryptic digest	1102	198+903[His-Trp-Leu-Ser-Phe-Ser-Lys]+H
	612	611[Gly-Glu-Pro-Met(O)-Tyr]+H
Chymotryptic digest	653	198+464[His-Trp-Leu]+H
	253	252[Ser-Phe]+H
	366	365[Leu-Ser-Phe]+H
	826	825[Ser-Lys-Gly-Glu-Pro-Met(O)-Tyr]+H

N-Terminal His was not detected by the dansyl method, but by the Edman procedure; PTH-His was identified as N-terminal amino acid. This evidence suggests that the N-terminal His must be modified somewhat in the peptide. FD mass spectrometric analysis gave the results shown in Table 1. αk Substance gave the ion [M+H] at m/z 1696 which is 198 mass unit larger than that of the peptide with His as N-terminus. In the spectra of trypsin and chymotrypsin digests, the ion from the N-terminal part of the fragments showed values 198 unit larger than that expected for a peptide with a His N-terminus. These results supported the proposed amino-acid sequence and revealed the presence of an unknown residue at N-terminal His. Thus, we proposed the structure for αk substance with an unknown residue (X) at the N-terminus as shown below (8).

X-His-Trp-Leu-Ser-Phe-Ser-Lys-Gly-Glu-Pro-Met(O)-Tyr-OH

αk Substance

αk Substance, thus isolated from the culture of α cells of *S. kluyveri* as the active principle inducing sexual agglutinability in *a* cells of *S. cerevisiae*, was found to induce morphological change in the opposite mating type *a* cells of *S. kluyveri*. Therefore αk substance was shown to be a mating pheromone of *S. kluyveri* and the existence of cross interaction of mating pheromones between *S. kluyveri* and *cerevisiae* was confirmed.

MATING PHEROMONE OF RHODOSPORIDIUM

In 1967, the yeast *Rhodotorula glutinis* was found by Banno (9) to have a sexual reproduction stage in its life cycle and was reclassified as *Rhodosporidium toruloides*, which belongs to *Heterobasidiomycetes*. Two haploid cells of opposite mating types are called *A* and *a* . In the mating process of these haploid cells, mating tubes are formed in each cell and two mating type cells are fused through the mating tubes to form a filamentous dikaryotic mycelium as shown in Fig. 4. Abe and her co-workers (10) showed that in the first stage *A* cells secrete a diffusible substance, named *A* factor, to induce mating tube formation in the opposite mating type *a* cells. The biological activity of *A* factor was detected by exposing *a* cells in agar film to a medium containing active principles for 5 hr and observing mating tubes under a microscope as shown in Fig. 5.

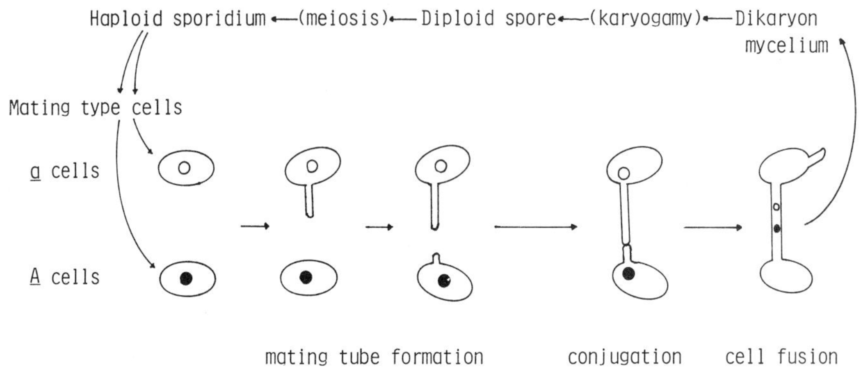

Fig. 4. Life cycle of *Rhodosporidium toruloides*

Isolation of rhodotorucine *A*

The active principle in the culture filtrate of *A* cells of *R. toruloides* was found to be extractable by n-butanol and extracts from a 300 liter culture filtrate were purified as shown in Fig. 6 to obtain 7.5 mg of pure *A* factor. The substance, named rhodotorucine *A*, showed biological activity in induction of mating tube formation in *a* cells at a concentration of 4 - 8 ng/ml, and showed chemical behavior characteristic of peptide.

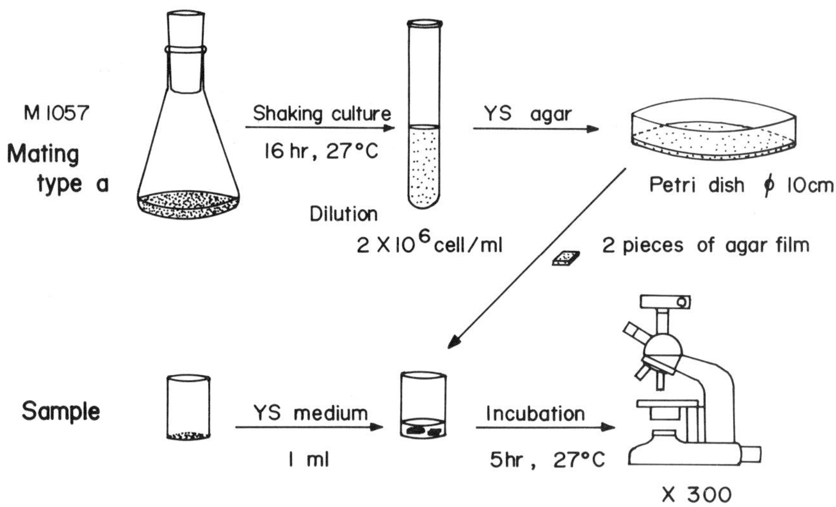

Fig. 5. Bioassay procedure for detection of biological activity in mating tube formation in *a* cells of *Rhodosporidium toruloides*

Chemical structure of rhodotorucine *A*

Amino acid analysis of the acid hydrolyzate gave equimolar amount of Asp, Thr, Ser, Glu, Pro, Gly, Ile, Tyr, Trp and Arg. Besides these amino acids, 0.16 molar equivalent of cystine was detected, suggesting the presence of a modified Cys residue in the peptide. Rhodotorucine *A* was subjected to sequence analysis by micro-scale Edman-dansyl and direct Edman degradations and revealed as having the sequence:

Culture filtrate (300 liters)
↓
Extracted with n-BuOH
↓
Partitioned between benzene-MeOH-H_2O (10:8:2)
↓
Gel filtration on Sephadex LH-20 with MeOH
↓
Gel filtration on Sephadex LH-20 with MeOH-buffer* (7:3)
↓
Countercurrent distributions (9 transfers) with n-BuOH-benzene-MeOH-buffer* (1:2:1:2)
↓
Countercurrent distributions (9 transfers) with benzene-n-PrOH-EtOH-buffer* (4:1:1:2)
↓
Gel filtration on Sephadex LH-20 with MeOH-buffer* (7:3)
↓
Gel filtration on Sephadex LH-20 with MeOH-buffer* (6:4)
↓
Precipitation at 4°C
↓
Reprecipitation from MeOH-H_2O (6:4) at 4°C
↓
Rhodotorucine A (7.3 mg)

*0.01 M ammonium acetate (pH 7.0)

Fig. 6. Isolation procedure for rhodotorucine *A*

H-Tyr-Pro-Glu-Ile-Ser-Trp-Thr-Arg-Asn-Gly-X

Digestion with trypsin gave two peptide fragments; the N-terminal part was an octa-peptide (Tr-1) and C-terminal part a tri-peptide (Tr-2). When the digest was extracted with n-butanol, Tr-2 containing the unknown residue (X) was extracted into the n-butanol phase and was obtained as pure crystals. The FT-PMR and CI-mass spectrometric analyses of Tr-2 disclosed the presence of a novel lipophilic amino acid, S-farnesyl cystein, as the unknown residue (X). Thus, the structure of H-Asn-Gly-Cys(S-farnesyl)-OH was proposed for Tr-2.

The structure of rhodotorucine *A* was thus established as shown below (11). The total synthesis of this novel lipopeptide has been accomplished by Kitada and Fujino (12). Through synthetic studies on rhodotorucine *A* , the peptide without a farnesyl side chain was found to be completely inactive, indicating that the presence of the side chain is essential for biological activity (13).

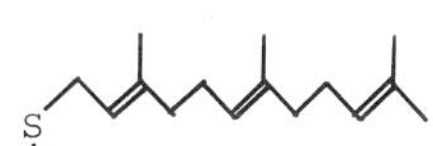

H-Tyr-Pro-Glu-Ile-Ser-Trp-Thr-Arg-Asn-Gly-Cys-OH

Rhodotorucine *A*

Sakagami and his co-workers (14, 15) isolated tremerogens A-10 and a-13 as the mating pheromones of *Tremella mesenterica* which belongs to *Heterobasidiomycetes*. These mating pheromones are also peptides with amino acid sequences different from rhodotorucine *A*, but are found to have the same S-farnesyl cystein residue at their C-terminus. There are no cross interactions in the pheromones between *Rhodosporidium* and *Tremella*, but it is worthy of note that the pheromones in *Heterobasidiomycetes* have a common lipopeptide structure.

Metabolism of rhodotorucine *A*
When rhodotorucine *A* was added to the cell suspension of *a* cells of *R. toruloides*, the biological activity of the supernatant disappeared within a few minutes, suggesting that the peptide is completely adsorbed on *a* cells or metabolized to an inactive form by *a* cells. To study this phenomena, radioactive rhodotorucine *A*s were prepared in the following way. When radioactive amino acids such as [^{35}S] cystein, [^{3}H] tyrosine and [^{14}C] arginine were incubated with *A* cells of *R. toruloides*, each amino acid was incorporated into the peptide, and Cys-labeled, Tyr-labeled and Arg-labeled rhodotorucine *A*s were obtained. Cys-labeled rhodotorucine *A* was rapidly metabolized when it was incubated with *a* cells, and the radioactive metabolite was found to be identical with the peptide fragment Tr-2, obtained by the digestion of rhodotorucine *A* with trypsin. In the case of Tyr-labeled and Arg-labeled rhodotorucine *A*s, the radioactive metabolite formed by *a* cells was identical with the peptide fragment Tr-1 (16). Thus, rhodotorucine *A* was shown to be hydrolyzed by *a* cells to two inactive peptide fragments as shown in Fig. 7. This conversion was specific to *a* cells, since the pheromone remained unchanged on incubation with *A* cells.

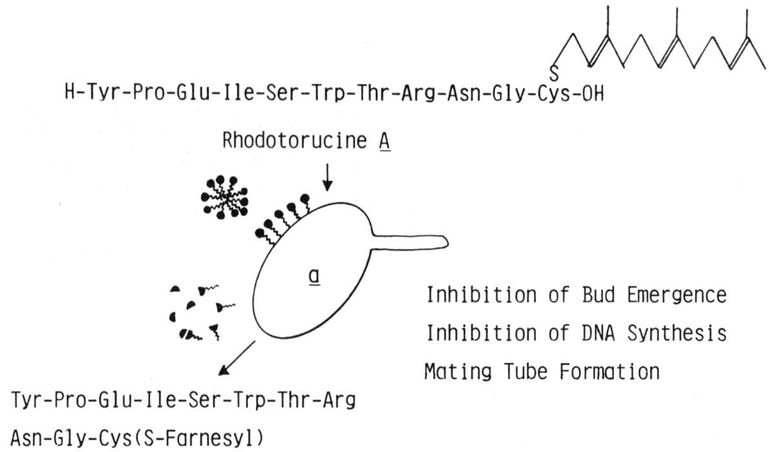

Fig. 7. Metabolism of rhodotorucine *A* by *a* cells of *Rhodosporidium toruloides* and early events of mating process

REFERENCES

1. H. van den Ende, *Sexual Interactions in Plants*, Academic Press, London (1976)
2. J. D. Levi, *Nature*, 177, 753 (1956)
3. D. Stötzler and W. Duntze, *Eur. J. Biochem.*, 65, 257 (1976)
4. K. Sakai and N. Yanagishima, *Arch. Microbiol.*, 84, 191 (1972)
5. A. Sakurai, S. Tamura, N. Yanagishima and C. Shimoda, *Agric. Biol. Chem.*, 40, 255 (1976); 41, 389 (1977)
6. D. Stötzler, H-H Kiltz and W. Duntze, *Eur. J. Biochem.*, 69, 397 (1976)
7. A. Sakurai, Y. Sato, K-H. Park, N. Takahashi, N. Yanagishima and I. Banno, *Agric. Biol. Chem.*, 44, 1451 (1980)
8. Y. Sato, A. Sakurai, N. Takahashi, Y-M. Hong, Y. Shimonishi, C. Kitada, M. Fujino, N. Yanagishima and I. Banno, *Agric. Biol. Chem.*, 45, 1531 (1981)
9. I. Banno, *J. Gen. Appl. Microbiol.*, 13, 167 (1967)
10. K. Abe, I. Kusaka and S. Fukui, *J. Bacteriol.*, 122, 710 (1975)
11. Y. Kamiya, A. Sakurai, S. Tamura, N. Takahashi, E. Tsuchiya, K. Abe and S. Fukui, *Agric. Biol. Chem.*, 43, 363 (1979)
12. C. Kitada, M. Fujino, Y. Kamiya, A. Sakurai, S. Tamura, N. Takahashi, E. Tsuchiya, K. Abe and S. Fukui, *Experientia*, 35, 1275 (1989)
13. Y. Kamiya and A. Sakurai, *Naturwiss.*, 68, 128 (1980)
14. Y. Sakagami, A. Isogai, A. Suzuki, C. Kitada and M. Fujino, *Agic. Biol. Chem.*, 43, 2643 (1979)
15. Y. Sakagami, M. Yoshida, A. Isogai and A. Suzuki, *Science*, 212, 1525 (1981)
16. Y. Kamiya, A. Sakurai and N. Takahashi, *Biochem. Biophys. Res. Comm.*, 94, 855 (1980)

MASSCULTURE OF MARINE PHYTOFLAGELLATES: AN APPROACH TO NEW SOURCES OF BIOLOGICALLY ACTIVE COMPOUNDS

Tomotoshi Okaichi, Sachio Nishio and Yukiya Imatomi

Marine Research Laboratory and Department of Agricultural Chemistry, Faculty of Agriculture, Kagawa University, Kagawa Prefecture 761-07, Japan

Abstract The massculture of marine phytoflagellates such as *Protogonyaulax catenella*, *Prorocentrum minimum* and *Chattonella antiqua* in 10 *l* or 100 *l* glass tanks have been examined. Filtered sea water or commercial sea salt solution, fortified with nutrients, vitamins and EDTA-Fe and -Mn was used as the culture medium after filter sterilization. Culture temperatures are 20-23°C and light intensity supplied by white fluorescent lamps was about 5000 lux under conditions of 14 hrs. light and 10 hrs. dark. The 100 *l* tank was equipped with a pH controller supplying CO_2 gas to keep the pH of the medium from 8.2 to 8.7. In the latter period of the exponential phase of the cell growth, half or three quarters of the culture was harvested and fresh medium was supplied aseptically. The cell yield of *P.catenella* was 33.2 g(dry basis) in 39 days with 400 *l*. The total PSP toxicities were 329,000 MU; of *P.minimum*, 32 g in 33 days with 410 *l* media; of *C.antiqua*, $1.2x10^{10}$ cells corresponding to 194 g on wet basis in 42 days with 440 *l*. These materials are now being used in chemical analyses.

INTRODUCTION

Investigations of bioactive substances in marine organisms continues to attract the interest of scientists in natural organic chemistry, as they are one of the main unexplored sources. The diversity of marine organisms enhances the possibilities of finding new types of organic substances in the future. Recent studies on gonyautoxins(1) and breve toxins(2) have served to encourage marine chemists. The morphological and ecological diversity in unicellular algae, including 13,000 species together with the phytoflagellates, seems to augur well for success in this field. The difficulties of collecting enough sample to promote studies, however, are always present.

In Japan, particularly in the Seto Inland Sea, large and dense red tides, mainly due to phytoflagellates, have occurred annually for more than ten years, causing mass mortality in fish and shellfish poisoning. Prevention of the red tide outbreaks and chemical studies on toxic substances are very serious problems. In the course of studies on red tides, some ten species of phytoflagellates have been isolated and cultured in unialgal or axenic states. Physiological conditions for the cultures of these species have also been thoroughly examined.

The authors proposed to promote massculture of red tide organisms, based on these backgrounds. This paper deals with the massculture system and the results of the cultures for three species.

EXPERIMENTAL

Organisms

The culture of 10 species were examined in 10 *l* glass bottles and of these three species, described below, were used for massculture. *Protogonyaulax catenella* (WHEDON & KOFOID) TAYLOR was isolated in Owase Bay in January of 1975. *Prorocentrum minimum* (PAVILLARD) SCHILLER was obtained in Harima Nada in May of 1975. *Chattonella antiqua* (HADA) ONO appeared as a dense red tide in June of 1978 and killed cultured yellowtail fish in Harima Nada, the Seto Inland Sea. The strain was separated from the red tide.

Medium and culture conditions

The composition of the medium used for preservation of the strains and for preculture was as follows: $NaNO_3$ 120 mg, K_2HPO_4 5 mg(or glycerophosphate 10 mg), cyanocobalamine 10 µg, thiamin 100 µg, biotin 1 µg, EDTA-Fe 260 µg, EDTA-Mn 330 µg, soil extract 50 ml and tris(hydroxymethyl) aminomethane 1 g in 1000 ml of filtered sea water or commercial sea salt solution. In the massculture medium, the soil extract and tris(hydroxymethyl) aminomethane were omitted. Before addition of vitamins the medium was first sterilized by UV irradiation and then filtered through a 0.2 µm membrane filter.

Light intensities were kept at 4000-5000 lux by white fluorescent lamps under 14 hrs. light and 10 hrs. dark condition. Culture bottles and tanks were kept in a constant temperature room at 20°C for of *P.catenella* and *P.minimum*, 23°C for *C.antiqua*.

Culture systems

This is shown in Fig. 1. Each of the 10 *l* bottles is connected through a silicone stopper to the medium supply / culture outlet line (stainless steel or teflon, 10 mm O.D.) and to the gas supply line (3 mm O.D.). The common medium supply line connects the bottles and is in turn connected to the medium supply line through a membrane sterilization filter. Aeration through the gas supply line is maintained at 50 ml min^{-1} in each bottle, CO_2 being supplied to maintain the pH in the range 8.0-8.7. In addition, each bottle carries a gas outlet and small sample collection outlet.

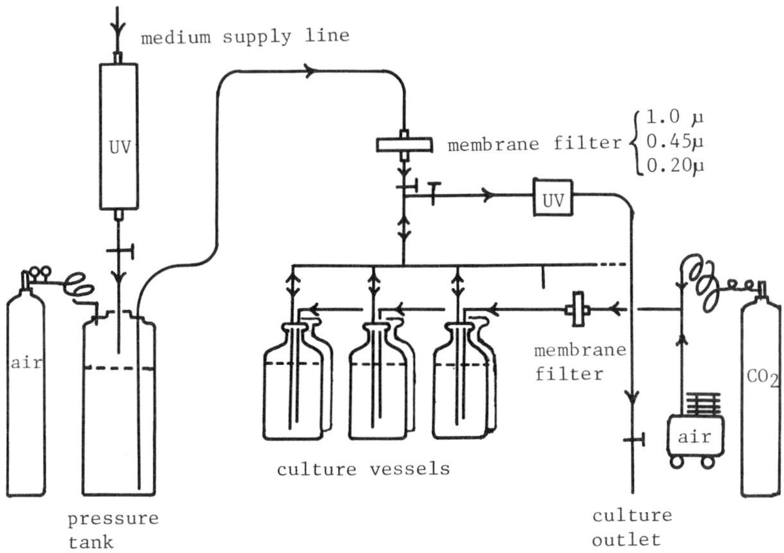

Fig.1 Phytoflagellates culture system using 10 *l* bottles.

A culture system using a 100 *l* tank is illustrated in Fig. 2. The tank and cover are made of thick hard glass; the cover is fixed to the tank by teflon packing and iron bolts to maintain axenic condition. The tank is equipped with automatic pH controller (Tokyo Rika Co. Ltd.) and the pH is controlled by CO_2 gas as in 10 *l* bottles. Sterilization of the tank is carried out by ethylene oxide. The medium is mixed by pressurized and filtered air at the rate of 1000 ml min^{-1} ; A sealed stirrer is also available for strong mixing.

Harvesting of the organisms

Armoured phytoflagellates such as *P.catenella* and *P.minimum* were collected by continuous centrifuge at 7000 rpm, with a flow rate of 30-50 *l* min^{-1}. For harvesting unarmoured species such as *C.antiqua*, the organisms were precipitated to the bottom of the tank by standing the bottles at 4°C over night or decreasing the pH to about 6.

In the latter period of the exponential phase of cell growth, 50-75 % of the culture were taken out through the main pipe and were replaced by fresh medium. Usually 3-5 days were needed for one harvest with these three species.

RESULTS

pH control with CO_2 gas and its growth promoting effect.

In the culture of *Chlorella* and marine macro algae CO_2 gas is continuously supplied as carbon source in admixture with air at 0.2-5 % concentration. As marine phytoflagellates are very sensitive to decrease in pH and to agitation of the medium, this method is not applicable. A slow supply of pure CO_2 gas when the pH rises to near 9.0 seemed to be more suited to our purpose.

Fig. 3 shows the result on the culture of *P.minimum* of supplying CO_2 gas once a day during the logarithmic growth stage. The initial cell density was 200 cells ml^{-1}. The pH began to increase when the cell density reached 10^4 cells ml^{-1} and reached to 8.7 at 10^5 cells. Seven days after inoculation, CO_2 gas was added to decrease the pH to 8.4, but after light irradiation of 12 hrs. it again rose to 8.8. The addition of CO_2 gas was repeated for 4 days as the arrows show in Fig. 3. Before the maximum cell yield was obtained, the increase of pH stopped. The growth of *P.catenella* was also influenced by the supply of CO_2 gas, in spite of the limited pH rise to 8.5 in the medium. The culture with CO_2 supply yielded $5.5x10^4$ cells ml^{-1} which was 2.5 times as much as that of the control culture.

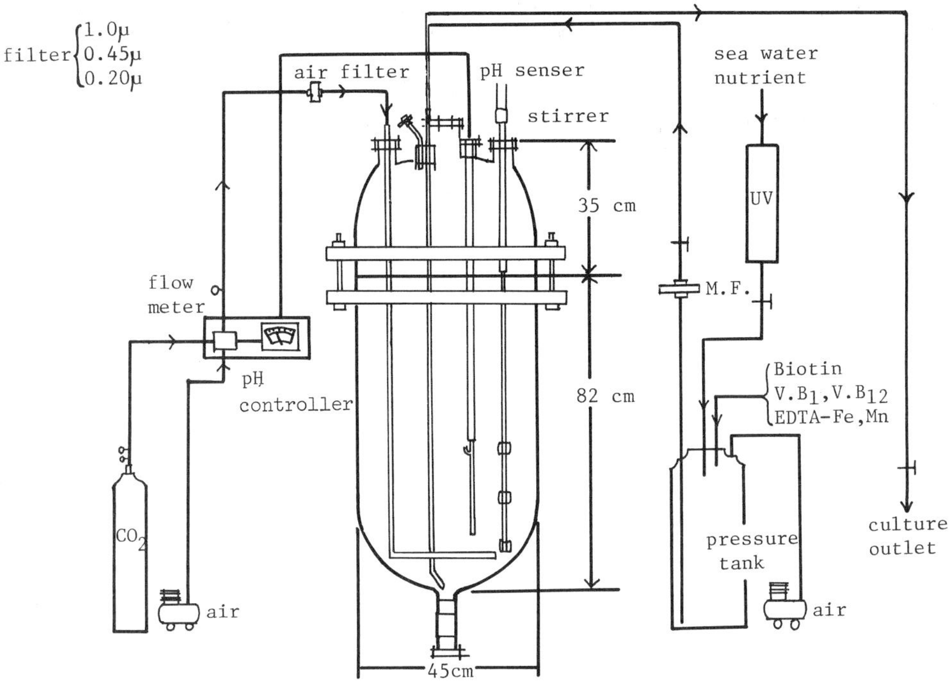

Fig.2 Intermittent harvesting culture system using 100 l tank

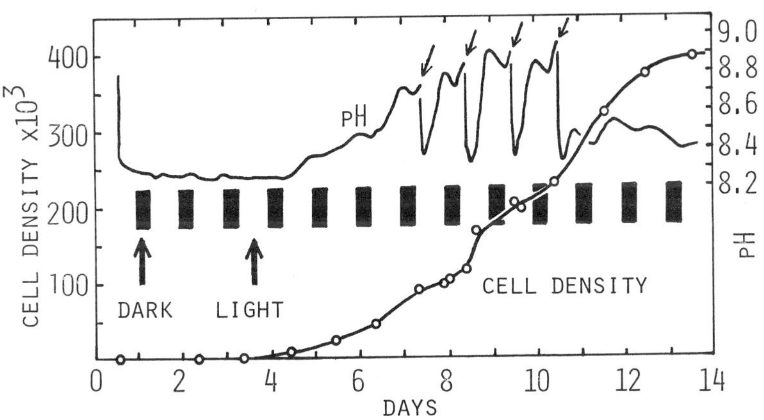

Fig.3 Culture of *Prorocentrum minimum* with pH control by CO_2
Arrows on the pH curve show the addition of CO_2

Massculture

P.catenella was cultured in a combination of 12 bottles of 10 l. Initially, 850 ml of inocula were added to 9.25 l of the medium and the pH was adjusted from 7.9 to 8.1 by CO_2 gas. On harvest, about 8.5 l of culture were taken out from each bottle and replaced by sterilized fresh medium. The cultures were continued for 4 harvests intermittently. Through these 4 intermittent cultures 305 g(wet weight, 33.2 g dry) of *P.catenella* were produced from 400 l. The toxicity of paralytic shellfish poison (PSP) was examined by the method adopted in A.O.A.C.(3). The effect on PSP accumulation of standing in darkness before harvest is shown in the culture experiments 2,3 and 4 of Table 1. The dark effect on accumulation of PSP was rather remarkable. The total toxicity estimated was 329,000 MU.

The cultures of *P.minimum* were examined both in 10 l bottle system and in 100 l tank. In the 10 l bottle system *P.minimum* was collected 9 times in 54 days using 12 bottles. Total volume of the medium was 490 l and the cell yield was 40 g on dry basis (Table 2). In the 100 l tank method the pH control (adjusted from 8.1 to 8.4) worked very well. The volumes taken out in one harvest were 75 l. In 33 days, 32 g of dry matter were obtained from 410 l culture.

C.antiqua was also cultured with 100 l tank. As it is difficult to collect the species by continuous centrifuge, the results are shown in cell numbers in Table 3. Seven cultures carried out in 42 days produced 1.2×10^{10} cells corresponding to 194 g on wet basis from the cell volume estimated under microscope.

Table 1. Intermittent harvesting culture of *Protogonyaulax catenella* using 10 *l* bottles.

Culture No.	Days	Medium Vol.(*l*)	Cell Density cells ml^{-1}	Yield (wet g)	Yield (dry g)	Total MU	Dark hours before harvest
1	14	100	47,000	103.2	11.2	35,000	-
2	10	100	67,000	67.0	7.1	82,000	46
3	8	100	65,000	86.0	9.1	128,000	48
4	7	100	32,000	49.2	5.8	84,000	48

Table 2. Intermittent harvesting culture of *Prorocentrum minimum* using 10 *l* bottles

Culture No.	Days	Medium Vol.(*l*)	Yield dry g
1	10	70	5.1
2	6	50	3.9
3	3	50	3.4
4	4	70	5.0
5	4	30	2.5
6	4	30	2.1
7	6	30	2.0
8	5	40	3.4
9	12	120	12.5
Total		490	39.9
yield per 100 *l*			8.1

Table 3. Intermittent harvesting culture of *Chattonella antiqua* using 100 *l* tank

Culture No.	Days	Medium Vol.(*l*)	Cell number ml^{-1}
1	7	60	21,600
2	6	60	17,000
3	8	60	16,700
4	5	60	24,700
5	5	60	36,000
6	5	60	40,000
7	4	80	29,000
Total		440	1.2×10^{10}
yield per 100 *l*			2.7×10^{9}

DISCUSSION

The intermittent harvesting of cultures of marine phytoflagellates was carried out successfully under pH control with CO_2 gas. In particular the 100 *l* tank cultures are recommended for use in the laboratory, because of the easy handling and high yield compared to the 10 *l* bottle system, as seen in the case of *P.minimum*. Although rather longer periods are needed to get maximum cell numbers than with other microbes, massculture of marine phytoflagellates seems not to be difficult, if the precultures are kept in good condition and infection by microbes are prevented. The latter is particularly important in the 100 *l* tank culture. The use of UV lamps on the harvest tube serves to aboid contaminations; in the 10 *l* bottle system it is possible to eliminate the contaminated bottle from the system. This may be one of the merits of 10 *l* bottle system. The medium composition now used is very simple. The artificial media thus far reported (4) are also available but the cell yields are inferior to sea water medium. The cultured materials were used in chemical studies of gonyautoxins (5) and the toxic activities of *P.minimum* (6). Chemical investigation of the cause of fish kill due to *C.antiqua* is now in progress.

REFERENCES

1. Y.Shimizu, M.Alam, Y.Oshima and W.E.Fallon, *Biochem.Biophys.Res.Commun.,* 66,731 (1975).
2. Y.Y.Lin, M.Risk, S.M.Ray, D.V.Engen, J.Clardy, J.Golik, J.C.James and K.Nakanishi, *J.Am. Chem.Soc.,*103, 6773, (1981)
3. W.Horwitz ed., Official methods of analysis of A.O.A.C.,24th ed., 319 (1975).
4. J.McLachlan, Handbook of phycological methods, Culture methods and growth measurements ed by J.R.Stein, Cambridge at the University Press, 25,(1973).
5. Y.Oshima, Y.Shimizu, S.Nishio and T.Okaichi, *Bull.Jap.Soc.Sci.Fish.*,44,395 (1978).
6. T.Okaichi and Y.Imatomi, Toxic Dinoflagellates Blooms ed.by D.Taylor and H.Seliger,Elsevier North Holland Inc, 385 (1979).

SYSTEMATIC ULTRA-MICRO ANALYSIS OF PLANT GROWTH REGULATORS

Isomaro Yamaguchi, Sachiko Fujisawa and Nobutaka Takahashi

Department of Agricultural Chemistry, The University of Tokyo, Bunkyo-ku, Tokyo 113, Japan

Abstract - Methods for qualitative and quantitative analysis of gibberellins, abscisic acid and cytokinins were examined. A systematic method, consisting of six steps for analysing gibberellins and abscisic acid and one of five steps for analysing cytokinins were established. A combination of these two methods permitted analysis for gibberellins, abscisic acid and cytokinins in the same process. These methods were applied to analyze the plant hormones in some organs of Pharbitis nil.

INTRODUCTION

In many aspects of plant growth, plant hormones and other plant growth regulators play important roles. There have been many investigations (Ref. 1-8) of the relationship between changes in endogenous plant growth regulators and physiological processes in plant growth, as well as isolation and characterization of new plant growth regulators. To facilitate further intensive research in this field, it is necessary to minimize the amount of plant material required and to shorten the analysis time and to this end we planned to devise systematic methods for analysis of gibberellins (GAs), abscisic acid (ABA) and cytokinins. At present, the most sensitive and reliable method for analysis of minute amounts of known free GAs and of some physiologically important cytokinins is considered to be gas chromatography - selected ion monitoring (GC-SIM), while that for ABA is gas chromatography - electorn capture detection (GC-ECD). Both analysis methods require some pre-purification, for which high performance liquid chromatography (HPLC) has been shown to be very effective: We therefore directed our attention to application of HPLC for purification prior to GC-SIM or GC-ECD analysis and to development of a systematic analysis for GAs, ABA and cytokinins which did not require bioassay.

RESULTS AND DISCUSSION

Gibberellins and abscisic acid.
The procedure, consiting of the following six steps, was designed for the purification and analysis of GAs and ABA. (1) Solvent fractionation to obtain an ethyl acetate-soluble acidic fraction. (2) Sephadex LH-20 column chromatography. (3) Reversed phase partition chromatography on Lichrosorb RP-18. (4) Gel permeation chromatography on Shodex A-801. (5) Chromatography on Nucleosil $N(CH_3)_2$. (6) GC-SIM for GAs and GC-ECD for ABA.

Steps 1-4 are designed to concentrate GAs and ABA, taking advantage of their chemical similarities. Step 5 effectively groups GAs by differences in functionality. Step 6 is a GC-SIM method to identify and quantify GAs, in which as little as 10-100 pg of GA can be analysed. In steps 1-4, ABA is fractionated into the same fraction as GAs. In the analysis of ABA, step 5 is unnecessary. ABA is analyzed by GC-ECD in the range of 50-100 pg. Recovery of GAs and ABA in purification steps 2-5 was examined using various GAs and ABA, as shown in Fig. 1.

Step 1 This is the conventional solvent fractionation, by which most GAs and ABA are fractionated into an ethyl acetate-soluble acidic fraction (Ref. 9).

Step 2 In this step, several solvent systems such as MeOH, MeOH-Me_2CO (1:1), MeOH-$CHCl_3$ (1:1) and Me_2CO-$CHCl_3$ (1:1) were examined. When MeOH-Me_2CO (1:1) was used, ABA and most of the GAs tested were eluted in a narrow range (0.7-1.0) of Ve (elution volume)/Vt (total volume), and teir recovery was reasonably high (Table 1). Step 2 works as rough gel permeation chromatography, and is effective in removing dusty material which would interfere with subsequent HPLC purification steps.

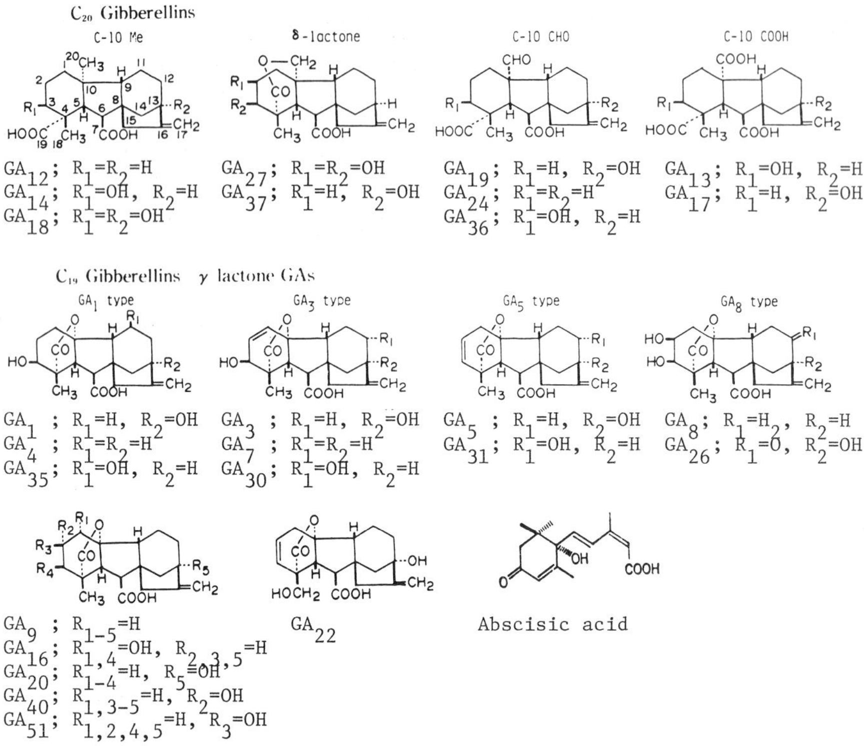

Fig. 1. ABA and types of basic skeletones of GAs used as authentic samples

TABLE 1. Elution pattern and recovery (%) of GAs and ABA in step 2

Ve/Vt	0.6	0.7	0.8	0.9	1.0	1.1	1.2	Total
GA_3	0	3.5	84.4	6.4	0	0		94.3
GA_5	0	40.6	69.2	0	0	0		109.8
GA_9	0	40.4	43.6	0	0	0		84.0
GA_{14}	0	0	19.5	59.9	1.1	0		80.5
GA_{17}	0	0	12.0	63.9	2.6	0		78.5
GA_{36}	0	0	4.8	96.0	8.5	0		109.3
GA_{37}	0	0	48.2	54.3	0.9	0		103.4
ABA	0	2.1	79.4	1.8	0	0		83.3

column size; 260 x 16 mm. sample size; 10 μg of each GAs and 5 μg of ABA

Step 3 In this step, two solvent systems were tested for elution of all GAs and ABA in relatively small volumes. In the procedure using solvent system 1, GAs and ABA dissolved in 60% MeOH were injected through a loop injector onto a column in a flow of 5 mM phosphate buffer (pH 3.2) containing 10% MeOH, and after 45 ml of effluent was collected the eluent was switched to H_2O (20 ml), 60% MeOH (90 ml), and 100% MeOH successively. In the second procedure using solvent system 2, GAs and ABA in 60% MeOH were injected onto a column in a flow of 0.05 mM formic acid (pH 2.9) containing 10% MeOH, and after 45 ml of effluent was collected, the eluent was switched to 0.01 mM formic acid (pH 5.2) containing 60% MeOH, and 100% MeOH (45 ml) successively. In both procedures, fractions eluted with solvents containing 60% MeOH were regarded as the GAs and ABA fractions, and their recovery was examined (Table 2).

TABLE 2. Recovery (%) of GAs and ABA in step 3

Solvent system	GA_1	GA_3	GA_5	GA_8	GA_9	GA_{37}	ABA
1	-	98.3	113.9	-	0	102.0	-
2	85.3	-	-	83.6	87.4	-	82.6

column size; 200 x 8 mm. sample size; 5 μg of each GA and ABA.
-; not tested

With solvent system 1, GAs possessing hydroxyl group(s) were recovered in reasonable yield. GA_9, however, was not recovered, suggesting that this procedure is unsuitable for purification of samples containing less polar GAs such as GA_9, GA_{12}, GA_{15} etc. On the other hand, GA_9 and other GAs were recovered in good yield in the procedure employing solvent system 2, which is, therefore, to be preferred.

Step 4 A prepacked column, Shodex A-801 (500 x 8 mm. made for gel permeation chromatography), was used with THF as eluant at a flow rate of 1.0 ml/min. R_t and recovery of GAs and ABA in step 4 are listed in Table 3. GAs were eluted in a very narrow range, showing that this column works in a gel permeation mode, with partition and adsorption on the gel being negligible. Step 4 effectively concentrates GAs and ABA with no recovery problems.

TABLE 3. R_t (min) and recovery (%) of GAs and ABA in step 4

Number of OH	C_{19}-GAs & ABA	R_t	Recovery	C_{20}-GAs	R_t	Recovery
none	GA_9	13.7	-	GA_{24}	13.0	-
mono	GA_5	12.9	93.9	GA_{13}	12.0	110.9
	GA_{20}	12.9	-	GA_{14}	12.6	-
	ABA	12.2	92.4	GA_{19}	12.2	-
				GA_{36}	12.3	79.2
di	GA_1	12.2	102.5	GA_{27}	12.8	-
	GA_3	12.3	-	GA_{41}	11.8	-
tri	GA_8	11.9	-			

column size; 500 x 8 mm. solvent; THF, 1.0 ml/min. detection; RI and UV (254 nm). 40 μg of each GA and 5 μg of ABA.

Step 5 Nucleosil $N(CH_3)_2$ columns were used with methanol containing 0.05% acetic acid as an eluant. The R_t of GAs and ABA on one of the columns are shown in Table 4.

TABLE 4. R_t (min) of GAs and ABA on Nucleosil $N(CH_3)_2$

Number of OH	ABA	Types of GAs: C-10 Me	δ-lactone	C-10 CHO	C-10 COOH	γ-lactone	
none		GA_{12} 10.7		GA_{24} 32.4		GA_9 27.0	
mono	c-ABA 15.1	GA_{14} 11.4	GA_{37} 13.8	GA_{36} 31.4	GA_{13} 28.0	GA_4 27.8	GA_5 38.2
	t-ABA 15.8			GA_{19} 41.6	GA_{17} 21.4	GA_7 27.8	GA_{20} 30.0
						GA_{31} 37.6	GA_{40} 28.0
di		GA_{18} 11.7	GA_{27} 15.6			GA_1 22.0	GA_3 28.9
						GA_{16} 25.6	GA_{22} 49.0
						GA_{26} 48.2	GA_{30} 28.6
tri						GA_8 26.0	

column size; 250 x 6 mm. particle size; 10 μm. column temp; 50°C.
solvent; 0.05% AcOH in MeOH, 2 ml/min. sample size; 20 μg of each GAs and 5 μg ofABA.
detection; UV (205 and 254 nm)

Introduction of hydroxyl group(s) into ent-gibberellane skeleton generally causes an increase in R_t; an exception is introduction of 3β-hydroxyl groups in C_{19}-GAs and C-10 CHO GAs, which decrease R_t — a tendency that seems to be common to δ-lactone GAs. This suggests that 3β-hydroxyl group in these GAs supress dissociation of the C-6 carboxyl group. While, the 3β-hydroxyl groups in C-10 COOH GAs and C-10 Me GAs seem to increase R_t. Interestingly, pairs such as GA_1/GA_3, GA_4/GA_7, GA_5/GA_{20}, GA_1/GA_{38}, GA_{20}/GA_{44} and GA_{27}/GA_{34}, which are all difficult to separate by conventional methods, can be clearly separated in step 5. The recovery of GAs and ABA in step 5 is reasonable (Table 5).

TABLE 5. Recovery (%) of GAs and ABA in step 5

	c-, t-ABA	GA_3	GA_5	GA_{13}	GA_{36}
Recovery	88.7	98.9	92.1	90.8	82.3

The elution pattern of GAs is summerized in Fig. 2. Based on the R_t, GAs can be divided into three groups: group I (R_t, 10-18 min); group II (R_t, 18-30 min); and group III (R_t, 30-52 min). Group I contains C-10 Me GAs and δ-lactone GAs , group II C-10 COOH GAs and most of the C_{19}-

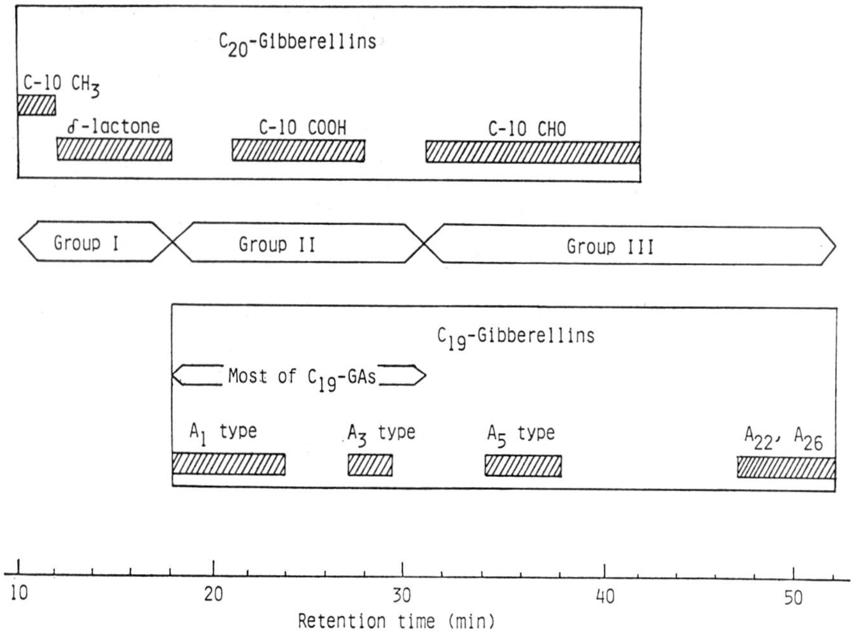

Fig. 2. Diagrams of the elution pattern of GAs in step 5

GAs, group III C-10 CHO GAs and C_{19}-GAs such as GA_5 type in ring A, GA_{22} and GA_{26}. Such groupings assist in the selection of ions to be monitored in GC-SIM (step 6).

As described above, steps 2-5 were examined using authentic GAs and shown to work well as pre-purification methods for GC-SIM analysis of GAs. In some practical purification procedures, some of the steps can be omitted. For example, when the content of GAs in a sample is relatively high, as in immature seeds of _Pharbitis nil_ (Ref. 9) and _Phaseolus vulgaris_ (Ref. 10), and a small sample is enough for analysis, steps 2 and 3 may be unnecessary.

Cytokinins

Ammong the many cytokinins characterized from plant sources, _cis_- and _trans_-zeatin (_c_- and _t_-Z), isopentenyladenine (i^6-Ade) and their ribosides (_c_-RZ, _t_-RZ and i^6-Ado) are the most common, and are expected to be concerned with many aspects of plant growth. Therefore, we concentrated on development of a convenient method of analysis for these six cytokinins, and devised a procedure consisting of the following 5 steps. Step 7. Toyopearl HW-40 (Fine) column chromatography. Step 8. HPLC on Hitachi Gel 3011-C. Step 9. GPC on Shodex A-801. Step 10. HPLC on ODS. Step 11. GC-SIM. The behavior of authentic cytokinins in each step was examined and their recovery was calculated.

Step 7 Toyopearl HW-40 (Fine) was suspended and swollen in 5% MeOH, then packed in a glass column in the same solvent. A mixture of authentic cytokinins, GAs and ABA dissolved in 20-40% MeOH was charged onto this column and the column was eluted with 5% MeOH. After collection of the effluent as much as the total volume (100 ml), the solvent was changed to 70% MeOH, and the effluent was collected in 10 ml fractions. Aliquots of each fraction were submitted to HPLC on ODS; the elution pattern and recovery of the authentic samples are shown in Table 6.

TABLE 6. Elution pattern and recovery (%) of cytokinins, ABA and GAs in step 7

Ve/Vt	1.6	1.7	1.8	1.9	2.0	2.1	2.2	Total
_t_-Z	0	2.1	84.2	2.4	0	0		89.7
_t_-RZ	0	6.8	86.1	0	0	0		92.3
i^6-Ade	0	0	28.3	61.0	0	0		89.3
i^6-Ado	0	0	40.1	59.4	0	0		99.5
_c_-, _t_-ABA	0	0	8.2	73.8	1.1	0		83.1
$GA_{3,4,7}$	±	+	+	+	±	±		

sample size; 5 µg of each cytokinin and ABA and 10 µg of each GA.
detection; UV (254 nm) and TLC.

All cytokinins, ABA and GAs were eluted in the range 1.6-2.1 Ve/Vt. Since there is a possibility that elution of cytokinins, ABA and GAs is affected by pH of the plant extracts, the use of buffer of pH 5.5 instead of distilled water is recommended. As long as the pH of plant extracts is between 4.0 and 6.0, however, the elution pattern of thses plant hormones seems not to be affected.

Step 8 In this step, a stainless steel column (200 x 8 mm) with a precolumn (50 x 8 mm) both packed with Hitachi Gel 3011-C (10 um) (a polystyrene-divinylbenzene copolymer containing carboxyl groups) was used. As eluant, 4.2 mM ammonia water-MeOH (4:6, v/v) was used at a flow rate of 3 ml/min, and samples were dissolved in 60% MeOH for loading. The behavior of authentic cytokinins, GAs and ABA are shown in Table 7 with their recoveries. Both conjugated and non-conjugated GAs and ABA were eluted earlier than adenine, while c- and t-Z, i^6-Ade and their ribosides were eluted later. In this step, plant hormones are grouped into three; group I containing GAs and ABA, group II containing c- and t-Z and their ribosides and group III containing i^6-Ade and i^6-Ado. Their recoveries are within reasonable limits (Table 7).

TABLE 7. R_t (min) and recovery (%) of cytokinins, ABA and GAs in step 8

	R_t	Recovery		R_t	Recovery
t-Z	5.0	88.9	c-,t-ABA	2.1	82.4
t-RZ	5.4	81.0	GA_3	2.1	84.4
i^6-Ade	14.0	85.6	GA_8	2.1	92.8
i^6-Ado	15.2	95.6	GA_9	2.2	83.2
Adenine	5.0	-			

Step 9 This step, GPC on shodex A-801, was carried out in quite the same manner as for GAs. As shown in Table 8, c-Z, t-Z and i^6-Ade are respectively separated from their ribosides.

TABLE 8. R_t (min) and recovery (%) of cytokinins in step 9

	R_t	Recovery		R_t	Recovery
c-, t-Z	12.0	94.6	i^6-Ade	12.5	98.3
c-, t-RZ	11.0	98.8	i^6-Ado	11.2	100.1

sample size; 500 ng of each cytokinin.

Step 10 A prepacked ODS column (Sensyu pack ODS, 250 x 6 mm, carbon content 20% in weight) was used with MeOH-H_2O mixtures as eluting solvent. For the separation of c- and t-RZ, 15% MeOH was used, and 20% MeOH for the setaration of c- and t-Z. The fractions containing i^6-Ade and i^6-Ado were also purified by this step. As eluants, 25% MeOH was used for i^6-Ado and 30% MeOH for i^6-Ade. The recovery of each cytokinin in this step is shown in Table 9.

TABLE 9. Recovery (%) of cytokinins in step 10

	t-Z	t-RZ	i^6-Ade	i^6-Ado
Recovery	88.8	96.9	82.9	100.8

Step 11 Cytokinins purified by step 10 were submitted to GC-SIM analysis as TMSi derivatives. Trimethylsilylation was performed by heating samples with the mixture of acetonitrile-BSA-TMCS-pyridine (10:5:2:2) at 70°C for 30min. Under these condition, the secondary amino group on C-6 is also trimethylsilylated.

Simultaneous analysis of GAs, ABA and cytokinins

As described above, GAs and ABA are analyzed together in the same procedure, while cytokinins are dealt with separately. As long as sufficient material is available, it is better to divide it into two portions, one for GAs and ABA analysis and the other for cytokinins. However, if the amount of sample is inadequate for separate analysis of GAs, ABA and cytokinins, these plant hormones can be analyzed as follows. The analysis of cytokinins is carried out exactly as described above. After separation of GAs and ABA from cytokinins by step 8, the GAs/ABA fraction is submitted to the procedure of steps 1-6 to be analyzed. In the simultaneous analysis procedure, however, steps 1-3 are often unnecessary.

Practical application

The systematic methods were applied to the analysis of GAs, ABA and cytokinins in *Pharbitis nil*. GAs, ABA and cytokinins in immature seeds were analyzed separately. In case of flower buds, pistils and anthers, only GAs were analyzed. GAs were analyzed by the procedure of step 1-6 where steps 2 and 3 were often omitted. The results are summerized in Table 10.

TABLE 10. Content of GAs in orgnas of _P. nil_ (μg/kg fr. wt)

	GA_3	GA_5	GA_{17}	GA_{19}	GA_{20}	GA_{26}	GA_{27}	GA_{29}	GA_{53}
Immature seeds	19	100	(+)	32	190	1200	176	40	0.8
Flower buds	0.2	0.6	(+)	1	1	0.04	2	1	7
Pistils	0.6	5.2	(+)	2	3	2.6	3.1	7.8	25
Anthers	+	3.8	(+)	0.2	0.8	-	-	0.4	-

amount of materials used for analysis; immature seeds 1.25 g, flower buds 5.0 g, pistils 0.4 g, anthers 1.6 g. (+); detected but the content was not determined because of failure in peak centering. +; too little to determine the content. -; not detected.

The content of GAs (except for GA_{53}) in immature seeds is notably high compared to other organs. The content of GAs with high degree of oxidation, such as GA_8 and GA_{26}, is particularly high. In contrast with this observation, GA_{53}, which is the first GA biosynthesized from steviol, is found to be high in pistils and flower buds. In anthers, the content of GAs is very low, and GA_{26} and GA_{27}, which were detected in other organs, were undetected.

Cytokinins in immature seeds were analyzed by the procedure of step 7-10, and the results are shown in Table 11. Cytokinins in immature seeds were mainly ribosides, and the content of _c_-Z, _t_-Z and i^6-Ade was very low. The glycosidation activity is expected very high in immature seeds.

TABLE 11. Content (μg/kg) of cytokinins in immature seeds of _P. nil_

	_t_-Z	_c_-Z	i^6-Ade	_t_-RZ	_c_-RZ	i^6-Ado
Content	trace	trace	trace	31.2	14.8	2.4

2.5 g of immature seeds were used for the analysis.

ABA was analyzed by the procedure of step 7-10, and the amount was tentaively determined by UV absorption in step 10. The amount of _c_-ABA in immature seeds (8 days after flowering) was approximately 16 μg/kg.

In this study, the effectiveness of the systematic analytical methods for the known GAs, ABA and cytokinins has been demonstrated. It is especially noteworthy that the amount of material required for analysis is greatly reduced in comparison with conventional methods. By the use of isotopically labelled internal standards, it will be possible to achieve even more accurate quantitative analysis.

REFERENCES

1. V. M. Frydman, P. Gaskin and J. MacMillan, _Planta 118_, 123-132 (1974)
2. I. Yamaguchi and N. Takahashi, _Plant Cell Physiol. 17_, 611-614 (1976)
3. S. Kurogochi, N. Murofushi, Y. Ota and N. Takahashi, planta 146, 185-191 (1979)
4. J. D. Metzger and A. D. Zeevaart, _Plant Physiol. 66_, 844-846 (1980)
5. A. Crozier and D. R. Reeve, _Plant Growth Regulation. Proceeding of the 9th International Conference of Plant Groth Substances_. (Pilet, P.-E.,ed.) p.67. Springer, Berlin.
6. I. Yamaguchi, T. Yokota, S. Yoshida and N. Takahashi, _Phytochemistry 18_, 1699-1702 (1979)
7. M. G. Jones, J. D. Metzger and A. D. Zeevaart, _Plant Physiol. 65_, 218-221 (1980)
8. G. W. M. Barendse, P. H. Van De Werken and N. Takahashi, _J. Chromatogr._ 198, 449-455 (1980)
9. T. Yokota, N. Murofushi, N. Takahashi and S. Tamura, _Agric. Biol. Chem. 38_, 2521-582 (1971)
10. K. Hiraga, S. Kawabe, T. Yokota, N. Murofushi and N. Takahashi, _Agric. Biol. Chem._ 38, 2521-2527 (1974)

PYRETHROID INSECTICIDES: BIOLOGICAL ACTIVITY, MODE OF ACTION, METABOLISM AND TOXICOLOGY

PYRETHRUM: 100 YEARS IN JAPAN

Minoru Nakajima

Department of Agricultural Chemistry, College of Agriculture, Kyoto University, Kyoto 606, Japan

Abstract - Natural pyrethrin has been widely used in domestic insecticides because of its strong insecticidal activity, rapid knock-down effect, and low mammalian toxicity. The introduction of *Chrysanthemum cinerariaefolium* into Japan about one hundred years ago might be described as accidental. The early history of the Japanese pyrethrum industry, a unique and convenient use of pyrethrum, and synthetic pyrethroids developed in Japan are reported.

Natural pyrethrin has been widely used in domestic insecticides because of its strong insecticidal activity, rapid knock-down effect, and low mammalian toxicity. It is, however, unstable and expensive to use for pest control in the field. Since the first successful development of the synthetic pyrethrin, allethrin by Dr. La Forge in 1947, a number of workers have modified natural pyrethrin which has resulted in remarkable changes in its properties. In particular, potent and photostable pyrethroids have been disclosed by researchers in Great Britain and Japan and these will be available for use for agricultural pest control on a large scale in the near future. Thus, the pyrethrin industry is now making remarkable progress in the world.

Incidentally, it has been over a hundred years since the first pyrethrum was planted and bloomed beautifully in Japan. It is of great significance to hold the centennial symposium on pyrethroids at the occasion of the 5th International Congress of Pesticide Chemistry. In this symposium, biological activity, mode of action, metabolism and toxicological effects of pyrethroids are extensively discussed. First, the early history of pyrethrum industry in Japan is summarized.

Pyrethrum flowers are of the genus *Chrysanthemum* and the most important commercial species is *cinerariaefolium*. The practical use of pyrethrum probably originated in Persia. It is difficult to determine the actual date when the plant's insecticidal activity was discovered but we do know that the species *C. cinerariaefolium* was cultivated in Dalmatia in about 1840, replacing a Persian species, *C. roseum*. Although accounts of the discovery of the toxicity to insects vary, it is fairly certain that pyrethrum was in use in Europe as an insecticide in the early nineteenth century and in Persia considerably earlier; Gnadinger(1936) reported importation of "insect powder" into the United States about 1860 and later dried flowers called "insect flowers" were also imported. When and how, then, was pyrethrum imported to Japan?

Opinion is divided on the circumstances of the earliest importation of pyrethrum seeds into this country. In 1885, Dr. K. Tamari, Professor of the Imperial University, carried back some seeds from the United States and planted them in the farm of the University. About that time, an Austrian consul in Japan advised the government to cultivate pyrethrum here. The Ministry of Agriculture issued a pamphlet on cultivation of pyrethrum and sent seeds to several prefectures for testing. Also about this time, Mr. H. Armour, an American who was interested in plant collections of the world, was on a visit to the Far East and happened to call on a Japanese living in Wakayama Prefecture. Mr. Eichiro Ueyama, the founder of Dainihon Jochugiku Co., Ltd., invited him to see his orchards, and during his visit they promised each other to exchange plants grown in their own countries. Among these seeds, there was a quantity of pyrethrum, which were carefully cultivated in

Wakayama, and in due time the plants gave abundant flowers. Mr. Ueyama exerted all his efforts in encouraging the cultivation of pyrethrum and, because of this, cultivation was extended to the Chugoku(Midlands) district of Okayama, Hiroshima, and Ehime Prefectures in 1889. About ten years later, the cultivation of pyrethrum succeeded in Hokkaido after years of hard trial, and by the 1930s about half of Japan's crop was harvested in Hokkaido. The production of pyrethrum reached a maximum of about 13,000 metric tons in 1931 and about half of this was exported to the United States. Cultivation, however, rapidly decreased with the outbreak of World War II and also due to replacement of natural pyrethrins with synthetic pyrethroids.

On the contrary, English growers in Kenya have cultivated pyrethrum plants since 1928, and the pyrethrin content of the African flowers was found superior to that of Japanese flowers. At present, Kenya is a major grower of pyrethrum flowers producing about 13,000 metric tons of dried flowers per year, which corresponds to about 70% of the world's total. There is now, however, a general decline in pyrethrum production throughout the world due to the development of new synthetic pyrethroids.

In 1909, Mr. K. Fujitani obtained a transparent yellowish oily syrup from the neutral fraction of alcohol extract of powdered pyrethrum flowers; this was found to be an ester with strong insecticidal activity and was called "pyrethron". Prof. R. Yamamoto hydrolyzed this ester and identified a transcaronic acid in 1923. He recognized some features in the structures of pyrethrins necessary for insecticidal activity, and knew that the constituent alcohols and acids were only active when combined with one another.

Important scientific studies on pyrethrum were made by Staudinger and Ruzicka in the period 1910 to 1916 but no publication of the work was made until 1924. They separated and partially identified the two primary active principles, Pyrethrin I and Pyrethrin II, and in a series of papers published in Helv. Chimica Acta, they established the scientific foundation for the present progress of pyrethrum chemistry.

Early analytical methods of pyrethrins were reviewed by Gnadinger(1936) and were divided into three types: (a) Acid analysis, in which the pyrethrins are saponified followed by isolation of the chrysanthemic acids, which are estimated either together or separately; (b) formation of the pyrethrin semicarbazones followed by estimation of the nitrogen content; (c) reduction methods using either an alkaline copper solution of potassium ferricyanide. Prof. S. Takei(1932) analyzed the pyrethrin content at each stage of development of the flower head using the modified acid method which was used in the commodity market to analyze both extracts and flowers. Before publication of his study, pyrethrum flowers were evaluated only by their external appearance but not by pyrethrin content. The establishment of the analytical method was useful to avoid trouble in the commodity market and contributed to the scientific development of the Japanese pyrethrum industry. We can truly say that Prof. R. Yamamoto and Prof. S. Takei are the eminent pioneers of this industry in Japan.

In olden times, we used mosquito net or "kayari"(mosquito repellents) to protect us from mosquito bites. To repel the insects, the dried leaves of various plants such as Kaya(miscanthus), Yomogi(sage), nezu(juniper) were burned in summertime. The idea of incense sticks was applied to make a burnable stick mixed with pyrethrum powder and this was patented by Mr. K. Ito in 1889. About six years later, the pyrethrum stick was changed to a coil form in order to prolong the burning time. The coil were marketed as mosquito coils and were widely used for mosquito control. The advantage of mosquito coils is that they release pyrethrins continuously for seven to eight hours(overnight). This has been used very conveniently for the control of flying insects in the hot summer months, particularly in rooms with open windows both in Japan and in other countries with tropical and subtropical climates. Last year about one hundred fifty million boxes(each box containing 5 double coils) were produced in Japan. At present the synthetic pyrethrum allethrin, is being used as an active ingredient in the mosquito coil since it is more stable than the natural pyrethrins when burned.

Recently an electric mosquito killer has been developed instead of the smoky mosquito coils. Mr. K. Kitagawa(1953) of the Fumakilla Co., Ltd., studied the thermal stability and volatility of allethrins and found that allethrin was slowly vaporized without decomposition by heating at about 200°C for 6-10hrs, while the natural pyrethrins were rapidly decomposed by heating at

70-80°C. The maximum volatility of allethrin was observed at about 165°C. With these experimental data, he has developed a new method of mosquito control using an electric vaporizer. In the new device 40mg of allethrin or a mixture of allethrin and the volatile pyrethroid, furamethrin, are impregnated in a paper mat mixed with a kind of evaporation regulator of pyrethroids. The paper disk is heated at 165-170°C on an electric heating plate so that the active ingredients continue to vaporize for about 10 hours. The rate of evaporation, 3mg pyrethroids per hour, is sufficient to exert strong insecticidal activity. Last year about two thousand million paper mats were produced and about half of them were exported.

Finally, recent progress of synthetic pyrethroids is briefly described. Among many synthetic pyrethroids, some of the most promising was developed in Japan. Tetramethrin reported by Dr. T. Kato in 1964 knocks insects down rapidly when incorporated into aerosols and comparable formulations. In 1966 resmethrin was developed by Dr. M. Elliot and this was the first compound which had properties superior to those of the natural esters. This suggested that the investigation of the esters of furylmethyl alcohol would be likely to lead to further practical insecticides. Furamethrin is one of these which was developed by Dr. Y. Katsuda as a useful constituent of aerially dispersed insecticidal sprays or an active ingredient of the electric mosquito killer. A further advance in the development of synthetic pyrethroids was made independently in Great Britain and Japan in 1971. Phenothrin is a 3-phenoxybenzyl ester which is highly active against insects: 3-phenoxybenzyl alcohol is accessible by a variety of synthetic routes and is less expensive.

An outstanding advance was achieved by Sumitomo group in 1973. They discovered a new class of substituted 2-phenyl-alkanoates which is unique in that they lack the cyclopropane ring, though hitherto presence of the cyclopropane ring was thought to be essential to reveal insecticidal activity. The most important compound is fenvalerate. Owing to the highly enhanced insecticidal power and persistency in the field, these synthetic pyrethroids are very useful for controling a variety of harmful insects with less than one-tenth of the usual dosage of the conventional insecticides such as organic phosphates and carbamates.

PRESENT STATUS AND FUTURE PROSPECTS FOR SYNTHETIC PYRETHROIDS

Geoffrey G. Briggs, Michael Elliott and Norman F. Janes

Rothamsted Experimental Station, Harpenden, Hertfordshire, AL5 2JO, UK

Abstract - The potential number of insecticidally active variations of compounds with a discernible relationship to pyrethrin I is continually increasing as new acid, alcohol, and other components, many of them asymmetric, are discovered. Knowledge of how structure affects activity for important practical uses (activity against pest species, acaricidal activity, selectivity between pests and beneficial species, persistence on crops and in the environment, rapidity of action, antifeedant or repellent properties, toxicity to mammals, birds and fish, etc.) is being rapidly accumulated. Although strictly such information can only be obtained by direct testing of many related compounds, broad conclusions about the physical properties that influence the behaviour of pyrethroids in the environment can be predicted from their structures. As with applications of such procedures to other groups of pesticides, most results are precise only within an order of magnitude but these nevertheless provide a basis for valuable generalisations. The prospects for developing pyrethroids with properties especially appropriate for particular insect control applications are therefore encouraging, and the scope of pyrethroids may become comparable with those of the longer established groups of insecticides.

INTRODUCTION

Early accounts of the activity against insects of preparations (powdered flower heads, or extracts from them) from Tanacetum cinerariaefolium stressed the impressive rapidity of knockdown rather than kill (Ref. 1). Procedures such as the Peet-Grady and Campbell turntable methods with houseflies assessed both rapidity of action and kill and were used to standardise natural pyrethrum extracts and in developing synthetic analogues of the natural pyrethrins (eg. 1A, 2A, 1B) such as allethrin (1C) and tetramethrin (1M). Consequently, knockdown rather than kill characterised these early synthetic pyrethroids, the first developed commercially (Ref. 2 & 3).

When the separated constituents of pyrethrum extract became available by chromatography (Ref. 4) or reconstitution (Ref.5), Sawicki demonstrated that esters of pyrethric acid (pyrethrin II and cinerin II) were outstandingly potent for both knockdown and kill against houseflies, whereas against insects other than the housefly (eg. the mustard beetle) pyrethrin I was more active than pyrethrin II and also much superior to allethrin (Ref. 4). Pyrethrin I (1A) rather than allethrin thus became the prototype for development of a number of synthetic pyrethroids. Amongst these bioresmethrin (cf 1N) had greater insecticidal activity combined with very low mammalian toxicity and permethrin (5K), cypermethrin (5R), deltamethrin (6R) and fenvalerate (11R), photostability adequate to protect agricultural crops. Fenvalerate (Ref. 6) was important in showing that the gem-dimethyl group was not necessarily supported on a cyclopropane ring, a feature present in all earlier pyrethroids; deltamethrin (Ref. 7) demonstrated the great potency against insects attainable when structural features and geometrical and optical configurations were optimised. These developments were based on screening series of compounds against insects which were not only readily accessible, but were also considered to represent a wide spectrum of pests, to determine requirements for greatest potency. When the initial range of compounds was tested more widely, valuable activity was recognised to extend to species not initially investigated. Very significant progress has now been made since the original compounds were developed in expanding the range of structural features within which insecticidal activity is retained and indeed may be increased to a level barely conceived as possible a decade ago, and considerably exceeding the potencies attained in the organochlorine, organophosphate and carbamate groups of insecticides. Subtle structural variations in the pyrethroids have been shown greatly to influence potency either generally or against particular species of insects or mites. A whole range of pyrethroids with activities optimised for particular applications (improved acaricidal activity, diminished fish toxicity, outstandingly rapid knockdown activity, greatly increased efficacy against soil pests, etc.) is now therefore practicable - some examples are described for the first time at this Congress. Each segment of the parent pyrethroid molecule (Ref. 8) can now be replaced by an equivalent group; even some non-esters have significant activity (Ref. 9). However, in all these compounds a relationship with either pyrethrin I or pyrethrin II can still be discerned by direct comparison of structures and by similarity in physical properties and types of biological activity. Pyrethroids therefore now constitute a complex and formidable group of insecticides with a broad range of structural features.

The purpose of this communication is to survey the generalisations possible, with accumulated experience, that can give useful guidelines to the properties and performance of members of the group. These are most valuable in relation to behaviour in the environment, persistence in soil, volatility, water solubility etc. but are probably not yet adequate to predict biodegradability, and thence toxicity, in living organisms, especially mammals where there are many variables and precision is of overriding importance. For these there is, at present, no substitute for practical investigations.

PHYSICAL PROPERTIES AND PYRETHROID BEHAVIOUR

The response of insects to insecticides is governed by the intrinsic activities of the toxicants and by physical and chemical interactions which regulate transport, distribution and persistence within the organism. The widely differing biological activities of geometrical and optical isomers which have close or identical physical properties show that shape is the dominant factor determining the intrinsic potency of pyrethroids. If all centres of isomerism in pyrethroids are optimized for activity, other properties influence ability to reach and persist at sensitive sites in invertebrates and vertebrates, and behaviour in plants and in the environment. To measure these properties for all pyrethroids is not feasible, but many aspects of behaviour depend on physical properties such as partition coefficients, which can either be measured directly for key compounds, or calculated with sufficient precision using pi or fragment constants (Ref. 10 & 11). Air-water and air-soil distributions can also be estimated directly from structures, as can vapour pressures and water solubilities if melting points are known. Thus prediction of many aspects of pesticide behaviour is possible from simple accessible physical constants. Such calculations have already been made for many established pesticides (Ref. 11) and are here extended to a range of pyrethroids representing the principal compounds at present available. The resulting values listed in the table agree to within factors of 2-3 with the limited number of measured constants published.

The lipid water partition behaviour (represented by $Log_{10}K_{OW}$) and water solubilities explain some aspects of the behaviour of pyrethroids to birds and to fish. In birds, generally high lipophilic character leads to partition into phases where metabolism and detoxification is rapid, so that avian toxicities of pyrethroids are low. In contrast, as with other lipophilic insecticides such as the organochlorine compounds, pyrethroids in water partition directly into the gills and thence the blood stream of fish where they exert a powerful action. The calculated water solubilities in the table are theoretically valuable parameters for comparisons and estimations even though, with these extremely insoluble compounds, practical assessments of these properties are complicated by strong adsorptions of pyrethroids on the walls of containers. The high fish toxicities measured in the laboratory indicate a much greater hazard to fish than are experienced in practice, because strong adsorption onto lipoid particles (soil, plants, etc.) greatly diminishes the effects of any adventitious contamination of open water.

Behaviour of pyrethroids in soil

The compounds in the table have lipophilicities, indicated by Log K_{OW} values, which although they range over about four orders of magnitude, are sufficiently high to lead to strong absorption by soil (Ref. 11), supporting the earlier conclusion (Ref. 12) that undesirable dispersion of pyrethroids throughout the environment by leaching is very improbable; deposits on soils will be limited to regions directly treated and will persist only until the insecticides have been decomposed by soil microorganisms.

The balance between stability on the crop and lack of persistence in soil, necessary for an environmentally acceptable yet sufficiently active insecticide, has been achieved in the currently marketed photostable pyrethroids, but there are indications in the Table that the same balance should not be assumed for all subsequent compounds. For instance, the predicted half-life for FCR 1622 is much longer than those of most of the other compounds. Under appropriate conditions, even compounds such as permethrin can persist adequately to be useful against soil pests. On the waxy outer coating of wheat seeds, its low water solubility and rate of dissolution enable it to survive the winter and thus diminish attack by the larvae of the wheat bulb fly (Ref. 13).

Nicholls et al. (14) have recently investigated the optimum water solubilities, vapour pressures, soil adsorption coefficients and octanol-water, air-water and air-wet soil partition coefficients in a group of organophosphate insecticides for efficient action in a range of soils. Soil active pyrethroids will need physical properties comparable to those

Physical Properties of Pyrethroids

Name and reference[a]		Structure	Log K_{ow}	Calculated solubility in pure water(ppm)	Vapour pressure mm.Hg	Concentration ratio air/wet soil Kas	Predicted half life in soil (days)
pyrethrin I		1A	5.9	0.2	2×10^{-5}	9×10^{-6}	<5
pyrethrin II		2A	4.3 [b]	9	4×10^{-7}	3×10^{-8}	<5
cinerin I		1B	5.6	0.6	4×10^{-5}	1×10^{-5} [c]	<5
allethrin		1C	5.0	2	7×10^{-5}	1×10^{-5}	<5
benzylnorthrin		1D	5.8	0.3	6×10^{-7}	3×10^{-7}	<5
barthrin		1E	4.9	3	1×10^{-5}	1×10^{-6}	<5
dimethrin		1F	6.0	0.2	5×10^{-4}	2×10^{-4}	<5
trimethrin		1G	6.5	0.1	3×10^{-4}	3×10^{-4}	<5
ABC		1H	6.3	0.1	3×10^{-4}	2×10^{-4}	<5
DMABC		1J	7.3	0.01	8×10^{-5}	2×10^{-4}	<5
tetramethrin		1M	4.2	5	1×10^{-7}	6×10^{-9}	<5
resmethrin		1N	5.9	0.2	9×10^{-6}	4×10^{-6}	<5
ethanoresmethrin		3N	6.8	0.03	3×10^{-6}	4×10^{-6}	<5
kadethrin		4N	5.4	1	4×10^{-8}	1×10^{-8}	<5
kikuthrin		1P	5.0	3	6×10^{-4}	1×10^{-4}	<5
furamethrin		1Q	4.5	9	1×10^{-3}	1×10^{-4}	<5
phenothrin		1K	7.4	0.01	4×10^{-6}	1×10^{-5}	<5
permethrin		5K	6.8	0.03	3×10^{-7}	4×10^{-7}	10
cypermethrin		5R	6.2	0.1	3×10^{-8}	2×10^{-8}	30 [d]
deltamethrin	(7)	6R	6.4	0.01	1×10^{-9}	8×10^{-10}	40
baythroid	(15)	5S	6.3	0.1	3×10^{-8}	2×10^{-8}	40
cyhalothrin	(16)	7R	6.6	0.05	1×10^{-7}	1×10^{-7}	60
cypothrin	(17)	15R	7.4	0.006	3×10^{-9}	8×10^{-9}	60
NRDC 173		8N	4.6	8	7×10^{-5}	7×10^{-6}	<5
terallethrin	(18)	10C	4.3	15	2×10^{-4}	1×10^{-5}	<5
fenvalerate	(6)	11R	6.8	0.01	1×10^{-9}	3×10^{-9}	80
fluorocythrin	(19)	12R	6.8	0.01	1×10^{-9}	3×10^{-9}	80
fenpirithrin	(20)	5T	5.6	0.7	1×10^{-8}	3×10^{-9}	20
FCR 1622	(15)	9S	8.6	0.0003	1×10^{-10}	1×10^{-9}	>150
fenpropathrin	(18)	10R	6.0	0.2	1×10^{-6}	5×10^{-7}	50
fenfluthrin	(21)	5L	5.2	2	2×10^{-4}	3×10^{-5}	25
tralomethrin	(22)	14R	6.9	0.01	3×10^{-11}	4×10^{-11}	(cf 6R)
fluvalinate	(23)	13R	6.4	0.01	3×10^{-10}	2×10^{-10}	40
GH 380	(24)	16K	7.0	0.02	3×10^{-10}	5×10^{-10}	20
S 3243	(18)	5U	5.4	0.4	4×10^{-4}	1×10^{-4}	5

a For primary references to early compounds, see Ref. 8.

bcd Underlining of entries indicates values considered appropriate for b: knockdown; c: soil fumigant activity; d: sufficient soil stability.

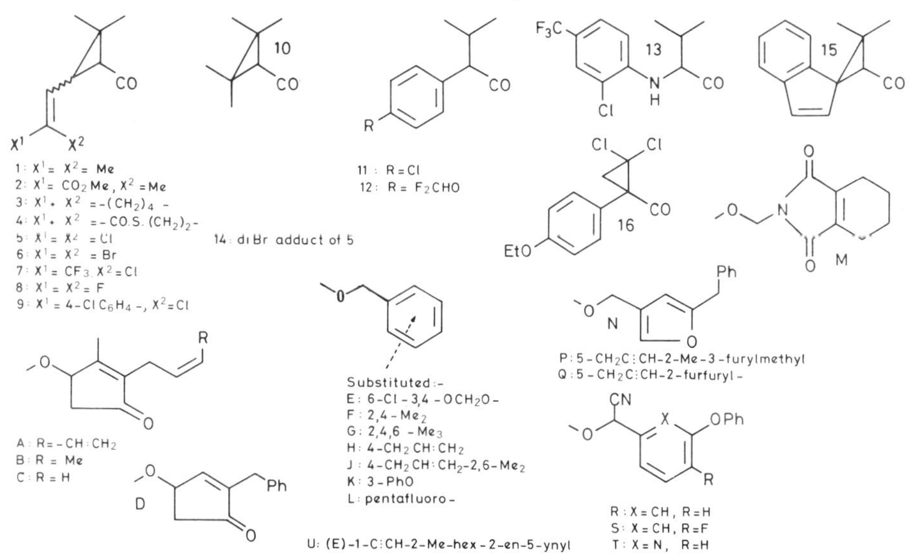

of the organophosphates (air-wet soil partition coefficients greater than 1×10^{-5}, implying vapour pressures greater than 1×10^{-4}mm; octanol-water partition coefficients ($\text{Log}_{10} K_{OW}$) greater than 4.0) to maintain sufficient concentrations of toxicants in the air phase in the soil; the compounds should also have adequate insecticidal activities and stability against soil microorganisms. Few pyrethroids are likely to possess a full combination of optimum properties but the pentafluorobenzyl ester, 5L and related compounds which have recently been patented as insecticides active against soil pests (Ref. 21) represent significant progress.

Behaviour in plants

The lipophilicity and low vapour pressure of pyrethroids in general limits their action against insects to direct contact effects, and possibly some stomach poison activity. Under most conditions, the insecticide is adsorbed onto the waxy cuticles of leaves and thereby protected from metabolism; pyrethroids used in practice so far show little or no translaminar activity. The possibility of systemic activity by pyrethroids is frequently discussed, but such activity in plants is generally restricted to compounds with log K_{OW} in the range -0.5 to + 3.5 with an optimum for upward movement of ca.2 (Ref. 25), outside the range for active pyrethroids (Ref. 26). Graham-Bryce (27) has discussed how chemical formulation might be used to confer systemic properties, by incorporating a group which could be metabolised, after transport, to give a less polar, active, compound. However, the extreme lipophilicity of active pyrethroids excludes many possibilities.

Knock-down activity

Following Sawicki's initial demonstration (Ref. 28) that pyrethrin II (2A) (a compound with a methoxycarbonyl substituent) knocked houseflies down almost twice as quickly as pyrethrin I (1A) (with a methyl group) even at one third the concentration, further informative comparisons between compounds have been recognised. The structures of those pyrethroids with rapid knockdown have some features in common with compounds effective for kill, but there are also significant differences. The former group of compounds (2A, 1C, 10C, 4N, 1P, 1Q, 5L) are nearly all more polar (less lipophilic) than the latter, so the higher polarity may be necessary for more rapid penetration to sites affected in knockdown (Ref. 29). Possibly coincidentally, some good knockdown compounds (eg. 2A) have sites at which they can be rapidly detoxified (by esteratic activity in the case of pyrethrin II). Smith *et al.* (30) have recently speculated that reversible Michael addition with a critical *thiol* in the pyrethroid receptor site might contribute to the unique potency and transient character of the neurotoxicity of tetramethrin (1M). Other compounds in Table 1 with good knockdown action may have structural features similarly capable of fast reversible interaction with thiol groups.

A minor, but significant and interesting application of pyrethroids with adequate volatility and rapidity of action is in mosquito coils. Originally the residues of the natural pyrethrins remaining in the flower marc when most of the insecticidal esters had been solvent extracted were mixed with wood chips to give a suitably slow burning coiled formulation. The more volatile pyrethrin I, cinerin I and jasmolin I were vaporised by the glowing tip before they could be thermally decomposed; the less volatile (II) esters were incinerated and wasted. Subsequently the even more volatile and more stable compound S-bioallethrin was found to be very effective in the traditional formulation and also in suitable heated pads. Volatility, heat stability, rapid action and high intrinsic potency to flying pests are important characteristics in this application (Ref. 31), for which kikuthrin (1P) and NRDC 173 (8N) are therefore potentially valuable.

STABILITY OF PYRETHROIDS IN LIGHT

The first photostable pyrethroids (Ref. 8) were developed in investigations of the extent to which the structures of the natural esters and allethrin, and subsequently of resmethrin and bioresmethrin, could be modified with retention or enhancement of their potency. In chrysanthemates the demonstration that replacing the methyl groups of the isobutenyl side chain by halogen increased insecticidal activity suggested that photostability might be examined, because this centre might be less sensitive to the photo-oxidative processes that Casida (32) had identified at this site in such esters. Comparably, esters of 3-benzylbenzyl and 3-phenoxybenzyl alcohols, discovered as effective alcoholic components when investigating compounds sterically equivalent to 5-benzyl-3-furylmethyl alcohol, proved, on the basis of general chemical reactivity, to be more photostable, as they did not contain the sensitive furan ring. Similar considerations applied to esters of substituted α-isopropylphenyl acetates when these were shown to be effective acidic components by Ohno *et al.* (6).

The types of reaction by which pyrethroids decompose in air and light can now, following Casida's extensive work, be recognised to fall into two chemically distinct categories which involve, or do not involve, activated forms of oxygen.

The isobutenyl side chains of chrysanthemates are oxidised rapidly under appropriate conditions by singlet or triplet oxygen, or by ozone, but the reactivity of the corresponding dihalovinyl compounds is such that comparable reactions do not take place with them. The furan ring in derivatives of 5-benzyl-3-furylmethyl alcohol (resmethrin, bioresmethrin, kadethrin) reacts rapidly with singlet oxygen to form a Diels-Alder type adduct, in contrast to the inert aromatic systems in 3-phenoxybenzyl alcohol derivatives. In compounds where decomposition is not dominated by such bimolecular reactions, photo-stability will be influenced by the intensity of light energy absorption by the chromophores in the structure and by whether the energy causes decomposition or can be dissipated (the quantum yield). For instance, rearrangements of the cyclopropane ring, and of the side chain of cyclopentenolones and cleavage of benzyl esters are probably due to intramolecular transfer of absorbed light energy.

The photostability of pyrethroids is therefore determined by whether groups susceptible to reaction with activated oxygen are present, by the intensity with which chromophores absorb, and by the efficiency of intramolecular energy transfer. The applicability of these principles has been demonstrated in the range of pyrethroids which are sufficiently stable for agricultural use, and indicate how otherwise suitable compounds found to be unduly stable or unstable could be modified for specific applications.

Formulations of photolabile pyrethroids may be stabilised on the shelf by adding antioxidants or selective absorbers of ultraviolet light, and by excluding oxygen and light. Stabilisation of a pyrethroid as a residue after it has been sprayed on the crop is much more difficult, not least because with conventional methods of formulation an unrealistically high initial concentration of stabiliser would be necessary to counter the dilution involved in spraying.

RESISTANCE AND SELECTIVITY

Present situation

The extent to which economically important insect pests, predators and parasites tolerate, or develop resistance to, pyrethroids under practical conditions will profoundly influence the future application of these insecticides. So far only 40 of the 350 species of arthropods with strains resistant to one or more insecticides have been shown to resist at least one pyrethroid in laboratory experiments (Ref. 33). Of these only about a third have led to control difficulties in the field. Thus with a few notable exceptions all key pests are at present effectively controlled with pyrethroids. Almost all pyrethroid resistance detected so far appears to have arisen through cross-resistance from the prolonged exposure of pest populations to other groups of insecticides (Ref. 34). Thus in *Blatella germanica* selection with diazinon or propoxur resulted in the development of resistance to these insecticides and to pyrethroids, while DDT used to control *Musca domestica* on Danish pig farms selected *kdr* (knock-down resistance), a mechanism conferring strong resistance to DDT and the pyrethroids.

The restricted use of photolabile pyrethroids (the natural pyrethrins, allethrin and isomers, tetramethrin, resmethrin and bioresmethrin) mainly against domestic and medical pests resulted in relatively low levels of resistance, but since 1976, the widespread application of photostable pyrethroids has exposed in some insects the potential to develop very strong pyrethroid resistance eg: x 2000, *Spodoptera exigua*; x 2800, *Plutella xylostella*; x 30,000, *M. domestica*; x 6000, *Culex quinquefasciatus*. These examples have prompted detailed investigations of the factors involved.

Resistance mechanisms

Several mechanisms have been shown to confer pyrethroid resistance. In most insects examined so far pyrethroid resistance is polyfactorial. Of the mechanisms involved some do not confer resistance directly but augment the influence of other factors, eg. *Pen*, a factor delaying penetration of insecticides. Others, eg. *kdr* involve the insensitivity of the site of action of pyrethroids, while esterases such as E4 which in *Myzus persicae* (Ref. 35) preferentially hydrolyses the *1S-trans* isomer of permethrin, or oxidases as those in resistant strains of *Sitophilus granarius* which attack the isobutenyl mechanism of chrysanthemates on the pentadienyl group in pyrethrin I are more active or present in larger amounts in the resistant insects. *Pen* can be recognised directly by measuring penetration and the metabolic resistance mechanisms by their response to synergists such as piperonyl butoxide (for pyrethroids) and FDMC (for DDT).

Kdr

Pyrethroids and DDT are considered to affect the passage of sodium ions across membranes in the insect nervous systems by related mechanisms but at greatly different concentrations; the kdr mechanism diminishes the sensitivity of the nervous receptor. Kdr is now implicated in the resistance of *Anopheles stephensi*, *Spodoptera littoralis*, *Boophilus microplus*, *B. germanica* and *M. persicae*, as well as *M. domestica*. Its presence is still demonstrable only by indirect means, eg. resistance to both pyrethroids and DDT in the presence of the appropriate synergists, but electrophysiological tests at present being developed should enable the direct detection of insensitivity to pyrethroids. This would facilitate the confirmation of kdr in insects other than the housefly, where it was first recognised. Sawicki (33) considers that widespread resistance to pyrethroids in insects not previously exposed to these insecticides is probably associated with kd resistance selected by worldwide application of DDT.

Practical implications

The mechanisms reviewed above, and possibly others, alone or in combination can explain many cases of development of resistance to the pyrethroids, both in the laboratory and in the field. Some results (resistance to permethrin, but not to fenvalerate, and the much greater levels of resistance inducible to deltamethrin than to permethrin) may be explained by mechanisms specifically affected by α-cyano substituents; others, such as the different levels of resistance produced by selection with one of the four isomers of permethrin, by pharmacodynamic and neurophysiological phenomena (Ref. 35). The kdr mechanism gives various levels of resistance with different pyrethroids and at present no correlation with structure can be discerned. Potential for resistance may also be correlated with the physical properties of the pyrethroid, such as polarity, in relation to the physiology of the species and stage of development. As well as the properties of the insecticide itself, the interaction of possible resistance mechamisms, the responses of the various species to be controlled and the whole range of environmental and ecological factors render the possibility of control in any one situation difficult to predict and potentially variable from season to season. However with a number of important species such as S. littoralis, Heliothis virescens and H. zea to which relatively high levels of resistance are demonstrated in the laboratory, comparably resistant field strains and failure of control at economically acceptable rates of application have not yet been encountered.

Sawicki (33) concludes that multidisciplinary investigations are needed to establish the most promising regimes for application of selected compounds, or combination of compounds and to preserve the value of pyrethroids or of other promising groups of insecticides. For example, the use of photostable pyrethroids to control populations of houseflies on pigfarms has led very quickly in some instances to the development of resistance. In this case, with the understanding consequent on a detailed study, sparing use of sprays of photolabile pyrethroids such as bioresmethrin has been shown to control successfully even houseflies with a proven potential for strong resistance without detectably increasing it further, because such treatments do not continuously select resistance mechanisms.

Selectivity

As with resistance, tolerance of particular species to pyrethroids (assessed on a ug/g basis, compared with other species) may be associated with variations in the rates of the essentially similar biochemical processes which are present within organisms to interact with pesticides (Ref. 36). For instance, Casida (37) has shown that the tolerance of lacewings Chrysopa carnea to pyrethroidal esters, especially the normally more potent cis forms, is due tc a high esterase activity, including a specific powerful cis-esterase which cleaves cis-permethrin and cis-cypermethrin 2-3-times faster than the corresponding trans isomers. In a study ranging over a wider variety of pyrethroidal structures, selective action against a pest (Ephestia kuehniella) rather than its parasite (Venturia canescens) had a factor between 2 and 150 fold (Ref. 38). Such a large difference in the selectivity factor for different compounds suggests that for any chosen pair of insects, at least some level of selectivity may be attainable with appropriate pyrethroids. Selectivity favouring the beneficial species, Apis mellifera (the honeybee) is an additional advantageous property of deltamethrin over bioresmethrin (Ref. 39), increased in practice by the repellency of deltamethrin.

RECENT DEVELOPMENTS

The original four photostable pyrethroids (permethrin 5K, cypermethrin 5R, deltamethrin 6R, and fenvalerate 11R) were sufficiently active to be effective in the field at application rates one fifth to one tenth those of the earlier major groups of insecticides. Since these products were introduced, no structural modifications have been reported which give substantial economic advantages over these established photostable pyrethroids. Graham-Bryce (27) doubts whether improvements in intrinsic activity may always be fully exploitable in practice.

In current products, refinements have optimised the proportions of the most potent optical and geometrical isomers, and substitutions have modified insecticidal activities. In es-fenvalerate (Ref. 40) both acidic and alcoholic chiral centres are resolved, and in cypermethrin the fully resolved chloro analogue (NRDC 182) of deltamethrin (6R) is induced to co-crystallise with its optical antipode to give a stereoisomeric mixture of very high insecticidal potency without involving a resolving agent (Ref. 41). The relative of fenvalerate in which a difluoromethoxy group replaces the 4-chlorosubstituent, fluorocythrin, 12R, has the enhanced activity associated with an optically active acid (Ref. 19); derived from the natural (active) amino acid valine, the acid in fluvalinate (13R) is also resolved (Ref. 23). The related 2-fluoro-4-trifluoromethyl compound is even more active than 13R. Modifications of activity are also produced by a 4-fluorosubstituent on α-cyano-3-phenoxy benzyl alcohol in the ester "cyfluthrin" (5S) (Ref. 15) and by incorporating a pyridoxy ring (Ref. 20 & 42) eg. in the analogue DOW 417 (5T). In [1R]-cis-2,2-dimethylcyclopropane carboxylates, replacement of the E-, but not the Z-chlorine of a 2,2-dichlorovinyl sidechain with trifluoromethyl (cyhalothrin isomer, 7R) gives enhanced activity against most species (Ref. 16). Both cyhalothrin, and the ester in which the same chlorine is replaced by a 4-chlorophenyl group (FCR 1622,9S) (Ref. 15) are effective acaricides.

The compounds above, some being introduced or strongly considered for practical aplication, were derived, like numerous others (Ref. 15) from extensive synthesis and testing programmes. The diversity of species investigated and the range of test methods used render general conclusions on structure-activity relationships difficult, but some are possible, for example that in active pyrethroids containing chiral centres, the epimeric forms of both acidic and alcoholic components give esters of greatly different potency - factors of more than 20 are common. Esters from [1R]-cyclopropane carboxylic acids and [1S]-α-isopropylphenyl acetic acids (or their chiral equivalents) are without exception much more active than those from their optical antipodes. An apparent exception to this generalisation has recently been reported in the compounds tralomethrin and tralocythrin, which are dibromo adducts of deltamethrin (5R), and of the corresponding isomer (NRDC 182) in cypermethrin (5R). The potencies of each of the 2-diastereomer mixtures obtained by adding bromine are the same (within a factor of 1.5) as those of the parent compounds, for both deltamethrin (against *Musca domestica*, and *Phaedon cochleariae*) (Ref. 43) and for NRDC 182 (against *Heliothus virescens*) (Ref. 44). There is substantial evidence from several sources that these compounds owe their insecticidal activity primarily to regeneration of the parent compound, rather than that they achieve these high levels of activity as intact structures: (i) The two separated diastereomers which are epimeric at C_1', have, in each case, about equal insecticidal activities (Ref. 22 & 44) a fact which is obviously fundamentally associated with their mode of action. This contrasts with previous experiences (above) of the potencies of epimeric pyrethroids, especially because the acid side chain is a site at which small changes usually produce profound modifications in activity (Ref. 8). A more likely explanation of the present results, therefore, is that the two forms react chemically at similar rates (losing bromine) to form the active species, rather than retaining the additional chirality, when they act, as this would be expected to lead to widely dissimilar activities. (ii) Loss of bromine has been identified as a substantial metabolic process when the compounds are applied to insects (Ref. 45). (iii) The compounds also lose bromine readily by photochemical processes on glass (Ref. 46) and leaves (Ref. 47). (iv) In an earlier investigation (Ref. 48) of esters of acids with either of two halogenated side chains ($ClCMe_2CH_2$- and $BrCF_2CH_2$) only the latter which is more able to generate the parent unsaturated compound was substantially potent. The concept of chemical formulation by using propesticides, is already well established in other classes of pesticides (Ref. 27) and with this first example in pyrethroids, further cases may confidently be expected to follow.

To investigate the relationships governing the effects of α-substitution, esters containing over 40 different α-substituents have recently been compared (Ref. 49). The results show a tendency for smaller substituents to give more active esters; the substitutions fell into four categories, linear (sp hybridised) substituents, those with C_1 sp^2 hybridised and bearing a hydrogen atom, other sp^2 and all sp^3 cases, and disubstitution (in decreasing order of the insecticidal activity conferred). The α-fluoro compound was therefore of interest, but when tested was not particularly active.

CONCLUSIONS

One outstanding characteristic of some of the recent synthetic pyrethroids has been potency one or even two orders of magnitude greater than that of established insecticides of other classes. Structure-activity investigations to explore the potential of molecular modifications continue to provide the basis for new discoveries and may be expected to lead to a wider range of novel applications. Such investigations may in future be increasingly guided by consideration of how physical properties influence behaviour of the pesticide in practice, using principles such as those discussed here.

Acknowledgement We thank R.M. Sawicki for helpful discussions on resistance.

REFERENCES

1. C.B. Gnadinger, Pyrethrum Flowers and Supplement (1936-1945) (690 pp) McLaughlin Gormley King, Minneapolis (1936 and 1945).
2. R.C. Roark, Digest of Information on Allethrin U.S.D.A. Paper E-846, 58pp (1952).
3. T. Kato, K. Ueda and K. Fujimoto, Agric. Biol. Chem. 28, 914-915 (1964).
4. J. Ward, Chem. and Ind. 586-587 (1953).
5. R.M. Sawicki, M. Elliott, J.C. Gower, M. Snarey and E.M. Thain, J. Sci. Fd. Agric., 13, 172-185 (1962).
6. N. Ohno, K. Fujimoto, Y. Okuno, T. Mizutani, M. Hirano, N. Itaya, T. Honda and H. Yoshioka, Pestic. Sci. 7, 241-247 (1976).
7. M. Elliott, A.W. Farnham, N.F. Janes, P.H. Needham and D.A. Pulman, Nature, 248, 710-711 (1974).
8. M. Elliott and N.F. Janes, Chem. Soc. Rev. 7, 473-505 (1978).
9. M.J. Bull, J.H. Davies, R.J.G. Searle and A.C. Henry, Pestic. Sci., 11, 249-256 (1980).
10. C. Hansch and A.J. Leo, Substituent Constants for Correlation Analysis in Chemistry and Biology, Wiley, New York (1979).
11. G.G. Briggs, J. Agric. Food Chem. 29, 1050-1059 (1981).
12. M. Elliott, N.F. Janes and C. Potter, Ann. Rev. Entomol. 23, 443-469 (1978).
13. D.C. Griffiths, Pestic. Sci. 8, 258-263 (1977).
14. P. Nicholls, A.W. Farnham and B. Buxton, Proc. Brit. Crop Protection Conf. - Pests and Diseases, 175-187 (1981).
15. K. Naumann, Chemie der synthetischen pyrethroid - Insektizide, Springer-Verlag, Berlin (1978).
16. P.D. Bentley, R. Cheetham, R.K. Huff, R. Pascoe and J.D. Sayle, Pestic. Sci. 11, 156-164 (1980).
17. D.G. Brown and R.W. Addor, Advances in Pesticide Science (IUPAC Conference, Zurich) 190-195 (1978).
18. T. Matsuo, T. Nishioka, M. Hirano, Y. Suzuki, K. Tsushima, N. Itaya and H. Yoshioka, Pestic. Sci., 11, 202-218 (1980).
19. W.K. Whitney and K. Wettstein, Proc. Brit. Crop Protection Conf. Pest and Diseases, 387-394 (1979).
20. S.K. Malhotra, J.C. van Heertum, L.L. Larson and M.J. Ricks, J. Agric. Food Chem. 29, 1287-1289 (1981).
21. Bayer, European Patent, 10154 (1978).
22. Roussel-Uclaf, Ger. Offen. 2,742,546 (1977).
23. C.A. Henrick, B.A. Garcia, G.B. Staal, D.C. Cerf, R.J. Anderson, K. Gill, H.R. Chinn, J.N. Labovitz, M.M. Leippe, S.L. Woo, R.L. Carney, D.C. Gordon and G.K. Kohn, Pestic. Sci., 11, 224-241 (1980).
24. G. Holan, D.F. O'Keefe, C. Virgona and R. Walser, Nature, 272, 734-736 (1978).
25. G.G. Briggs, R.H. Bromilow, R. Edmondson and M. Johnston, in Herbicides and Fungicides - Factors affecting their Activity. (Chem. Soc. Spec. Pub. No. 29) 128-134 (1977).
26. G.G. Briggs, M. Elliott, A.W. Farnham, N.F. Janes, P.H. Needham and S.R. Young, Pestic. Sci. 7, 236-240 (1976).
27. I.J. Graham-Bryce, Pestic. Sci., in press.
28. R.M. Sawicki and E.M. Thain, J. Sci. Food Agric. 5, 292-297 (1962).
29. G.G. Briggs, M. Elliott, A.W. Farnham and N.F. Janes, Pestic. Sci. 5, 643-649 (1974).
30. I.H. Smith, E.J. Wood and J.E. Casida, J. Agric. Food Chem. 30, 600-602 (1982).
31. P.R. Chadwick, Mosquito News, 30(2), 161-170 (1970).
32. R.L. Holmstead, J.E. Casida and L.O. Ruzo in Synthetic Pyrethroids (ACS Symposium Series No. 42) ed. M. Elliott pp. 137-146 (1977).
33. R.M. Sawicki, Feuilles d'Information du CILDA, in preparation.
34. R.M. Sawicki, Proc. 8th Brit. Insect. Fungic. Conf. 799-811 (1975).
35. A.L. Devonshire and G.D. Moores, Pestic. Biochem. Physiol, in press, (1982).
36. J.R. Corbett, Proc. Brit. Crop Protection Conf. - Pests and Diseases, 717-730 (1979).
37. I. Ishaaya and J.E. Casida, Environ. Entomol., 10, 681-684 (1981).
38. M. Elliott, N.F. Janes, J.H. Stevenson and J.H.H. Walters, in preparation.
39. J.H. Stevenson, Plant Pathology, 27, 38-40 (1978).
40. Sumitomo, Ger. Offen. 2,830, 031 (1977).
41. Shell, U.K. Patent Appl. 2,064,528 and 2,075,011 (1979).
42. M. Elliott, N.F. Janes and D.A. Pulman, Rothamsted Report for 1979, Part 1, 112.
43. M. Elliott, N.F. Janes and A.W. Farnham, unpublished results.
44. P. Ackermann, F. Bourgeois and J. Drabek, Pestic. Sci. 11, 169-179 (1980).
45. L.O. Ruzo, L.C. Gaughan and J.E. Casida, Pestic. Biochem. and Physiol., 15, 137-142 (1981).
46. L.O. Ruzo and J.E. Casida, J. Agric. Food Chem. 29, 702-706 (1981).
47. M. Elliott et al., Rothamsted Report for 1981, Part 1, 126-127; L.O. Ruzo, L.C. Gaughan and J.E. Casida, Abstracts of 180th ACS Symposium, (August 1980), No. 122.
48. M. Elliott, A.W. Farnham, N.F. Janes, P.H. Needham and D.A. Pulman, Pestic. Sci. 7, 492-498 (1976).
49. M. Elliott, A.W. Farnham, N.F. Janes and B.P.S. Khambay, Pestic. Sci., in press.

CHIRALITY AS A MAJOR FACTOR IN THE SELECTION OF HIGHLY ACTIVE COMPOUNDS IN PYRETHRINOID SERIES

Jacques J. Martel

Centre de Recherches Roussel-UCLAF, 102 route de Noisy, 93230 Romainville, France

It has already been stressed by us (1) and by others (2) that asymmetric centers of pyrethrinoids are playing a predominant role in the never ending search for compounds even more active than the existing ones. Furthermore as indicated in the title of this lecture the search for highly active compounds may take advantage of a systematic study of chiral changes at the various available asymmetric fragments of the molecule: at the alcoholic part on the one hand, and at the acidic part on the other hand.

CHIRAL CHANGES OF THE ALCOHOLIC PART

As a general rule, one and only one of the enantiomeric forms leads to active insecticidal esters. The other one gives rise to less active or inactive compounds even if, in a few cases, the occurrence of some kind of synergism between two diastereoisomeric esters may somewhat obscure the preceding clear-cut statement.
Let us focus our attention on the alcoholic components : as shown below, if we leave aside, for the moment, the last alcohol, at the bottom of the slide, for all other active alcoholic components there is only one spatial disposition that appears suitable, as far as a good level of activity is concerned.

Fig. 1. Spatial disposition of the alcoholic part

Allethrolone

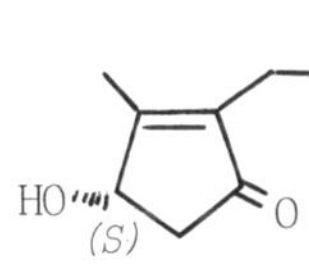

m-Phenoxybenzylic α-substituted alcohols

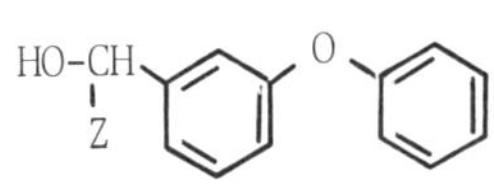

	Configuration leading to insecticidal esters	
Z = CN	S	same spatial disposition
Z = CH_3 , C≡CH	R	
Z = C(=O)-NH_2 , C(=S)-NH_2	S	

Dow alcohol

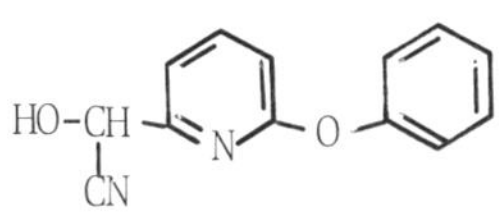

Turning now to the Dow alcohol (α-cyano-(6-phenoxy-2-pyridinyl) methyl alcohol), at first sight an apparent exception to the former statement, let us note that both enantiomers combined with the same acid lead to esters with similar insecticidal properties.

This last observation might mean that also in the case of Dow alcohol, activity is connected with the S configuration but then why is the other enantiomeric ester active too?. We can imagine that a fast racemization of the asymmetric center takes place in vivo and therefore the measured insecticidal activity would correspond, in fact, to that of a (RS) ester. Furthermore, no matter what the original ester is (R or S) the measured activity would correspond to that of the (RS) ester, due to this postulated fast "in vivo" racemization of the asymmetric center. In support of this assumption it has been found that "in vitro" racemization of "Dow esters" is much easier than the corresponding phenocyanol esters.

CHIRAL CHANGES OF THE ACIDIC PART

As it is already well established there are two prerequisites for any insecticidal activity of esters, namely a hydrogen must be present on asymmetric carbon 1, the configuration of which has to be (R).
The configuration of carbon 3, on the other hand, allows several variations. Depending on the nature of the alcoholic component of the pyrethrinoid, the substituent at carbon 3 may be either *trans* or *cis* with respect to the carboxyl at 1 in order to yield the compound endowed with the highest activity.
Thus the *trans* disposition appears more favorable for esters of allethrolone and 5-benzyl-3-furyl methanol whereas the *cis* disposition supplies especially active esters of m-phenoxybenzylic alcohols, substituted or not at the α-carbon.
Consonant with our previous assumptions is the fact that the esters of tetramethyl cyclopropane carboxylic acid which has built in *cis* and *trans* substituents are also active.
It is difficult at present to foresee which geometry whether the 1R, *cis* or the 1R, *trans* would give the best results and the more so that the activity may depend on the tested species, at the very least there are many opportunities for a modulation of activity.

VARIATIONS THROUGH THE CREATION OF A NEW ASYMMETRIC CENTER

There are several methods to induce more chirality into our molecules and two of them are presented now :
- halogen addition to the double bond

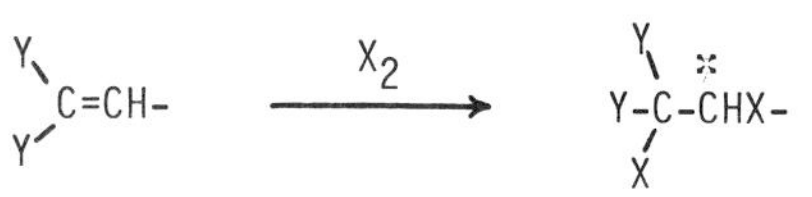

Halogen addition to the double bond yields a diastereoisomeric mixture of two isomers if the reaction is performed on a enantiomerically pure ester. It has been established by our group at Roussel Uclaf (3) and by Ciba-Geigy (4) that when X is Br and Y is Cl or Br, the activities of both diastereoisomeric forms do not significantly differ, be it, either in the (1*R*, *trans*) or in the (1*R*, *cis*) series.
- enhancing the asymmetry of the double bond
This type of asymmetry is widely known since Mother Nature has already prepared pyrethric acid and the corresponding esters but it was, nevertheless, interesting to look further into this area.
Resuming the pyrethric structures and combining them with (S) phenocyanol gives rather disappointing results, since the activities remain at best at a modest level.

Fig. 2. Insecticidal activity of pyrethric esters

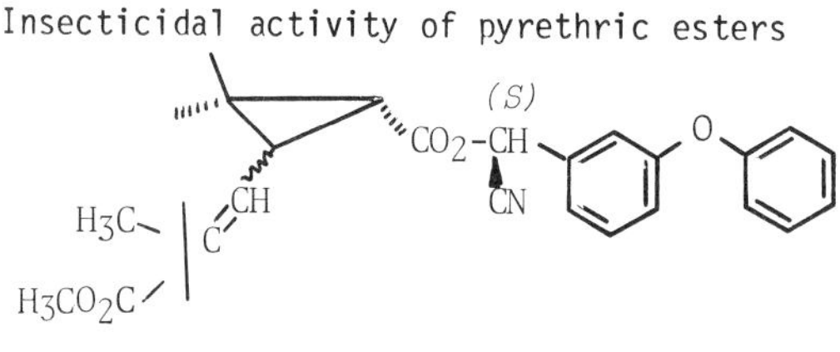

	Insecticidal activity/M.d topical application (deltamethrin = 100)
1*R*, *cis* E	2
1*R*, *cis* Z	4
1*R*, *trans* E	7
1*R*, *trans* Z	2

By contrast, when the vinylic methyl is missing there is a distinct improvement of the looked for activity for the (1R, cis)-Z (5) compound. Only hypotheses can be formulated as to the origin of this enhancement of activity. It seems difficult to ascribe it only to the 1R, cis Z geometry since it was shown on a former slide that the (1R, cis)-Z pyrethrate derivative has a low level of activity; but we cannot exclude the importance of the vinylic hydrogen on the compound with (1R, cis)-Z geometry.

Fig. 3. Insecticidal activity of nor-pyrethric esters

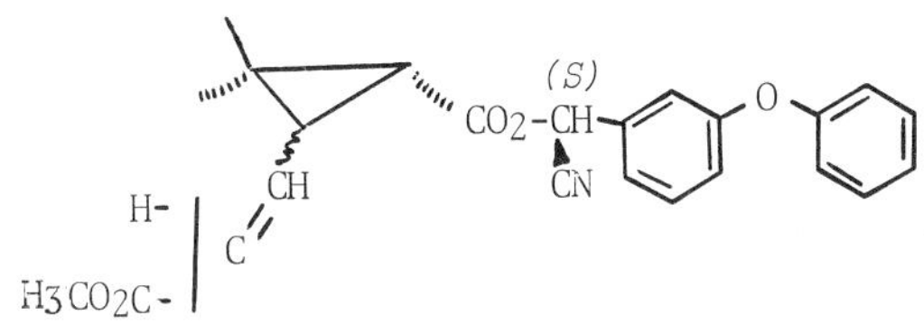

	Insecticidal activity/M.d. topical application (deltamethrin = 100)
1R, cis E	2
1R, cis Z	29
1R, trans E	2
1R, trans Z	2

To further clear up this point, let us analyse the following results.

Fig. 4. Insecticidal activity of a few esters of "phenocyanol" (S-α-cyano m-phenoxybenzylic alcohol)

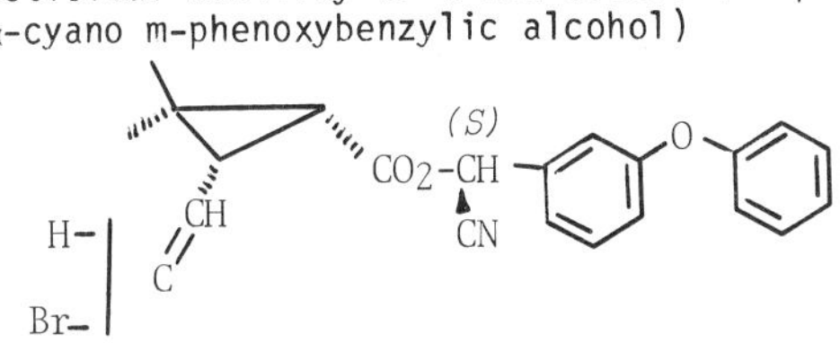

	Insecticidal activity/M.d. topical application (deltamethrin = 100)
1R, cis E	4
1R, cis Z	12

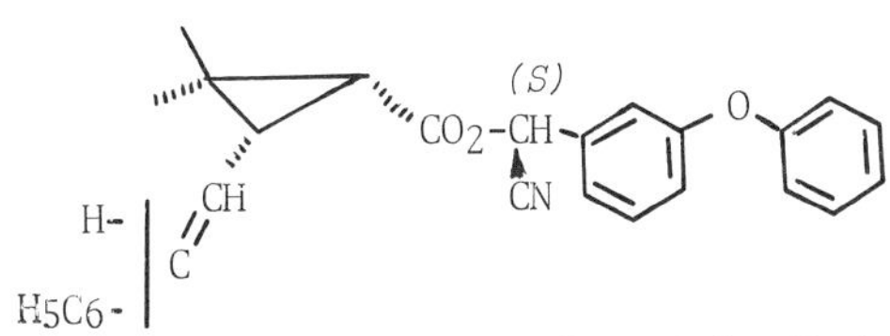

	Insecticidal activity/M.d. topical application (deltamethrin = 100)
1R, cis E	3
1R, cis Z	18

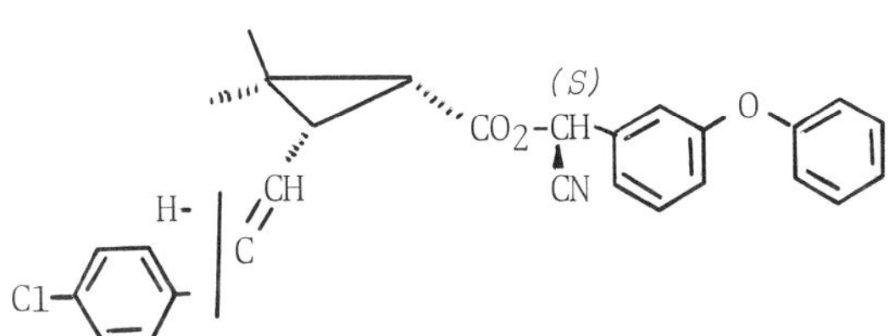

	Insecticidal activity/M.d. topical application (deltamethrin = 100)
1R, cis E	2
1R, cis Z	42

Even though it is much less active after the loss of one bromine, the more efficient derivative still belongs to the (1R, *cis*)-Z series. In support of this view, it is worthwhile to reproduce here the results of a study conducted by us on oxime derivative mixtures described by the Shell Group (6).

Fig. 5. Insecticidal activity of a few oxime derivatives

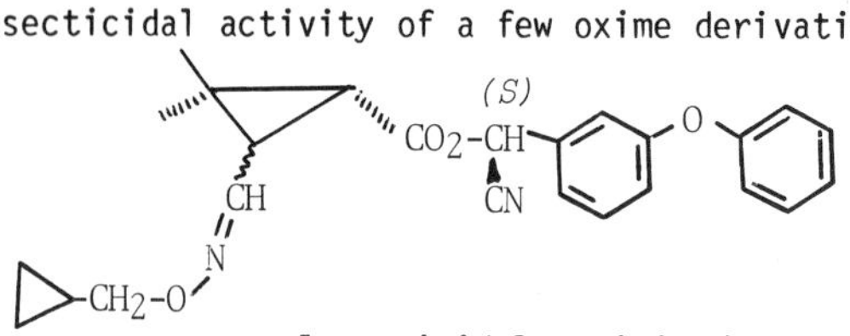

	Insecticidal activity/M.d topical application (deltamethrin = 100)
1R, *cis* E (anti)	4
1R, *cis* Z (syn)	65
1R, *trans* E (anti)	22
1R, *trans* Z (syn)	5

Again in this case (1R, *cis*)-Z outweighs all the others but the (1R, *trans*)-E derivatives does not fall so far behind. The last examples do not allow a definite conclusion since it can be said that either a hydrogen or a lone pair of electrons are required in order to observe strong differences of activity between isomers. Another piece of information to be added to the reflexion is the fact that when the double bond is disubstituted (R_1 and $R_2 \neq$ H), as in the pyrethic series, activities are of a low level, the same is true when R_1 and R_2 are part of a ring as in the following case).

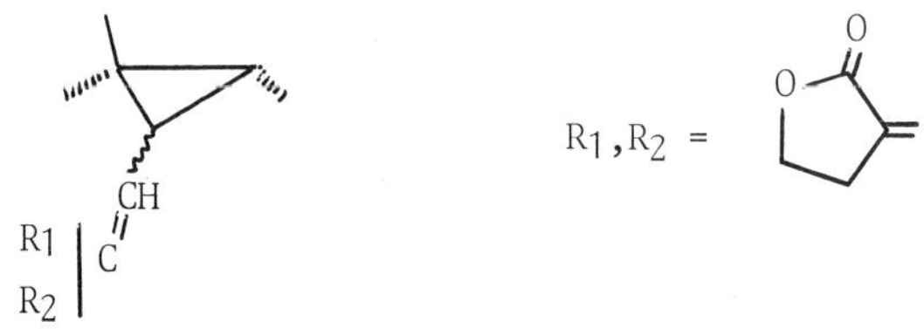

Furthermore there are quite a few examples that clearly show that the geometry of the double bond is able to strongly influence the level of activity even in the absence of hydrogen on the unsaturated terminal carbon end. Here are a few instances.

Fig. 6. Compared insecticidal activity of esters of phenocyanol and fluoro phenocyanol

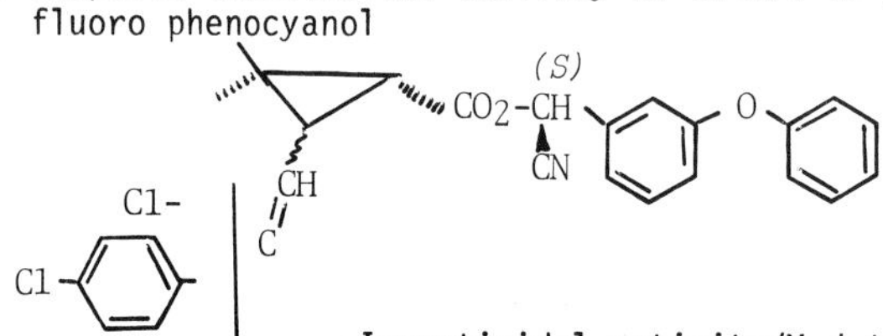

	Insecticidal activity/M.d topical application (deltamethrin = 100)
1R, *cis* E	14
1R, *cis* Z	< 1
1R, *trans* E	< 1
1R, *trans* Z	37

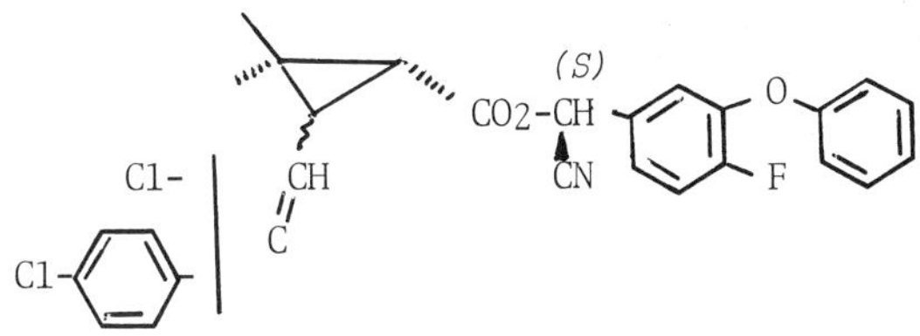

	Insecticidal activity/M.d topical application (deltamethrin = 100)
1R, *cis* E	22
1R, *cis* Z	1
1R, *trans* E	1
1R, *trans* Z	59

In the above example, not only the (1R, *cis*)-E outclasses the isomeric (1R, *cis*)-Z but the isomer that confers the best activity belongs to the trans series.

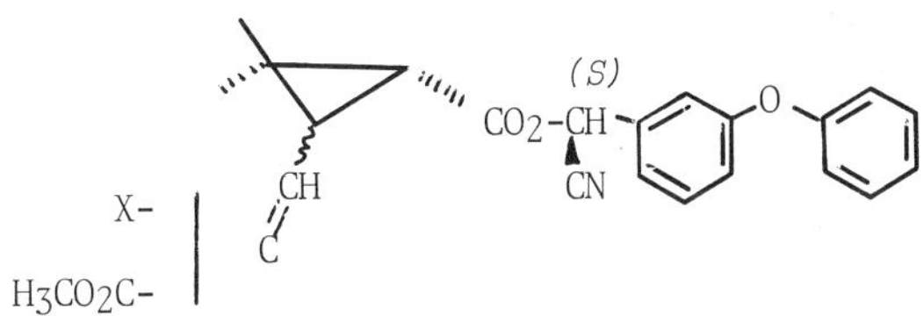

		Insecticidal activity M.d. topical application (deltamethrin = 100)(7)
X = F	1R, *cis* E	37
	1R, *cis* Z	<1
	1R, *trans* E	1
	1R, *trans* Z	2
X = Cl	1R, *cis* E	20
	1R, *cis* Z	<1
X = Br	1R, *cis* E	10
	1R, *cis* Z	1

CONCLUSION

Thus it seems fairly well established that, in a few cases, a dissymmetric disubstitution of the end of the double bond induces an unexpected enhancement of activity but this statement cannot be taken as a general one. Activity is the sum of many complex factors. Besides geometric and steric factors, many others whether polar or electronic do come into play and contribute to the overall activity. Only through a thorough evaluation of the relative importance of all these factors and a better understanding of the mechanisms involved can the pyrethrinoid chemist reach its objective: to find derivatives that out-perform all the preceding ones.

Fig. 7. Influence of the geometry of the double bond on the activity

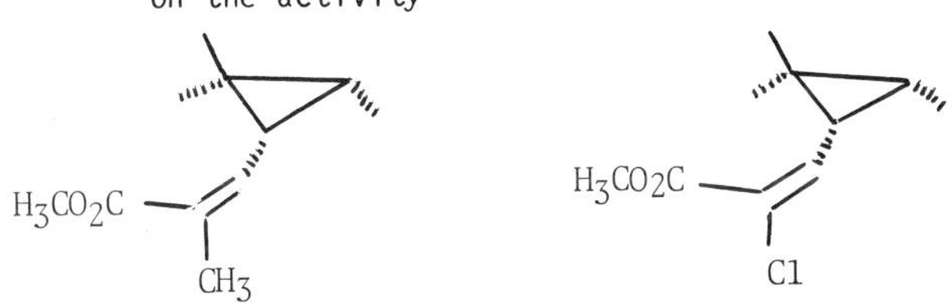

not much active (4) active (20)

(deltamethrin = 100)

REFERENCES

(1) J. MARTEL and J. BUENDIA, Synthesis of New Potent Pyrethroids, VII International Symposium on Chemistry of Natural Products, Riga (1970)
J. MARTEL, Stereocontrolled Synthesis of Some Natural Products, Kyoto (1980), Kyushu (1980)
(2) cf. for instance, M. ELLIOTT and N.F. JANES, Chem Soc. Rev. 1978, 7, 473-505
(3) Roussel-UCLAF, French Patent 2.364.884
(4) P. ACKERMANN, F. BOURGEOIS and J. DRABEK, Pest. Sci. 1980, 11, 169-179
(5) Roussel-UCLAF, E.P. 0038271
(6) Shell USP 4.211.792 and 4.282.249
(7) Roussel-UCLAF, E.P. 0050534

QUANTITATIVE STRUCTURE-ACTIVITY RELATIONSHIPS OF PYRETHROIDS

Toshio Fujita, Keiichiro Nishimura, Shoji Nakagawa and Minoru Nakajima

Department of Agricultural Chemistry, Kyoto University, Kyoto 606, Japan

Abstract - Convulsive and lethal activities of a set of substituted benzyl (1R)-*trans*-chrysanthemates against American cockroaches were determined by injection with and without application of synergists as inhibitors of metabolism. The neuroexcitatory and neuroblocking activities also were determined in terms of minimum effective concentrations to induce repetitive train of impulses and conduction blockage, respectively, to central nerve cords excised from the cockroaches. Each symptomatic activity from which the effect of metabolism is eliminated was found to be quantitatively analyzable by means of a linear combination of indices for two types of neurophysiological activity when the transport factor is separated by use of the hydrophobicity parameter. Neuroblocking activity is more responsible for the convulsive effect than the neuroexcitatory activity, while both neurophysiological effects operate together on the cockroach resulting in paralysis and death. The substituent effects on the neuroexcitatory activity were highly specific to substituent positions, whereas those on the neuroblocking activity were not. Steric effect of substituents represented by van der Waals volume was found to play the most significant role in determining the variation in the neuroexcitatory activity. Peculiar substituent effects depending upon the bulkiness and position of substituents, which had been observed in the toxicity of this class of compounds, can be rationalized by the present analysis indicating that the optimum van der Waals volume of substituents is largest at the ortho and smallest at the para position.

INTRODUCTION

The most distinctive aspect of pyrethroid insecticides is that they exhibit lethal as well as knockdown effects, particularly, against flying insects (1). It has been acknowledged that these toxic effects are due to their action on the nerve function (2). A number of attempts have been made to identify the site(s) of action of the knockdown and lethal effects and to determine relationships between symptomatic and neurophysiological activities using house flies (3-5), American cockroaches (6, 7) and other insects (8).

We have been studying on the structure-activity correlations of pyrethroids using a set of variously substituted benzyl (1R)-*trans*-chrysanthemates (Fig. 1) and related compounds. We have determined pyrethroid levels which

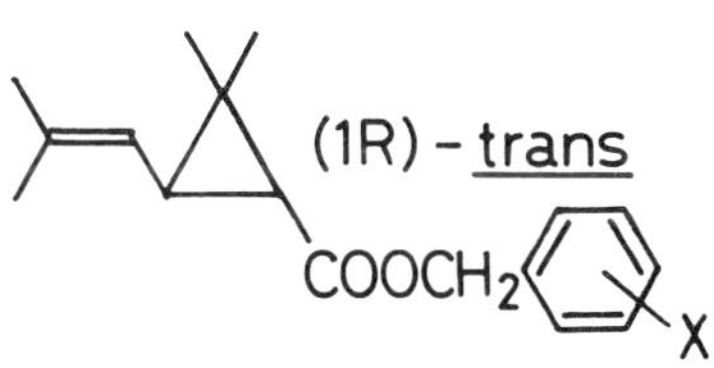

Fig. 1. Substituted benzyl (1R)-*trans*-chrysanthemates, where X is o- , m- and p- alkyl, alkoxy, halogen, phenoxy etc.

induce convulsions as well as cause death in American cockroaches, with and without synergists as metabolic inhibitors. Neuroexcitatory and neuroblocking activities also were determined using the central nerve cords excised from the cockroaches. We have quantitatively analyzed correlations between symptomatic and neurophysiological activities with the aid of physicochemical parameters of the molecule. To understand structural factors determining the variations in the neurotoxicity of the compounds, the neurophysiological activities also were quantitatively analyzed in terms of the substituent effects using physicochemical substituent parameters and regression analysis (9, 10). Here, we summarize the results and discuss the significance of the quantitative analyses.

MATERIALS AND METHODS

Convulsive and Lethal Activities: These symptomatic activities were determined against male adult American cockroaches, *Periplaneta americana* by injection of methanol solution of the compounds. From the observation of symptoms at 20(±1)°C, the minimum dose above which the cockroaches convulse within 30 min (MCD in mol/insect) and that above which the cockroaches are killed after 24 hr (MLD in mol/insect) were determined (5, 11). The paralyzed but not completely killed insects were counted as being dead. The log(1/MLD) and log(1/MCD) values were used as indices of respective activities. In order to determine the "intrinsic" lethal activity, MLD value also was determined by eliminating metabolic detoxication factors, with synergists such as piperonyl butoxide (PB) and NIA 16388 (NIA) as inhibitors of oxidative and hydrolytic metabolism, respectively. The effect of synergists was shown to be insignificant for the convulsive activity determined 30 min after injection. Thus, the unsynergized MCD value was used for the analysis of the convulsive activity.

Neurophysiological Activities: Neuroexcitatory and neuroblocking activities were determined by means of an extracellular technique using the excised central nerve cord of the male adult American cockroach at 20(±1)°C. The response of the nerve cord to an electric stimulus was recorded at certain time intervals after starting the immersion in Ringer's solution containing ≤1% methanol and various concentrations of each compound as shown in Fig. 2 for the p-NO_2 derivative. By increasing the concentration, the repetitive

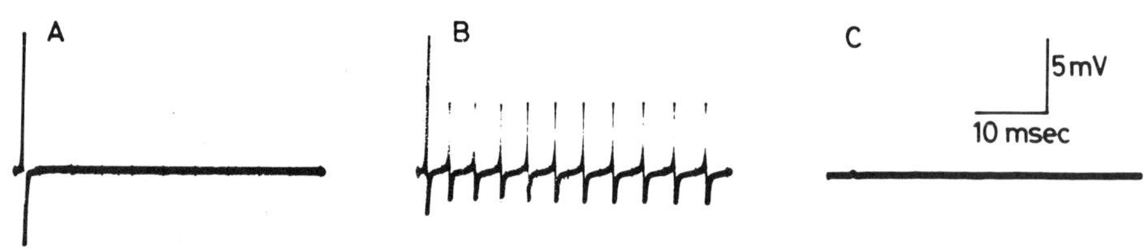

Fig. 2. Action potentials induced by a single stimulus, recorded (A) before the treatment and after the treatment with (B) 6.6×10^{-8}M p-nitrobenzyl (1R)-*trans*-chrysanthemate for 30 min and (C) 2.0×10^{-5}M p-nitrobenzyl chrysanthemate for 60 min.

train of impulses emerged (Fig. 2B). By increasing the concentration further, the nerve conduction was blocked (Fig. 2C). The minimum concentration above which the nerve cord exhibits repetitive discharges after stimulation of 600 mV and 0.1 msec was determined within 30 min after starting the immersion (MEC in M). Similarly, the minimum concentration above which action potential did not exceed 1 mV, even with the stimulation of 900 mV and 0.1 msec within 1 hr, was determined (MBC in M). The log(1/MEC) and log(1/MBC) values were used as indices for the excitatory and blocking activities, respectively. The standard error involved in these indices was less than ±0.1.

Correlation Analyses: First, we examined the relationship between symptomatic and neurophysiological activities according to equations of the type of eq. 1,

$$\log(1/C_1) = a \log(1/C_2) + b \log P + \text{const.} \quad (1)$$

where $\log(1/C_1)$ and $\log(1/C_2)$ are indices of two types of activity, symptomatic and neurophysiological, respectively. Log P is the hydrophobic parameter of the molecule, where P is the 1-octanol/water partition coefficient, and was used to examine the difference in the role of hydrophobicity between the two types of activity. Other physicochemical parameters such as the steric and electronic constants, in place of and in addition to log P, were found to be insignificant. The coefficients a and b were determined by regression analysis and the level of significance was examined by the t-test. Unless otherwise noted, each of the terms in the correlation equations is justified above the 0.95 level of significance in this study.

Difficulty was anticipated in the experimental determination of the P value for each compound, since the log P values of this series of compounds roughly estimated by means of the additivity principle (12) were very high, being at least about 5. Thus, we determined directly the log P value only for a few compounds such as m-NO_2 and p-CN derivatives by means of a published procedure at 25°C (13). Then, the hydrophobicity parameter π for substituents on the benzyl alcohol benzene ring defined by eq. 2, where P_X and P_H are the partition coefficients of substituted and unsubstituted derivatives, respectively (13), were calculated.

$$\pi = \log P_X - \log P_H \qquad (2)$$

The π values of the substituents of these compounds were close to those reported for monosubstituted benzenes (12). Therefore, the log P values of other substituted benzyl chrysanthemates were estimated as the sum of the value of the unsubstituted benzyl chrysanthemate and the π value of the substituent from the monosubstituted benzenes throughout this study.

Second, the variations in each of the biological activities were analyzed with the benzyl alcohol substituent parameters according to eq. 3., where C is either MEC or MBC. σ is the Hammett constant for the electron withdrawing effect.

$$\log(1/C) = \rho\sigma + a\pi - b\pi^2 + c\Delta Vw - d\Delta Vw^2 + \text{const.} \qquad (3)$$

For ortho substituents, the corresponding σ(para) values were used (14). ΔVw is the group van der Waals volume relative to that of H defined as eq. 4 where Vw(X) and Vw(H) are those of X-substituents and H, respectively, calculated according to Bondi (15).

$$\Delta Vw = Vw(X) - Vw(H) \ (cm^3/mol) \qquad (4)$$

The ΔVw value used here is scaled by 0.1 to make the size comparable to that of other parameters. ρ, a, b, c and d are regression coefficients determined by the least square method and their level of significance was examined by the t-test. The squared parameter terms are added to examine the optimum in respective physicochemical effects so that $b,d \geq 0$.

RESULTS

Relationships between Lethal and Neurophysiological Activities: Since the lethal activity determined with PB and NIA is considered to be the activity from which metabolic factors are eliminated as far as possible, it is expected to correlate with neurophysiological activities. In Fig. 3 and 4, the unsynergized and synergized lethal activity indices are plotted against the neuroexcitatory activity index. Although variation in lethal activity is in general correspondence with excitatory activity when synergists are used, a direct relationship does not seem to exist between the two activities as shown in Fig. 4B. However, if the hydrophobic parameter log P is combined with the neuroexcitatory activity index (abscissa), an improved relationship is evident as shown in Fig. 5. The situation for 41 benzyl chrysanthemates is formulated as eq. 5 and 6 for Fig. 4B and 5, respectively. Without one or both of the synergists, the corresponding correlations are much poorer.

$$\log[1/MLD(PB + NIA)] = \underset{(\pm 2.226)}{1.739} + \underset{(\pm 0.350)}{0.835} \log(1/MEC)$$

$$n = 41 \quad s = 0.822 \quad r = 0.611 \qquad (5)$$

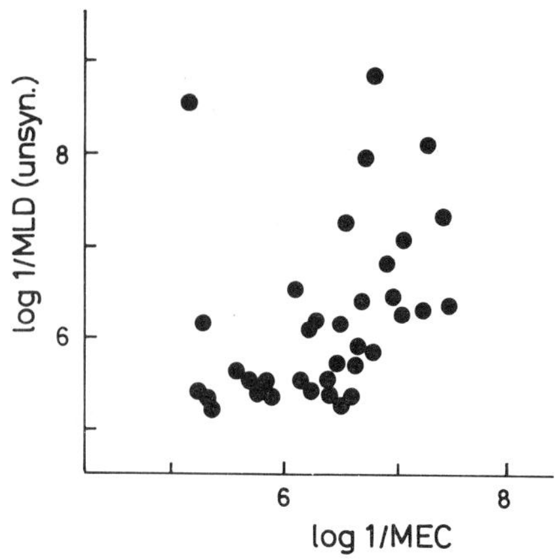

Fig. 3. Relationship between lethal activity determined without the synergists and neuroexcitatory activity of substituted benzyl (1R)-*trans*-chrysanthemates.

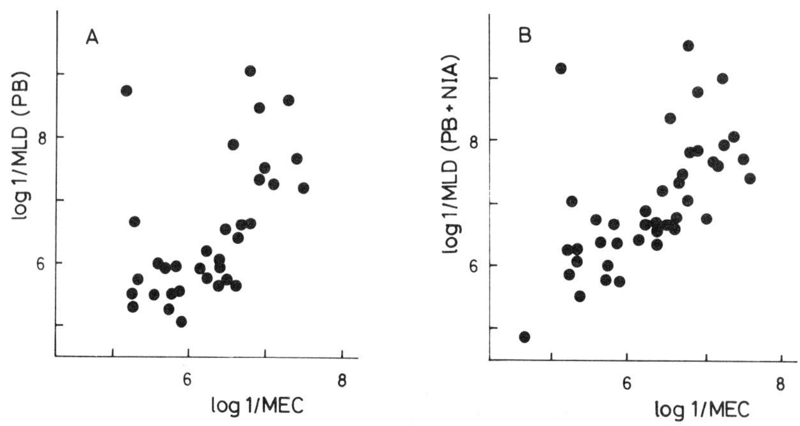

Fig. 4. Relationship between lethal activity determined with PB(A) or PB plus NIA(B) and neuroexcitatory activity of substituted benzyl (1R)-*trans*-chrysanthemates.

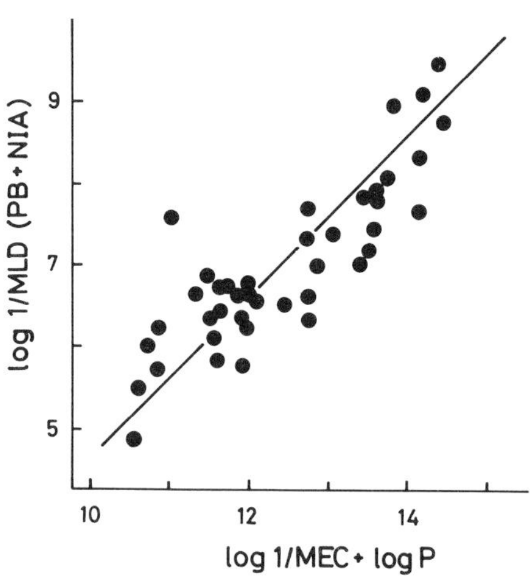

Fig. 5. Relationship between lethal activity (determined with PB and NIA) and neuroexcitatory activity combined with hydrophobicity parameter of substituted benzyl (1R)-*trans*-chrysanthemates.

$$\log[1/\mathrm{MLD(PB + NIA)}] = \underset{(\pm 1.913)}{-2.906} + \underset{(\pm 0.228)}{0.931} \log(1/\mathrm{MEC}) + \underset{(\pm 0.180)}{0.664} \log P$$

$$n = 41 \quad s = 0.530 \quad r = 0.864 \qquad (6)$$

Similar calculations with neuroblocking activity index for 19 benzyl esters whose log(1/MBC) values were available yield eq. 7 and 8.

$$\log[1/\mathrm{MLD(PB + NIA)}] = \underset{(\pm 4.055)}{0.901} + \underset{(\pm 0.899)}{1.415} \log(1/\mathrm{MBC})$$

$$n = 19 \quad s = 0.843 \quad r = 0.627 \qquad (7)$$

$$\log[1/\mathrm{MLD(PB + NIA)}] = \underset{(\pm 3.411)}{-2.032} + \underset{(\pm 0.672)}{1.280} \log(1/\mathrm{MBC}) + \underset{(\pm 0.335)}{0.615} \log P$$

$$n = 19 \quad s = 0.623 \quad r = 0.829 \qquad (8)$$

Although the addition of the log P term in eq. 6 and 8 is justified at better than the 99.5% level, the correlations are far from complete, showing fairly large standard deviations. We expected that the indices, log(1/MEC) and log(1/MBC), can be used together to analyze the lethal activity and formulated eq. 9-11 for the 19 compounds where both activity indices are determinable.

$$\log[1/\mathrm{MLD(PB + NIA)}] = \underset{(\pm 3.232)}{-3.110} + \underset{(\pm 0.437)}{1.026} \log(1/\mathrm{MEC}) + \underset{(\pm 0.298)}{0.619} \log P$$

$$n = 19 \quad s = 0.555 \quad r = 0.868 \qquad (9)$$

$$\log[1/\mathrm{MLD(PB + NIA)}] = \underset{(\pm 3.026)}{-4.282} + \underset{(\pm 0.463)}{0.733} \log(1/\mathrm{MEC}) + \underset{(\pm 0.634)}{0.721} \log(1/\mathrm{MBC}) + \underset{(\pm 0.263)}{0.598} \log P$$

$$n = 19 \quad s = 0.486 \quad r = 0.907 \qquad (10)$$

$$\log[1/\mathrm{MLD(PB + NIA)}] = \underset{(\pm 5.680)}{7.146} + \underset{(\pm 0.310)}{0.604} \log(1/\mathrm{MEC}) + \underset{(\pm 0.416)}{0.714} \log(1/\mathrm{MBC}) - \underset{(\pm 1.730)}{3.099} \log P + \underset{(\pm 0.147)}{0.316} (\log P)^2$$

$$n = 19 \quad s = 0.317 \quad r = 0.964 \qquad (11)$$

The correlation represented by eq. 9 is almost identical to its counterpart, eq. 6, indicating that the contribution of each term to lethal potency is unchanged even when the number of compounds is reduced. The addition of the log(1/MBC) term to eq. 9 as well as that of the log(1/MEC) term to eq. 8 are highly significant at the 97.0 and 99.5% level, respectively, leading to eq. 10. The simple correlation coefficient between log(1/MEC) and log(1/MBC) is r=0.562, which is much lower than that expected from similar correlation equations such as eq. 8 and 9. Interestingly, the addition of the $(\log P)^2$ term to eq. 10 leads to a far better correlation as shown in eq. 11. The sign of the $(\log P)^2$ term is positive, suggesting that there might be a competitive process reducing the effective concentration at the target site by accumulating the compounds in non-target phases. For this competitive process, the parabolic dependence on the hydrophobicity may exist with the optimum log P value about 4.9.

<u>Relationships between Convulsive and Neurophysiological Activities</u>: Since the metabolic factors for the convulsive activity are not significant, the convulsive activity index determined without the synergists was analyzed similarly.

$$\log[1/\mathrm{MCD(alone)}] = \underset{(\pm 2.491)}{0.626} + \underset{(\pm 0.313)}{0.702} \log(1/\mathrm{MEC}) + \underset{(\pm 0.203)}{0.389} \log P$$

$$n = 43 \quad s = 0.646 \quad r = 0.663 \qquad (12)$$

$$\log[1/\text{MCD(alone)}] = \underset{(\pm 3.465)}{0.236} + \underset{(\pm 0.722)}{1.176} \log(1/\text{MBC}) + \underset{(\pm 0.332)}{0.392} \log P$$

$$n = 20 \quad s = 0.677 \quad r = 0.747 \qquad (13)$$

$$\log[1/\text{MCD(alone)}] = \underset{(\pm 5.137)}{14.013} + \underset{(\pm 0.409)}{1.101} \log(1/\text{MBC}) - \underset{(\pm 1.684)}{4.464} \log P + \underset{(\pm 0.147)}{0.426} (\log P)^2$$

$$n = 20 \quad s = 0.381 \quad r = 0.932 \qquad (14)$$

$$\log[1/\text{MCD(alone)}] = \underset{(\pm 5.252)}{12.658} + \underset{(\pm 0.351)}{0.263} \log(1/\text{MEC}) + \underset{(\pm 0.473)}{0.903} \log(1/\text{MBC}) - \underset{(\pm 1.636)}{4.276} \log P + \underset{(\pm 0.143)}{0.409} (\log P)^2$$

$$n = 20 \quad s = 0.363 \quad r = 0.942 \qquad (15)$$

Eq. 12 shows that the convulsive activity is not significantly related to the neuroexcitatory activity alone. The addition of $(\log P)^2$ term to eq. 12 did not improve the situation much. Eq. 13 and 14 indicate, however, that the activity variation is nicely delineated by the neuroblocking activity index when the log P and $(\log P)^2$ terms are introduced in the analysis. The addition of the neuroexcitatory index improves the correlation slightly as shown in eq. 15, although it is justified at a level slightly less than 90% (86.9%). Again, the sign of the $(\log P)^2$ term is positive, similar to that in eq. 11. The magnitude of the coefficient larger than that in eq. 11 shows a parabolic dependence more conspicuous than that in eq. 11. As speculated for eq. 11, there might be a competitive process reducing the effective concentration at the target site also for this convulsive activity.

Substituent Effects on Neuroexcitatory Activity: Since substituent effects which were highly specific to their positions were expected by preliminary examinations, the analyses by means of eq. 3 have been performed for sets of ortho, meta and para derivatives separately. The unsubstituted compound is included in each of the sets as the reference. Eq. 16-18 are derived for the neuroexcitatory activity of the ortho, meta and para substituted derivatives, respectively.

Ortho derivatives:

$$\log(1/\text{MEC}) = \underset{(\pm 0.480)}{5.501} - \underset{(\pm 0.673)}{1.011}\sigma - \underset{(\pm 0.332)}{0.301}\pi^2 + \underset{(\pm 0.332)}{0.405}\Delta Vw$$

$$n = 14 \quad s = 0.372 \quad r = 0.878 \qquad (16)$$

Meta derivatives:

$$\log(1/\text{MEC}) = \underset{(\pm 0.459)}{5.454} + \underset{(\pm 0.397)}{0.654}\Delta Vw - \underset{(\pm 0.066)}{0.066}\Delta Vw^2$$

$$n = 17 \quad s = 0.325 \quad r = 0.850 \qquad (17)$$

Para derivatives (omitting alkoxy derivatives):

$$\log(1/\text{MEC}) = \underset{(\pm 0.578)}{5.775} - \underset{(\pm 0.205)}{0.344}\pi + \underset{(\pm 0.522)}{1.132}\Delta Vw - \underset{(\pm 0.098)}{0.260}\Delta Vw^2$$

$$n = 18 \quad s = 0.398 \quad r = 0.933 \qquad (18)$$

Eq. 16 indicates that the larger the van der Waals volume, the more favorable are the ortho substituents to the excitatory activity on the nerve cord. Since the activity of the o-α-naphthoxy derivative, of which $\Delta Vw = 7.21$, was not detected, it seems to exist an optimum ΔVw value between 4.65 (for the o-phenoxy group which is the bulkiest among substituents included in the correlation) and 7.21. Electron withdrawing effect of the ortho substituents deteriorates the activity. The activity varies parabolically with the π value, the optimum of which is about $\pi = 0$, although the π^2 term in this equation is justified only at the 93% level of significance.

Eq. 17 shows that an optimum van der Waals volume exists for the meta substituents, which is located at about $\Delta Vw = 4.9$. No electronic and hydrophobic substituent effects are significant in determining the activity variations in the m-substituted derivatives. Except for the alkoxy derivatives, the steric effect of para substituents is somewhat similar to that of meta substituents. The optimum volume for the para substituents is calculated as $\Delta Vw = 2.2$ from eq. 18. The hydrophobicity of substituents is not favorable to the activity at the para position. Even with combinations of independent variables other than those used in eq. 18, the activity of the p-OEt and -OPr(i) derivatives could not be accommodated. Some detrimental factor due to the alkoxy oxygen must be in operation.

Substituent Effects on Neuroblocking Activity: In contrast to the effect on excitatory activity, substituent effects on blocking activity were not specific to substituent positions. With the position-independent hydrophobic and steric parameters, eq. 19 is formulated for 20 compounds including those used for eq. 7-11 and the m-SO_2Me derivative the finite activity indices of which are available.

$$\log(1/MBC) = \underset{(\pm 0.240)}{3.972} + \underset{(\pm 0.138)}{0.370}\Delta Vw - \underset{(\pm 0.158)}{0.283}\pi^2$$

$$n = 20 \quad s = 0.284 \quad r = 0.812 \qquad (19)$$

The correlation coefficient of eq. 19 seems rather low but the correlation was highly significant at a level better than 99.5%. This is mainly due to the fact that the variation in the potency is not very large for 20 compounds. Eq. 19 reveals that the bulkier the substituents the more potent the blocking activity. There is an optimum hydrophobicity value at about $\pi = 0$.

DISCUSSION

As far as the benzyl chrysanthemates are concerned, the above analyses indicate that, after eliminating the metabolic effects and after separating the hydrophobic factors required for transport processes, the variations in the whole body symptomatic effects are delineated by the linear combination of two neuroactivity indices.

The convulsive activity was determined within 30 min after injection. Within such a short period, distribution of the compounds in the insect should not be even. Local concentration of the compound should be high and enough to block the nerve conduction in the vicinity of the site of injection. The more distant the location from the site of injection, the lower is the concentration of insecticides which induces nerve excitation. In the convulsive symptom, cockroaches were unable to regain their feet. This may be due to conduction blockage in some parts of the nervous system. The quivering movement of feet seems attributable to the excitation of other parts of the nervous system. In eq. 15, the log(1/MBC) term outweighs the log(1/MEC) term, showing that the neuroblocking activity is more responsible for the convulsive effect than the neuroexcitatory activity. This may be due to the fact that the lower concentration zone is not widely developed within 30 min.

For the lethal effect as represented by eq. 11, the coefficients of the log(1/MBC) and log(1/MEC) terms are almost equivalent. This may be rationalized as follows. Since the lethal activity was determined 24 hrs after injection, the insecticide should be distributed more evenly and the lower concentration zone should be developed more widely than within the shorter convulsion test period. Therefore, the relative significance of the neuroexcitatory effect should increase with the passage of time. The two types of neurophysiological effects eventually operate together on the cockroach resulting in paralysis and death.

In Fig. 6, the neuroexcitatory activity is expressed as the function of the ΔVw value at each position according to eq. 16-18. It is easily understood that, other factors being equal, the sequence of the activity among positional isomers varies from para > meta > ortho to meta > ortho > para with increase in the bulkiness of substituent from nitro to phenoxy. Essentially the same position-specific effect of substituents was observed for the two types of symptomatic activity (10). The steric restriction of substituents seems to be highest at the para position and lowest at the ortho position for suitable interaction of the molecule with the target site. Actually, position-specific electronic and hydrophobic substituent effects overlap the

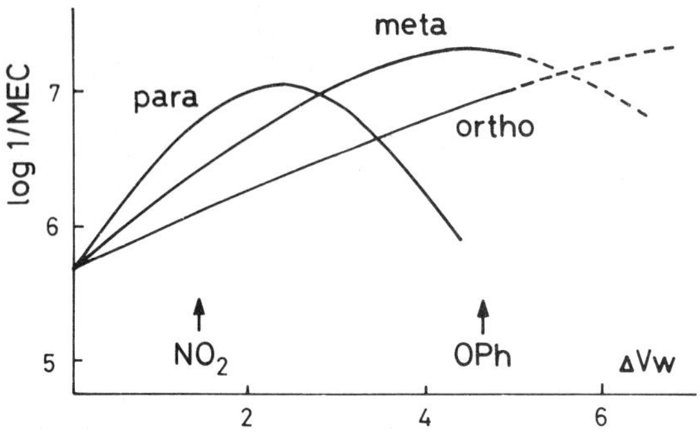

Fig. 6. Effect of substituent volume on the neuroexcitatory activity of substituted benzyl (1R)-*trans*-chrysanthemates.

topographical effect in determining the variation of the neuroexcitatory and lethal activities. Similar position specific steric effect of substituents was observed for the neuroexcitatory activity of lindane analogs although the mode of action is different from that of pyrethroids (16).

The neuroblocking activity of benzyl chrysanthemates related to the position-independent hydrophobicity is rather similar to that of structurally unrelated compound set including lindane isomers and alkanols which perhaps belongs to a type of physical toxicity (17). The fact that the blocking activity of chrysanthemates also is related to the bulkiness of substituents, however, suggests a mode of action more specific to structural factors.

The present work clearly indicates the versatility of the quantitative procedure using substituent parameters and regression analysis in analyzing the structure-activity relationships of pyrethroid insecticides. Although further examinations are required to draw a comprehensive picture, we expect a possibility to extend the present procedure to structure-activity study of various subsets of pyrethroids.

Acknowledgment - This investigation was supported in part by Grants-in-Aid for Scientific Research and for Special Project Research awarded by the Ministry of Education, Science and Culture.

REFERENCES

1. e.g., R.D. O'Brien, *Insecticides, Action and Metabolism*, Academic Press, New York, N.Y., p.164 (1967).
2. T. Narahashi, *Adv. Insect Physiol.*, 8, 1 (1971).
3. T.A. Miller and M.E. Adams, *ACS Symp. Ser.*, 42, 98 (1977).
4. M.E. Adams and T.A. Miller, *Pestic. Biochem. Physiol.*, 11, 218 (1979).
5. P.E. Burt and R.E. Goodchild, *Pestic. Sci.*, 5, 625 (1974).
6. P.E. Burt and R.E. Goodchild, *Pestic. Sci.*, 8, 681 (1977).
7. D.W. Gammon, *Pestic Sci.*, 9, 79 (1978).
8. A.N. Clements and T.E. May, *Pestic. Sci.*, 8, 661 (1977).
9. S. Nakagawa, N. Okajima, T. Kitahaba, K. Nishimura, T. Fujita and M. Nakajima, *Pestic. Biochem. Physiol.*, 17, in press (1982).
10. S. Nakagawa, N. Okajima, K. Nishimura, T. Fujita and M. Nakajima, *Pestic. Biochem. Physiol.*, 17, in press (1982).
11. P.R. Chadwick, *Pestic. Sci.*, 10, 32 (1979).
12. C. Hansch and A.J. Leo, *Substituent Constants for Correlation Analysis in Chemistry and Biology*, John Wiley and Sons, New York, N.Y., p.13 (1979).
13. T. Fujita, J. Iwasa and C. Hansch, *J. Amer. Chem. Soc.*, 86, 5175 (1964).
14. T. Fujita and T. Nishioka, *Prog. Phys. Org. Chem.*, 12, 49 (1976).
15. A. Bondi, *J. Phys. Chem.*, 68, 441 (1964).
16. M. Kiso, T. Fujita, N. Kurihara, M. Uchida, K. Tanaka and M. Nakajima, *Pestic. Biochem. Physiol.*, 8, 33 (1978).
17. M. Uchida, N. Kurihara, T. Fujita and M. Nakajima, *Pestic. Biochem. Physiol.*, 4, 260 (1974).

NEUROPHYSIOLOGICAL STUDY OF PYRETHROIDS: MOLECULAR AND MEMBRANE MECHANISM OF ACTION

Toshio Narahashi

Department of Pharmacology, Northwestern University Medical School, 303 East Chicago Avenue, Chicago, Illinois 60611, USA

Abstract - We have previously shown that allethrin and tetramethrin cause a marked prolongation of membrane sodium current thereby increasing the depolarizing after-potential to the level of threshold for repetitive excitation. This accounts for the symptoms of poisoning in animals. Our recent voltage clamp studies indicate that a population of sodium channels is modified by the pyrethroids to give rise to a very slow opening and closing. A kinetic model has been proposed in which the pyrethroid molecules bind to the sodium channels in their closed and open configurations. Both (+)-trans and (+)-cis isomers of tetramethrin are highly potent in modifying the sodium channel, whereas (-)-trans and (-)-cis isomers bind to channel sites without any effect thereby preventing the action of the subsequently applied (+) isomers. Thus tetramethrin binds to a trans site, a cis site or a negative allosteric site in the sodium channel depending on its optical and geometrical configurations. In contrast to the pyrethroids that do not contain a cyano group at α-carbon position (type I) such as tetramethrin and allethrin, the pyrethroids that contain an α-cyano group (type II) cause a large depolarization of the membrane. The time courses of opening and closing of the modified sodium channel are much slower. Despite such apparent differences in action, the kinetic model described for type I pyrethroids is still applicable to type II pyrethroids with modifications of rate constants and voltage dependence for various reactions. We have recently developed patch voltage clamp techniques to record opening and closing of individual sodium channels from cultured neuroblastoma cells. In support of the observations of "macroscopic" or "compound" sodium currents in giant axons, pyrethroids have been found to modify a population of sodium channels in an all-or-none manner. The modified channel opens for a much longer period of time than the normal channel.

INTRODUCTION

The mechanism of action of pyrethroids has been studied by many investigators. Most pyrethroids cause hyperactivity, ataxia, convulsions, and paralysis in animals, and there is no doubt that the major and primary target site is the nervous system (Ref. 1-3). They affect both nervous conduction and synaptic transmission, and induce repetitive discharges. Several questions must be answered in order to complete a picture of the mechanism of action of pyrethroids on the nervous system. First, where is the origin of repetitive discharges observed in pyrethroid-poisoned nerves? Second, how are the repetitive discharges produced at the site of their origin? Third, what is the cellular, membrane and molecular mechanism underlying the repetitive discharges? We have performed a systematic investigation to answer these questions, and come up with explanations close to the molecular level.

SITE OF REPETITIVE DISCHARGES

Pyrethrins, allethrin and other pyrethroids are known to cause repetitive discharges in a variety of regions of the nerve and muscle system. This includes nerve fibers (Ref. 4-6), neuromuscular junctions (Ref. 7-9), sensory cells (Ref. 10-11), and the central nervous system (Ref. 12-14). The effective concentration for this effect varies widely in different preparations and for different pyrethroids, ranging from micromolar to picomolar levels. However, it is generally lower for preparations containing synapses than nerve fibers.

Experiments with frog neuromuscular junctions have clearly shown that repetitive end-plate responses induced by a nerve stimulus in the presence of pyrethroids originate in presynaptic nerve terminals (Ref. 7-9). The end-plate potential and spontaneous miniature end-plate potentials were unaffected by the pyrethroids, but each of the focally recorded repetitive end-plate potentials as induced by a single nerve stimulus is prededed by a nerve terminal potential. This clearly indicates that the repetitive postsynaptic responses are due to repetitive excitation in the presynaptic nerve terminal. Similar results and conclusions were obtained for DDT type compounds (Ref. 15). Thus the next step was to find out how repetitive discharges are produced in nerve terminals. For this purpose, giant axon preparations were used as a model, because the large size permitted measurements of a variety of parameters that govern excitability.

MECHANISM OF REPETITIVE DISCHARGES

The action potential recorded from the cockroach giant axon is composed of a large spike phase, a small undershoot immediately following the spike, and a small and prolonged depolarizing (negative) after-potential that follows the undershoot. After application of allethrin, the depolarizing after-potential increased in amplitude and eventually attained the threshold level for repetitive discharges (Ref. 16). Similar effects were observed in tetramethrin-poisoned crayfish giant axons (Ref. 17). Therefore the next question is how the depolarizing after-potential is increased by pyrethroids.

MECHANISM OF DEPOLARIZING AFTER-POTENTIAL INCREASE

Mechanism of nerve excitation

In order to study the mechanism underlying the pyrethroid-induced increase in depolarizing after-potential, we have to know how the normal action potential is generated. Nerve excitation occurs as a result of membrane permeability changes to sodium and potassium (Ref. 18). In the resting condition, the membrane is almost exclusively permeable to potassium. The potassium concentration is much higher in the axoplasm than in the outside. Therefore, the resting membrane potential is close to the equilibrium potential for potassium calculated by the Nernst equation. Depolarization of the membrane causes a rapid increase in membrane sodium permeability in a regenerative manner. Thus the membrane becomes almost exclusively permeable to sodium, changing the membrane potential from its large negative resting value to a value close to the equilibrium potential for sodium at a large positive value. This forms the rising phase of the action potential. The increased sodium permeability starts decreasing by a mechanism called sodium inactivation and at about the same time the membrane potassium permeability starts increasing beyond the resting level. Thus the membrane again becomes almost exclusively permeable to potassium bringing back the membrane potential toward the resting level. Sodium ions rush in the axon during the rising phase of the action potential according to their electrochemical gradient, and potassium ions rush out the axon during the falling phase according to their electrochemical gradient. However, the change in internal ionic concentration as a result of one action potential is very small, being in the order of 1/1000 for an axon with a diameter of 1 μm. No matter how small the change may be, it must be restored. This is accomplished by the Na-K pump driven by metabolic energy.

Based on the above metioned scheme of the action potential production, any change in the shape of the action potential could be explained in terms of changes in membrane ionic permeabilities. A decrease in the amplitude of the action potential could be due to an inhibition of the sodium permeability increase mechanism. A change in the falling phase of the action potential including those in the depolarizing after-potential could be due to a change in the sodium inactivation mechanism and/or the potassium permeability increase mechanism. Of course a change in action potential could result from a metabolic inhibition, but many chemicals acting on nerve fibers exert their effects through alterations of membrane ionic permeabilities. It should be pointed out that these membrane ionic permeability mechanisms are totally independent of metabolic energy. Therefore we have to examine the effects of pyrethroids on the membrane ionic permeabilities. Such measurements can best be done by voltage clamp methods.

Voltage clamp experiments

When a step depolarizing pulse is applied to a giant nerve fiber under voltage clamp conditions, the membrane current recorded is composed of four components, i.e. capacitative current, peak transient current, steady-state current, and leakage current. The capacitative currents occur upon depolarizing and repolarizing steps, and are very brief in duration. These currents are the result of charging and uncharging the membrane capacity, and are not carried by ions. The leakage current goes through non-specific pathways of the membrane, and is carried by various ions. The peak transient current is carried mostly by sodium ions passing through the sodium channel. It flows in the inward direction at the membrane potentials more negative than the sodium equilibrium potential and in the outward direction at the potentials more positive than that. The steady-state current is carried primarily by potassium ions passing through the potassium channel. This current flows in the outward direction as the potassium equilibrium potential is usually more negative than the resting membrane potential. Figure 1 illustrates a family of membrane currents associated with step depolarizations from the holding potential of -100 mV to various levels indicated in a squid giant axon (control record).

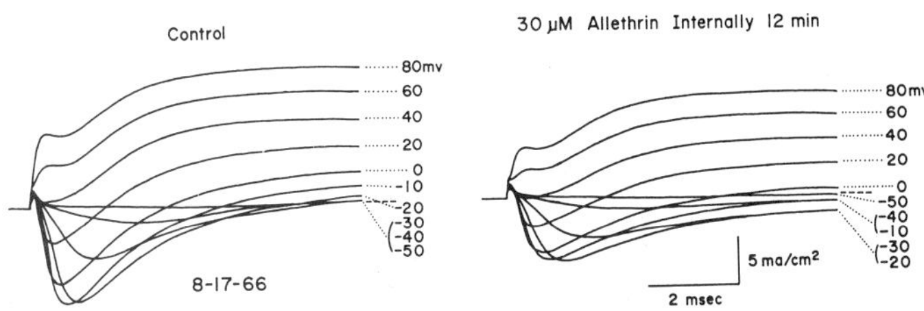

Fig. 1. Membrane currents associated with step depolarizations from the holding potential of -100 mV to the levels indicated in an internally perfused, voltage clamped squid giant axon before and during exposure to 30 μM allethrin internally. The broken line on the right of the records (between -10 mV and -20 mV in control, and between 0 mV and -50 mV in allethrin) indicates the zero membrane current level (from Ref. 19).

Effects of pyrethroids on membrane ionic currents

When applied to the squid giant axon either internally or externally, allethrin exerted three effects on the sodium and potassium currents (Ref. 19, 20): 1) The peak sodium current was suppressed; 2) the steady-state potassium current was suppressed; and, 3) the falling phase of sodium current was prolonged. An example of the effect of 30 μM allethrin applied internally is shown in Fig. 1. Further experiments clearly indicated that the membrane parameter most sensitive to pyrethroids is the falling phase of sodium current or the sodium inactivation. This effect accounts for the observed increase in depolarizing after-potential. Therefore more recent studies were carried out to elucidate the mechanisms whereby the sodium inactivation is inhibited by pyrethroids.

In order to measure the sodium inactivation the sodium and potassium components of membrane current must be separated. There are several specific channel blocking agents which can be used to eliminate one of the membrane current components. For example, tetrodotoxin blocks the sodium channel at very low concentrations in a highly specific manner (Ref. 21, 22). Tetraethylammonium (Ref. 23), 4-aminopyridine (Ref. 24, 25) and cesium (Ref. 26) block the potassium channel. Another method to eliminate an ionic current component is to remove the ion from external and/or internal medium. Internal perfusion techniques developed in the early 1960's allow us to change the ionic compositions of both external and internal perfusates at will (Ref. 27). In choosing the method for current separation, it should be borne in mind that each of the sodium and potassium channels is not completely selective for an ion. For example, the sodium channel is slightly permeable to potassium, and the potassium channel is slightly permeable to sodium. Therefore, the best way is to combine the two methods. In order to measure the sodium current passing through the sodium channel, potassium ions are eliminated from the internal perfusate and are replaced by cesium ions, a potassium channel blocker.

A family of membrane currents associated with various step depolarizations in a crayfish giant axon perfused internally with K-free cesium solution is illustrated in Fig. 2A.

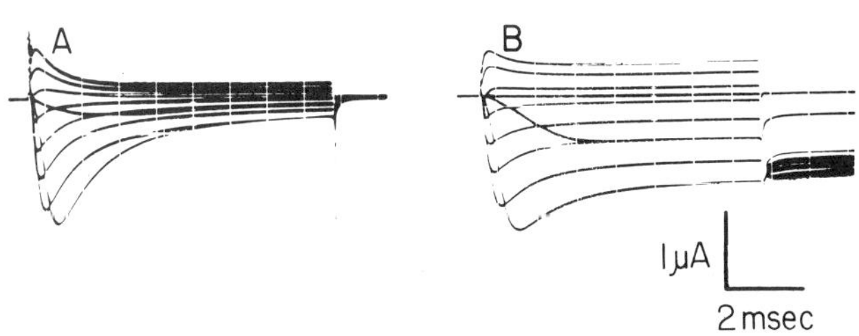

Fig. 2. Membrane sodium currents recorded from an internally perfused crayfish giant axon in response to step depolarizations to various levels before (A) and after (B) internal perfusion of 20 μM tetramethrin. Internal K was replaced by Cs to eliminate potassium current through potassium channel.

The peak transient sodium currents are followed by steady-state currents which are quickly terminated upon repolarization of the membrane. The currents were blocked by tetrodotoxin indicating that they were flowing through the sodium channel. Internal application of 20 μM tetramethrin drastically altered the sodium current (Fig. 2B) (Ref. 17). The peak amplitude was not changed, but the steady-state sodium current was markedly increased. Furthermore, the tail current associated with step repolarization of the membrane was greatly increased and decayed very slowly. If a very prolonged depolarizing pulse was applied, the slow component of the sodium current was seen to increase slowly with a time course of several hundred milliseconds and decay extremely slowly with a time course of a few seconds. The tail current associated with step repolarization also decayed very slowly. Allethrin had similar effects on the sodium current. Prolonged tail current was also observed in vertebrate nodes of Ranvier poisoned with allethrin and DDT (Ref. 28, 29).

Modification of sodium channel by pyrethroids

The observations described above suggest that the sodium channel is modified by tetramethrin to give rise to a slow opening and a very slow closing. In order to characterize the process by which the sodium channel is modified, detailed voltage clamp analyses have been performed (Ref. 17, 30). The tail current produced by repolarizing the membrane during the slow sodium current in the presence of tetramethrin is a measure of the open (conducting) modified sodium channel. Thus when a series of depolarizing pulses of a constant amplitude but of varying durations is applied, the time course of development of the tail current amplitude represents the time course of development of the modified open channel. Examples of such current records are shown in Figs. 3A, B and C. The black dots on each current record indicate the initial amplitudes of the slow compenent of tail current, and their conductance values are plotted as a function of pulse duration in Fig. 3D. Also shown in Fig. 3D is the time course of sodium conductance during a prolonged step depolarization (open circles). As expected these two conductances go parallel with each other except during the peak sodium current.

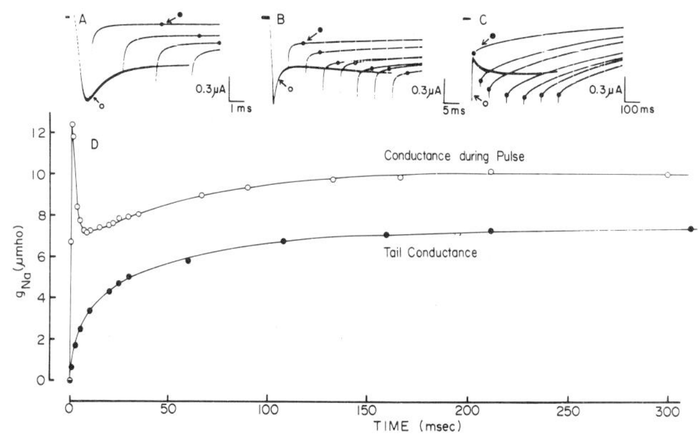

Fig. 3A, B and C. Families of membrane sodium currents and tail currents recorded from a crayfish giant axon internally perfused with 20 μM tetramethrin in response to step depolarizations to -20 mV with varying durations. The initial amplitudes of slow tail currents were measured at the points marked by filled circles. Note the different time scales in A, B and C. D. Sodium conductance (g_{Na}) during depolarizing pulses (open circles) and those at the beginning of the slow tail currents (filled circles) (from Ref. 17).

The time course of development of the modified open state was further analyzed using squid giant axons (Ref. 30). It was clearly shown that the modified open state developed with a dual exponential time course, one with a time constant of 1.3 msec and the other with a time constant of 24.3 msec. The slow phase disappeared after internal application of pronase, an agent that blocks the sodium inactivation. Thus the slow phase is somehow related to the sodium inactivation.

From these and other observations, a kinetic model has been developed to account for the modification of the sodium channel by pyrethroids (Fig. 4). Upon depolarization of the membrane, the closed (or non-conducting) sodium channel (C) opens to become O which is conducting. During a prolonged depolarization, the open sodium channel is inactivated (I). Pyrethroid can bind to the open sodium channel to convert it to O* which is also conducting. Pyrethroid can also bind to the closed sodium channel to yield C* which is not conducting. The modified open channel is slowly inactivated to become I* during a prolonged depolarization. Since pronase blocks the sodium inactivation (from O to I) and eliminates the slow phase of the modified open channel development, this slow phase must be derived from the route of I to O* via O. In the pronase-treated axon, tetramethrin causes a secondary, slowly developing sodium current to appear. This is due to a slow opening of C* to yield O*. The final, steady-state amplitude of sodium current in the pronase-treated axon is increased by tetramethrin. This change is due to the fact that more amount of O becomes available to yield O* due to the absence of I. Myelinated nerve fibers are somewhat different from giant axons in terms of behavior of sodium current in response to pyrethroids (Ref. 28, 29). Upon repolarization of the membrane, the tail current increases in

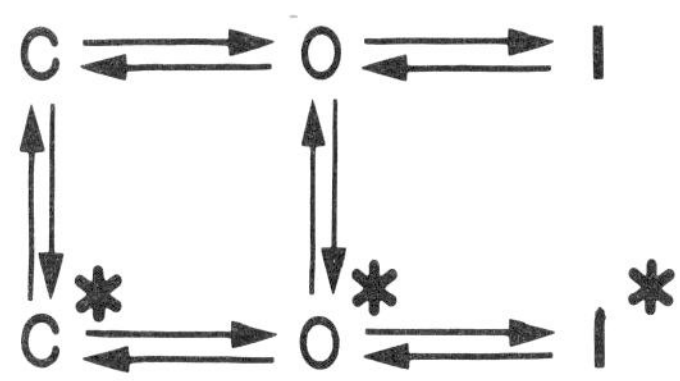

Fig. 4. A kinetic model for the action of pyrethroids on sodium channels. C, closded state of sodium channel; O, open and conducting state; O*, pyrethroid-bound open and conducting state; I*, pyrethroid-bound inactivated state. See text for further explanation.

amplitude, attains a maxiumum, and then decays slowly. This effect is interpreted as being due to a slow closing of the m gate of sodium channel rather than changes in the h gate.

It should be noted that only a very small fraction of sodium channel population needs to be modified by pyrethroids for repetitive discharges to be produced. It was estimated that the fraction of channels which must be modified to produce a 10 mV depolarizing after-potential is in the order of 0.1% (Ref. 33). The concentration of tetramethrin to cause this effect is approximately 20 nM (Ref. 33). This is compatible with the observations that very small doses of pyrethroids are generally needed to produce symptoms of poisoning charcterized by hyperactivity and ataxia.

Pyrethroid-tetrodotoxin antagonism

Tetrodotoxin is known to block the sodium channel in a highly specific manner (Ref. 21, 22). Block occurs only when tetrodotoxin is applied externally, and no effect is observed with internal application (Ref. 31). It was proposed that tetrodotoxin plugs the sodium channel at its external mouth (Ref. 32). Because of its very specific and potent sodium channel blocking action, tetrodotoxin is now widely being used as a powerful probe to study the sodium and potassium channels (Ref. 22). Thus tetrodotoxin is a useful probe for determining the site of action of pyrethroids.

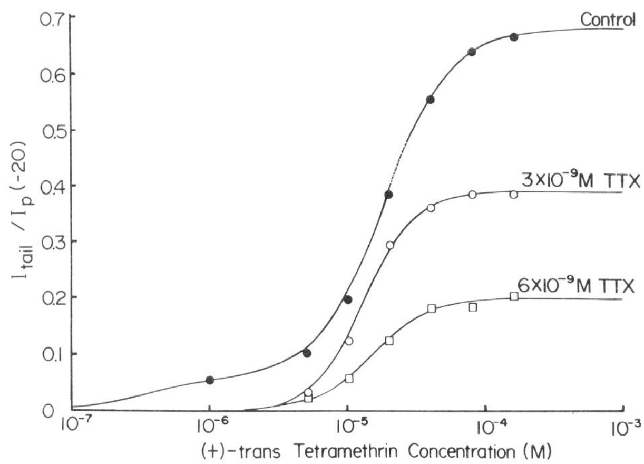

Fig. 5. Dose-response relationships for (+)-trans tetramethrin in the absence and presence of tetrodotoxin (TTX) at concentrations of 3 X 10^{-9}M and 6 X 10^{-9}M in a crayfish giant axon. The slow tail current (I_{tail}) amplitude was normalized to the peak current recorded at -20 mV (I_p (-20)), and was taken as a measure of response (from Ref. 33).

The slow component of tail current was measured as an index of the modified open channel in the presence of tetramethrin. In order to normalize the value, the slow tail current amplitude was divided by the peak current amplitude. This ratio is plotted against the tetramethrin concentration in Fig. 5 (control). Tetrodotoxin at concentrations of 3 nM and 6 nM decreased the tail current without changing the apparent dissociation constant, indicating a non-competitive antagonism. Thus tetramethrin and tetrodotoxin act on separate sodium channel sites (Ref. 33).

Effects of pyrethroid isomers: the sites of action

A pyrethroid can exist in geometrical and opitcal isomers. The potency in affecting the nerve is vastly different among the isomers (Ref. 34, 35). This provides us with an excellent opportunity to study the sites of action of pyrethroids on the sodium channel. Figure 6 is an example of a series of experiments in which the interaction of (-)-trans tetramethrin which is totally inactive by itself and (+)-trans tetramethrin which is highly potent (Ref. 33).

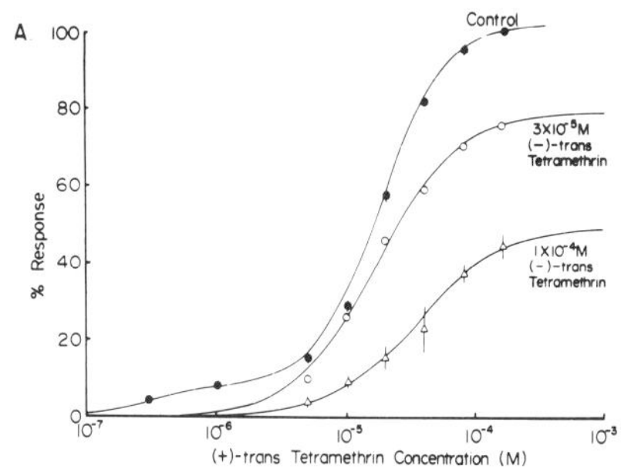

Fig. 6. Dose-response relationships for (+)-trans tetramethrin and antagonism by 3 X 10^{-5}M and 1 X 10^{-4}M (-)-trans tetramethrin in crayfish giant axons. The percent response was calculated in the same way as that for Fig. 5 (from Ref. 33).

The normalized slow tail current amplitude is plotted in the ordinate as a measure of response. (-)-trans tetramethrin was found to antagonize the action of (+)-trans tetramethrin in a non-competitive manner. Similarly, (-)-trans tetramethrin antagonized the active (+)-cis tetramethrin, and the inactive (-)-cis tetramethrin antagonized (+)-trans tetramethrin, both in a non-competitive manner. (-)-cis tetramethrin also antagonized the active (+)-cis tetramethrin, but the antagonism was competitive in nature.

A model for tetramethrin binding sites has been developed based on these observations (Fig. 7) (Ref. 33). It assumes three different sites to which tetramethrin can bind. The active (+)-trans and (+)-cis isomers bind to a trans agonistic site and a cis agonistic site, respectively, to modify the sodium channel. In order to account for

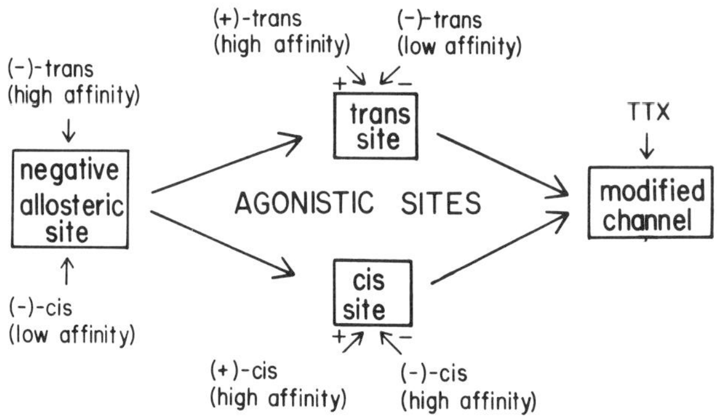

Fig. 7. A hypothetical model for the interactions of tetramethrin isomers with the sodium channel. See text for explanation (from Ref. 33).

non-competitive antagonism, a negative allosteric site is assumed. Thus binding of an inactive (-) isomer to an agonistic site would cause a competitive antagonism, whereas binding of an inactive (-) isomer to a negative allosteric site would cause a non-competitive antagonism. Tetrodotoxin binds to the tetramethrin modified sodium channel (as well as the normal sodium channel), thereby causing a non-competitive antagonism.

Two types of pyrethroids

The effects of allethrin and tetramethrin on the action potential and the sodium channel as described in the preceding sections have also been found with some other pyrethroids including phenothrin, permethrin, resmethrin and proparthrin (Ref. 29, 36). However, some other pyrethroids have been found to exert different effects. These pyrethroids include deltamethrin, cyphenothrin (S2703), and fenvalerate, all of which have a cyano group at the α-carbon position. Thus pyrethroids are classified into two groups (Ref. 37). Type I pyrethroids do not have an α cyano group, and cause repetitive discharges, an increase in depolarizing after-potential, a slow sodium current during depolarizing step, and a large tail current upon repolarization. Type II pyrethroids have an α cyano group, and cause membrane depolarization without repetitive discharge, no increase in depolarizing after-potential, only a small slow current, and a small but long-lasting tail current (Ref. 36). Deltamethrin has been found to cause a similar type II action on the frog myelinated nerve fiber (Ref. 38). The same classification of pyrethroids was also proposed based on the effects on the cockroach at a gross level (Ref. 39). Despite apparent differences in the action of type I and type II pyrethroids, it is clear that they both exert qualitatively the same effect on the sodium channel with differences only at the quantitative level (Ref. 36, 37).

Effects of tetramethrin on single sodium channels

The voltage clamp experiments described above allow us to measure membrane ionic currents from which membrane ionic conductances can be calculated. These measurements provide us with the basis on which a variety of changes in action potential can be explained. However, the membrane ionic current observed is a sum of the activity of a large number of ionic channels. Recently, techniques have been developed whereby opening and closing of individual ionic channels can be directly observed. Neher and Sakmann (Ref. 40) successfully recorded opening and closing of ionic channels associated with extrajunctional acetylcholine receptors in the denervated muscle. This technique was later improved to give a gigaohm resistance sealing between the capillary tip wall and the membrane, thereby permitting observations of very small currents occurring in a limited number of channels (Ref. 41, 42).

In short a glass capillary with a tip inner diameter of less than 1 μm and containing a physiological solution is placed against the membrane surface with a negative pressure applied to the inside of the capillary. The sealing resistance at the capillary tip wall is increased to as high as 10 gigaohm. Thus a very small area of the cell membrane is electrically insulated from the rest of the membrane. This enables us to measure ionic currents as a result of opening of ionic channels present in the membrane patch. This patch clamp technique has been successfully applied to a variety of cells and ionic channels, including the ionic channel associated with acetylcholine receptor (Ref. 43, 44), the sodium channel (Ref. 45-47), the calcium dependent potassium channel (Ref. 48, 49), the potassium channel that causes delayed rectification (Ref. 50), and the calcium channel (Ref. 51).

We began our patch clamp single channel recording experiments using cultured neuroblastoma cells in the early 1981, and have now reached the stage at which the interactions of a variety of specific agents with ionic channels can be studied in great detail (Ref. 45, 46, 50, 52). Neuroblastoma cells are an excellent material for such experiments, because the density of sodium channels is low and also because no connective tissues or Schwann cells are present around the cell membrane. Therefore, the interaction of tetramethrin with the sodium channel was studied by this technique (Ref. 53).

Opening of individual sodium channels was observed during step depolarization of the membrane from a holding potential of -90 mV to -50 mV. The channel opened abruptly and closed abruptly with an average open time of approximately 2 msec at 10°C. The current amplitude was of the order of 1-1.3 pA, and the single channel conductance calculated from the current-voltage relationship was of the order of 10-15 pS. Tetramethrin at a concentration of 60 μM dramatically increased the mean open time to as much as 20 msec without appreciable change in single channel current amplitude and conductance. All these currents before and after application of tetramethrin were abolished by 1 μM tetrodotoxin indicating that they passed through the sodium channel. The observed prolongation of the open time is compatible with the conventional "macroscopic" or "compound" sodium current measurement. It is also important to note that in the presence of tetramethrin the sodium channels can clearly be divided into two groups based on the open time, one showing the normal open time Poisson distribution and the other showing a Poisson distribution with much prolonged open times. Thus it can be concluded that tetramethrin modified the sodium channels in an all-or-none manner, the modified channels exhibiting a prolonged open time. This gives a firm support to our previous hypothesis of an all-or-none modification of sodium channels by tetramethrin.

Acknowledgements - This work was supported by a grant from the National Institutes of Health (NS 14143). I thank Janet Henderson for secretarial assistance.

REFERENCES

1. T. Narahashi, In: Advances in Insect Physiology, ed. J.W.L. Beament, J.E. Treherne and V.B. Wigglesworth, Vol. 8, p. 1-93, Academic Press, London and New York (1971).
2. T. Narahashi, In: Insecticide Biochemistry and Physiology, ed. C.F. Wilkinson, p. 327-352, Plenum Publ. Corp., New York (1976).

3. W. Wouters and J. van den Bercken, Gen. Pharmacol. 9, 387-398 (1978).
4. T. Narahashi, J. Cell. Comp. Physiol. 59, 61-65 (1962).
5. T. Yamasaki and T. Ishii (Narahashi), Oyo-Kontyu 7, 157-164 (1952).
6. J. van den Bercken, L.M.A. Akkermans and J.M. van der Zalm, Europ. J. Pharmacol. 21, 95-106 (1973).
7. J. van den Bercken, Pesticide Sci. 8, 692-699 (1977).
8. M.H. Evans, Pesticide Biochem. Physiol. 6, 547-550 (1976).
9. W. Wouters, J. van den Bercken and A. van Ginneken, Europ. J. Pharmacol. 43, 163-171 (1977).
10. L.M.A. Akkermans, J. van den Bercken and M. Versluijs-Helder, Pesticide Biochem. Physiol. 5, 451-457 (1975).
11. J. van den Bercken, A.B.A. Kroese and L.M.A. Akkermans, In: Neurotoxicology of Insecticides and Pheromones, ed. T. Narahashi, p. 183-210, Plenum Publ. Corp., New York (1979).
12. K. Takeno, K. Nishimura, J. Parmentier and T. Narahashi, Pesticide Biochem. Physiol. 7, 486-499 (1977).
13. P.E. Burt and R.E. Goodchild, Entomol. Exp. Appl. 14, 179-189 (1971).
14. G. Camougis, In: Pyrethrum, The Natural Insecticide, ed. J.E. Casida, p. 211-222, Academic Press, New York (1973).
15. J.M. Farley, T. Narahashi and G. Holan, Neurotoxicology 1, 191-207 (1979).
16. T. Narahashi, J. Cell. Comp. Physiol. 59, 67-76 (1962).
17. A.E. Lund and T. Narahashi, Neurotoxicology 2, 213-229 (1981).
18. A.L. Hodgkin and A.F. Huxley, J. Physiol. London 117, 500-544.
19. T. Narahashi and N.C. Anderson, Toxicol. Appl. Pharmacol. 10, 529-547 (1967).
20. C.M. Wang, T. Narahashi and M. Scuka, J. Pharmacol. Exp. Ther. 182, 442-453 (1972).
21. T. Narahashi, J.W. Moore and W.R. Scott, J. Gen. Physiol. 47, 965-974 (1964).
22. T. Narahashi, Physiol. Rev. 54, 813-889 (1974).
23. I. Tasaki and S. Hagiwara, J. Gen. Physiol. 40, 859-885 (1957).
24. J.Z. Yeh, G.S. Oxford, C.H. Wu and T. Narahashi, J. Gen. Physiol. 68, 519-535 (1976).
25. H. Meves and Y. Pichon, J. Physiol. London 268, 511-532 (1977).
26. W.K. Chandler and H. Meves, J. Physiol. London 180, 788-820 (1965).
27. P.F. Baker, A.L. Hodgkin and T.I. Shaw, Nature London 190, 885-887 (1961).
28. J. van den Bercken and H.P.M. Vijverberg, In: Insect Neurobiology and Pesticide Action, p. 79-85, Society of Chemical Industry, London (1980).
29. H.P.M. Vijverberg, J.M. van der Zalm and J. van den Bercken, Nature London 295, 601-603 (1982).
30. A.E. Lund and T. Narahashi, J. Pharmacol. Exp. Ther. 219, 464-473 (1981).
31. T. Narahashi, N.C. Anderson and J.W. Moore, J. Gen. Physiol. 50, 1413-1428 (1967).
32. B. Hille, Biophys. J. 15, 615-619 (1975).
33. A.E. Lund and T. Narahashi, Neurotoxicology, In press (1982).
34. T. Narahashi, K. Nishimura, J.L. Parmentier, K. Takeno and M. Elliott, In: Synthetic Pyrethroids, ed. M. Elliott, ACS Symposium Series, No. 42, p. 85-97, American Chemical Society, Washington, D.C. (1977).
35. K. Nishimura and T. Narahashi, Pesticide Biochem. Physiol. 8, 53-64 (1978).
36. A.E. Lund and T. Narahashi, unpublished observations (1982).
37. T. Narahashi, In: Pyrethroids Insecticides: Chemistry and Action, Table Ronde Roussel Uclaf, No. 37, ed. J. Mathieu, p. 15-17, Roussel Uclaf, Romainville, France (1980).
38. H.P.M. Vijverberg and J. van den Bercken, Europ. J. Pharmacol. 58, 501-504 (1979).
39. D.W. Gammon, M.A. Brown and J.E. Casida, Pesticide Biochem. Physiol. 15, 181-191 (1981).
40. E. Neher and B. Sakmann, Nature London 260, 779-802 (1976).
41. O.P. Hamill, A. Marty, E. Neher, B. Sakmann and F.J. Sigworth, Pflügers Arch. 391, 85-100 (1981).
42. F.J. Sigworth and E. Neher, Nature London 287, 447-449 (1980).
43. O.P. Hamill and B. Sakmann, Nature London 294, 462-464 (1981).
44. D.C. Ogden, S.A. Siegelbaum and D. Colquhoun, Nature London 289, 596-598 (1981).
45. F.N. Quandt and T. Narahashi, Soc. Neurosci. Abstr. 7, 902 (1981).
46. F.N. Quandt and T. Narahashi, In preparation (1982).
47. J. Patlak and R. Horn, J. Gen. Physiol. 79, 333-351 (1982).
48. A. Marty, Nature London 291, 497-500 (1981).
49. H.D. Lux, E. Neher and A. Marty, Pflügers Arch. 389, 293-295 (1981).
50. F.N. Quandt and T. Narahashi, Soc. Neurosci. Abstr. 8, In press (1982).
51. E. Neher, A. Marty and F.J. Sigworth, VII Internat. Biophys. Congr. and III Pan-American Biochem. Congr. Abstr. p. 297 (1981).
52. F.N. Quandt, J.Z. Yeh and T. Narahashi, Biophys. J. 37 (No. 2, Part 2), 319a (1982).
53. D. Yamamoto, F.N. Quandt and T. Narahashi, Soc. Neurosci. Abstr. 8, In press (1982).

NOVEL ASPECTS OF METABOLISM OF PYRETHROIDS

John E. Casida

Pesticide Chemistry and Toxicology Laboratory, Department of Entomological Sciences, University of California, Berkeley, California 94720, USA

Abstract - The relative importance of detoxification and target site specificity in determining pyrethoid structure-activity relationships is considered with three examples, i.e.: houseflies and rethronyl chrysanthemates and analogs with various unsaturated side chains in the acid and alcohol moieties affecting the ease of synergism by piperonyl butoxide; American cockroaches and the trans- and cis isomers of tetramethrin, phenothrin and permethrin of high potency for inducing repetitive discharges in the cercal sensory nerve but not always of parallel toxicity; mice and the trans- and cis isomers of resmethrin, ethanomethrin, phenothrin and cyphenothrin varying from exceptionally low to moderately high intraperitoneal and intracerebral toxicity. There are large differences in the contribution of esterases and oxidases to detoxification and in the optimal synergist depending on the pyrethoid and species involved. Recent studies on pyrethroid metabolic chemistry have identified 12 conjugates of 3-phenoxybenzoic acid in plants, insects, birds and 13 species of mammals and three bile acid conjugates of the fluvalinate acid moiety in chickens, rats and cows. trans-Tetramethrin is decarboxylated via the epoxychrysanthemate and undergoes reduction of the tetrahydrophthalimide fragment possibly via the glutathione conjugate. Several of the fluvalinate and flucythrinate metabolites are now identified. Derivatizations of the oxime ether and dihalovinyl substituents of potent pyrethroids provide the first examples of propyrethroids undergoing bioactivation.

INTRODUCTION

Advances in understanding pyrethroid metabolism, since our review covering studies to mid-1979 (1), are principally in the areas of the influence of detoxification on structure-activity relationships, the importance of esterases and oxidases in detoxification, and the identification of new metabolites from examining additional pyrethroids and focusing on specific conjugates. Other recent reviews are either general (2) or emphasize mammals (3), insects (4), or plants and soils (5).

RELATIVE IMPORTANCE OF DETOXIFICATION AND TARGET SITE SPECIFICITY IN PYRETHROID STRUCTURE-ACTIVITY RELATIONSHIPS

Pyrethroid structure-activity relationships are conveniently examined with various biological end points (e.g., neurophysiological activity and toxicity to normal insects or insects treated with synergists to minimize detoxification) and analyzed by several physicochemical criteria (e.g., substituent parameters and conformational analysis). Structure-activity studies based on direct nerve response and toxicity to synergist-treated organisms are assumed to most closely approximate the optimization of structure for fit at the relevant neuroreceptor. Frequently-used synergists are piperonyl butoxide and NIA 16824 as mixed-function oxidase (MFO) inhibitors and DEF, profenofos and PSCP as esterase inhibitors.

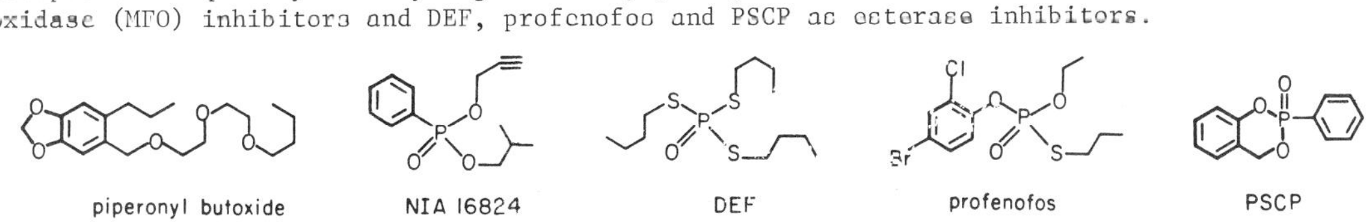

Influence on Housefly Toxicity of 3-Substituent of Acid Moiety and Side Chain of Alcohol Moiety of Rethronyl Chrysanthemates and Their Analogs

Pyrethrin I and allethrin are readily metabolized at the isobutenyl substituent of the acid moiety (6) and probably also at the pentadienyl and allyl groups of the alcohol moiety (7). Recent studies (8) revealed that the PB-synergized potency is the same for R= $-CH=CH_2$ and R= $-CH=CF_2$ analogs and differs less than 2-fold for the (1R,trans)-chrysanthemates, (1R,cis)-3-(2,2-dibromovinyl)-2,2-dimethylcyclopropanecarboxylates and 2,2,3,3-tetramethylcyclopropanecarboxylates, suggesting that these structural modifications have little effect on the intrinsic activity. All of these compounds are synergized to similar extents indicating that other detoxification sites are utilized when the unsaturated substituents of the acid and alcohol moieties are no longer susceptible to oxidation. However, pyrethrin I is much more potent than other compounds in this series to PB-synergized flies.

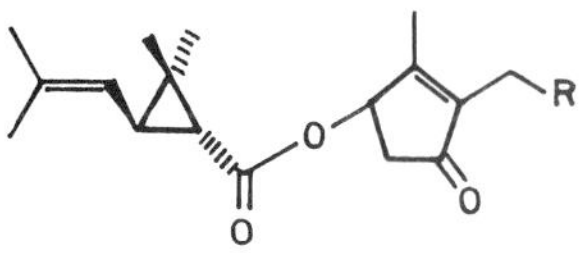

rethronyl chrysanthemates

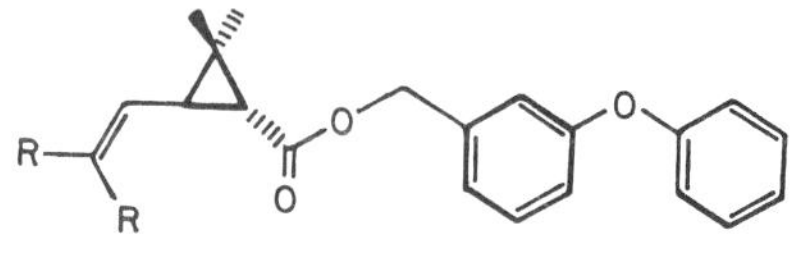

phenothrin R = - CH_3
permethrin R = - Cl

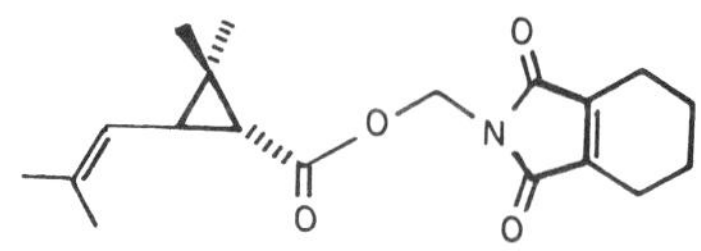

tetramethrin

Influence on Neuroactivity and American Cockroach Toxicity of 3-Substituent of Phenothrin, Permethrin and Tetramethrin and of Tetrahydrophthalimide Group of Tetramethrin

The *trans*- and *cis*-isomers of phenothrin and permethrin are of similar potency for inducing repetitive firing in cercal sensory nerves indicating that the 3-substituent within this series has no marked effect on intrinsic neuroactivity (Table 1). These findings parallel the similar toxicity to cockroaches of *trans*- and *cis*-phenothrin and *trans*-permethrin (Table 1). The toxicity of *trans*-phenothrin and *trans*-permethrin is moderately synergized by PB plus an NIA 16824 analog and in the case of *trans*-phenothrin there is also some synergism by PB alone (10). The 7-fold toxicity difference for *trans*- and *cis*-permethrin may be due in part to the relative ease of hydrolytic metabolism since injected *trans*-permethrin is metabolized slightly faster than *cis*-permethrin (11). The remarkable neuroactive potency of both *trans*- and *cis*-tetramethrin may contribute to their knockdown activity. Their brief duration of action when applied directly to the cercal sensory nerve is probably due to rapid detoxification of the very low levels in the nerve, *e.g.* tetramethrin is metabolized by an oxidase in the cockroach abdominal nerve cord (9). A possible contributing factor to the neuroactivity of the tetramethrin isomers is the potential ability to undergo Michael addition with thiols (discussed later) such as at a relevant neuroreceptor (12). The inactivity of *cis*- relative to *trans*-tetramethrin in the American cockroach (Table 1) is also apparent in the German cockroach where the isomeric specificity is probably not associated with detoxification but instead may be related to a pyrethroid nerve receptor which does not accept *cis*-tetramethrin (13, 14).

Influence on Mouse Toxicity of 3-Substituent of Acid Moiety of Resmethrin, Ethanomethrin, Phenothrin and Cyphenothrin and of α-Cyano Group of Cyphenothrin

Comparative intraperitoneal (ip) and intracerebral (ic) LD_{50} values for mice (Tables 2 and 3) and relative metabolism rates by mouse liver microsomes (Table 4) provide a basis for speculation on the relative importance of detoxification and target site sensitivity in determining the toxicity of the resmethrin, ethanomethrin, phenothrin and cyphenothrin isomers. *trans*-Resmethrin and *trans*- and *cis*-phenothrin are of very low toxicity or are nontoxic both on ip administration even to synergist-treated mice and on ic administration. This appears to be primarily due to an inability to interact at the relevant target site. The low toxicity of the *trans*-isomers of ethanomethrin and cyphenothrin is attributable in large part to rapid detoxification, *i.e.* they are highly toxic administered ic and their ip toxicity is greatly increased by PB and DEF. A seemingly small change in the 3-substituent of *trans*-resmethrin, *i.e.* to give *cis*-resmethrin and *trans*-ethanomethrin, is apparently enough for greatly enhanced receptor interaction. The greater toxicity of *cis*- than of *trans*-cyphenothrin is due both to higher potency for target site interaction in the brain (18) and to slower detoxification. The poisoning syndrome for cyphenothrin (Type II) which acts primarily in the brain differs from that for the other three compounds (Type I) which may have a greater peripheral component in their action.

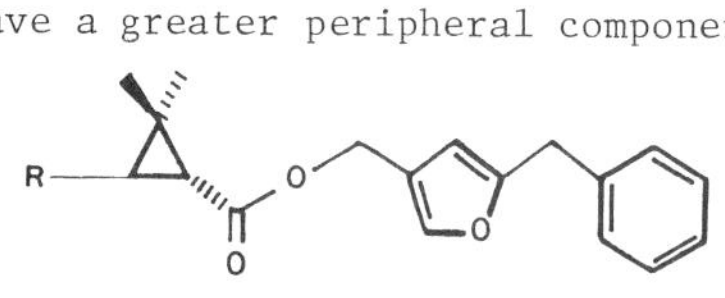

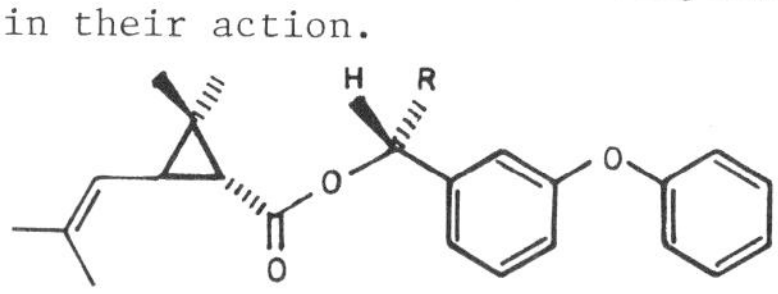

resmethrin R = $(CH_3)_2C$ = CH-

ethanomethrin R =  = CH-

phenothrin R = -H

cyphenothrin R = -CN

RELATIVE IMPORTANCE OF ESTERASES AND OXIDASES IN DETOXIFICATION

Esterases from most species hydrolyze the *trans* isomers of permethrin, cypermethrin and related cyclopropanecarboxylates much faster than the corresponding *cis* isomers (15, 17, 19, 20). Interesting exceptions include common green lacewing larvae, important biological control agents, which hydrolyze *cis*-isomers faster than *trans*-isomers (21) and human liver which not only hydrolyzes the *trans* and *cis* isomers of cypermethrin at almost equal rates but also is more active than comparable preparations from rat liver microsomes (22). The rat liver microsomal pyrethroid esterase in partially purified form is proposed to be the same as

Table 1. Sensitivity of American Cockroaches and Their Cercal Sensory Nerves to *trans*- and *cis*-Isomers of Phenothrin, Permethrin and Tetramethrin

	Nerve response, M[a]		LD_{50}, µg/g[a]	
(1R)-Pyrethroid	*trans*	*cis*	*trans*	*cis*
Phenothrin	8×10^{-9}	9×10^{-9}	0.7	0.7
Permethrin	8×10^{-9}	7×10^{-9}	0.6	0.09
Tetramethrin	3×10^{-13}	3×10^{-13}	57	~500

[a]Induction of repetitive firing following a single electrical stimulus and topical LD_{50}; data from ref. 9.

Table 2. Sensitivity of Mice to *trans*- and *cis*-Isomers of Resmethrin and Ethanomethrin Administered Intraperitoneally and Intracerebrally

	LD_{50}, mg/kg[a]			
	(1R)-Resmethrin		(1R)-Ethanomethrin	
Synergist	*trans*	*cis*	*trans*	*cis*
	Intraperitoneal, relative to body weight			
None	>1500	320	>1500	10
PB	>1500	13	25	2.1
DEF	>1500	29	8	2.4
	Intracerebral, relative to brain weight			
None	>8600	41	14	7

[a]Intraperitoneal data from ref. 15 and intracerebral data from ref. 16.

Table 3. Sensitivity of Mice to *trans*- and *cis*-Isomers of Phenothrin and Cyphenothrin Administered Intraperitoneally and Intracerebrally

	LD_{50}, mg/kg[a]			
	(1R)-Phenothrin		(1R,αRS)-Cyphenothrin	
Synergist	*trans*	*cis*	*trans*	*cis*
	Intraperitoneal, relative to body weight			
None	>1500	>1500	>500	58
PB	>1500	>1500	25	8
DEF	>1500	>1500	25	19
	Intracerebral, relative to brain weight			
None	>8600	>4300	12	4

[a]Intraperitoneal data from ref. 15 and intracerebral data from ref. 16

Table 4. Metabolism Rates of *trans*- and *cis*-Isomers of Resmethrin, Ethanomethrin, Phenothrin and Cyphenothrin Incubated with Mouse Liver Microsomal Enzymes

	Relative metabolism rate[a]			
	Esterase		Oxidase	
(1R)-Pyrethroid	*trans*	*cis*	*trans*	*cis*
Resmethrin	79	< 3	20	29
Ethanomethrin	19	< 3	12	21
Phenothrin	59	< 4	27	37
(αRS)-Cyphenothrin	3	< 3	5	8

[a]Esterase + oxidase metabolism of (1R)-resmethrin = ~ 100; data from ref. 17.

malathion carboxyesterase (20) but selective inhibition studies point to a more complex situation with several pyrethroid-hydrolyzing esterases differing in substrate specificity (23).

Many types of compounds are active as MFO inhibitors (24) and esterase inhibitors (25), in addition to those structurally defined above, giving a considerable range for optimization of synergists. Organophosphates are obvious candidates as synergists because their inhibition of pyrethroid-hydrolyzing esterases persists long after the organophosphate is dissipated, a useful feature in control. Care must be taken in selecting synergists for pyrethroids to make sure that their favorable toxicity for mammals and non-target species is not compromised. Rethronyl chrysanthemates including allethrin and pyrethrin I are metabolized primarily by the MFO system and so oxidase inhibitors such as PB are effective synergists, particularly in some dipterous insects (6, 7). The other commercial pyrethroids are esters of primary alcohols and α-cyano-3-phenoxybenzyl alcohol detoxified by either esterase or oxidase attack, depending on the particular pyrethroid and species involved, and synergized by esterase or oxidase inhibitors or both. Thus, PB is an excellent synergist for pyrethrin I in houseflies (18- to 325-fold) (7, 8), NIA 16824 for cis-tetramethrin in houseflies (65-fold) (13), DEF for (1R,trans)-ethanomethrin in mice (> 188-fold) (Table 2) (15), profenofos for cis-cypermethrin in cabbage looper larvae (20-fold) (19) and PSCP for trans-permethrin in lacewing larvae (68-fold) (21).

RECENT ADVANCES IN PYRETHROID METABOLIC CHEMISTRY

The rapidly expanding use of pyrethroids has been paralleled by increasing knowledge on their fate in various organisms and environments (1-5). Three areas of significant recent progress are the identification of conjugates, the metabolism of new pyrethroids, and the bioactivation of propyrethroids.

New Conjugates of Pyrethroid Metabolites

The principal pyrethroid metabolites are alcohols or phenols from hydroxylation and carboxylic acids from ester cleavage or further oxidation of intermediate alcohols. These phase I metabolites are converted in animals and plants to a variety of conjugates of interest for their diversity and species specificity. 3-Phenoxybenzoic acid has been most extensively examined, because of its importance as a metabolite of many pyrethroids, leading to 12 identified conjugates.

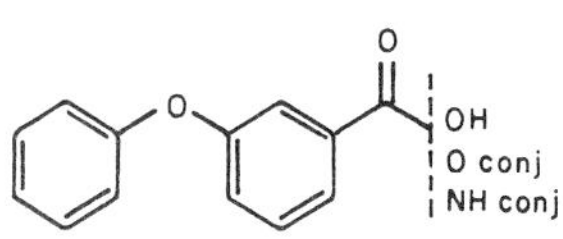

conjugates of 3-phenoxybenzoic acid

Type of moiety	Species and ref.
Amino acids and dipeptides	
glycine	housefly (11), looper (11), rat (26-29), dog (30), cow (31), goat (32), 9 other mammals (29), duck (29)
glutamic acid	housefly (11), cockroach (11), cow (31), goat (32)
glutamine	cockroach (11)
α-N-acetylornithine	chicken (33)
taurine	mouse (34, 35), 5 other mammals (29)
glycylvaline	duck (36)
triglycerides	
2- and 3-dipalmitins	rat skin (37)
glucuronide and glycosides	
glucuronic acid	10 mammals (26, 28, 29, 31, 34), duck (29)
glucose	plants (5, 38), housefly (11), looper (11)
glycosylarabinose and glycosylxylose	plants (5, 38)

Bile acid conjugates are major (5-12%) metabolites of fluvalinate in the feces of cows, chickens and rats (39) as shown on the next page.

Metabolism in Rats of Tetramethrin, Flucythrinate and Fluvalinate

Reexamination of tetramethrin metabolism in rats and mouse liver MFO systems establishes that sites sensitive to oxidation are either of the isobutenyl methyl groups, the isobutenyl double bond, and the alcohol moiety before and after cleavage and reduction (40, 41). Metabolic decarboxylation involves sequential enzymatic isobutenyl epoxidation, hydrolysis of the epoxychrysanthemate, and a nonenzymatic concerted decarboxylation and oxirane-ring opening reaction (41). Tetramethrin and its tetrahydrophthalimide metabolite readily undergo Michael addition with glutathione (GSH) under physiological conditions (12). The GSH conjugate of

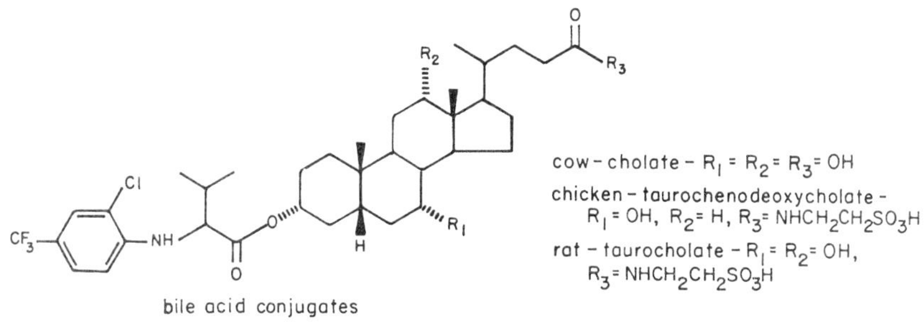

tetramethrin is also formed in the presence of mouse liver and housefly homogenate fractions but probably as a nonenzymatic reaction; this conjugate and the corresponding mercapturic acid are not detected as metabolites in the bile or urine of tetramethrin-treated rats and mice (12). The mechanism for reduction of the tetrahydrophthalimide might involve an NADPH-dependent reductase (40) or could proceed via the GSH conjugate.

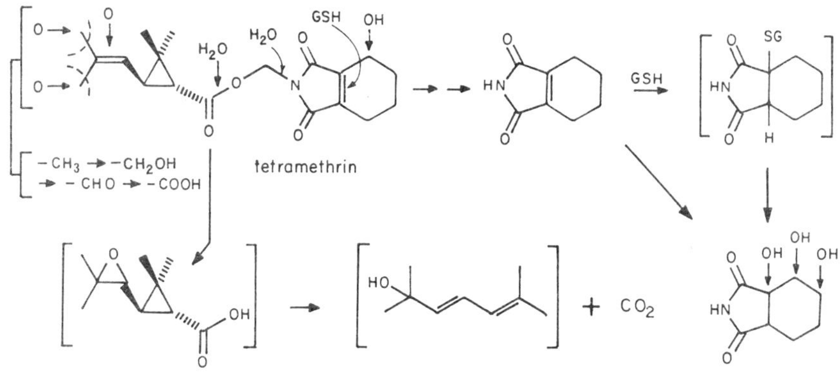

Flucythrinate and fluvalinate are derived from acid moieties not previously subjected to metabolic investigations. Flucythrinate yields 3-phenoxybenzoic acid and its 4'-hydroxy derivative (free and conjugated) and p-(difluoromethoxyphenyl)-3-methylbutyric acid and its hydroxylated derivatives in the urine and a metabolite from hydrolysis of the difluoromethoxy group of the parent in the fat (42). The acid moiety from hydrolysis of fluvalinate undergoes methyl-group hydroxylation and in addition is excreted free and as conjugates not only with cholic acid derivatives as above but also with glycine, threonine, serine and valine (43).

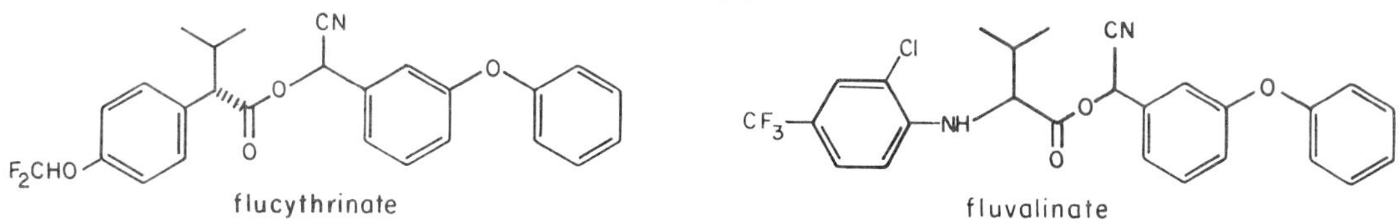

Propyrethroids

Most pyrethroids undergo metabolic detoxification rather than activation, but there are exceptions. The epoxychrysanthemates are formed under some metabolic conditions (41) but are generally of relatively low insecticidal activity. No attempt has been made to systematically assay pyrethroid metabolites in relevant neurophysiological systems. Suitable protective groups allow the conversion of some known pyrethroids to propyrethroids. Thus the indicated oxime ether can be reduced and converted to a formamide, a process reversed in insects where hydrolysis and oxidation regenerates the insecticidal oxime ether (44). Tralomethrin and tralocythrin undergo nonenzymatic debromination in the presence of biological thiols to yield deltamethrin and cypermethrin, respectively, thereby serving as propyrethroids (45,46); this conversion is very efficient so tralomethrin and tralocythrin are highly effective insecticides.

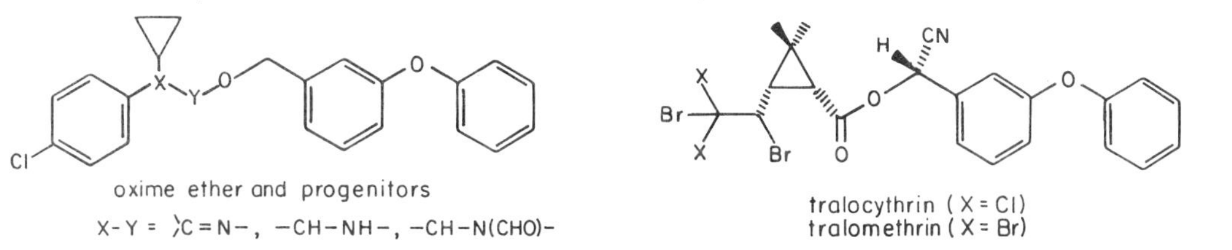

Acknowledgments - Studies from the Berkeley laboratory were supported in part by the National Institutes of Health (Grant P01 ES00049). D. H. Hutson provided helpful suggestions.

REFERENCES

1. J. E. Casida and L. O. Ruzo, Pestic. Sci. 11, 257-269 (1980).
2. J. Miyamoto, K. I. Beynon, T. R. Roberts, R. J. Hemingway, and H. Swaine, Pure & Appl. Chem. 53, 1967-2022 (1981).
3. D. H. Hutson, Prog. Drug Metab. 3, 215-252 (1979).
4. D. M. Soderlund, J. R. Sanborn and P. W. Lee, Prog. Pestic. Biochem., in press (1982).
5. T. R. Roberts, Prog. Pestic. Biochem. 1, 115-146 (1981).
6. I. Yamamoto, E. C. Kimmel and J. E. Casida, J. Agric. Food Chem. 17, 1227-1236 (1969).
7. I. Yamamoto, in Pyrethrum The Natural Insecticide, Ed. J. E. Casida, Academic Press, N. Y., pp. 195-210 (1973).
8. T. Ando and J. E. Casida, unpublished results.
9. D. W. Gammon, M. A. Brown and J. E. Casida, Pestic. Biochem. Physiol. 15, 181-191 (1981).
10. S. Nakagawa, N. Okajima, T. Kitahaba, K. Nishimura, T. Fujita and M. Nakajima, Pestic. Biochem. Physiol. 17, 243-258 (1982).
11. T. Shono, T. Unai and J. E. Casida, Pestic. Biochem. Physiol. 9, 96-106 (1978).
12. I. H. Smith, E. J. Wood and J. E. Casida, J. Agric. Food Chem. 30, 598-600 (1982).
13. L. T. Jao and J. E. Casida, Pestic. Biochem. Physiol. 4, 456-464 (1974).
14. L. T. Jao and J. E. Casida, Pestic. Biochem. Physiol. 4, 465-472 (1974).
15. D. M. Soderlund and J. E. Casida, in Synthetic Pyrethroids, Ed. M. Elliott, Amer. Chem. Soc. Symp. Ser. 42, 162-172 (1977).
16. L. J. Lawrence and J. E. Casida, Pestic. Biochem. Physiol., in press (1982).
17. D. M. Soderlund and J. E. Casida, Pestic. Biochem. Physiol. 7, 391-401 (1977).
18. L. J. Lawrence and J. E. Casida, unpublished results.
19. I. Ishaaya and J. E. Casida, Pestic. Biochem. Physiol. 14, 178-184 (1980).
20. T. Suzuki and J. Miyamoto, Pestic. Biochem. Physiol. 8, 186-198 (1978).
21. I. Ishaaya and J. E. Casida, Environ. Entomol. 10, 681-684 (1981).
22. A. Croucher and C. J. Logan, 184th Amer. Chem. Soc. National Meeting, Abstract 39, Kansas City, MO, September (1982).
23. D. M. Soderlund, Y.A.I. Abdel-Aal and D. W. Helmuth, Pestic. Biochem. Physiol. 17, 162-169 (1982).
24. B. Testa and P. Jenner, Drug. Metab. Rev. 12, 1-117 (1981).
25. M. Eto, Organophosphorus Pesticides: Organic and Biological Chemistry, CRC Press, Cleveland, OH, 387 pp (1974).
26. L. C. Gaughan, T. Unai, and J. E. Casida, J. Agric. Food Chem. 25, 9-17 (1977).
27. K. R. Huckle, G. H. Tait, P. Millburn and D. H. Hutson, Xenobiotica 11, 635-644 (1981).
28. K. R. Huckle, J. K. Chipman, D. H. Hutson and P. Millburn, Drug. Metab. Dispos. 9, 360-368 (1981).
29. K. R. Huckle, D. H. Hutson and P. Millburn, Drug. Metab. Dispos. 9, 352-359 (1981).
30. D. H. Hutson, unpublished results.
31. L. C. Gaughan, M. E. Ackerman, T. Unai and J. E. Casida, J. Agric. Food Chem. 26, 613-618 (1978).
32. G. W. Ivie and L. M. Hunt, J. Agric. Food Chem. 28, 1131-1138 (1980).
33. K. R. Huckle, G. Stoydin, D. H. Hutson and P. Millburn, unpublished results.
34. D. H. Hutson, L. C. Gaughan and J. E. Casida, Pestic. Sci. 12, 385-398 (1981).
35. D. H. Hutson and J. E. Casida, Xenobiotica 8, 565-571 (1978).
36. K. R. Huckle, I. J. G. Climie, D. H. Hutson and P. Millburn, Drug. Metab. Dispos. 9, 147-149 (1981).
37. J. V. Crayford and D. H. Hutson, Xenobiotica 10, 349-354 (1980).
38. J. E. More, T. R. Roberts and A. N. Wright, Pestic. Biochem. Physiol. 9, 268-280 (1978).
39. G. B. Quistad, L. E. Staiger and D. A. Schooley, Nature 296, 462-464 (1982).
40. H. Kaneko, H. Ohkawa and J. Miyamoto, J. Pesticide Sci. 6, 425-435 (1981).
41. I. H. Smith and J. E. Casida, Tetrahedron Lett. 22, 203-206 (1981).
42. J. Zulalian, E. Orloski, H. Berger, S. Stout and P. Gingher, 184th Amer. Chem. Soc. National Meeting, Abstract 35, Kansas City, MO, September (1982).
43. L. E. Staiger, G. B. Quistad and D. A. Schooley, Second Chemical Congress of the North American Continent, Abstract 116, Las Vegas, CA, August (1980).
44. M. A. Brown and J. E. Casida, Second Chemical Congress of the North American Continent, Abstract 118, Las Vegas, CA, August (1980).
45. L. O. Ruzo, L. C. Gaughan and J. E. Casida, Pestic. Biochem. Physiol. 15, 137-142 (1981).
46. L. M. Cole, L. O. Ruzo, E. J. Wood and J. E. Casida, J. Agric. Food Chem., 30, 631-636 (1982).

DEGRADATION OF PYRETHROID INSECTICIDES IN THE FIELD

Junshi Miyamoto and Nobuyoshi Mikami

Research Department, Pesticides Division, Sumitomo Chemical Co. Ltd., Takarazuka 665, Japan

Abstract - Permethrin, cypermethrin, deltamethrin, fenvalerate and fenpropathrin are highly insecticidal pyrethroids currently used for agriculture. The pyrethroids are photodecomposed mainly by isomerization of the cyclopropane ring and αR/αS epimerization in water and on plant foliage, with subsequent cleavage of the ester bond in water, except for fenvalerate which primarily undergoes photodecarboxylation and ester bond cleavage. The pyrethroids are metabolized in plant by hydrolysis, and by oxidation at the 2'- and the 4'-positions of the alcohol moiety and at the gem-dimethyl group of the acid moiety of permethrin and deltamethrin, and to a lesser extent by hydration of the cyano substituent to the corresponding amide. These sites are also involved in metabolism of the pyrethroids in soil and of fenvalerate in the aquatic model ecosystem consisting of soil, fish, daphnia, snail and algae. The hydrolytic products and their oxidized derivatives are further degraded in soil ultimately leading to carbon dioxide from radiolabels in various positions of the molecule, and are converted in plants to a variety of glycoside conjugates. These plant conjugated metabolites are bioavailable in rats. The aglycones liberated due to microbial attack in the intestine are rapidly metabolized followed by complete excretion. Conjugation with glucose lowers the acute oral toxicity in mice.

INTRODUCTION

The usefulness of the natural pyrethrins and their closely related compounds is limited primarily due to their easy decomposition by air and sunlight. So, more stable compounds with better biological performance have been desired, particulary in horticulture and agriculture (Ref. 1). During the past decades, extensive efforts have been made to obtain the pyrethroids for agricultural use by replacing substituents susceptible to photochemical or metabolic degradation with alternative groupings that confer greater overall stability in the molecule. Consequently, the newer pyrethroids which have greatly improved potency and stability in the field, are successfully developed (Ref. 2,3).

In common with other insecticides, the pyrethroids should be protected from undue abiotic degradation and insect metabolism but susceptible to metabolism in mammals and environmental systems. Since the stabilized compounds may be persistent in mammals and act as environmental contaminants, the environmental movement and fate including mammals have been extensively studied over the past few years (Ref. 4,5,6). The comparative metabolism mainly in mammals and insects of the pyrethroids derived from 3-phenoxybenzyl and α-cyano-3-phenoxybenzyl alcohols was reviewed by Casida et al (Ref. 7). In the present article, degradation of the pyrethroids in the field with emphasis in plant, soil and aquatic environment is discussed. The findings are useful in evaluating their safety and in understanding their effective use as well as their biodegradability.

Abbreviation : PBalc [3-phenoxybenzyl alcohol], PBald [3-phenoxybenzaldehyde], PBacid [3-phenoxybenzoic acid], Cl_2CA [2,2-dimethyl-3-(2,2-dichlorovinyl) cyclopropanecarboxylic acid], Br_2CA [2,2-dimethyl-3-(2,2-dibromovinyl)cyclopropanecarboxylic acid], Cl-Vacid [α-isopropyl-4-chlorophenylacetic acid], TMCA [tetramethylcyclopropanecarboxylic acid].

PHOTODEGRADATION

Photochemical reactions play a role in degrading permethrin (Ref. 8), deltamethrin (Ref. 9) and fenvalerate (Ref. 10,11,12,) to various degrees depending upon the chemical structures and environmental conditions. The photolysis study by sunlight in distilled water (Ref. 13) or on cotton plant (Ref. 14) indicate that the photodegradation rates decreased in the order of deltamethrin>cypermethrin>permethrin>fenvalerate. The *cis* isomers were by ~1.5 fold more photolabile than the *trans* isomers. Either replacement of one of the hydrogen atoms of the benzyl methylene group of permethrin with a cyano group, or replacement of chlorine atoms of cypermethrin with bromine led to the more photolabile compound. The half-life of disappearance in water ranged from 1.4 days to 10 days (TABLE 1), each of which was in good accord with that computed according to the methods of Zepp *et al* (Ref. 15). Photostability of fenvalerate as compared with other pyrethroids is attributed to the lower quantum yield as well as the lower rates of specific sunlight absorption.

TABLE 1. Half-life of disappearance for pyrethroid insecticides in distilled water under natural sunlight (September) at 40 degree north latitude

compound		$\Phi^{a)}$	Half-life (days) Calcd.[b)]	Found	Relative rates[c)]
Deltamethrin	[1R, *cis*, αS]	0.28	2.2	1.4	1.0
	[1R, *trans*, αS]	0.18	3.4	2.4	1.7
Cypermethrin	[1R, *cis*, αS]	0.12	5.5	4.2	3.0
	[1R, *trans*, αS]	----	---	4.4	3.1
Permethrin	[1R, *cis*]	0.51	7.5	4.9	3.5
	[1R, *trans*]	----	---	5.2	3.7
Fenvalerate	[2S, αS]	0.08	9.3	10.0	7.1

a) disappearance quantum yield
b) calculated half-life according to the equation [$T_{1/2}=0.639/\Phi\cdot ka$]
c) relative to deltamethrin [1R, *cis*, αS] isomer

The major photochemical reactions occurring in the pyrethroids were divided into seven categories by Holmstead *et al* (Ref. 16).

A) isomerization of the cyclopropane ring (1R/1S, *trans*/*cis*)
B) αR/αS epimerization
C) ester bond cleavage
D) oxidation of the cleavage products
E) photoelimination of carbon dioxide
F) reductive dehalogenation including those encountered with halovinyl substituent
G) dimerization of free radicals

Among these reactions, the pyrethroids either in water or on plant foliage under sunlight underwent primarily isomerization of the cyclopropane ring together with αR/αS interconversion in the case of α-cyano esters except for fenvalerate which underwent only a limited extent of epimerization at the benzylic carbon in the alcohol moiety but none in the acid moiety (Ref. 13). With permethrin, up to ca. 23 % of *cis* to *trans* and ca. 16 % of *trans* to *cis* interconversions occurred on cotton plant. In water, the more thermodynamically stable *trans* isomers constituted ca. 65 % of the equilibrium mixture. Although a single stereoisomer of deltamethrin or cypermethrin gave the respective eight possible isomers, the [1R, *cis*, αS] compounds yielded the *trans* isomers by ~1.6 fold more than the αR epimers, while the [1R, *trans*, αS] compounds gave the αR epimers in a slight preference to the *trans* isomers. The resulting isomer mixtures underwent further photodecomposition in water to yield more polar products (40-50 %) including mainly PBald, PBalc and PBacid from the alcohol moiety, and Cl_2CA and Br_2CA from the acid moiety via ester cleavage reaction. However, relatively small amounts of polar photoproducts (<10 %) including the ester cleavage products were formed on cotton plant even on prolonged irradiation. On the other hand, fenvalerate underwent photodecarboxylation and ester bond cleavage to yield decarboxy-fenvalerate, and PBacid and Cl-Vacid in greater amounts in water (Ref. 12) but in only limited amounts on cotton leaf (Ref. 14). HCN released on cleavage at the ester bond of fenvalerate was rapidly transformed by sunlight to mainly CO_2 together with a small amount of more polar products (Ref. 12).

On/in soil relatively little isomerization at the cyclopropane ring of permethrin (Ref. 8) and αR/αS epimerization in the case of fenvalerate (Ref. 12) was encountered as compared with the photolysis in water and on plant foliage. In addition, photodecarboxylation of fenvalerate as well as photo-induced cleavage at the ester bond of permethrin and fenvalerate appears to be of little importance on soils tested. However, sunlight accelerated the formation of the amide analog of fenvalerate resulting from hydration of the cyano group. The amide analog was subsequently converted to a lesser extent into the corresponding carboxylic acid and desphenyl derivatives as in the case of metabolism in soil discussed later.

Smaller or trace amounts monochloro-permethrin (Ref. 8) and dechlorinated decarboxy-fenvalerate (Ref. 11) were formed respectively on soil and in water, but reductive dehalogenation was a minor photo-reaction as compared with other reactions. The carbon-halogen bond strengths of the pyrethroids seemed to be relatively rigid so that other reactions might take place over the photo-dehalogenation reaction. With this respect, a more extensive dehalogenation was expected with deltamethrin than with permethrin and fenvalerate (Ref. 17). The halogen-substituted double bond of the acid moiety including monodehalogenated derivatives of permethrin and deltamethrin appears to be quite resistant to photooxidation (Ref. 16).

Irradiation (>290 nm) of deltamethrin in hexane (Ref. 9) and of fenvalerate in various solvents (Ref. 11) led to dimers of free radicals generated during the photolysis process. The main dimeric products were formed from deltamethrin via coupling of α-cyano-3-phenoxybenzyl radical and from fenvalerate by recombination of the α-cyano-4-chlorobenzyl radical resulting from decarboxylation reaction discussed later. Again, these dimeric products were not detected or if any in minor amounts in dilute aqueous solutions or on cotton plant under sunlight (Ref. 13,14).

As with the dimerization, most of the photochemical reactions proceeded through free-radical intermediates. Holmsted and Fuller postulated that photo-decarboxylation of α-cyano esters occurred via discrete radical intermediates which were formed by the stepwise loss of carbon dioxide with subsequent recombination of the radicals within a solvent cage (Ref. 10). In consisting with the hypothesis, α-cyano-3-phenoxybenzyl and α-isopropyl-4-chlorobenzyl radicals were identified to be the intermediates of photoelimination process of fenvalerate by ESR using a spin trapping method which enabled the short-lived free radicals to convert into the more stable ones (spin adducts). Since UV irradiation of fenvalerate in benzene in the presence of nitroso-durene as a spin trapping reagent yielded a mixture of at least two spin adducts, separation was also performed by HPLC equipped with ESR prior to characterization (Ref. 17). The mechanism excluded the posibility of decarboxy-fenvalerate formation in biological systems.

METABOLISM IN PLANTS

In the parallel outdoor experiments, about 65 % (permethrin), 50 % (cypermethrin) and 20 % (deltamethrin and fenvalerate) of the applied radiocarbon was lost probably due to evaporation from the cotton plant after one week in similar proportion to their inherent vapor pressure. On the other hand, penetration of the radiolabel into the plant tissues occurred to almost the same degree (13-25 %) during the same period. As a result of metabolism in plant, vapor loss and photolysis on plant foliage as discussed earlier, the pyrethroid residues in/on cotton leaves decreased in the order of fenvalerate >cypermethrin≥deltamethrin>permethrin. The *cis* isomers were a little more persistent than *trans* isomers (Ref. 14).

Although it is difficult to make valid detailed comparison of metabolism in plants due to variation of plant species and environmental conditions tested, the sites of metabolic attack on pyrethroids are summarized in Fig. 1. There is extensive ester cleavage for each pyrethroid with ~2.8 fold *trans/cis* difference in the case of permethrin isomers (Ref. 18,19,20) but not so extensive in cypermethrin isomers (Ref. 21). A major reaction was hydroxylation at the gem-dimethyl group of permethrin isomers, and the 2'- and the 4'-positions of alcohol moiety of fenvalerate before or after hydrolysis. The more stable *cis* isomer of permethrin was by ~2.5 fold more oxidized than the *trans* isomer. Hydroxylation at the 2'- and the 4'-positions of permethrin, the 4'-position of cypermethrin, and the gem-dimethyl group and the 4'-position of deltamethrin also occurred but to lesser extents. The hydroxy ester appears to be detected in minor amounts. There was a considerable specificity for hydroxylation of the methyl group *cis* to the carboxyl with *trans*-permethrin, but this specificity was not so prominent with *cis*-permethrin. The metabolites hydroxylated at the methyl group *cis* to the carboxyl readily underwent cyclization to form γ-lactone as in mammalian metabolism (Ref. 22). With deltamethrin,

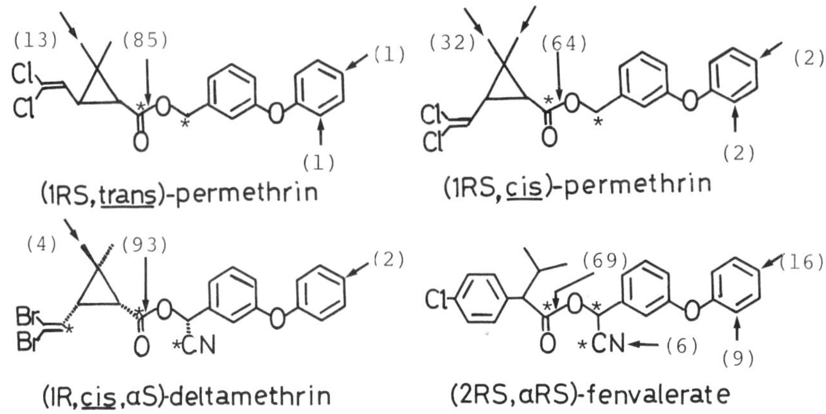

Fig. 1 Metabolic sites of four pyrethroids in plants.
Data are relative per cents to the total metabolites in cotton (permethrin and deltamethrin) and in bean plant (fenvalerate). No detailed quantitative data are available from cypermethrin. Reference - permethrin (20), deltamethrin (26), fenvalerate (27).

the trans methyl group relative to the carboxyl group was only hydroxylated. An additional metabolites of fenvalerate and cypermethrin were the amide analog resulting from hydration of the cyano substituent. Little translocation of the pyrethroids and their metabolites to the untreated parts of the plant occurred.

The cleavage products or oxidized derivatives were usually converted to a variety of glycoside conjugates. The major metabolites were PBalc and PBacid, and acid moiety such as Cl_2CA, Br_2CA and Cl-Vacid which also occurred mainly in conjugated form. PBacid and PBalc were similary converted in cotton plants to mono-glucoside and disaccharides, particularly the glucosylarabinose and glucosylxylose coujugates (Ref. 23,24). In bean and cucumber plants and cabbage, the malonylglucoside of PBacid was mainly formed. In tomato, not only (1-6)-triglucoside ester but trisaccharide with varying substitution position of glucose moiety was formed. The latter saccharide as well as the gentiobioside conjugate was predominant. Cl_2CA and Cl-Vacid formed nearly the same glycosides as those from PBacid (Ref. 25). The malonylglucosides of PBacid and Cl-Vacid were resistant to β-glucosidase hydrolysis but were completely cleaved by cellulase while other conjugates were readily hydrolyzed by β-glucosidase (Ref. 25). In addition, some evidence of formation of small amounts of cyanohydrin glucoside conjugates was obtained with deltamethrin (Ref. 26) and fenvalerate (Ref. 27).

Although the tissue distribution of the glucosides and of enzymes involved has not been clarified, some cyanogenic glucoside was found to be located entirely in the epidermal layers of the leaf blade, whereas the two enzymes responsible for its catabolism were present almost exclusively in the mesophyll tissue. The uridine diphosphate glucose; glucosyltransferase catalyzing final step of the biosynthesis was found in both mesophyll and epidermal tissues (Ref. 28,29).

The cyano group was released as HCN on hydrolysis of α-cyanobenzyl alcohol or its hydroxy derivatives. Although metabolites derived from HCN was not identified yet, Miller and Conn suggested that HCN was converted at least in part to β-cyanoalanine followed by asparagine which could then be incorporated into the general biosynthetic routes of the plant, and/or to thiocyanate by rhodanase which occurred far less commonly in plants (Ref. 30).

Only a limited amount of Cl_2CA and a cyclopropane dicarboxylic acid were shown to be present in sugar beet grown in soil treated with permethrin. It is likely that both carboxylic acids are formed in soil and are subsequently taken up by the plant (Ref. 31). When bean plants were grown in soil treated with fenvalerate, very little uptake of radioactive residues resulted (Ref. 24). Based upon the available information, the terminal residues of the pyrethroids in plants are likely to be mainly unchanged parent compounds, possibly with some free and conjugated metabolites derived from the acid and alcohol moieties.

DEGRADATION IN SOIL

Fenvalerate was degraded more rapidly under aerobic conditions than under anaerobic conditions, and was hardly decomposed in sterilized soils (Ref. 32). Under waterlogged, anaerobic conditions degradation of permethrin (Ref. 33), cypermethrin (Ref. 34) and fenpropathrin (Ref. 35) occurred at a slower rate than under aerobic conditions. Degradation of the pyrethroids appears to be mainly mediated by soil microorganisms. In consistent with the foregoing results, the isolated or mixed microbial culture solutions actively decomposed fenvalerate (Ref. 32) and permethrin isomers (Ref. 33).

Under similar upland conditions, the degradation rates in two Japanese soil decreased in the order of permethrin>cypermethrin>deltamethrin>fenpropathrin> fenvalerate. The time necessary for loss of a half of the chemicals ranged from 4-95 days depending upon the chemical structure of the compound and the soil type (TABLE 2). It is interesting that either dichlorovinyl replacement for the dibromovinyl, substitution of a cyano group with one of the benzyl-methylene proton of permethrin or removal of the dihalovinyl group from cypermethrin and deltamethrin reduced the overall degradation rates. Where the isomers existed, the <u>trans</u> isomers were degraded more rapidly than the <u>cis</u> isomers and the αS epimers were decomposed faster than the αR antipodes. With cypermethrin and deltamethrin, the [1R, <u>trans</u>, αS] compounds were degraded most rapidly followed in decreasing order by [1R, <u>trans</u>, αR], [1R, <u>cis</u>, αS] and [1R, <u>cis</u>, αR] isomers. Both <u>trans/cis</u> and αR/αS interconversions did not occur in soil, or if any, to only a limited extent (Ref. 36).

TABLE 2. Half-life of disappearance for pyrethroid insecticides in soil under aerobic upland conditions

compound		Half-life (days)[a] Kodaira soil[b]	Azuchi soil[c]
Permethrin	[1R, <u>trans</u>]	4.2	7.2
	[1R, <u>cis</u>]	7.7	12.6
Cypermethrin	[1R, <u>trans</u>, αS]	6.3	9.1
	[1R, <u>trans</u>, αR]	14.7	15.4
	[1R, <u>cis</u>, αS]	18.2	23.1
	[1R, <u>cis</u>, αR]	25.2	44.8
Deltamethrin	[1R, <u>trans</u>, αS]	8.8	12.6
	[1R, <u>trans</u>, αR]	21.7	23.8
	[1R, <u>cis</u>, αS]	23.1	41.3
	[1R, <u>cis</u>, αR]	34.3	56.0
Fenpropathrin	[αSR]	24.5	38.5
Fenvalerate	[2S, αS]	29.4	67.9
	[2S, αR]	53.2	94.5

a) average of duplicate experiments(25°C)
b) light clay (40 % H_2O) c) sandy clay loam (40 % H_2O)

Except for fenpropathrin, both hydrolytic and oxidative reactions were involved in the initial metabolism (Fig. 2). Hydroxylation occurred at the 4'-position of the alcohol moiety and at the gem-dimethyl group of the acid moiety before or after hydrolysis. The hydroxymethyl derivative of Cl_2CA was further oxidized to the carboxylic acid (Ref. 37). There was no significant steric preference in the oxidation of both methyl groups in the acid moiety. Another degradation route of fenvalerate not reported in studies with other pyrethroids was ether cleavage resulting in formation of des-phenyl fenvalerate which might be derived from hydroxylation at the 2'-position of the alcohol moiety as was suggested by Ruzo <u>et al</u>(Ref. 38). Fenvalerate was also degraded by hydration of the cyano substituent to the corresponding amide analog, a portion of which was abiologically formed by action of clay minerals such as Kaolinite and montomorinate (Ref. 32). Fenpropathrin underwent only hydrolysis at either the ester linkage or the cyano group, in the latter case yielding the amide and carboxylic acid analogs (Ref. 35). The major ester metabolites included 4'-OH-permethrin which was present in greater amounts from the <u>cis</u> isomer than the <u>trans</u> isomer (Ref. 39), and des-phenyl fenvalerate. A major reaction for each pyrethroid was hydrolysis of the ester bond leading to the formation of PBalc and PBacid, the acidic half of the molecule such as Cl_2CA, TMCA and Cl-Vacid, and their hydroxy derivatives. The <u>trans</u> and αS isomers were hydrolyzed more rapidly than the <u>cis</u> and αR isomers, respectively, so that the hydrolytic products were formed in relatively large amounts from the <u>trans</u> and αS isomers than the corresponding counterparts. The difference in hydrolysis rate influenced the overall biodegradability of each isomer in soil.

Under aerobic conditions, further extensive degradation of the hydrolysis products including hydrogen cyanide occurred with the formation of $^{14}CO_2$ from radiolabels incorporated in various positions of the molecule (Fig. 2). With

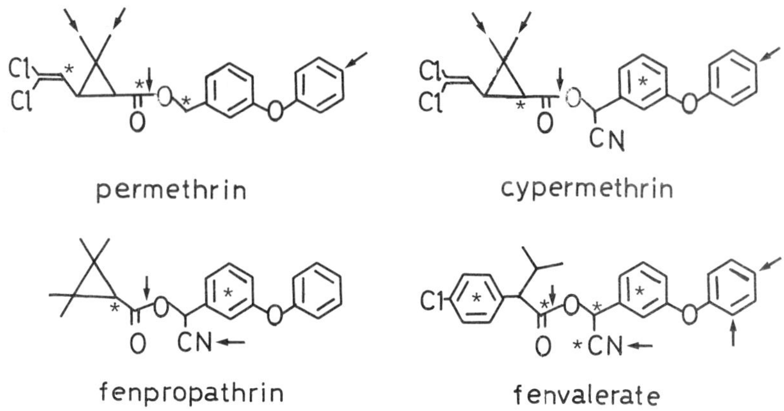

Fig. 2. Labeled positions of the pyrethroids used for soil study. (⟼) indicates the initial metabolic sites in soil

fenvalerate, large amounts of $^{14}CO_2$ were produced from the cyano radiolabel as compared with other labeled compounds (Ref. 32). The initial rate of evolution of $^{14}CO_2$ was more rapid from the alcohol moiety than from the acid moiety. Bearing in mind that the positions of radiolabelling were in the cyclopropyl- and phenyl-rings with α-cyano esters, this $^{14}CO_2$ evolution was evidence for ring opening followed by degradation of the products formed. Under anaerobic conditions, some hydrolysis products were degraded slowly and there was little evolution of $^{14}CO_2$.

The ester and/or cleavage products formed the unextractable "bound" residues which were mainly distributed in the soil organic matter fractions such as fulvic acid, humic acid and humin. With cypermethrin, small amounts of PBacid, 4'-OH-PBacid and Cl_2CA were detected in the fulvic acid fraction (Ref. 37). $^{14}CO_2$ was released at a slow but steady rate from the "bound" residues arising from cypermethrin (Ref. 34) and fenvalerate (Ref. 40) by mixing with fresh soil. It is likely that the "bound" residues are degraded further. There appears to be little likelihood of persistency of the pyrethroids or their metabolites for lengthy periods in soil.

Although trace amounts of 4'-OH-permethrin, PBacid, Cl_2CA (Ref. 41) and Cl-Vacid (Ref. 32) were eluted by water from soil columns which had been pre-treated and aged before elution, very little movement for each intact pyrethroid occurred through soil. PBalc was only slightly mobile. Soil pH seemed to be the primary factor affecting mobility of organic acid chemicals in soil, and both Cl_2CA and PBacid were less mobile in acid soil than in alkaline soil (Ref. 41).

DEGRADATION IN THE AQUATIC ENVIRONMENT

In aquatic model ecosystem, the bioacumulation ratios for fenvalerate in carp (67-117) were by 10-20 fold less than those for DDT and DDT-R (sum of DDT, DDE and DDD), and were lower than in snails, daphnids and algae. Fenvalerate underwent primarily hydrolysis at the ester bond together with hydroxylation at the 2'- and the 4'-position of alcohol moiety and hydrolysis at the cyano group in four species of aquatic organisms in the ecosystem. It appears that fish is most active in the metabolism of fenvalerate among four species.
No metabolites which accumulated to higher degrees in comparison with fenvalerate were formed in fish. Fenvalerate appears not to be accumulated by fish to a high degree from food, i.e., through food chains in the aquatic environment (Ref. 42). Both *trans*- and *cis*-permethrin were similary taken up from water and eliminated by rainbow trout. Urine appeared to be a minor excretion route of permethrin. The metabolites were mainly excreted into the bile as a glucuronide of 4'-OH-permethrin, and to a lesser extent into the urine at least in part as sulfate conjugates (Ref. 43). Although carp and trout liver microsomes hydrolyzed *trans*-permethrin much more extensively than the *cis*-permethrin *in vitro*, no significant hydrolysis occurred *in vivo* with both isomer (Ref. 44,45).

BIOAVAILABILITY OF CONJUGATED PLANT METABOLITES

When administered orally to rats, the glucoside conjugate of PBacid was rapidly absorbed and eliminated as a mixture of metabolites very similar to those derived from PBacid (Ref. 46). The principal urinary metabolite was the sulfate ester of 4'-OH-PBacid. The enterohepatorenal disposition of PBacid was confirmed by suppression on the gut microflora with antibiotics *in vivo*, which drastically reduced the extent of deconjugation of biliary glucuronides and hence reabsorption of the free benzoic acids (Ref. 47). There were considerable species variations in conjugation of PBacid. The most striking examples were the large amounts of the glucuronic acid conjugates of PBacid and 4'-OH-PBacid in marmoset, rabbit, guinea pig and hamster, of the O-sulfate conjugate of 4'-OH-PBacid in rat, of the taurine conjugate of PBacid in mice, and of the glycylvaline dipeptide in mallard duck (Ref. 48,49). Upon single oral administration of PBalc and its mono-, di- and tri-β-glucosides with (1-6) glucoside linkage to intact and bile duct-cannulated rats, ca. 40 % of the dose of each compound was excreted in bile after 1 day, and 70 % in urine and 10-30 % in feces after 7 days. The major metabolites in urine was found to be the O-sulfate ester of 4'-OH-PBacid, whereas glucuronide conjugates of PBalc and 4'-OH-PBalc were predominant in bile. The glucoside conjugates of PBalc and PBacid were not enzymatically cleaved to a significant extent *in vitro* in saliva, gastric juice, bile, pancreatic juice and urine. However, extensive deconjugation occurred by microflora in the gut. Thus, although the glucoside conjugates may provide a bioavailable source of exogeneous compounds if consumed in the diet of man and animals, the liberated aglycones were rapidly metabolized followed by complete excretion. Conjugation of PBacid, PBalc and Cl-Vacid with glucose significantly lowered the acute oral toxicity in mice (TABLE 3) (Ref. 50).

TABLE 3. Mouse oral LD_{50} values for PBacid, PBalc and Cl-Vacid, and their glucoside conjugates

	LD_{50} mmol/kg		LD_{50} mmol/kg
PBacid	3.25	PBalc	3.45
PBacid-α-Glu	5.37	PBalc-β-Glu	6.96
PBacid-β-Glu	6.17	PBalc-β-Glu-Glu[a)]	6.26
(+)Cl-Vacid	2.28	PBalc-β-Glu-Glu-Glu[a)]	14.5-21.8
(+)Cl-Vacid-α-Glu	9.79		
(+)Cl-Vacid-β-Glu	6.02		

α: α-glycoside β: β-glycoside Glu: glucose
a) (1-6) glycoside linkage

CONCLUSION

The pyrethroids discussed in this review are readily subjected to various types of biotic and abiotic degradation in the environment. Together with the lower application dosage, possible environmental contamination by the pyrethroids would be minimal and negligible in most cases. However, certain degradation products like decarboxy-fenvalerate may be persistent as compared with the parent compound. In such case more extensive investigation in respect to their ultimate environmental fate will be desirable.

Only little information up to date is available on the behavior of the pyrethroids in the aquatic environment. The studies on accumulation and/or metabolism in aquatic organisms are important under circumstances where river, pond and sea water could be contaminated with residues of pyrethroids and their degradation products. These informations might be useful in providing insight into the development of the new type of pyrethroids with low toxicity in fish.

REFERENCES

1) J. Miyamoto; Environ. Health. Perspect. 14, 15-28 (1976)
2) M. Elliott; ACS Symp. Ser. 42, 1-28 (1977)
3) N. Itaya, T. Mastuo, H. Ohno, T. Mizutani, F. Fujita and H. Yoshioka; ACS Symp. Ser. 42, 45-54 (1977)
4) J. Miyamoto, K. I. Beynon, T. R. Roberts, R. J. Hemingway and H. Swaine; Pure & Appl. Cheml., 53, 1967-2022 (1981)
5) T. R. Roberts; in "Progress in Pesticide Biochemistry" vol. 1, p.115-146, D. H. Hutson and T. R. Roberts, eds. John Wiley & Sons (1981)
6) D. H. Hutson; in "Progress in Drug Metabolism" vol. 3, p.215-252 J. W. Bridges and L. F. Chausseaud, eds. John Wiley & Sons (1979)

7) J. E. Casida, L. C. Gaughan, L. O. Ruzo; in "Advance in Pesticide Science" p.182-189. H. Geissbuehler, G. T. Brooks and P. C. Kearney. eds. Pergamon Press (1979)
8) R. L. Holmstead, J. E. Casida, L. O. Ruzo and D. G. Fuller; J. Agric. Food Chem., 26, 590-595 (1978)
9) L. O. Ruzo, R. L. Holmstead and J. E. Casida; J. Agric. Food Chem., 25, 1385-1934 (1977)
10) R. L. Holmstead and D. G. Fuller; J. Agric. Food Chem., 25, 56-58 (1977)
11) R. L. Holmstead, D. G. Fuller and L. O. Ruzo; J. Agric Food Chem., 26, 954-959 (1978)
12) N. Mikami, N. Takahashi, K. Hayashi and J. Miyamoto; J. Pesticide Sci., 5, 225-236 (1980)
13) N. Mikami, N. Takahashi, H. Yamada and J. Miyamoto; unpublished observation
14) N. Mikami, N. Wakabayashi, H. Yamada and J. Miyamoto; unpublished observation
15) R. G. Zepp and D. M. Cline; Environ. Sci. Technol., 11, 359-366 (1977)
16) R. L. Holmstead, J. E. Casida and L. O. Ruzo; ACS Symp. Ser., 42, 137-146 (1977)
17) N. Mikami, N. Takahashi, H. Yamada and J, Miyamoto; unpublished observation
18) H. Ohkawa, H. Kaneko and J. Miyamoto; J. Pesticide Sci., 2, 67-76 (1977)
19) L. C. Gaughan, T. Unai and J. E. Casida; ACS Symp. Ser., 42, 186-193 (1977)
20) L. C. Gaughan and J. E. Casida; J. Agric.Food Chem., 26, 525-528 (1978)
21) A. N. Wright, T. R. Roberts, A. J. Dutton and M. V. Doig; Pestic. Boichem. Physiol., 13, 71-80 (1980)
22) D. M. Soderlund and J. E. Casida; ACS Symp. Ser., 42, 173-185 (1977)
23) J. E. More, T. R. Roberts and A. N. Wright; Pestic. Biochem. Physiol., 9, 268-280 (1978)
24) T. R. Roberts and A. N. Wright; Pestic. Sci., 12, 161-169 (1981)
25) N, Mikami, N. Shibano, H. Yamada and J. Miyamoto; Abstract of papers present at 6th Annual Meeting of Pesticide Science Society of Japan No. 242 (1981)
26) L. O. Ruzo and J. E. Casida; J. Agric. Food Chem., 27, 572-575 (1979)
27) H. Ohkawa, K. Nambu and J. Miyamoto; J. Pesticide Sci., 5, 215-233 (1980)
28) M. Kojima, J. E. Poulton, S. S. Thayer and E. E. Corn; Plant Physiol., 63, 1022-1028 (1979)
29) S. S. Thayer and E. E. Corn; Plant Physiol., 67, 617-621 (1981)
30) J. M. Miller and E. E. Corn; Plant Physiol., 65, 1199-1202 (1980)
31) J. P. Leachey and P. K. Carpenter; Pestic. Sci., 11, 279-289 (1980)
32) H. Ohkawa, K. Nambu, H. Inui and J. Miyamoto; J. Pesticide Sci., 3, 129-141 (1978)
33) D. D. Kaufman, S. C. Hayes, E. G. Gordon and A. J. Kayser; ACS Symp. Ser., 42, 147-161 (1977)
34) T. R. Roberts and M. E. Standen; Pestic. Sci., 8, 305-319 (1977)
35) T. R. Roberts and M. E. Standen. Pestic. Sci., 8, 600-610 (1977)
36) N. Mikami, S. Sakata, H. Yamada and J. Miyamoto; unpublished observation
37) T. R. Roberts and M. E. Standen; Pestic. Sci., 12, 285-296 (1981)
38) L. O. Ruzo, T. Unai and J. E. Casida; J. Agric. Food Chem., 26, 918-925 (1978)
39) H. Kaneko, H. Ohkawa and J. Miyamoto; J. Pesticide Sci., 3, 43-51 (1978)
40) N. Mikami, S. Sakata, H. Yamada and J. Miyamoto; unpublished observation
41) D. D. Kaufman, B. A. Russel, C. S. Helling and A. J. Kayser; J. Agric. Food Chem., 29, 239-245 (1981)
42) H. Ohkawa, R. Kikuchi and J. Miyamoto; J. Pesticide Sci., 5, 11-22 (1980)
43) A. H. Glickman, A. A. R. Hamid, D. E. Richert and J. J. Lech; Toxicol. Appl. Pharmacol., 57, 88-98 (1981)
44) A. H. Glickman, T. Shono, J. E. Casida and J. J. Lech; J. Agric. Food Chem., 27, 1038-1041 (1979)
45) A. H. Glickman and J. J. Lech; Toxicol. Appl. Pharmacol., 60, 186-192 (1981)
46) J. V. Crayford and D. H. Hutson; Xenobiotica, 10, 355-364 (1980)
47) K. R. Huckle, J. K. Chipman, D. H. Hutson and P. Millburn; Drug Metab. Dispos., 9, 360-368 (1981)
48) K. R. Huckle, I. J. G. Climie, D. H. Hutson and P. Millburn; Drug Metab. Dispos., 9, 147-149 (1981)
49) K. R. Huckle., D. H. Hutson and P. Millburn; Drug Metab. Dispos., 9, 352-359 (1981)
50) N. Mikami, J. Yoshimura, H. Kaneko, H. Yamada and J, Miyamoto; unpublished observation

PHOTOOXIDATION REACTIONS OF PYRETHROID INSECTICIDES

Luis O. Ruzo

Pesticide Chemistry and Toxicology Laboratory, Department of Entomological Sciences, University of California, Berkeley, California 94720, USA

Abstract - The reactions of a variety of pyrethroids with triplet and singlet oxygen and with ozone have been studied. The principal identified oxidation processes of pyrethroids involve allylic oxidation, epoxidation, hydroperoxide formation and cleavage of the alkene substituent on the cyclopropane ring. Secondary reactions are detected during and after ester cleavage. A mutagenic photoproduct of allethronyl esters is described. It is formed by di-π-methane rearrangement of the allyl group, followed by epoxidation of the double bond in the cyclopentenolone ring.

Introduction

The natural pyrethrins are potent insecticides which can be rapidly deactivated by exposure to air and light. This lack of photostability severely limits their usefulness for agricultural purposes. Attempts at stabilizing the natural pyrethrins with combinations of antioxidants and ultraviolet screening agents have met limited success (Ref. 1). The pyrethroids that are derivatives of chrysanthemic acid contain an isobutenyl group which is very susceptible to biological and photochemical degradation (Ref. 2 and 3), modifications being detected in the chrysanthemic acid moiety. Irradiation of purified pyrethrum extract also yield chrysanthemic acids upon hydrolysis (Ref. 4). Photolyzed mixtures from pyrethrin I, allethrin, tetramethrin and dimethrin yield oxidized forms of chrysanthemic acid upon saponification (Ref. 5) (Fig. 1), but the primary products were not identified.

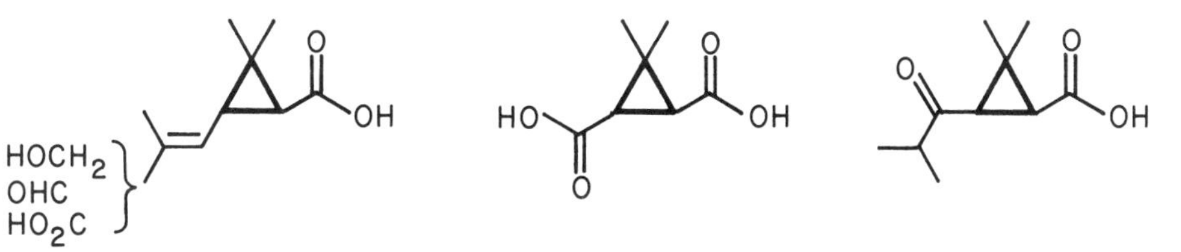

Fig. 1. Oxidized products obtained from synthetic analogs of pyrethrin I.

The isobutenyl group has also been reported to readily form oxetanes when irradiated in the presence of sensitizer ketones (Ref. 6), a finding that establishes the possibility of photocycloaddition reactions at this site.

The new synthetic pyrethroids are considerably more resistant to oxidation processes, because of deactivation to electrophilic reactions by halogen substituents and by the stability of the 3-phenoxybenzyl moiety. Several comparative studies of pyrethroid photoreactivity have been reported. Resmethrin is more stable than allethrin when irradiated as a thin film on glass, but more reactive on silica gel (Ref. 7). The acid moiety of the potent knockdown agent kadethrin destabilizes the ester to a greater extent than the analogous lactone-substituted chrysanthemate, the pyrethrate or the chrysanthemate when their 2-octyl esters are photosensitized by acetone or isobutyrophenone (Ref. 8). A series of quantum yields (ϕ) determined in oxygenated methanol for six pyrethroids at 300 nm vary 3-10 fold between compounds with a cyclopentenone chromophore (allethrin) as compared with the phenoxybenzyl-substituted compounds. It is evident that a large portion of the absorbed radiation in the latter results is no net reaction since ϕ is greater for the methyl ester of 2,2-dimethyl-3-(2,2-dibromovinyl)cyclopropanecarboxylic acid (Ref. 9) than for deltamethrin.

This oxidation is enhanced with allethrin by photolysis in the presence of aromatic ketones which may act as oxygen transfer agents (Ref. 10 & 12). The products shown in Fig. 2 closely resemble those obtained upon metabolism of chrysanthemates (Ref. 2).

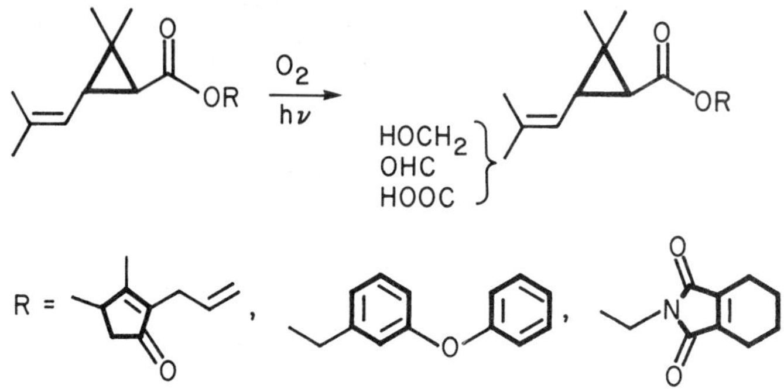

Fig. 2. Allylic oxidation in several chrysanthemates.

Epoxidation Reactions

Studies with allethrin (Ref. 10), tetramethrin and phenothrin (Ref. 11), kadethrin (Ref. 8) and resmethrin (Ref. 7), establish the generality of epoxidation reactions in the chrysanthemate group. In all cases two isomers are obtained, corresponding to triplet oxygen addition from above and below the plane of unsaturation. The possible participation of ozone in this process (Fig. 3) is unlikely since epimeric epoxides are obtained in similar yields, a result not expected with ozone in view of its normal stereospecificity (13).

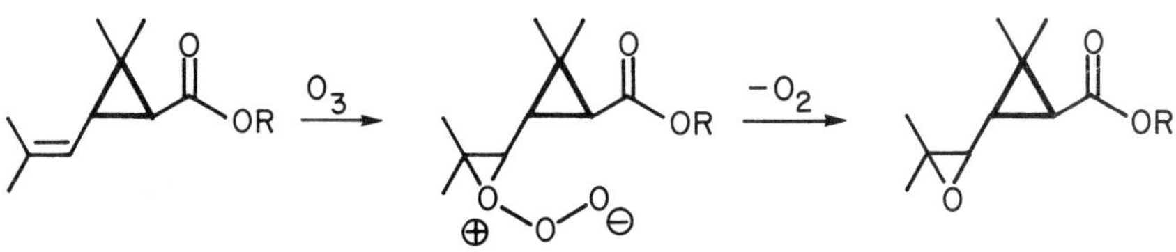

Fig. 3. Possible role of ozone in chrysanthemate epoxidation.

Epoxides constitute ~ 10% of reacted allethrin and phenothrin, ~ 15% of decomposed tetramethrin, < 5% of resmethrin and are only found in trace amounts from kadethrin. The yield of allethrin epoxides can be enhanced when solutions are photolyzed in the presence of the diketone benzil (Ref. 10). Such diketones have been reported to act as oxygen transfer agents in addition to their traditional role as sensitizers (Ref. 12) (Fig. 4).

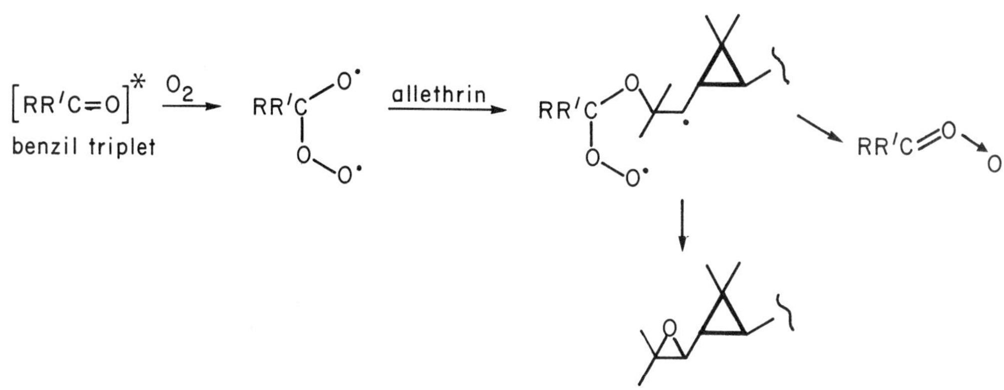

Fig. 4. Epoxidation of allethrin with benzil.

Epoxychrysanthemic acid has not been detected among the ester cleavage products of chrysanthemates, probably because upon formation it decomposes rapidly to the dienol, liberating CO_2 (Fig. 5) as shown in a metabolic study of tetramethrin (Ref. 14).

Epoxidation has also been detected in the cyclopentenolone ring of allethrin and terallethrin. This product arises from di-π-methane rearrangement of the propenyl side-chain (Ref. 10 & 15), followed by oxidation (Ref. 16) (Fig. 6). It is obtained in low yields (~ 1%) when these

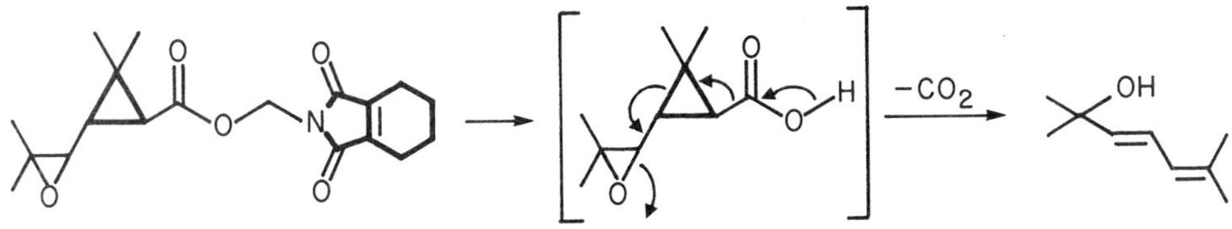

Fig. 5. Decomposition of epoxychrysanthemic acid.

pyrethroids are irradiated as thin films on glass with sunlight or at 360 nm by ultraviolet light, and exhibits moderate mutagenic activity in the Ames test. A mutagenic epoxide from allethrin was isolated and characterized by chemical ionization-mass spectrometry (CI-MS). and nucleomagnetic resonance (NMR). The analogous epoxide arising from terallethrin was identified by comparison of its chromatographic and spectroscopic properties with those of authentic material synthesized by reaction with *m*-chloroperoxybenzoic acid (MCPBA). Dichloro-allethrin appears to yield a similar product (CI-MS).

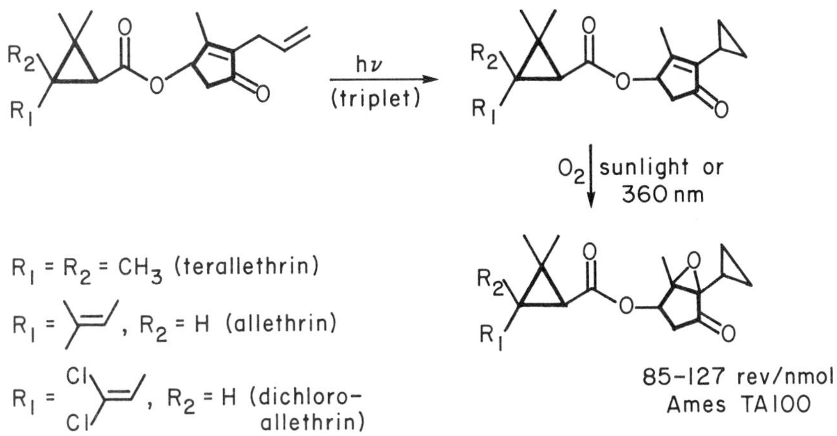

Fig. 6. Formation of mutagenic epoxides from allethronyl esters.

Several factors may be responsible for the low yields obtained. The di-π-methane rearrangement is relatively inefficient at long wavelengths, the α,β-unsaturated ketone is stable towards electrophilic reaction, and the cyclopropyl group may provide steric hindrance to oxidation. The recovered yields are also low due to the instability of the epoxides. These mutagens may be minor mfo metabolites of the cyclopropyl derivatives since they are active on S9-activation. Other mutagenic products were detected in allethrin and terallethrin photolysates but were not isolated or characterized. Several commercial pyrethroids examined yield sunlight photoproduct mixtures with no more than 10% of the mutagenic activity of photodecomposed allethrin and terallethrin (Ref. 16).

The dihalovinyl-substituted pyrethroids have not been found to undergo photoepoxidation, but monochloro-permethrin is slowly epoxidized by *m*-chloroperoxybenzoic acid (Ref. 17). Furthermore, methyl 2,2-dimethyl-3-(2,2-dibromovinyl)cyclopropanecarboxylate is converted to a bromomethoxy-epoxide derivative in low yields in methanol solution irradiated at 300 nm. Presumably this product forms by initial nucleophilic substitution by solvent followed by oxidation (Ref. 9). Haloethylene oxides have been previously reported as products of photooxidation, peroxide and peroxyacid reactions (Ref. 18). Thus, the formation of such oxides may be expected from dihalovinyl-pyrethroids under appropriate conditions.

Singlet Oxygen Reactions

Most photosensitized oxygenations are now established to involve an excited singlet state of molecular oxygen (Ref. 19). Only the $^1\Delta_g$ state (22.5 Kcal/mole) has a sufficiently long lifetime in solution to be responsible for chemical reactions. Singlet oxygen ($^1O_2$) is commonly generated by dye sensitization, but other energy donors can effect the excitation. The chemistry of singlet oxygen has been related to a variety of processes such as air pollution, photocarcinogenicity and chemiluminescence, and it has been shown to form in natural waters as a result of sensitisation by humic acids (Ref. 20). The reactions of $^1O_2$ most commonly involve ene reactions yielding hydroperoxides and 2 + 2 additions to alkenes producing dioxetanes.

Early studies of pyrethroid photoreactivity suggested that hydroperoxides were formed upon exposure to light and air (Ref. 21), but the products were not characterized. The benzyl furylmethyl group of resmethrin and kadethrin is extensively oxidized in solution or thin film irradiation yielding an endoperoxide which decomposes further as shown in Figure 7 (Refs 7 & 8).

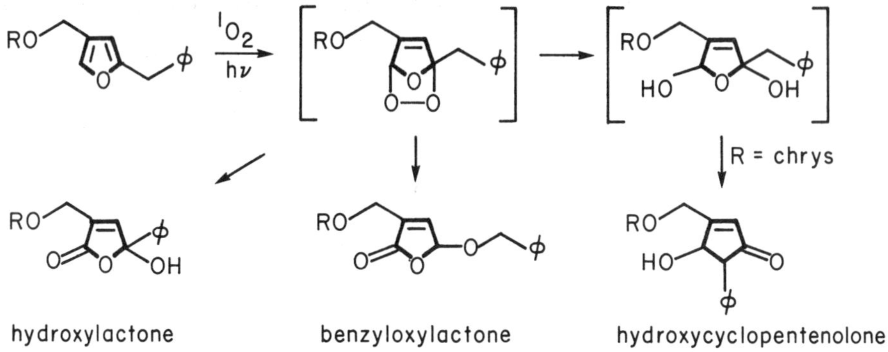

Fig. 7. Singlet oxygen reactions of resmethrin and kadethrin.

Involvement of $^1O_2$ is established by reaction of resmethrin with oxygen in methanol solution containing the dye rose bengal, leading to formation of the same products obtained on direct irradiation (Ref. 7). The isobutenyl group in allethrin, phenothrin and tetramethrin (Ref. 10 & 11) reacts with $^1O_2$ yielding hydroperoxides by the ene mechanism. The racemic hydroperoxides are significant products (6-22%) of phenothrin and tetramethrin irradiated in thin films or benzene solution (~ 30% conversion), reacting further to the corresponding alcohol and ketone (Fig. 8). Quenching of the reaction with 2,5-dimethylfuran results in sharply decreased hydroperoxide formation, supporting $^1O_2$ involvement. The tertiary hydroperoxide, an alternative product is not favored and is not detected. *S*-bioallethrin is converted to the hydroperoxides on reaction with $^1O_2$, but these products are not detected on direct irradiation (Ref. 10).

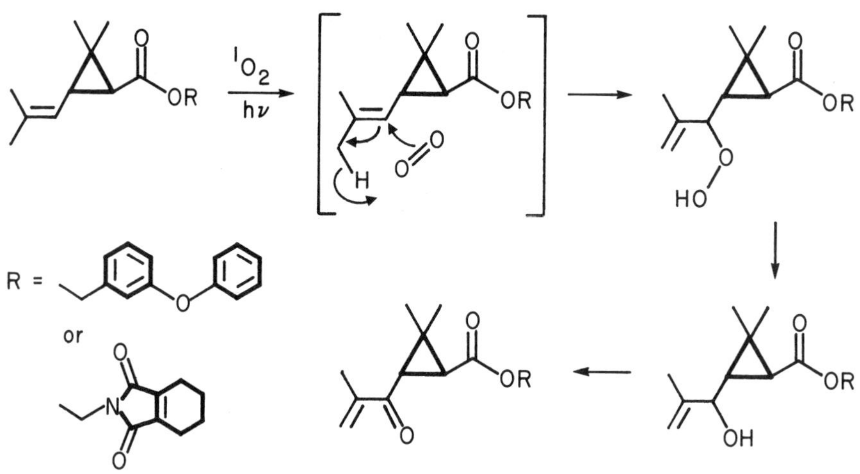

Fig. 8. Reaction of phenothrin and tetramethrin with singlet oxygen.

Treatment of deltamethrin or cypermethrin with $^1O_2$ generated with rose bengal in methanol gives only very low yields of ester cleavage products which probably arise from direct absorption by the pyrethroid (Ruzo and Casida, unpublished results).

Oxidative cleavage of vinyl substituents

Caronic acid is obtained on hydrolysis of photolysates from pyrethrin I, allethrin, tetramethrin and dimethrin (Ref. 5) (Fig. 1). Phenothrin is converted to an ozonide on plant surfaces (Ref. 22), a possible intermediate in oxidative cleavage. Phenothrin and tetramethrin photolyze to caronaldehyde derivatives (1-10%) in solution and thin film irradiations. The photoproducts characterized (Ref. 11) suggest the intervention of ozone or intermediacy of dioxetanes from oxygen addition (Fig. 9). Disproportionation leads to caronaldehyde esters which on further oxidation produce caronic acid derivatives.

In a recent study on the comparative photoreactivity with sunlight of thin films of 3-benzoylbenzyl-, 3-phenylbenzyl- and 3-phenoxybenzyl-pyrethroids (Ref. 23), esters of caronic acid were obtained in several cases, although always in lower yields with the 3-phenoxybenzyl-

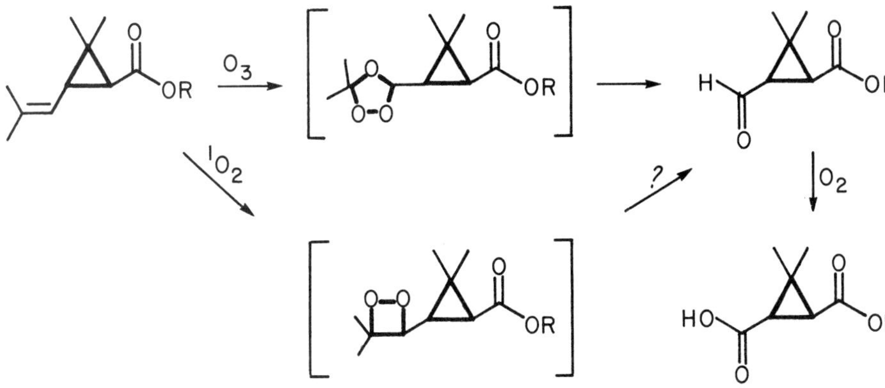

Fig. 9. Cleavage of the isobutenyl group in phenothrin and tetramethrin

compounds. Treatment of 3-phenylbenzyl-3-(2,2-dichlorovinyl)-2,2-dimethylcyclopropane-carboxylate with ozone resulted in release of phosgene, trapped in solution as the carbonate (Ref. 23). The interaction of ozone with vinyl halides is well documented (Ref. 24 and 25) yielding epoxides, aldehyde, acyl halides and dihalocarbenes.

Secondary oxidation reactions

The further reactions of photooxidized primary products usually yield complex mixtures of polar materials which are very difficult to isolate and characterize. However, doubly oxidized products have been obtained from resmethrin (Ref. 7) and tetramethrin (Ref. 11) as shown below.

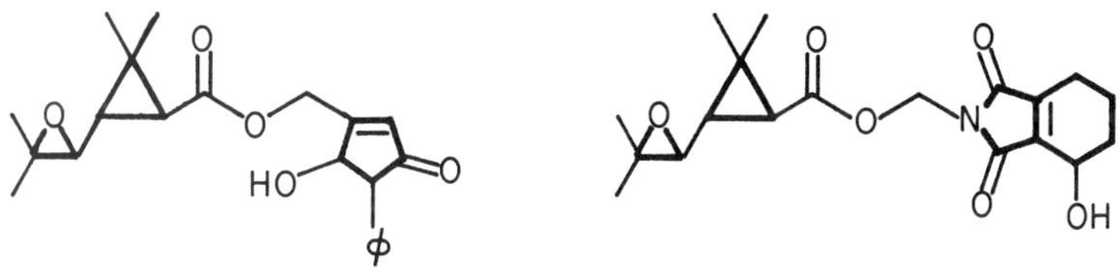

The 3-phenoxybenzyl-, 3-benzoylbenzyl- and 3-phenylbenzyl alcohols obtained from photolysis of the corresponding esters (Ref. 23) are subsequently oxidized to the aldehydes and acids. Likewise,benzyl alcohols from resmethrin and kadethrin are converted to benzaldehyde and benzoic acid (Ref. 7 and 8).

When α-cyano-3-phenoxybenzyl-pyrethroids are irradiated (300 nm) in oxygenated methanol the major ester cleavage products result from reaction of the initial radicals formed with molecular oxygen (Fig. 10) to yield 3-phenoxybenzoyl cyanide which in the presence of nucleophilic solvents yields the ester (MeOH) or acid (H_2O-CH_3CN). In thoroughly degassed solutions the major products from ester cleavage are the dihalovinyl-acid and 3-phenoxybenzyl nitrile. In all cases varying amounts of α-cyano-phenoxybenzyl alcohol are obtained. However, in the presence of oxygen several additional products are detected (Ruzo and Casida, unpublished results).

Compound *A* (R=Me) is only detected at early stages of conversion from the *cis-* but not *trans-* pyrethroids. After longer irradiation periods caronic acid derivatives became significant products. *A* is tentatively characterized by (^{1}H)NMR, CI-MS and FT-IR spectroscopy, and by diazomethane treatment of *A* (R=H) to yield *A* (R=Me).

Several forms of oxygen are now known to effect the degradation of pyrethroids, but the possible role of other oxidizing species, *i.e.* O_2^-, •OH and H_2O_2 is yet to be defined. The mechanism of oxidation and/or oxygenation processes arising during ester cleavage are also important, especially if there exists a correlation with metabolic processes. Furthermore, information is necessary regarding the importance of oxidation reactions in the activation of pyrethroids to toxic compounds.

Acknowledgment - The research carried out at the Pesticide Chemistry and Toxicology Laboratory was funded in part by the National Institute of Environmental Health Sciences (Grant NO. P01 ES00049). Prof. J. E. Casida provided useful suggestions for this report.

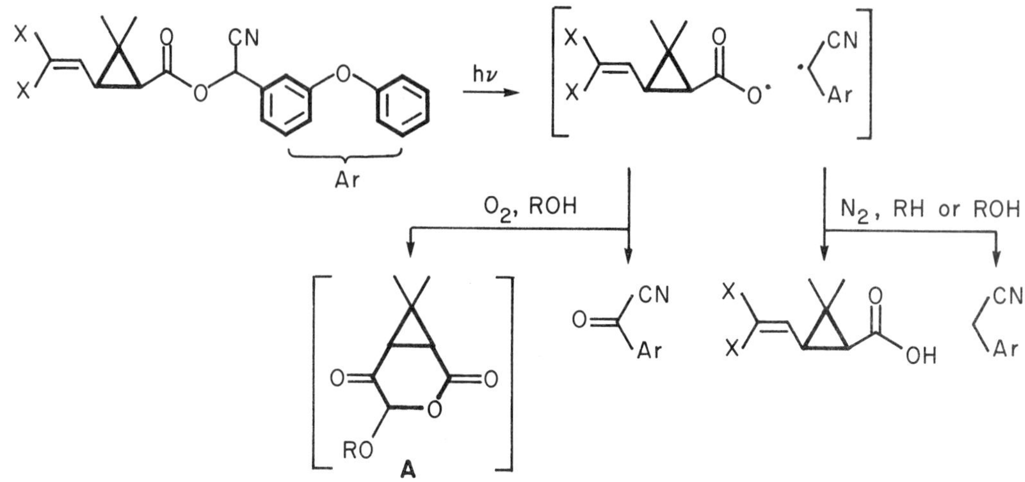

Fig. 10. Ester cleavage and subsequent oxidation of cypermethrin and deltamethrin.

References

1. R. P. Miskus and T. L. Andrews, *J. Agric. Food Chem. 20*, 313-315 (1972).
2. I. Yamamoto and J. E. Casida, *J. Econ. Entomol. 59*, 1542-15 (1966).
3. L. O. Ruzo, Photochemical Reactions of the Synthetic Pyrethroids in *"Progress in Pesticide Biochemistry"*, D. H. Hutson and T. R. Roberts, Eds., Wiley, 1982, in press.
4. A. Campbell and W. Mitchell, *J. Sci. Food Agr. 1*, 137-141 (1950).
5. Y. L. Chen and J. E. Casida, *J. Agric. Food Chem. 17*, 208-215 (1969).
6. T. Sasaki, S. Eguchi and M. Ohno, *J. Org. Chem. 33*, 676-679 (1968).
7. K. Ueda, L. C. Gaughan and J. E. Casida, *J. Agric. Food Chem. 22*, 212-220 (1974).
8. K. Ohsawa and J. E. Casida, *J. Agric. Food Chem. 27*, 1112-1120 (1979).
9. L. O. Ruzo and J. E. Casida, *J. Chem. Soc. Perkin I* 728-732 (1980).
10. L. O. Ruzo, L. C. Gaughan and J. E. Casida, *J. Agric. Food Chem. 28*, 246-249 (1980).
11. L. O. Ruzo, I. H. Smith and J. E. Casida, *J. Agric. Food Chem. 30*, 110-115 (1982).
12. N. Shimizu and P. D. Bartlett, *J. Amer. Chem. Soc. 98*, 4193-4200 (1976).
13. R. W. Murray and A. Suzui, *J. Amer. Chem. Soc. 95*, 3343-3348 (1973).
14. I. H. Smith and J. E. Casida, *Tetrahedron Lett. 22*, 203-206 (1981).
15. M. J. Bullivant and G. Pattenden, *Tetrahedron Lett. 22*, 3679-3680 (1973).
16. E. C. Kimmel, J. E. Casida and L. O. Ruzo, *J. Agric. Food Chem.* in press (1982).
17. R. L. Holmstead, J. E. Casida, L. O. Ruzo and D. G. Fullmer, *J. Agric. Food Chem. 26*, 590-595 (1978).
18. S. A. Kline, J. J. Solomon and B. L. Van Duren, *J. Org. Chem. 43*, 3596-3600 (1978).
19. L. M. Stephenson, *Acc. Chem. Res. 13*, 419-415 (1980).
20. R. G. Zepp, G. L. Baughman and D. F. Schlotzhauer, *Chemosphere 10*, 109-117 (1981).
21. E. Stahl, *Arch. Pharm. 293*, 531-537 (1960).
22. K. Nambu, H. Ohkawa and J. Miyamoto, *Nippon Noyaku Gakkaishi 5*, 177-197 (1980).
23. L. O. Ruzo and J. E. Casida, *J. Agric. Food Chem.* in press (1982).
24. K. Griesbaum and J. Brüggeman, *Adv. in Chem. 112*, 50-65 (1972).
25. T. S. Huh, J. Neumeister and K. Griesbaum, *Canadian J. Chem. 59*, 3188-3191 (1981).

CHARACTERISATION OF THE PRINCIPAL MAMMALIAN TOXICOLOGICAL AND BIOLOGICAL ACTIONS OF SYNTHETIC PYRETHROIDS

Melville H. Litchfield

Imperial Chemical Industries PLC, Central Toxicology Laboratory, Alderley Park, Cheshire, UK

Abstract - Studies have been undertaken with permethrin and cypermethrin to investigate the toxicological and biological actions of synthetic pyrethroids in the rat with particular emphasis on their reversibility and reaction to prolonged administration. Acute and sub-acute studies showed that the principal changes were observed as clinical signs of neurotoxicity at high dose level and by liver hypertrophy. Detailed study showed that both changes were rapidly reversible. Prolonged administration of permethrin in the rat over two years revealed that neither type of change lead to an altered or increased effect. The consequences of these observations to the practical usuage of these compounds is discussed.

INTRODUCTION

Since their more general commercialisation from the mid-nineteen seventies the synthetic pyrethroids have been the subject of an intensive investigation of their toxicological properties, which has resulted in more data being generated within a relatively short time span, about 5 years, than for any other class of compound previously. Some of the data produced by the Companies involved is becoming public knowledge, at least in summary form, by means of the monographs produced from FAO/WHO reviews. Also, publications have appeared in the scientific literature describing investigations into the mode of toxic action.

It is evident from a survey of the available published data that the two principal actions of synthetic pyrethroids in mammals take place in the nervous system and the liver. Whenever a toxic mode of action is described it needs to be put into context regarding the level of effect and its potential to cause more lasting or serious effect. This paper presents the results of a series of evaluations on the toxicological potential of permethrin and cypermethrin in order to deduce the reversibility of the effects and their reaction to the prolonged administration of the two compounds. Permethrin (1) and cypermethrin (2) are representative of the non α-cyano and α-cyano types of synthetic pyrethroid.

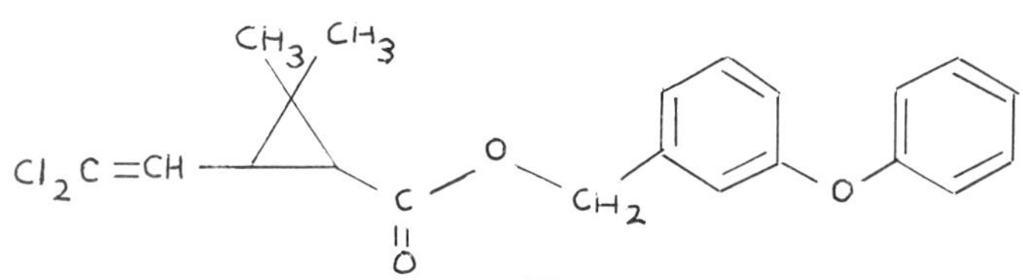

(1)

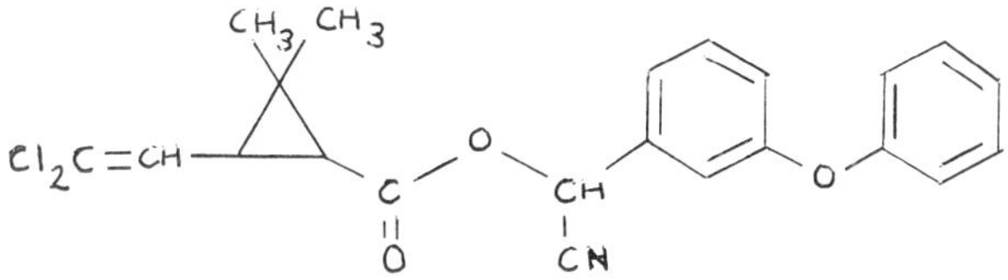

(2)

The isomeric ratio of the two compounds in the studies to be described was 40:60:cis:trans.

TOXICOLOGICAL INVESTIGATIONS

Acute toxicology

The acute oral LD50 of permethrin and cypermethrin has been determined in the rat using a variety of vehicles. Aqueous suspension has usually produced the least toxic results with values of 2000 - 4000mg/kg. Corn oil has been utilised as the more standard vehicle for pyrethroids providing values of about 500mg/kg for permethrin and 250mg/kg for cypermethrin. For both compounds the cis isomer is more toxic than the trans by an order of magnitude.

The clinical symptoms for these two compounds at lethal levels differ somewhat. Permethrin causes whole body tremors of varying degree from slight to convulsive, the latter being accompanied by salivation in some cases. Associated symptoms are hyperactivity and hypersensitivity to external stimuli. A major sign of cypermethrin toxicity is a splayed limb effect with the movement of the limbs being impaired in the more affected animals. Other clinical signs are hypersensitivity to external stimuli, staining of fur in the genital area, piloerection, disorientation and convulsions. A characteristic writhing type sign of toxicity with cypermethrin has been described as choreoathetosis and is the distinguishing feature between the toxic action of the α-cyano pyrethroids such as cypermethrin and the non α-cyano compounds such as permethrin (Barnes & Verschoyle (1) Ray & Cremer (2)).

Subacute and chronic studies

The neurotoxic signs noted in the acute toxicity studies for permethrin and cypermethrin are reflected sub-acutely and have been examined in some detail for the level of effect and their reversibility. Investigations have been made also during subchronic and chronic studies in order to elucidate their reaction to more prolonged administration. Hepatic changes noted in subacute studies similarly have been investigated for reversibility and reaction to longer term administration.

Nervous system changes

The neurotoxic action of both compounds has been studied in specially designed 14-day sub-acute feeding studies in the rat. The animals were fed paired control or high dose level diets and were observed for clinical symptoms daily during the course of the experiment. A gross post-mortem was carried out on all animals found dead or likely to die before the next observation and on all animals surviving at 14 days. The sciatic nerves taken at post-mortem were fixed in buffered formol saline, processed through to paraffin sections and stained with haematoxylin - eosin or with luxol fast blue - cresyl violet and in some cases by Palmgren's silver technique. Nerves selected for electron microscopy were processed through to 1 um Araldite sections. Selected areas were sectioned at 700 - 900 Å, and stained with uranyl acetate and lead citrate.

Permethrin was studied at a series of dose levels from 2500ppm to 7500ppm. Deaths occurred at the higher doses of 5000 and 7500ppm. Clinical signs of effect were seen at all doses and were similar to those described acutely although only mild tremoring was evident in the animals at 2500ppm. However it was notable that at all dose levels, and even on animals surviving 5000ppm for 14 days, that all signs of neurotoxic action had disappeared before the end of the study.

Histopathological and ultrastructural examination of the sciatic nerve was concentrated upon animals at the 2500 and 5000ppm dose levels. Microscopic evidence for an increase in the number of degenerating nerve fibres was seen only in the two rats surviving the full 14 day treatment at 5000ppm. None of the animals dying or killed before 14 days showed an increase in these changes, nor did any of the animals given 2500ppm. A variety of changes were observed ultrastructally in nerves from rats given 5000ppm; these included swelling and increased vesiculation of unmyelinated nerves, hypertrophy of Schwann cells, and fragmentation of myelinated axons. These changes were more marked than in the paired control animals. Nerves from animals receiving 2500ppm in diets for 14 days were comparable to their paired controls and represented the level at which no effect was seen for ultrastructural changes in the sciatic nerve for permethrin.

The dose levels used for cypermethrin were from 1250ppm to 5000ppm. Deaths occurred at the two higher levels of 2500 and 5000ppm. Clinical signs of an effect were seen at all dose levels and were similar to those described acutely. These effects diminished during the course of the study at the two lower levels of 1250 and 2500ppm. The histopathological and ultrastructural examinations were confined mainly to the animals in the 2500ppm group. Microscopic examination indicated that damage to the sciatic nerve was generally either absent or slight and in only one animal was there a marked increase in the number of degenerating nerve fibre fragments. Similarly, only this one rat showed evidence of ultrastructural changes in the form of axonal damage, the remaining animals in this group showing no differences from the paired controls.

Therefore both permethrin and cypermethrin induce only occasional evidence of an effect on peripheral nervous tissue from subacute administration and then only at lethal levels of the compounds.

The effects of both pyrethroids on the nervous system have been evaluated also by more prolonged administration. Cypermethrin was fed to rats over 90 days at dietary levels of 0, 75, 150 or 1500ppm. There were 16 male and 16 female rats per group. At termination a full post mortem was undertaken on all animals. The sciatic nerves were processed through to sections as described for the sub-acute study for histopathological and ultrastructural examinations. No clinical signs of neurotoxicity were seen at any dose level on this study and no changes were observed in the histopathological or ultrastructural examinations.

Permethrin was fed to groups of 60 male and 60 female rats for up to two years at dose levels of 0, 500, 1000 and 2500ppm. An interim kill at one year was undertaken on 12 males and 12 females per group. The sciatic nerves of animals from the interim and final two year kills were examined histopathologically and ultrastructurally following the processing techniques described previously. Clinical observations on all animals on study were made daily.

Tremors and hypersensitivity were noted on animals given 2500ppm during the first two weeks but not seen thereafter. No effects were seen in the sciatic nerves from either microscopic or electron microscopic examination at any dose level. These longer term studies on both compounds demonstrate that the neurotoxic effects seen at high dose level in sub-acute studies are not manifest as more pronounced or delayed effects from prolonged administration at what are still relatively high dose levels.

Hepatic changes

The hepatic changes caused by permethrin and cypermethrin have been evaluated for their reversibility in specially designed studies.

For permethrin, groups of female rats were fed 0 or 2500ppm of compound for 4 weeks. At the end of that period 12 animals from each group were killed for investigation, the remainder being maintained on control diet only, for a further 4 weeks at which time 12 animals from each group were killed for terminal investigations. A gross post-mortem examination was undertaken on all animals killed at each time period. The liver was removed immediately and weighed. A section was taken from the median lobe for electron microscopy. The liver remaining was put into a pot surrounded by ice for enzyme assay.

The pieces of liver taken from the median lobe were fixed in 3% glutaraldehyde in 0.1M phosphate buffer and then post fixed in 1% buffered osmium tetroxide, dehydrated and embedded in 'Araldite' resin. Sections 700 - 900 Å were cut with an LKB ultra-microtome stained with uranyl acetate and lead citrate and examined in an AEI EM6B electron microscope. Quantitation of the smooth endoplasmic reticulum (SER) findings was analysed following the procedure of Weibel and Knight (3).

The liver samples taken for biochemical measurements were analysed for the microsomal enzyme aminopyrine-N-demethylase activity (APDM) and cytochrome P-450 content by the methods of Gilbert and Golberg (4) and the modified method of McLean and Day (5) respectively.

The results of these examinations are shown in Table 1.

TABLE 1. Hepatic assays. Permethrin liver reversibility study

Assay	Liver wt (g)		APDM activity (μ mole AP/h/g)		P450 (n mole/g)		SER	
Dietary Permethrin (ppm)	0	2500	0	2500	0	2500	0	2500
4 weeks	8.6	9.3*	0.03	0.16**	23.5	38.3**	115	159*
4 weeks recovery	9.1	9.0	0.06	0.05	21.8	19.7	133	136

*P <0.05 **P <0.01

After 4 weeks administration at 2500ppm permethrin the 4 indices of liver changes were all increased above control values. After 4 weeks recovery the values in the group previously treated with permethrin had returned to the control levels.

This study showed that permethrin acts similarly to many other compounds which cause liver hypertrophy and microsomal enzyme induction which are readily reversible upon cessation of dosing.

The effect of cypermethrin upon the liver was investigated by a 13 week rat study incorporating a recovery component. Groups of 20 male and 20 female rats were fed diets containing 0 or 1500ppm cypermethrin. After 13 weeks 16 males and 16 females from each group were killed for terminal examination, the remaining animals being retained on control diet for a 4 week recovery period before termination. A gross post-mortem examination was undertaken on all animals killed at each time period. The livers were removed immediately and weighed and then portions were removed and processed as described above for electron microscopic examination and the assay of APDM activity. The results of these examinations are shown in Table 2. The results for females only are shown since the males showed a similar pattern of response.

TABLE 2. Hepatic assays. Cypermethrin liver reversibility study

Assay	Liver wt (g)		APDM activity (μ mole AP/h/g)		SER	
Dietary Cypermethrin (ppm)	0	1500	0	1500	0	1500
13 weeks	9.5	9.4	0.04	0.16**	118	138*
4 weeks recovery	9.3	9.0	0.03	0.04	115	123

*$P < 0.05$ **$P < 0.01$

In contrast to permethrin the administration of cypermethrin at high dose level did not cause an increase in liver weight in the rat. However there were definite increases for APDM activity and SER proliferation. After a 4 week recovery period the microsomal enzyme activity had returned to control value while the SER proliferation had substantially reverted to control value. Thus although the action of cypermethrin is similar in some respects to that of permethrin, it did not appear to cause liver enlargement as such at the dose level studied.

The effect of more prolonged administration of permethrin on the liver changes was studied during the course of a two year rat study. The compound was fed to groups of 60 male and 60 female rats for up to two years with an interim kill at one year on 12 males and 12 females per group. At termination at each of the time periods a gross post-mortem examination was undertaken on all animals, the livers were removed immediately and weighed, portions were removed and processed as described previously for electron microscopic examination and the assay of APDM activity. The results for the female control and highest dose level (2500ppm) are shown in Table 3. The males had a similar pattern of response.

TABLE 3. Hepatic assays. Permethrin two year rat study

Assay	Liver wt (g)		APDM activity (μ mole AP/h/g)		SER	
Dietary Permethrin (ppm)	0	2500	0	2500	0	2500
One year	10.4	11.8	0.04	0.17**	127	172**
Two years	12.8	14.0	0.05	0.16**	101	136*

The first point to note is that the results at one year are remarkably similar to those produced after only 4 weeks administration of permethrin as shown in Table 1. Secondly the results after two years are similar to but rather less than those at one year. Overall there is very little difference in the liver changes produced by permethrin, either over a relatively short period of administration or a more prolonged period. There is no indication that prolonged administration results in any increase in the hepatic effects.

DISCUSSION

Permethrin and cypermethrin as representatives of the non α-cyano and α-cyano- types of synthetic pyrethroids basically produce similar effects in mammals; however there are some differences to be noted. Acutely the clinical signs of neurotoxicity are characterised mainly by tremoring with permethrin and by the writhing or splay-legged action with cypermethrin. In sub-acute and longer term studies at high dose level these signs, if expressed, regress or disappear within two weeks of the commencement of the studies. Examination of the peripheral nerves in these studies at 2, 13, 52 or 104 week intervals show no effects on these tissues by light or electron microscopy.

Subacute and longer term studies cause liver enlargement, increased hepatic microsomal enzyme activity and SER proliferation with permethrin. Cypermethrin does not increase liver weight under these circumstances but does bring about the other changes. This difference in effect may not be significant since cypermethrin being comparatively more toxic than permethrin and therefore studied at comparatively lower dose levels may not be able to express the liver weight increase. It should be emphasised that both compounds anyhow are comparatively mild agents of these liver changes compared with many other compounds which produce these type of changes. Liver enlargement or hypertrophy is a well recognised effect caused by many compounds after shorter or longer term administration (Conney (6), Crampton et al (7), Golberg (8)). It is generally considered to be an adaptive response of no toxicological importance provided it is shown to be readily reversible (Feuer et al (9), Gilbert and Goldberg (4), Crampton et al (7)). This condition has been met by permethrin and cypermethrin and there is no indication to show that their prolonged administration alters the degree or type of response in the liver. Histopathological examination of the liver of the animals from the permethrin two year rat study showed that hypertrophy was the only microscopically observable change due to the compound.

The studies described in this paper have characterised the two main modes of toxicological and biological action of permethrin and cypermethrin in mammals after shorter or longer term administration. Both compounds have a low potency for causing these changes in mammals and this has been reflected by the experience of their safe usage as pesticides world-wide over several years with no significant problems for operator safety.

REFERENCES

1. J.M. Barnes and R.D. Verschoyle, Nature 248, 711 (1974)
2. D.E. Ray and J.E. Cremer, Pestic. Biochem. Physiol. 10, 333-340 (1979)
3. E.R. Weibel and B. Knight, J. Cell Biol. 21, 367 (1964)
4. D. Gilbert and L. Golberg, Fd. Cosmet. Toxicol. 3, 417-432 (1965)
5. A. McClean and P. Day, Biochem. Pharmacol. 23, 1173 (1974)
6. A.H. Conney, Pharmacol. Rev. 19, 317 (1967)
7. R.F. Crampton, T.J.B. Gray, P. Grasso and D.V. Parke, Toxicology 7, 289-306 (1977)
8. L. Golberg, Proc. Eur. Soc. Drug Toxicity 7, 171-184 (1966)
9. G. Feuer, L. Golberg and J. R. LePelley, Fd. Cosmet. Toxicol. 3, 235-249 (1965)

THE FATE AND IMPACT OF PYDRIN® INSECTICIDE (FENVALERATE) ON NON-TARGET SYSTEMS FOLLOWING FIELD APPLICATIONS

W. T. Reed, A. Ehmann, P. W. Lee, G. F. Barber and J. L. Bishop

Shell Development Company, P.O. Box 4248, Modesto, California 95352, USA

Abstract - PYDRIN® Insecticide (fenvalerate) is a broad spectrum synthetic pyrethroid insecticide used on a wide variety of crops. A principal mechanism of decomposition of PYDRIN following field application is through photolytic decomposition. Laboratory studies show the presence of a spectrum of different products, some of which are found following the analysis of PYDRIN treated crop materials. In all cases, the most prevalent photolytic product is the decarboxylated derivative. Evidence to date indicates that the formation of these products represents mechanisms of detoxication. Following the application of PYDRIN to the soil, extensive adsorption prevents significant leaching of the product. Following the application of radiolabeled PYDRIN to a soil column and the subsequent elution with water, little PYDRIN emerged from the column with the majority of the applied radioactivity being recovered in the top 3 cm of the soil. Soil dissipation data indicate the half-life of PYDRIN to be approximately 90 days under outdoor conditions. The degradation of PYDRIN in the soil environment was primarily by microbial action with the principal pathway being cleavage of the ester linkage. In addition, $CONH_2$- and 4-OH-PYDRIN were also detected. Soil metabolites formed did not accumulate to a significant level or present a problem in subsequent rotation crops. These rotation crops consisted of lettuce, beets, and wheat planted at 30, 60, 120-days and 1-year post soil treatment and were harvested at maturity. Finally, although PYDRIN has intrinsically high toxicity to a variety of aquatic organisms, field studies demonstrate that the toxicant is unavailable to the non-target organisms. Therefore, it has little or no impact on this system following the maximum allowed use rate of 2 lb a.i. per acre per year.

INTRODUCTION

Historically, pyrethrins and the early synthetic pyrethroids have had inadequate stability and excessively high manufacturing cost to permit their wide spread use as agricultural chemicals. The discovery of a new generation of synthetic pyrethroids with the metaphenoxybenzyl group as the alcohol moiety has led to a highly useful group of agricultural pesticides that are used at much lower rates than the previously used insecticide classes. One such compound, fenvalerate, was discovered by Sumitomo Chemical Company Ltd (Ref. 1) and is marketed by Sumitomo as Sumicidin, by Shell International Chemical Company as Belmark and by Shell Chemical Company (USA) as PYDRIN® Insecticide. The high insecticidal activity and longer residual life of PYDRIN, coupled with its relative safety to mammals, has been responsible for its becoming an important product for the control of a wide variety of insects on a large spectrum of crops. This wide use spectrum and the longer residual life, however, also raises the question as to the fate and impact of PYDRIN and its breakdown products on non-target organisms and thus its eventual effect on the environment.

It has been suggested that, as a class, the synthetic pyrethroids will not accumulate in wildlife, agricultural animals or humans (Ref. 2). This is because upon ingestion by mammals and birds, rapid degradation occurs by ester cleavage and oxidation with the resultant products possessing functional groups which can be readily conjugated and excreted. However, considering that pyrethrin has a 24 hour LC_{50} of 56 ppb to rainbow trout (Ref. 3), the increased relative stability of the newer synthetic pyrethroids raises the question of their impact on the aquatic ecosystem.

This report deals with the fate of PYDRIN in the environment and its impact on the biological communities with which contact would be anticipated. The principal thrust is to integrate the results of our studies with those of other researchers to describe the processes of PYDRIN decomposition including photolysis under laboratory and field conditions, plus leaching and aerobic and anaerobic microbial degradation in the soil environment. The relative toxicity of the resultant products to several different organisms is examined with particular attention being paid to the aquatic community. This information provides a basis for a qualitative and quantitative assessment of the impact of this pesticide on non-target organisms following its application under actual field conditions.

PHOTOCHEMISTRY

The half life of PYDRIN irradiated at 300 nm was 240 min when dissolved in hexane and 90 min in acetone as determined by GC (FID) and GC-MS. When exposed to natural sunlight in glass culture tubes, PYDRIN was more stable with a half life of 4-5 days in acetone while 80% of the parent in hexane remained after 30 days. By contrast, PYDRIN dissolved in acetone exposed to natural sunlight in quartz had a half life of only 4 hours. When ^{14}C chlorophenyl ring labeled PYDRIN was applied as a thin film to silica gel thin layer plates, exposed to natural sunlight and analyzed by LSC, GC and GC-MS, almost 90% of the initially applied radioactivity was still present at the end of 26 days. Similar studies conducted on soil thin layer plates demonstrated a light-dependent loss of radioactivity following exposure to artificial and natural sunlight amounting to 24% and 35% respectively, after 48 days. The rate of PYDRIN degradation followed pseudo-first order kinetics for the first 12 days with the corresponding half lives of 16 days (artificial light) and 6 days (natural sunlight). In contrast, the half lives of PYDRIN on the dark control soil thin layers were estimated at 53 and 33 days respectively. Essentially all (83-99%) of the applied radioactivity remained on the soil throughout the test.

The relative amounts of the degradation products formed in the solution photolysis studies are summarized in Table 1 with the thin layer photolysis studies being summarized in Table 2. The structural identity of PYDRIN and its metabolites are outlined in Fig. 1. Studies with a single treatment of radiolabeled PYDRIN at 0.25 lb ai/acre to the foliage of cotton, soybeans, tomatoes and sugarbeets plus developing cotton fibers, soybean pods and tomato fruits were conducted under natural sunlight. Here, 65-85% of the initially applied radioactivity was present at harvest (20-35 days later) and 80-95% of the radiolabeled residue was associated with the surface of application. The principal component was PYDRIN (80-95% of the residue) and there was no significant translocation from treated foliage to other parts of the plant. The average residues present consisted of compound 1, 4.5%; compound 4, 1.5%; compound 11, 2.4%; compound 6, 1.2%; compound 7, 1.0%, and compound 15, 1.1% in terms of the applied dose.

TABLE 1. PYDRIN solution photolysis

Compound	Artificial Sun (300 nm) for 5 hours		Natural Sunlight in Glass		Natural Sunlight in Quartz for 4 hours
	Acetone (%)	Hexane (%)	Acetone (5 days) (%)	Hexane (30 days) (%)	Acetone (%)
PYDRIN	3.4	48.2	38	82	64
Compound 1	49.0	28.1	40	9	17
Compound 2	14.9	6.3	13	6	6
Compound 3	12.6	4.6	1	0.3	6
Compound 4	8.3	3.0	6	2	5
Compound 5	2.7	1.3	...	...	...
Compound 6	2.2	2.4	...	...	...
Compound 7	2.0	1.1	2	0.5	1.5
Compound 8	1.4	0.8	...	...	...
Compound 9	0.5	0.5	...	...	...

TABLE 2. PYDRIN thin layer photolysis.

Compound	Silica Gel 26 days Exposure	Soil - 24 days Exposure Artificial Sun	Natural Sun	Dark
PYDRIN	68.6	41.4	18	72.3
Compound 1	19.1	0.2	0.8	...
Compound 6	3.1	.1	.4	...
Compound 7	2.1	...	...	...
Compound 10	...	5.8	7.8	6.1
Compound 11	...	4.3	5.1	...
Compound 12	...	2.6	1.5	1.8
Compound 13	...	1.5	2.7	...

It is apparent from an examination of these data and those of other workers (Ref. 4, 5, 6 and 7) that the photolysis of PYDRIN varies widely, both qualitatively and quantitatively, depending upon the conditions of the trial. The principal photodegradant, compound 1 (the decarboxylated material), is common throughout all studies. Some of the reported materials such as compounds 10, 11, and 12 may not even be photoproducts. If they are, they are also formed by other processes in addition to photolysis.

An effort was made to determine the relative stability of the most important PYDRIN photoproducts. Following irradiation for 5 hours at 300 nm, compound 1 demonstrated 1.8% decomposition; compound 4, 7.9%; compound 6, 97.6%; and compound 7, 6.5%. From these data, it was apparent that at least 3 of the PYDRIN photoproducts are more stable than PYDRIN itself.

Because of the wide variation in results from photolysis studies depending upon the conditions of the test, it was felt that accurate projections as to their presence in PYDRIN treated crops would be impractical. In order to properly determine the extent of their presence, crops where the highest residue was anticipated were sprayed with commercial application equipment at the maximum rate allowed on Shell's proposed label. Each crop was grown in the regions of the U. S. where the commercial production is most prevalent. Upon harvest, samples were frozen and sent to Shell's Biological Sciences Research Center for analysis by GC and HPLC. Data from typical crops are indicated in Table 3. From this, it is apparent that under actual use conditions, photoproducts are found only at very low levels. On food crops that are directly consumed by humans, only compound 1 has been found and that always below 0.1 ppm on the whole, unprocessed, agricultural commodity. The highest level of photoproducts found in these field studies was for animal feed crops such as alfalfa or field corn stover where essentially no growth dilution took place subsequent to treatment and where field drying of the crop occurred prior to harvest. Even here, the residue for all of the photoproducts combined have not exceeded 2 ppm.

SOIL DEGRADATION

In order to determine the leaching properties of PYDRIN in the soil environment, various soils were examined by column chromatography. Soils with an organic matter ranging from 0.23 to 2.0% and clay content from 7.0 to 32.4% were used. Radiolabeled PYDRIN was applied to the surface followed by elution with 50 cm of water. The combined aqueous effluents from each of the soil columns contained less than 3% of the initially applied radioactivity. Approximately 90% to 95% of the applied radiation was recovered in the first 3 cm of soil with the remainder principally occurring in the next 3 cm. Trace amounts were found up to 15 cm but no further. In a second leaching study, ^{14}C-labeled

PYDRIN was incubated aerobically for 30 days in Hanford sandy loam soil. Elution followed by the daily application of 1.3 cm water for 45 days. Approximately 92% of the applied radioactivity was recovered in the top 3 cm, with 6% in the remaining 27 cm of the soil column and 1% in the combined aqueous effluents.

This apparent lack of soil mobility was verified by soil thin-layer chromatography. By comparing with reference standards of known soil mobility (trichloroacetic acid, 2,4-D, DDT and atrazine), it was found that PYDRIN was immobile in all soils tested.

PYDRIN

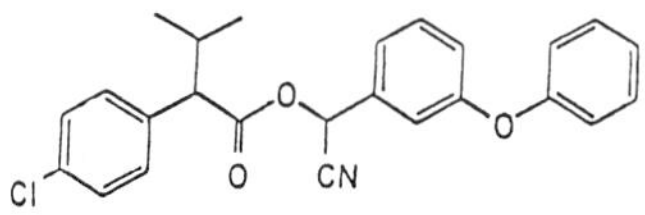

COMPOUND 1

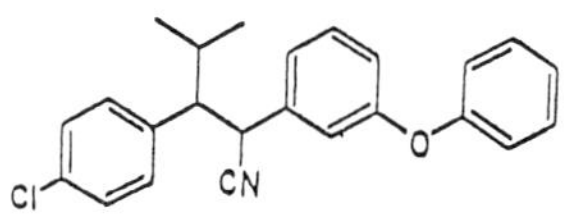

COMPOUND 2

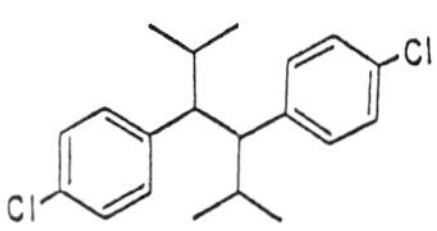

COMPOUND 3

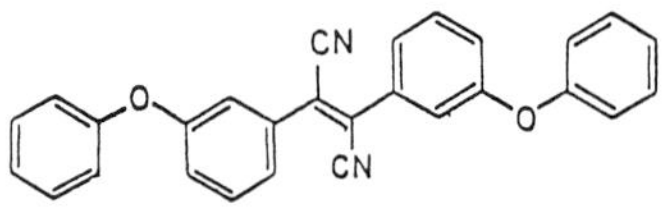

COMPOUND 4

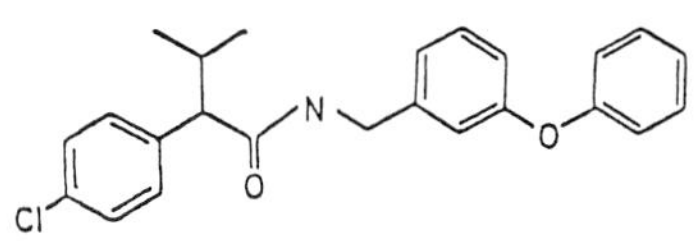

COMPOUND 5

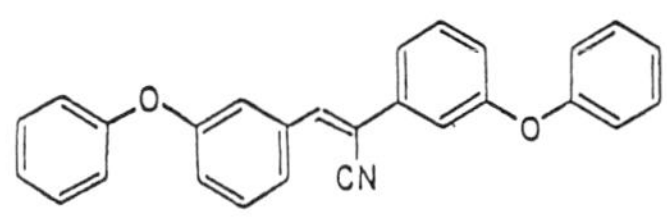

COMPOUND 6

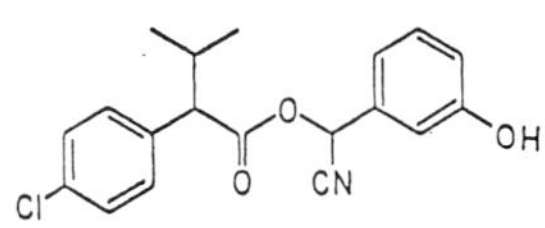

COMPOUND 7

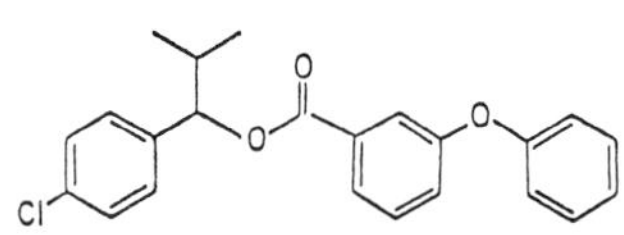

COMPOUND 8

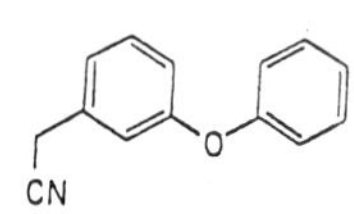

COMPOUND 9

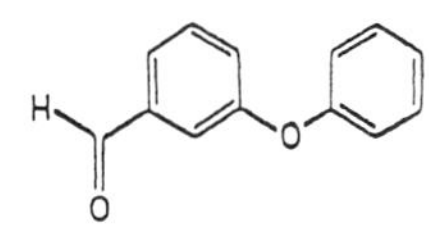

COMPOUND 10

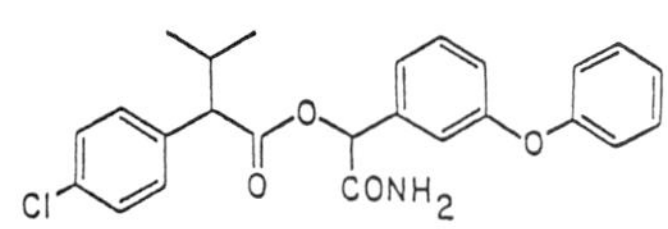

COMPOUND 11

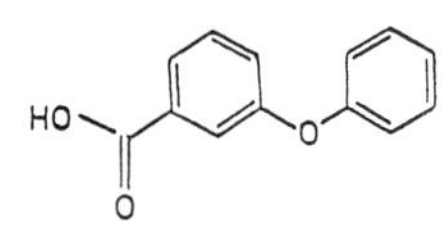

COMPOUND 12

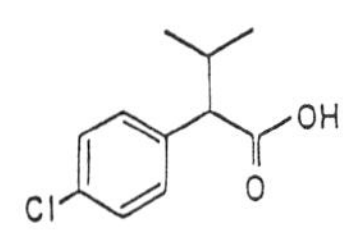

COMPOUND 13

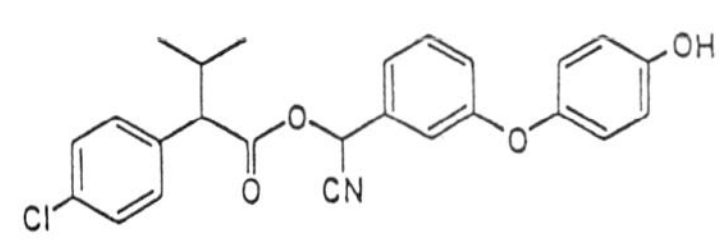

COMPOUND 14

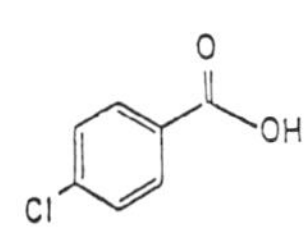

COMPOUND 15

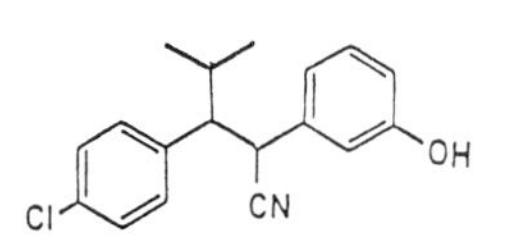

Figure 1. Structures of PYDRIN® Insecticide and its degradation products.

Laboratory aerobic and anaerobic soil degradations studies were conducted using ^{14}C-chlorophenyl-PYDRIN. Three different test soils were used (a sandy loam, silty loam and a silty clay loam). In all test soils, there was no meaningful qualitative and quantitative difference in the rate and the pattern of degradation between aerobic and anaerobic conditions. Approximately 50, 55 and 78% of the applied ^{14}C-PYDRIN was recovered unchanged after 90 days aerobic incubation from the sandy loam, silty loam and silty clay loam soil respectively. The major degradation pathways in the soil were the cleavage of the ester linkage leading to the formation of 4-chloro-α-(1-methyl-ethyl)-benzeneacetic acid (compound 12), the hydration of the CN-moiety to $CONH_2$ (compound 10), and the 4′-hydroxylation of the phenoxy-moiety of the parent PYDRIN molecule (compound 13). Further degradation of these metabolites was shown by the generation of $^{14}CO_2$ (equivalent to 50% of the applied radioactivity over the 12-month period) and a significant amount of the applied radioactivity (25%) was recovered as methanol unextractable soil bound residues (Fig. 2). Further, aqueous extraction of the soil bound residues resulted in the release of compound 12 as the major radiolabeled product. Under anaerobic conditions, compound 12 was also the major degradation product recovered in the water saturated fraction. Approximately 17% of the applied ^{14}C-PYDRIN was recovered unchanged in the sandy loam, 12% in the silty loam and 52% in the silty clay loam soil at the end of the 12-month period.

TABLE 3. PYDRIN and photoproduct residues following commercial applications of PYDRIN to crops under field conditions.

Crop	Number of Application	Rate (lb ai/acre)	Preharvest Interval (days)	Residues Detected (ppm) PYDRIN	Comp. 1	Comp. 7	Comp. 10	Comp. 4	Comp. 6
Field corn stover	5	0.2	23	12	0.64	0.09	0.13	0.13	0.04
Alfalfa	1	0.2	14	12	0.61	0.05	0.02	<0.02	<0.02
Apples	7	0.4	21	1.1	<0.02	<0.02	<0.02	<0.02	<0.02
Dry apple Pomace	7	0.4	21	10	0.56	0.04	nd	nd	nd
Pears	4	0.4	28	0.6	0.06	<0.02	<0.02	<0.02	<0.02
Pear peels	4	0.4	28	0.6	0.07	<0.02	nd	nd	nd
Peaches	5	0.4	14	2.6	0.02	<0.02	<0.02	<0.02	<0.02
Tomatoes	10	0.4	7	1.5	<0.02	<0.02	nd	nd	nd
Celery	15	0.2	1	3.1	0.05	<0.02	nd	nd	nd

nd - not determined

A soil metabolism study using sterilized sandy loam soil indicated that the degradation of PYDRIN in soil was predominantly because of microbial activity.

A rotation crop study in Hanford sandy loam soil was conducted outdoors using both ^{14}C-chlorophenyl and ^{14}C-phenoxyphenyl-PYDRIN. The initial concentration of PYDRIN in the soil sample was 0.25 ppm. Lettuce, beets, and wheat planted at 30, 60, 120-days and 1-year after soil treatment were harvested at various growing stages and at maturity and were analyzed for total ^{14}C-residues, parent and metabolites. Soil samples were analyzed similarly.

In the soil samples, a rapid dissipation of the applied ^{14}C-PYDRIN was observed. At the 120-day planting time, approximately 27% of the initial applied PYDRIN was recovered. In addition to undegraded PYDRIN, compound 13 and compound 10 were detected as soil degradation products for both ^{14}C-chlorophenyl and ^{14}C-phenoxyphenyl labeled PYDRIN. Compound 12 was detected as the major soil degradation product in the ^{14}C-chlorophenyl-PYDRIN treated soil. A trace amount of ^{14}C-chlorophenyl and ^{14}C-phenoxyphenyl-PYDRIN equivalent radioactivity was recovered as unextractable soil bound residues.

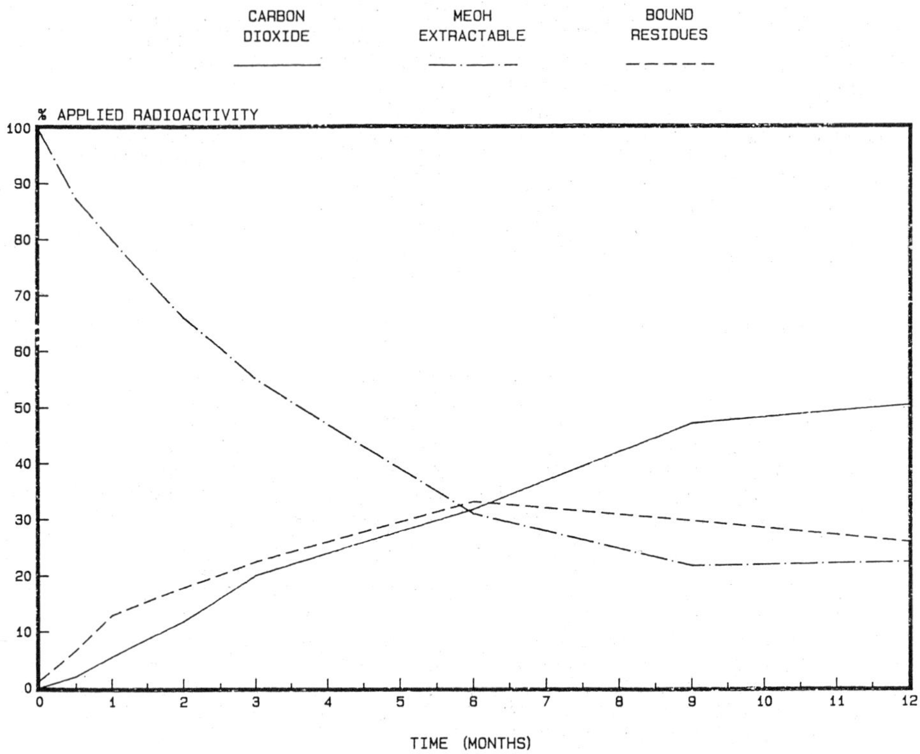

Figure 2. Degradation of ^{14}C PYDRIN in Soil

Analysis of the total residue in plant tissues indicated a low level of ^{14}C-residues (0.01-0.03 ppm) in the lettuce, beet and wheat samples. Approximately 0.06 ppm of ^{14}C-chlorophenyl-PYDRIN equivalent residue was detected in the wheat straw. Analysis of the 60-day wheat straw sample demonstrated that the majority of the ^{14}C-chlorophenyl-PYDRIN residue was the water-soluble conjugate of compound 12. Approximately 30% of the recovered radioactivity in the wheat straw was associated with the unextractable cellulose fraction. Trace levels of ^{14}C-phenoxyphenyl- PYDRIN equivalent residues (<0.01 ppm) were observed in all plant tissues throughout this study.

Results obtained from this study show that PYDRIN was relatively non-persistent in the soil environment. The rate of decomposition was somewhat slower than some studies (Ref. 8) although the products were the same with the exception that we did not detect any of the ether cleavage compound. We saw little difference between aerobic and anaerobic metabolic rate, however, in all cases the degradation in the soil was microbial. Differences in the degradation rate from one soil to another are not unexpected as variation in the soil environment have produced wide variations in pyrethroid stability (Ref. 9).

The soil immobility observed was consistent with other studies with surface applied fenvalerate remaining in the top few cm of soil (Ref. 10). In addition, these studies and others (Ref. 11) demonstrated that no meaningful residues of PYDRIN or its metabolites occur in rotation crops planted in PYDRIN treated soil.

TOXICITY OF PYDRIN PRODUCTS

The housefly toxicity of PYDRIN and its degradation products were determined by spraying 4 day old, mixed sex houseflies (NAIDM strain) with the product dissolved in No. 10 base oil. The toxicity was expressed as Toxicity Indices (TI) which equaled LC_{50} parathion x $100/LC_{50}$ toxicant. In this test, PYDRIN had a TI = 138, compound 13 had a TI = 51 and compounds 1, 4, 6, 7, 9, 10, 11, 12 and 14 had TI's = 0. Mouse IP LD_{50}'s demonstrated PYDRIN and compounds 1, 11 and 12 to be all greater than 500 mg/kg (Ref. 5). These limited data indicate that the degradation products are less toxic than PYDRIN except for 2 photolysis products of the alcohol moiety (Ref. 5) which were reported to be more toxic to mice than PYDRIN. We did not detect either of these in our studies. Because of this low toxicity, coupled with their low concentration in crop materials, it was felt that the PYDRIN degradation products did not constitute a hazard.

ENVIRONMENTAL IMPACT

PYDRIN's relatively low toxicity to mammals (acute oral LD_{50}, rats = 451 mg/kg) and birds (acute oral LD_{50}, pheasant, mallard duck and partridge >2,000 mg/kg) coupled with the lack of any long term effects in these animals, indicates that no adverse terrestrial ecological effects would be expected. Of greater potential concern, however, is the aquatic environment. Rainbow trout have demonstrated a 24 hr LC_{50} of 76.0 ppb for the technical product and 21 ppb for formulated material (Ref. 12) indicating that PYDRIN is intrinsically quite toxic to fish. PYDRIN is also intrinsically toxic to aquatic invertebrates, demonstrating a 96 hr LC_{50} of 0.14 ng/ml for lobster and a 0.04 ng/ml for shrimp (Ref. 13). In an effort to predict the impact of fenvalerate on the aquatic community, aquatic model ecosystem studies were conducted (Ref. 14). Here, the (S)-acid isomer of fenvalerate was compared to DDT. When carp were held in static water containing approximately 0.8 ppb toxicant, S,RS-fenvalerate residues were taken up more slowly and were eliminated more quickly (T 1/2 = 5 days) than DDT (hardly eliminated) when placed in clear water. S,RS-fenvalerate had bioaccumulation ratios from 69 to 117 in fish depending upon the location of the ^{14}C label. The bioaccumulation ratios for DDT and its degradation products were from 10 to 20 times greater. As fenvalerate did not tend to accumulate in fish, snails, daphnids or algae, it seems that the adverse impact that might have been inferred from the acute toxicity may not be as serious as anticipated following the direct application of fenvalerate to the aquatic environment.

To further assess the impact of fenvalerate on the estuarine environment, studies were conducted on laboratory and field colonized benthic communities exposed to this toxicant (Ref. 15). The effect of fenvalerate on laboratory-colonized communities was determined by comparing numbers and species of estuarine animals that grew from planktonic larvae in aquaria treated with fenvalerate for 8 weeks with those that grow in untreated aquaria. The effect of fenvalerate on benthic animal communities collected in the field was determined by placing sand-filled aquaria in the Santa Rosa Sound to be colonized by naturally occurring animals for approximately 8 weeks. The established communities were brought into the laboratory and exposed to 0.1, 1.0 and 10.0 ng/ml fenvalerate for 1 week. The abundance of living animals in contaminated and control aquaria was compared. In both field and laboratory-derived colonies, the community structure was altered significantly. In the laboratory-derived colonies, the number of species did not decrease but the abundance of organisms was reduced. In the field-derived colonies, the reverse was true. While the majority of the organisms were different between the two types of tests, it was concluded that low concentrations of fenvalerate could adversely impact the benthic communities.

These data suggest that if PYDRIN comes in contact with a variety of aquatic organisms, some are likely to be adversely affected. Data presented earlier on the leaching and soil adsorption of PYDRIN demonstrated that PYDRIN was bound tightly to soil particles and did not show a propensity to move. This indicates that the potential detrimental effect of PYDRIN on the aquatic ecosystem may be mitigated by the compound being prevented from reaching the organisms under proper use conditions. Because of the importance of this issue, it was felt that studies involving actual field trials in a potentially hazardous situation were warranted. It was believed that only in this manner could the impact of PYDRIN on the aquatic ecosystem be properly evaluated.

An aquatic ecological effect study following the aerial application of PYDRIN was conducted by EG&G, Bionomics under contract by Shell Development Company. A site was selected in the cotton growing region of northern Louisiana consisting of a treatment pond and a control pond several miles apart. The treatment pond bordered on a 65 hectare cotton field that was aerially sprayed 10 times with 0.2 lb ai/acre PYDRIN, the maximum amount of product allowed to be applied to a given piece of ground during a single season. This field drained into a pond rich in aquatic organisms (Fig. 3) permitting an intensive evaluation of both the qualitative and quantitative effects of a large PYDRIN treatment area draining into a relatively small aquatic ecosystem. To insure that exposure took place, mylar drift cards were placed strategically during the first, second and last pesticide application. Runoff from the cotton field into the pond was monitored. Appropriate samples were obtained before and after application for biological and chemical analysis. These samples consisted of benthic macroinvertebrates, zooplankton, water, sediment, and fish (both caged and wild). Observations are being made over a 1 year period following the first application. While the trial is not yet complete, some preliminary data indicate some distinct trends.

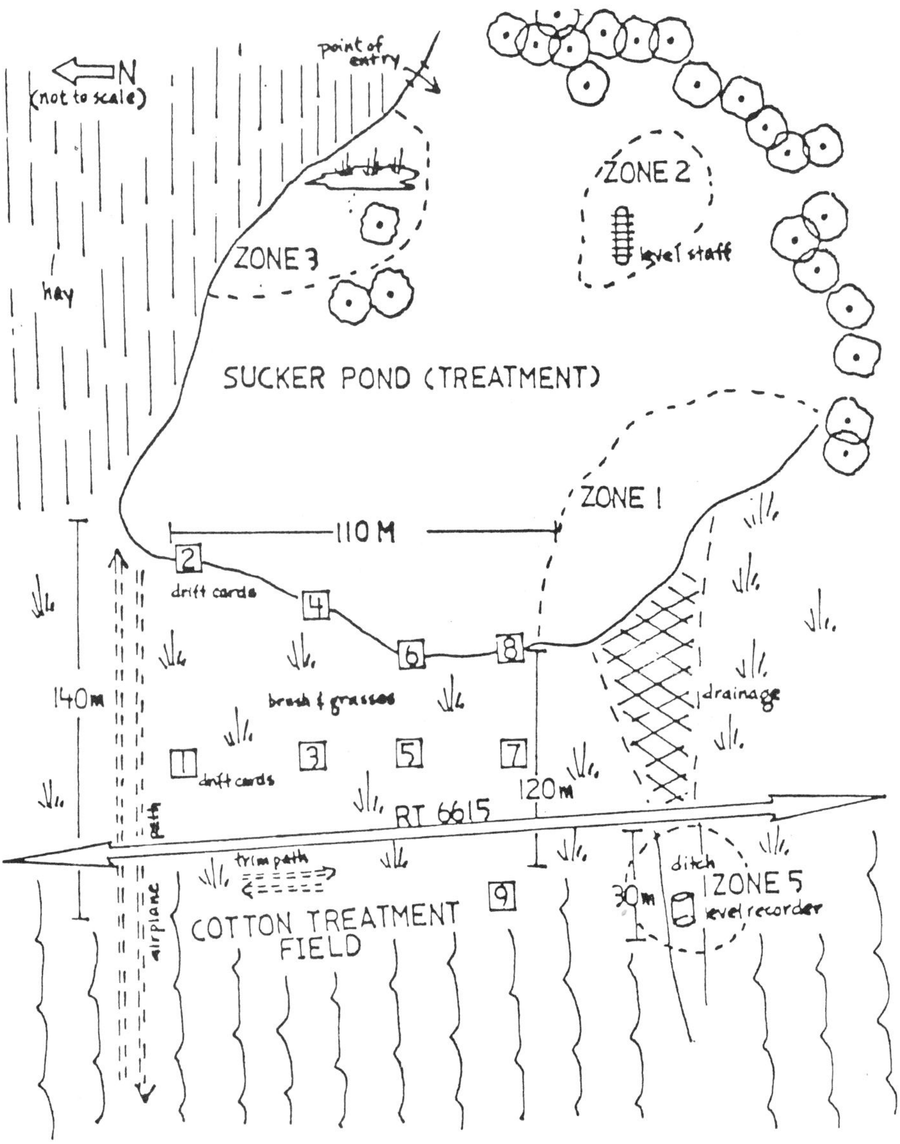

Figure 3. Diagram of treatment pond location illustrating relationship between primary sampling zones 1, 2 & 3 and the impacted zone 5 and position of drift cards during monitoring.

Residue analyses indicated that PYDRIN reached the aquatic environment by both drift and through runoff. By far, the greatest PYDRIN concentration in the water was recorded at zone 5 which was directly in the spray pattern. In this area, a significant portion of the macroinvertebrate community present was visibly stressed or moribund following PYDRIN applications. However, a partial recovery of the community present in this habitat had occurred after 3 weeks. At the other sampling sites, aquatic organisms remained abundant throughout the test and population fluctuations did not appear to be compound related. Final conclusions will be drawn at the completion of the test.

CONCLUSIONS

It is apparent from these studies that the effects of PYDRIN on non-target systems have been well investigated. The compound is degraded by photolysis as well as aerobic and anaerobic soil microorganisms. Data to date indicate that the products formed are less toxic than PYDRIN itself. While PYDRIN is intrinsically toxic to several aquatic organisms, it appears that the impact of the compound under proper use conditions is minimal. This is because the pesticide is rapidly made unavailable to those organisms along with simultaneous decomposition to less hazardous products.

REFERENCES

1. J. Hattori, Japan Pest. Info 33, 13-19 (1977).
2. J. D. Leahey, Outlook Agri. 10, 135-142 (1979).
3. O. Cope, Pesticide Widelife Studies, U.S. Dept. of Int., Fish and Wildl. Serv., Circ. 199 (1963).
4. R. L. Holmstead and D. G. Fullmer, J. Agric. Food Chem. 25, 56-58 (1977).
5. R. L. Holmstead, D. G. Fullmer and L. O. Ruzo, J. Agric. Food Chem. 26, 954-959 (1978).
6. H. Ohkawa, K. Nambu and J. Miyamoto, J. Pesticide Sci. 5, 215-223 (1980).
7. N. Mikami, N. Takahashi, K. Hayashi and J. Miyamoto, J. Pesticide Sci. 5, 225-236 (1980).
8. H. Ohkawa, K. Nambu, H. Inui and J. Miyamoto, J. Pesticide Sci. 3, 129-141 (1978)
9. I. H. Williams and M. J. Brown, J. Agric. Food Chem. 27, 130-132 (1979).
10. B. D. Hill, J. Agric. Food Chem. 29, 107-110 (1981).
11. R. A. Chapman and C. R. Harris, J. Environ. Sci. Health B16(5), 605-615 (1981).
12. J. R. Coats and N. L. O'Donnell-Jeffrey, Bull. Environm. Contam. Toxicol. 23, 250-255 (1979).
13. D. W. McLeese, C. D. Metcalfe and V. Zitko, Bull. Environm. Contam. Toxicol. 25, 950-955 (1980).
14. H. Ohkawa, R. Kikuchi and J. Miyamoto, J. Pesticide Sci. 5, 11-22 (1980).
15. M. E. Tagatz and J. M. Ivey, Bull. Environm. Contam. Toxicol. 27, 256-267 (1981).

NEW APPLICATIONS OF PYRETHROID INSECTICIDES

Yoshio Katsuda, Hajime Hirobe and Yoshihiro Minamite

Research Laboratory, Dainihon Jochugiku Co. Ltd., Toyonaka, Osaka 561, Japan

Abstract - Two new practical applications of pyrethroid insecticides are described. The pyrethrins/CD insecticides have been developed by including natural pyrethrins in β-cyclodextrin. The inclusion significantly improves the stability of pyrethrins in air, light and mineral dust without reducing the innate insecticidal activities. In Japan, dust and wettable powder formulations of the pyrethrins/CD complexes have been registered for agricultural use on teas, ornamental plants and rice plants. Field tests showed that Pyrethrins CD WP was more effective for control of tea leaf rollers than the non-included pyrethrins w.p. formulation, particularly with regard to their residual activity. The use of a dust formulation of the pyrethrins/CD complexes has been found to be practical from an economic standpoint when used in combination with carbaryl, showing excellent efficacy against the organophosphorus- and carbamate-resistant strains as well as the susceptible strains of green rice leafhoppers and planthoppers. Synthetic pyrethroids, such as d-phenothrin and permethrin, have been recognized as excellent insecticides for pest control use because of their rapid knockdown effect, low mammalian toxicity and sufficient residual activity. The ULV spraying, which has been mainly limited to outdoor use, can be applied indoors by utilizing recently developed water-based emulsifiable concentrates of pyrethroid insecticides. Such formulations have greatly decreased fire hazards, providing the most promising ULV techniques to control sanitary pests such as houseflies and cockroaches. The particles, when sprayed in ULV mists under practical conditions, were under 20μ, most of them being 1.5μ in diameter. In field tests, the ULV treatments with d-phenothrin and permethrin at a rate of $40mg/m^3$ and $20\text{-}30mg/m^3$ respectively gave rapid flushing effect and later satisfactory kill, reducing the number of resident cockroaches over a period of 60 days.

INTRODUCTION

Recent significant development in pyrethroid insecticides has led to various useful compounds and the field of application is expanding from indoor to outdoor use. Yet, few reports are available on research of formulations and application methods.

Pyrethrum, a natural insecticide, has been largely used for sanitary pest control by virtue of such excellent features as rapid knockdown effect, wide spectrum of insecticidal activity, low mammalian toxicity and efficacy against resistant insects. On the other hand, instability in air and light has limited its use as an agricultural insecticide. In order to overcome this disadvantage, we have investigated stabilized formulations of pyrethroids by preparing β-CD inclusion compounds (1,2,3). The practical applications of pyrethrins/CD insecticides are described.

Surface treatment with organophosphorus insecticides has been commonly used indoors to control crawling insects. Checks for the toxicants, however, have become necessary because of widespread resistance to these compounds and in view of safety hazards to operators. After learning that surface treatment alone would not always provide satisfactory pest control, we have taken notice of the needs for ULV treatment with pyrethroid insecticides, particularly in the cases where residual treatment is found to be troublesome in enclosed facilities such as restaurants, warehouses, and transport vehicles. Thus, water-based emulsifiable concentrates of d-phenothrin and permethrin have been developed. This paper describes the established indoor ULV techniques.

PYRETHRINS/CD INSECTICIDES FOR AGRICULTURAL APPLICATIONS

Pyrethrins/CD compounds

The β-cyclodextrin molecule (4) is a cyclic D-glucose polymer consisting of seven anhydroglucose units joined by α-1,4-glucosidic linkages. It is derived from the breakdown of starch or dextrin by the action of cyclodextrin glycosyl transferase of *Bacillus macerans*, *Bacillus* No.38-2 and recently the alkaliphilic *Bacillus* No.38-2 (5,6). Inclusion compounds are prepared when a molar excess of the complexants with a hydrophobic group are added to an aqueous solution of β-CD. The pyrethrins/CD possesses the following characteristics:

1. High stability in air and light
2. Applicability in powdery formulations
3. Retention of the innate properties of natural pyrethrins.

Since 1974, w.p. and dust formulations containing pyrethrins/CD have been tested in the field and have proved to have practical pest control efficacy against several agricultural pests. Pyrethrins CD 5% WP and Pyrethrins CDN Dust containing 0.1% pyrethrins plus 2% carbaryl have been put into practical use.

Pyrethrins CD 5% WP

Pyrethrins CD 5% WP has been registered for use against pests such as tea leaf rollers, yellow tea thrips and fall worms on tea and ornamental plants, which must be treated with non-hazardous insecticides. Particularly, insecticides for use in tea cultivation are limited in number from the standpoint of residue and effect on tea flavor.

Tea leaf roller control. Many insects are known as pests on tea plants and among them, the tea leaf roller has caused the most serious damage to green tea production in Japan. The larvae of this insect emerge mainly from May through July and roll the tea leaves, which are filled with their feces. This spoils the flavor and color of the tea, resulting in a grade reduction. Therefore, the control of this insect before leaf rolling is essential for successful tea production. The best time for effective application of insecticides is at the emergence of a new brood, 7-12 days after the time of peak adult populations. Although organophosphorus insecticides such as chlorfenvinphos and methidathion have been conventionally used for the tea leaf roller control, the following disadvantages in practical use have become serious in recent years: the use of organophosphorus insecticides is prohibited for a period of 14-20 days before the day of gathering tea leaves, and these compounds are ineffective in controlling any new brood which emerges a few days after the application because of their insufficient residual activity. Pyrethrins CD WP as well as cartap has proved to be one of the effective control measures; the withholding period has been shortened to 10 days and residual potency has improved. In the field test shown in Table 1, Pyrethrins CD WP provided excellent control efficacy, which is superior to that of chlorfenvinphos emulsifiable concentrate.

TABLE 1. Effect of Pyrethrins CD WP to tea leaf rollers, Mie Agri. Tech. Center, Tea Branch

Insecticide	A.I. (g/ha)	Number of rolled leaves	Withholding period before harvest (days)
Pyrethrins CD 5% WP	150	1.7	10
Chlorfenvinphos EC	720	4.7	20
Untreated	—	187.7	—

Recently, the simultaneous control of tea leaf rollers and yellow tea thrips, another major pest to tea plants, has become important as the demand to reduce the frequency of insecticide applications grows in view of environmental problems. The control potency of cartap to yellow tea thrips has been on the decline, although this compound is used effectively as a tea leaf roller larvicide. Pyrethrins CD WP which possesses high control efficacy against both pests is a promising candidate for this purpose. The combination of the pyrethrins/CD with another type of insecticides is under investigation in order to obtain still more satisfactory control.

Pyrethrins CDN Dust

Insecticides for the protection of rice plants have been applied commonly in dust formulations in Japan. Although formulations of natural pyrethrins as dusts were previously unsatisfactory, the β-CD inclusion has provided stabilized dust formulations, making them applicable to paddy fields. The registered Pyrethrins CDN Dust containing 0.1% pyrethrins plus 2% carbaryl is an effective insecticide in the control of organophosphorus- and carbamate-resistant strains as well as the susceptible strains of green rice leafhoppers and planthoppers.

Green rice leafhopper control. The green rice leafhopper causes serious damage to rice plants not only by sucking the juice but also by transmitting dwarf virus and yellow dwarf mycoplasma. In western Japan, this insect has developed a resistance to organophosphorus and carbamate insecticides. Pyrethrins/CD (3), as well as free pyrethrins, has been reported to have high insecticidal activity against resistant strains of this insect. Free pyrethrins are unsuccessful in green rice leafhopper control because of their rapid decomposition in the field. On the other hand, as shown in Fig. 1, pyrethrins/CD was sufficiently stable to maintain effectiveness against this insect in the field.

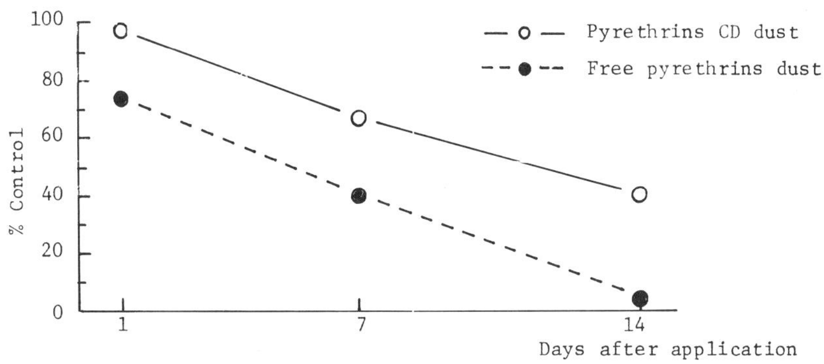

Fig. 1. Residual activity of pyrethrins/CD and free pyrethrins against green rice leafhoppers, Kagawa Agri. Exp. Stn.

The use of a dust formulation of pyrethrins/CD has been found to be practical from an economic standpoint when used in combination with carbaryl, showing excellent control efficacy against green rice leafhoppers. In the field tests shown in Table 2, Pyrethrins CDN Dust and some other common insecticides were applied and checks were made on the first and fifth day after application. The Pyrethrins CDN Dust treatments reduced the leafhopper populations rapidly, which is one of the excellent properties of pyrethroid insecticides, and thereafter provided higher residual effectiveness than other insecticides.

TABLE 2. Effect of Pyrethrins CDN Dust to green rice leafhoppers, Ehime Agri. Exp. Stn.

Insecticide	Active ingredient	Number of insects before appli.	One day after appli.		5 days after appli.	
			Number of surviving insects	Corrected* density index	Number of surviving insects	Corrected* density index
Pyrethrins CDN Dust	Pyrethrins 0.1% Carbaryl 2.0%	194	33	19	20	10
Diazinon Dust	Diazinon 3.0%	586	446	86	179	30
Carbaryl Dust	Carbaryl 2.0%	550	503	103	173	31
Untreated	——	187	166	100	191	100

*Corrected density index = Ta/Tb x Cb/Ca x 100

Cb = Number of insects in untreated plot before application
Ca = Number of insects in untreated plot after application
Tb = Number of insects in treated plot before application
Ta = Number of insects in treated plot after application

INDOOR ULV APPLICATIONS OF d-PHENOTHRIN AND PERMETHRIN

Unique formulations for ULV treatment

The ULV method (7) is based on breaking a liquid insecticide concentrate down into small droplets with a limited range of size from 1 to 20μ, and has been useful in field treatments because of a dramatic reduction in spraying rate. However, some requirements must be fulfilled before this technique can be expanded to indoor applications. They are as follows:

1. Active ingredients
   a. Must be safe to operators who are exposed to a mist of high concentrates.
   b. Must have rapid insecticidal activity and efficacy against organophosphorus- and carbamate-resistant strains of insects.

2. Formulations
   a. Must be nonflammable, because ULV mist remains airborne for a considerable length of time.
   b. Should prevent property damage and offensive odors.
3. Particle size
   Must be well controlled by ULV applicators for penetrating into cracks and crevices and impinging upon insects effectively.

Therefore, d-phenothrin and permethrin, which are sufficiently stable, were chosen as active ingredients. Effectiveness of these pyrethroid insecticides to resistant strains of houseflies is shown in Table 3.

TABLE 3. LD_{50} values of 4 insecticides to the various colonies of the houseflies by topical application method

Colony name	LD_{50} Value (μg/fly) Insecticide			
	Propoxur	Fenitrothion	d-Phenothrin	Permethrin
Wakayama	51.0 (300)	41.5 (1297)	0.059 (1.2)	0.034 (0.9)
Shiga(I)	38.0 (223)	42.3 (1322)	0.034 (0.7)	0.034 (0.9)
Shiga(II)	27.5 (162)	6.4 (200)	0.038 (0.8)	0.028 (0.8)
Hyogo	11.3 (66)	1.5 (47)	0.039 (0.8)	0.037 (1.0)
Takatsuki (Susceptible)	0.17 (1.0)	0.032 (1.0)	0.048 (1.0)	0.036 (1.0)

( ) : Resistance ratio

Recently developed water-based emulsifiable concentrates are composed of pyrethroid insecticide which is stable in water, emulsifier and deionized water. The new formulations have been proved to be outstanding in controlling crawling and flying insects, while reducing fire hazards greatly by not using organic solvent, and were registered in 1981 as unique insecticides for ULV treatment in Japan. Improvements of ULV applicators have been also made, taking into account particle size, noise and other factors.

ULV tests of 10% d-phenothrin and 5% permethrin water-based emulsifiable concentrates

ULV tests of new formulations were conducted in cockroach control using SUPER JET U-1, one of the ULV applicators. The application rates followed the label directions as below.

TABLE 4. Recommended spraying rates under practical conditions

Formulation	Spray volume (ml) per m^3	per m^2 (2.5m high)
10% d-Phenothrin water-based EC	0.4	1.0
2 times dilution (1:1)	0.8	2.0
4 " " (1:3)	1.6	4.0
5% Permethrin water-based EC	0.4-0.6	1.0-1.5
2 times dilution (1:1)	0.8-1.2	2.0-3.0
4 " " (1:3)	1.6-2.4	4.0-6.0

Flushing out. Cockroaches are flushed out and then move around more actively when treated with pyrethroids, but not with organophosphorus insecticides. This flushing-out action provides the following excellent advantages with regard to control efficacy:

1. Increases the opportunities for contact with the toxicant and gives better kill.
2. Indicates the hiding places of cockroaches, thus making it easier to use supplemental residual treatments.

Insecticide deposit rates and sites. The insecticide deposit rates and sites in ULV application, when sprayed in an area with $22m^2$ of floor space and 2.5m high ceiling, are illustrated in Fig. 2. The rates were determined by periodically analyzing the deposits on the sheets placed on the floor, one of the walls and the ceiling. The results indicate that most droplets settled on the floor in 3 hours. During a 6 hour period, the floor received 76% of the total dosages applied and the wall 1.6%. No insecticide was detected on the ceiling. Therefore, residual treatment of the walls in advance provides more effective control of cockroaches which are flushed out and creep up the walls.

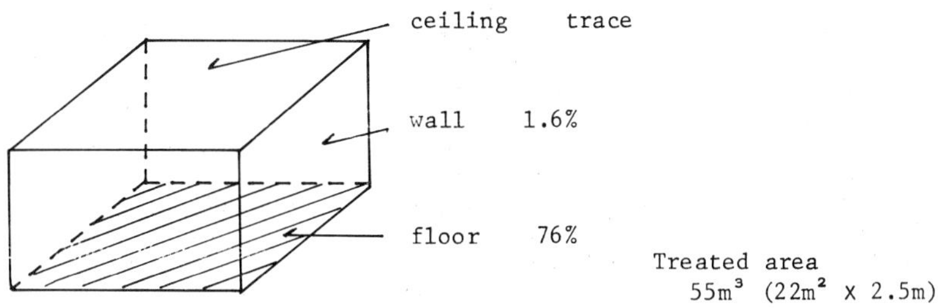

Fig. 2. Insecticide deposit rates of total dosages 6 hours after application of d-phenothrin at a rate of $40mg/m^3$.

Areal concentrations of active ingredients. Model tests were carried out in a glass chamber with a volume of $8m^3$. A ULV formulation was sprayed into the chamber and the mist was drawn through a trap apparatus by suction. The aerial concentrations of active ingredients were determined at a given time elapsed by analyzing the mist trapped with benzene. The highest concentrations of d-phenothrin and permethrin were recorded immediately after application, being $17.7\text{-}20.5mg/m^3$ and $11.2\text{-}17.1mg/m^3$, respectively. After half an hour, the rates declined to $2\text{-}6mg/m^3$ and were under $1mg/m^3$ after 3 hours.

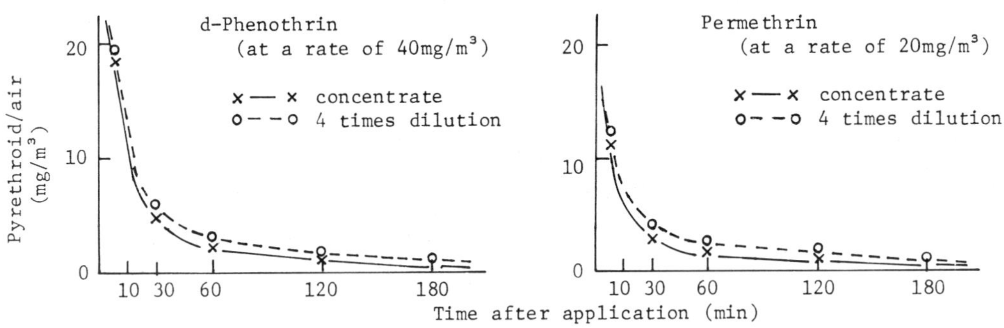

Fig. 3. Changes in aerial concentration of pyrethroids

The aerial concentrations reached in practical applications seem to be harmless, because our experimental results for acute inhalation toxicity indicated the non-toxic level of each pyrethroid is more than 20 times above the practical level. The dramatically shortened spraying time in ULV treatments is also one of the favorable factors for safety to the operators. For example, it requires only a few minutes to treat an area with a volume of $70m^3$ using the concentrates. Moreover, as can be seen in Fig. 2 and 3, the treated area should be closed for at least 3 hours, 6 hours preferably.

Droplet size. Droplet size can be measured in a variety of ways. Although lazer holography (8,9) has been reported as the most promising method, we used the modified settling method described by Mount (10) because of its convenience and simplicity. Glass slides coated with a silicone film were placed 60cm above the floor in the same chamber. The d-phenothrin concentrate and its 4 times dilution were applied at a rate of $40mg/m^3$. For permethrin, the application rate was $20mg/m^3$. Droplets of ULV mist were collected on the slides for microscopic examination. We measured the flattened droplet sizes by means of microphotography, and airborne particle diameters were determined according to Gessner's equations (11).

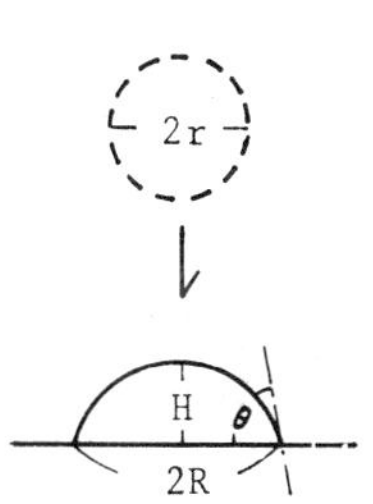

$$r = \sqrt[3]{H(3R^2 + H^2)/8} \quad (1)$$

$$\tan(\theta/2) = H/R \quad (\theta < 90°) \quad (2)$$

H: plano-convex height

2R: plano-convex width

2r: airborne particle diameter

θ : contact angle of droplet

Fig. 4. Gessner's equation

The distribution curves of particle size collected immediately after application are illustrated in Fig. 5. The particles were under 20μ under practical conditions and most of them were 1.5μ in diameter.

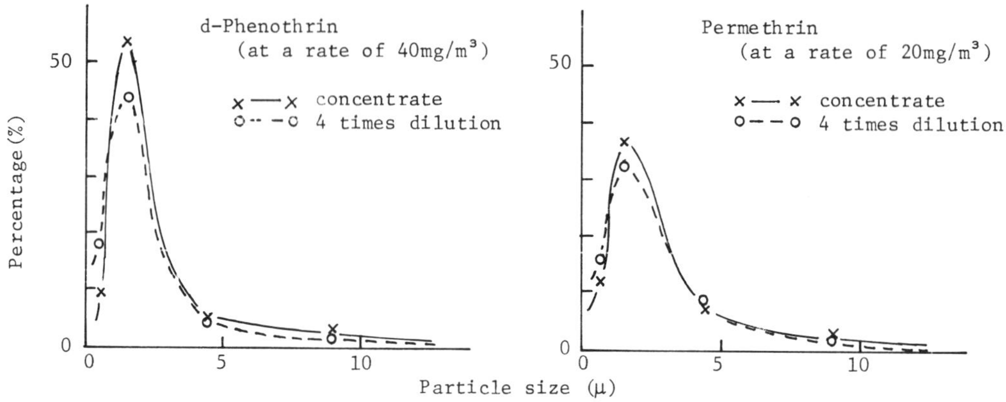

Fig. 5. Distribution curve of particle size immediately after application

Field tests for cockroach control

In field tests, d-phenothrin and permethrin were applied at a rate of 40mg/m³ and 20-30mg/m³, respectively. The change in the number of cockroaches before and after application was examined using trapping boxes in the area. All ULV treatments gave rapid flushing effects and satisfactory kills, and then reduced resident cockroaches over a period of 60 days. Therefore, ULV application of d-phenothrin and permethrin has been revealed to be highly effective in controlling sanitary pests such as cockroaches, together with reducing the application rates and shortening the time required.

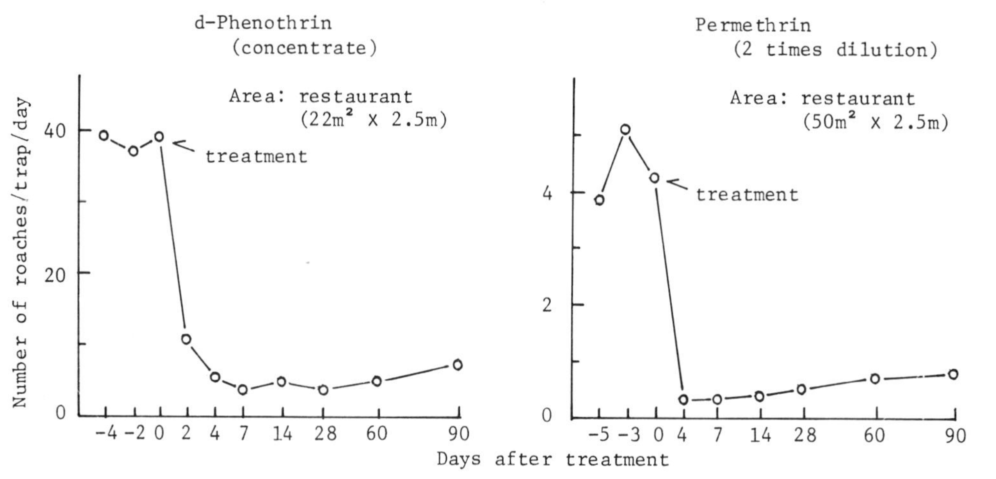

Fig. 6. Changes in the number of cockroaches by ULV treatment

The procedures of ULV treatment for satisfactory control are summarized in the following:

1. Open cupboards, drawers and lockers, and close ventilation fans and windows tightly.
2. Treat walls with residual insecticides beforehand.
3. Conduct ULV spraying, starting from the corner of the room and then moving toward the entrance. After completing the treatment, close off the room immediately.
4. Close the area for 3-6 hours or overnight preferably.

CONCLUSIONS

Two novel modes of application of pyrethroids, namely, the agricultural application of pyrethrins/CD inclusion compounds and the indoor ULV application with the water-based emulsifiable concentrates of d-phenothrin and permethrin, have proved to be effective in practice for pest control. We are sure that the pyrethroid insecticides will become much more promising by development of more effective application measures as well as inventions of new pyrethroids.

REFERENCES

1. I. Yamamoto, T. Unai, Y. Suzuki and Y. Katsuda, J. Pesticide Sci. 1, 41 (1976).
2. I. Yamamoto, K. Ohsawa and F.W. Plapp, Jr., J. Pesticide Sci. 2, 41 (1977).
3. I. Yamamoto and Y. Katsuda, Pestic. Sci. 11, 134 (1980).
4. D. French, Adv. Carbohydr. Chem. 12, 189 (1957).
5. N. Nakamura and K. Horikoshi, Agric. Biol. Chem. 40, 753 (1976).
6. N. Nakamura and K. Horikoshi, Staerke 27, 410 (1975).
7. R.C. Moore, J. Econ. Entomol. 70, 86 (1977).
8. C.B. Rathburn, Jr., Mosq. News 30, 501 (1970).
9. R.B. Roberts, R. L. Lyon, M. Page and R.P. Miskus, J. Econ. Entomol. 64, 533 (1971).
10. G.A. Mount and N.W. Pierce, Mosq. News 32, 586 (1972)
11. V.H. Gessner and L. Primavesi, Kolloid-Zeitschrift und Zeitschrift Polymere 182(1-2), 140 (1962).

NEW PYRETHROID INSECTICIDES FOR INDOOR APPLICATIONS

Tadahiro Matsunaga, Kiyofumi Yoshida, Goro Shinjo, Shigenori Tsuda, Yoshitoshi Okuno and Hirosuke Yoshioka

Pesticide Research, Institute for Biological Science, Sumitomo Chemical Co. Ltd., Takarazuka, Hyogo 665, Japan

Abstract The potencies of two novel pyrethroid stereoisomers, *d*-prallethrin and *d*-cyphenothrin, were evaluated for development in indoor applications under several test methods for control of housefly, mosquito and cockroach. *d*-Prallethrin, a propargyl analog of allethrin, generally showed a twice or more the knockdown and killing activities of *d*-allethrin against the pest insects, and *d*-cyphenothrin showed more than twice the killing activity of permethrin against cockroach. Both of them revealed an outstanding flushing-out activity against cockroach. The insecticidal potencies in practical formulations are also described in detail as associated with their physical and chemical properties.

INTRODUCTION

Extensive and continuing studies on the structure modification of natural pyrethrins which had been initiated by LaForge *et al.* (1, 2, 3) have resulted in a number of useful synthetic pyrethroids such as allethrin. Among them, the modifications from allethrin were of major trend in the past. It had been reported by Gersdorff *et al.* (4) that an analog of allethrin containing a propargyl group in place of the allyl group in the ketoalcohol moiety had a 0.6 times the lethal activity of allethrin against housefly. Katsuda (5) had also reported, as named propargylrethrin, a 1.2 times the toxicity over that seen for allethrin but further study had not been made for long on the analog mainly due to extremely limited availability by synthesis up till recent years, that now has become apparently improved by the work of Matsuo *et al.* (6).

On the other hand, cyphenothrin had been disclosed by Matsuo (7) as a most potent killing agent among synthetic pyrethroids of the chrysanthemate structure. Although cyphenothrin did not appear to be adequately persistent in agricultural fields, its potency for control of indoor pest insects has not been assessed yet from a practical point of view.

Both of the chrysanthemates can be supplied as stereoisomer mixtures consisting of *d*-*trans*, *cis* forms. Then, we now have conducted thorough reinvestigations on the analog of allethrin which we named *d*-prallethrin as a proposed common name for (*RS*)-2-methyl-3-(2-propynyl)-4-oxocyclopent-2-enyl (1*R*)-*cis*, *trans*-chrysanthemate (8) as knockdown agent, and on *d*-cyphenothrin or (*RS*)-α-cyano-3-phenoxybenzyl (1*R*)-*cis*, *trans*-chrysanthemate (9) as killing agent, and they have also been assessed in a variety of mixed formulations for most efficient control of major flying and crawling insects.

RESULTS AND DISCUSSION

Chemical and physical properties of d-prallethrin and d-cyphenothrin

The studies were made on each technical grade of *d*-prallethrin and *d*-cyphenothrin (90.1 % and 93.6 % purity respectively). The data are compiled in Table 1, 2 and Fig. 1.

Table 1. Physical and chemical properties of d-prallethrin.

Items	Properties
Chemical name	(RS)-2-methyl-3-(2-propynyl)-4-oxocyclopent-2-enyl (1R)-*cis*,*trans*-chrysanthemate
Structure	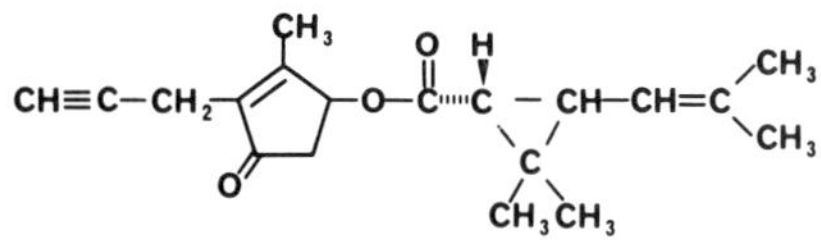
Empirical formula	$C_{19}H_{24}O_3$
Molecular weight	300.38
Appearance	Yellowish liquid
Specific gravity	d_{25}^{25} 1.021
Viscosity	284.2 cP at 30 °c
Vapor pressure*	9.97×10^{-5} mm Hg at 30 °c

*cf. d-allethrin: 1.25×10^{-4} mm Hg at 30 °c

Table 2. Physical and chemical properties of d-cyphenothrin.

Items	Properties
Chemical name	(RS)-α-cyano-3-phenoxybenzyl (1R)-*cis*, *trans*-chrysanthemate
Structure	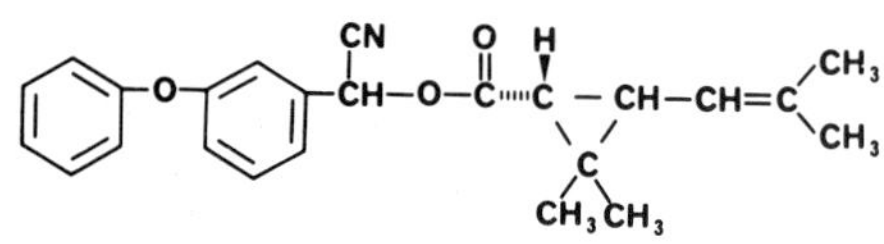
Empirical formula	$C_{24}H_{25}O_3N$
Molecular weight	375.45
Appearance	Yellowish viscous liquid
Specific gravity	d_{25}^{25} 1.083
Viscosity	808.8 cP at 30 °c
Vapor pressure	3.11×10^{-6} mm Hg at 30 °c

In addition, they were miscible with most of organic solvents but scarecely soluble in water (d-prallethrin : 2-3 ppm, d-cyphenothrin : 0.01-0.1 ppm at 25 °c), and they were stable in dry or wet air (60 °c, 6 months) and in most of organic solvents exept for lower alkanols (40 °c, 6 months) and in water-based aerosol (pH 4-5, 40 °c, 9 months). Therefore, they can be well compatible with a wide variety of practical formulations. The vapor pressure of d-prallethrin was very close to that of d-allethrin as determined by GLC method, and thus d-prallethrin appeared to be essentially applicable to the existing fumigation system for d-allethrin.

Fig. 1 shows the degradation of d-prallethrin and d-cyphenothrin under the light (0.35-2.7 μ) on the forced condition (5000 to 7000 lux at the level of irradiated specimens). The half life period of d-prallethrin was 2 to 3 days, which was similar to that of d-allethrin. d-Cyphenothrin showed a longer half life period of 2 weeks, but it was still less persistent than permethrin and was expected to be suitably residual on indoor applications.

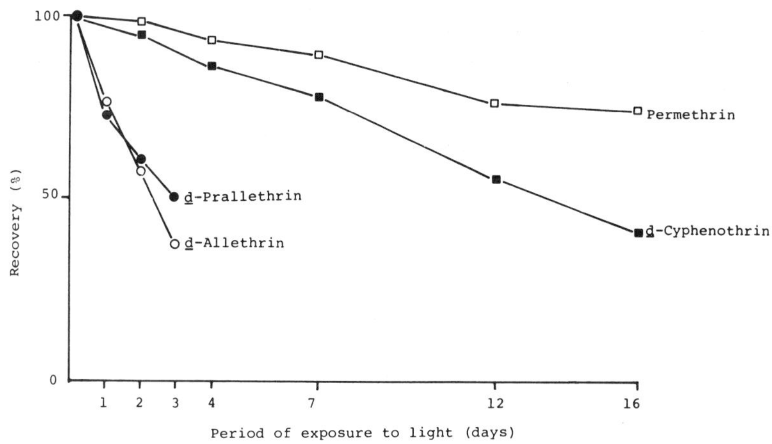

Fig. 1. Photostability of d-prallethrin and d-cyphenothrin in comparison with d-allethrin and permethrin.

Insecticidal activity of d-prallethrin and d-cyphenothrin against housefly, mosquito and cockroach

(i) d-prallethrin

d-Prallethrin was primarily characterized as knockdown agent by the KT50 values in Table 3, in which it was generally more than twice as effective as d-allethrin against housefly and mosquito, although it exhibited an excellent lethal activity against cockroach that was 2 to 4 times higher than that of d-allethrin and was equivalent to that of permethrin (see Table 4). Besides, d-prallethrin had a more than twice the lethal activity of d-allethrin against mosquito, and a 1.5 times the lethal activity of d-allethrin against housefly (Table 3) that was virtually concordant with the Katsuda's data already referred.

(ii) d-cyphenothrin

As shown in Table 3 and 4, d-cyphenothrin was most distinguished in the overall killing activities against the major nuisance insects. In particular, it had a twice the activity of permethrin against cockroach and was superior to propoxur and equivalent with fenitrothion.

Flushing-out activity against cockroach

Chadwick (11) and Shinjo *et al.* (12) recently introduced in detail the flushing-out effect on indoor application of pyrethroid insecticides against cockroach. d-Cyphenothrin and d-prallethrin were most dominated in the flushing-out effect over the rest of the conventional insecticides including the specific isomers of allethrin (Table 4). The flushing-out effect has a crucial importance in cockroach control since it can drive the hidden cockroaches out of their shelters and get them promptly exposed to the highly lethal pyrethroid mists or residues. In Table 4, the organophosphorus and carbamate insecticides did not show any flushing-out effect, which was in good concordance with the result by Ebert (13) indicating a poor control of cockroaches remaining in the shelter.

Thus, d-cyphenothrin and d-prallethrin can formulate a number of new and highly efficient recipes for cockroach control jointly with many of conventional insecticides.

Table 3. Insecticidal activity of d-prallethrin and d-cyphenothrin against housefly and mosquito in comparison with other pyrethroids for indoor fields.

Insecticide	LD50 (μg/insect): Topical application method		KT50 (min.): Glass chamber method (oil spray)(10)			
	Musca domestica	*Culex pipiens*	*Musca domestica*		*Culex pipiens*	
	Female	Female	0.05%	0.1%	0.05%	0.1%
d-Prallethrin	0.143	0.0143	1.3	0.9	1.5	1.1
d-Allethrin[a)]	0.220	0.0365	2.5	1.4	4.2	3.1
d-trans-(S)-[b)] Allethrin	0.121	0.0183	1.5	1.1	2.6	1.6
Pyrethrins	0.780	0.0229	4.2	2.0	5.3	2.9
d-Cyphenothrin	0.0141	0.00493	5.8	4.5	7.8	6.2
Permethrin	0.0133	0.00801	>10	10.2	9.2	7.4

a) (RS)-2-Methyl-3-(2-propenyl)-4-oxocyclopent-2-enyl (1R)-cis, trans-chrysanthemate
b) (S)-2-Methyl-3-(2-propenyl)-4-oxocyclopent-2-enyl (1R)-trans-chrysanthemate

Table 4. Insecticidal activity of d-prallethrin and d-cyphenothrin against cockroach (Blattella germanica) in comparison with other conventional insecticides.

Insecticide	LD50 (μg/insect): Topical application method		FT50 (min.)-%Mortality[a)]	
	Male	Female	0.25%	0.5%
d-Prallethrin	0.32	0.87	3.8-45	2.3- 90
d-Allethrin	1.40	2.20	8.7-22	5.0- 52
d-trans-(S)-Allethrin	0.76	1.50	4.9-46	3.1- 77
Pyrethrins	0.70	1.10	4.6-48	3.0- 79
d-Cyphenothrin	0.19	0.40	2.9-98	2.4-100
Permethrin	0.48	0.80	4.6-76	3.5-100
Fenitrothion	0.21	0.25	-	>10.0-(0)[b)]
Dichlorvos	0.18	0.28	-	>10.0-(6)
Propoxur	0.27	1.10	-	>10.0-(3)

a) Shinjo's method (10), Dosage: 4.2 ml of oil spray / 0.34 m^3.
FT50: Time required for 50 % of cockroaches flushed-out from a plywood shelter.
b) % Mortality in the shelter.

Evaluation of d-prallethrin for specific indoor applications

(i) Mosquito coil

d-Prallethrin and d-allethrin were impregnated in a supporting media designated as mosquito coil for assessment of their potencies against mosquito and housefly under the fumigation. As shown in Fig. 2, d-prallethrin exhibited about 2 times the knockdown activity of d-allethrin. Furthermore, the activity ratio of d-prallethrin, which was demonstrated on the test in a glass chamber (0.34 m^3), was retained on the test in a large chamber (28 m^3) as shown in Table 5, and was as active as d-trans-(S)-allethrin. d-Prallethrin was stable (40 °c, 3 months) in common supporting materials used for mosquito coil formulations.

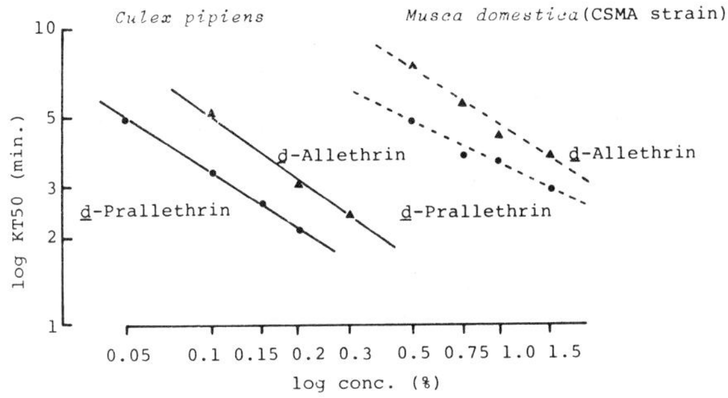

Fig. 2. Knockdown activity of mosquito coils containing d-prallethrin and d-allethrin against mosquito and housefly by the fixed amount smoking method (0.5 g / 0.34 m^3) (14).

Table 5. Knockdown activity of mosquito coils containing d-prallethrin, d-allethrin and d-trans-(S)-allethrin against mosquito (Culex pipiens) by the modified MacIver method (15) in a large chamber (28 m^3).

Insecticide:	d-Prallethrin			d-Allethrin	d-trans-(S)-Allethrin
Conc. (%) :	0.1	0.2	0.3	0.4	0.2
KT50 (min.):	24.8	16.9	14.0	21.0	20.0

(ii) Mosquito mat

Referring to the results of the mosquito coil fumigation, the test mat that contained d-prallethrin was compared with the d-allethrin mat of a doubled dosage regarding the efficacy to mosquito and housefly. As shown in Table 6, the efficacy of mosquito mat which contained 20 mg of d-prallethrin exhibited an equivalent performance to that containing 40 mg of d-allethrin. As illustrated in Fig. 3, the mosquito mats that contained d-prallethrin showed a very similar cumulative vaporization ratio to that seen for the d-allethrin mats of the doubled dosages on a conventional electric vaporizer designed for allethrin.

The results indicate that d-prallethrin is twice as active as d-allethrin on the current fumigation device. The thermal decomposition of the active ingredient could be minimized by addition of a suitable phenolic antioxidant.

Table 6. Knockdown activity of mosquito mats containing d-prallethrin and d-allethrin against mosquito and housefly by the glass chamber test method (0.34 m^3) (14).

Insecticide	Mg in mat[a)]	Preheating time 15 min.	2hr.	4hr.	6hr.	8hr.
				KT50(min.): Culex pipiens		
d-Prallethrin	20mg	3.7	3.4	3.7	3.7	3.7
d-Allethrin	40mg	5.7	4.2	4.1	3.8	3.8
				KT50(min.): Musca domestica		
d-Prallethrin	20mg	13.0	15.0	11.0	12.0	12.0
d-Allethrin	40mg	13.0	15.0	14.0	12.0	11.0

a) Examined mosquito mats were heated on a conventional electric vaporizer.

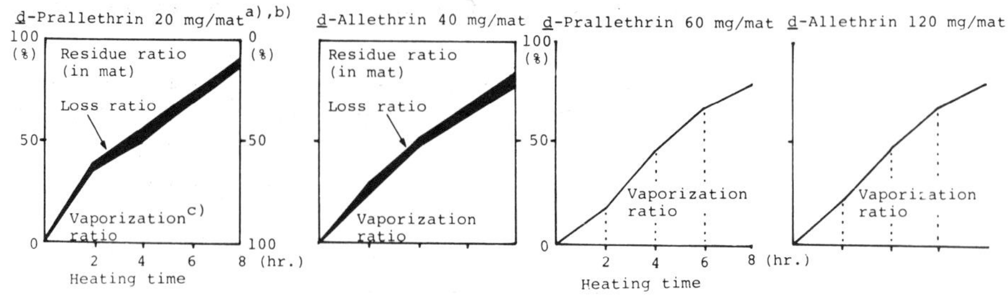

a) Mat (Woodpulp, 2.2 cm long and 3.5 cm broad): Thickness was 2.8 mm for d-prallethrin 20 mg and d-allethrin 40 mg mat, and 1.1 mm for d-prallethrin 60 mg and d-allethrin 120 mg mat.

b) Recipes in mat: Each test mat was prepared by adding the indicated amount of corresponding insecticide with a certain antioxidant and solvent.

c) Cumulative value.

Fig. 3. Vaporization of d-prallethrin and d-allethrin from mosquito mats on a conventional electric vaporizer.

(iii) Aerosol for flying insects

The aerosol formulation which contains pyrethroid insecticides generally consists of a knockdown agent and a killing agent (or a synergist). The water-based aerosols which contained d-prallethrin or d-allethrin as a knockdown agent and d-phenothrin or (RS)-3-phenoxybenzyl (1R)-cis, trans-chrysanthemate as a killing agent were prepared for the assessment. It is obvious in Fig. 4 that d-prallethrin also demonstrated in aerosol formulation the better performance than d-allethrin against housefly and mosquito at any mixing ratio with d-phenothrin.

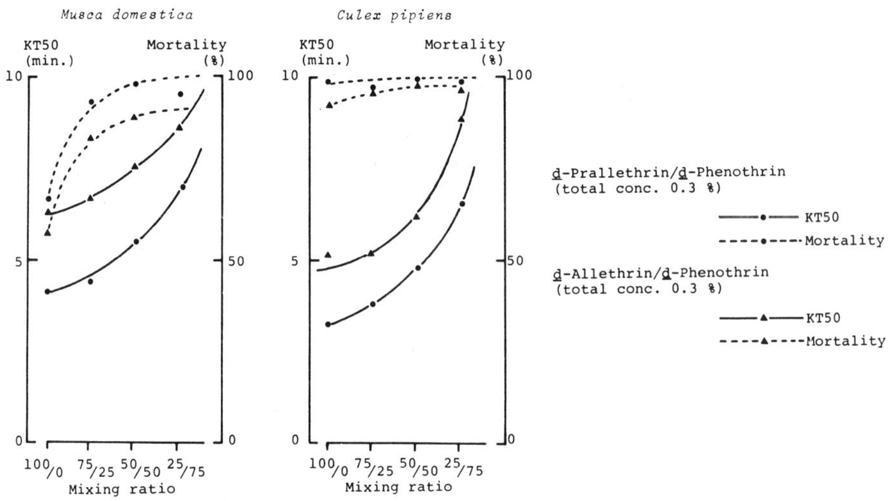

Fig. 4. Insecticidal activity of water-based aerosols containing d-prallethrin and d-phenothrin against housefly and mosquito in comparison with d-allethrin formulations by CSMA aerosol test method (16).

Evaluation of d-cyphenothrin for specific indoor applications

d-Cyphenothrin showed in Table 7 a lasting control of cockroach under the residual contact method using an EC formulation, in which d-cyphenothrin as well as permethrin demonstrated a complete control for longer period than that seen for fenitrothion. Moreover, it is also noteworthy in Table 7 that d-cyphenothrin had a notable knockdown effect to cockroach in comparison to permethrin. In addition, d-cyphenothrin appeared to be promising as a space fumigant evaporated from the specific fumigation device whose feature is given in Table 8.

Table 7. Insecticidal activity of emulsion formulations containing d-cyphenothrin against cockroach (Blattella germanica) in comparison with other insecticides.

Emulsifiable concentrate	Direct spray[a)]		Residual effect[b)]			
	KT50 (min.)-%Mortality at indicated dilution		Dosage (A.I.mg/m^2)	KT50 (min.)-%Mortality at ...weeks		
				Initial	2	4
d-Cyphenothrin 5% EC	x 20	4.9-100	125	3.8-100	5.4-100	6.8-100
	x 10	3.6-100	250	2.7-100	5.2-100	6.5-100
Permethrin 5% EC	x 20	10.8-100	125	7.4-100	32.0-100	54.0-100
	x 10	6.7-100	250	5.1-100	14.0-100	18.0-100
Fenitrothion 10% EC	x 40	>20.0-100	125	68.0-100	>120-100	>120- 47
	x 20	>20.0-100	250	34.0-100	>120-100	>120- 73

a) Cockroach spray test method (17), Dosage: 4.5 ml of dilution / CSMA chamber.

b) Confined contact method (18), Dosage: 50 ml of dilution / m^2. Test surface: Plywood panel overlaid with melamin resin (15 x 15 cm).

Table 8. Insecticidal activity of fumigant formulations containing d-cyphenothrin and permethrin against housefly, mosquito and cockroach in a large chamber (28 m^3).

Exposure time[a)]:90 min.

Insecticide	Dosage (a.i.mg/m^3)	KT50 (min.)-%Mortality			FT50 (min.):(KT50 (min.))[b)]-%Mortality
		Musca domestica	*Culex pipiens*	*Blattella germanica* in a glass dish	*Blattella germanica* in a plywood-shelter
d-Cyphenothrin	10	8.5-100	10.5-100	18.8-100	17.0 : (24.0)-100
	20	–	–	14.8-100	14.0 : (18.0)-100
Permethrin	10	9.0-100	15.0-100	24.0- 90	16.4 : (32.0)- 74
	20	–	–	16.2-100	12.2 : (17.5)-100

a) Insect cage: Four cages containing a group of 20 houseflies or mosquitoes were hung in the chamber.

Glass dish: A glass dish containing 10 cockroaches was placed on the floor.

Glass dish with plywood shelter: A plywood shelter containing 10 cockroaches was set on a glass dish, and then they were placed on the floor.

Fumigation device: A porous ceramic mat which had been impregnated with an active ingredient was heated at 300 °c on the specially designed electric vaporizer.

b) KT50: Time required for 50 % of cockroaches knocked-down after flushing-out.

Evaluation of d-prallethrin and d-cyphenothrin in the combined formulations

Taking the outstanding insecticidal potencies of the two new pyrethroid stereoisomers into account, we finally introduce in Table 9 a number of their efficient performances in the combination recipes for aerosol formulation containing 0.15 to 0.3 % of total active ingredients for control of the major nuisance insects in household. The knockdown activity against mosquito and housefly was still more enhanced by increasing the d-prallethrin ratio to d-cyphenothrin, while the killing activity was notably reinforced by increasing the ratio of the latter to that of the former. The increase of d-prallethrin ratio resulted in the higher flushing-out effect against cockroach and the killing effect was still remarkable even at the lowest d-cyphenothrin ratio, which is due to the high lethal activity of d-prallethrin against cockroach already referred.

The total amount of active ingredients can be significantly minimized by the new joint recipes in comparison to the conventional and very popular recipes consisting of, for example, tetramethrin and d-phenothrin as knockdown and killing agents whose total concentration often requires to be over 0.5 % for the better performances as multipurpose aerosol. The integrated potency that results from each of the essential insecticidal activities can be the most efficient tool especially for cockroach control in direct or ambushing application even in the lowest concentration of 0.075 % for each of the new active ingredients as featured by the most distinguished flushing-out effect.

Table 9. Insecticidal activity of the combined oil-based aerosol formulations of d-prallethrin and d-cyphenothrin.

		KT50(min.)-%Mortality[a)]		FT50(min.)[b)]	KT50(min.)-%Mortality[c)]
Aerosol	A.I.(%w/w)	*Musca domestica*	*Culex pipiens*	*Blattella germanica*	
d-Prallethrin/d-Cyphenothrin	0.225/0.075	4.3-85	4.7-90	4.2	2.5-100
total 0.3 %	0.15 /0.15	6.0-92	5.1-94	4.6	3.4-100
	0.075/0.225	6.4-97	6.2-98	5.4	4.8-100
total 0.15 %	0.075/0.075	6.8-82	6.3-88	5.6	4.8-100
Tetramethrin/d-Phenothrin	0.3 /0.15	6.0-86	7.1-89	5.7	5.4- 98
Propoxur/Dichlorvos	1.0 /0.5	9.1-69	7.7-87	(NE)	4.4-100
OTA: Pyrethrins/PBO	0.2 /1.6	9.2-79	11.0-80	9.5	8.7- 88

a) CSMA aerosol test method (16).
b) Shinjo's method (10), FT50: Time required for 50 % of cockroaches flushed-out from a plywood shelter.
Dosage: 1 g of aerosol spray / 0.34 m^3.
c) Direct spray method (14), Dosage: 400 mg of aerosol spray / cylinder (20 cm in diameter and 60 cm in height).

REFERENCES

1. LaForge, F. B. and H. L. Haller, J. Am. Chem. Soc. 58, p. 1777 (1936)
2. LaForge, F. B. and W. F. Barthel, J. Org. Chem. 10 (1945)
3. LaForge, F. B. and S. B. Soloway, J. Am. Chem. Soc. 69, p. 186 (1947)
4. Gersdorff, W. A. and P. G. Piquett, J. Econ. Ent. 54(6),p. 1250 (1961)
5. Katsuda, Y., The Second International Congress of Pesticide Chemistry IUPAC, p. 443 (1971)
6. Matsuo, T., T. Nishioka, M. Hirano, Y. Suzuki, K. Tsushima, N. Itaya and H. Yoshioka, Pestic. Sci. 11, p. 202 (1980)
7. Matsuo, T., N. Itaya, T. Mizutani, N. Ohno, K. Fujimoto, Y. Okuno and H. Yoshioka, Agr. Biol. Chem. 40(1),p. 247 (1976)
8. Sumitomo Chemical Co., Ltd., Japanese Patent 55-16402 (1980)
9. Sumitomo Chemical Co., Ltd., Japanese Patent 51-5450 (1976)
10. Shinjo, G., T. Yamaguchi, S. Tsuda, K. Yoshida and Y. Okuno Jap. J. Sanit. Zool. 32(3), p. 221 (1981)
11. Chadwick, P. R., International Pest Control Jan./Feb., p. 15 (1976)
12. Shinjo, G., K. Yoshida and Y. Okuno, Jap. J. Sanit. Zool. 29, p. 48 (1978)
13. Ebert, M. A., Aerosol Age Sept., p. 33 (1976)
14. Yamaguchi, T., G. Shinjo, S. Tsuda, K. Yoshida, E. Inaba and Y. Okuno Jap. J. Sanit. Zool. 32(1), p. 59 (1981)
15. MacIver, D. R., Pyrethrum Post 7, p. 7 (1964)
16. CSMA aerosol test method, Soap. Chem. Spec., BLUE BOOK, p. 161 (1971)
17. CSMA cockroach spray method, Soap. Chem. Spec., BLUE BOOK, p. 166 (1971)
18. Okuno, Y., T. Yamaguchi and Y. Fujita, Botyu-Kagaku 41, p. 42 (1976)

ANTIBIOTICS FOR AGRICULTURAL USE

RECENT STATUS AND FUTURE ASPECTS OF AGRICULTURAL ANTIBIOTICS

Tomomasa Misato

Institute of Physical and Chemical Research, Wako, Saitama 351, Japan

Abstract - Nowadays, use of agricultural antibiotics is not been limited only to controlling plant diseases, but is extended wider over various areas such as insecticidal and herbicidal uses, or as plant regulators in Japan. Here, the author intends to consider the reasons why so much is expected of antibiotics of microorganic origin as pesticides, and he also wishes to present a brief introduction to the present situation of antibiotic research and development in the country.

INTRODUCTION

In today's world where the population is constantly increasing, an increase in food production is essential. Pesticides have been playing epoch-making role in stabilizing and increasing crop yield. Yet, on the other hand, pesticides are accused of being possible source of environmental pollution with residual toxicity harmful to mammals, and wildlife. This soicial concern is urging the exploitation of non-polluting safe pesticides. Antibiotics are produced by soil microorganisms in the soil. The advantage of their being derived from and returned to the soil have made antibiotics model pesticides which do not cause environemtal problems.

Studies on the use of antibiotics for agricultural purposes were first started in Europe and the United States, stimulated by the remarkable progress in the medical field since the tank culture method for penicillin production was developed. The energetic efforts did not bear so much fruit as expected, leading only to the use of streptomycin (which had been used for medical purposes) combined with tetracyclin for the control of bacterial diseases of fruit trees and vegetable diseases. The consumption of cycloheximide (U.S.A.) and griseofluvin (U.K.), both developed as agricultural antibiotics, was also very limited.

In Japan, however, the above four antibiotics were put to practical use; blasticidin S was also successfully developed. This success stimulated exploitation of a series of new agricultural antibiotics such as kasugamycin, polyoxins, and validamycin. Antibiotics began to be used not only as fungicides but as miticides; tetranactin, for instance, has been put to practical use, and bialaphos recently appeared in the market as a herbicide and is regarded as promising by the major chemical industries of the world.

Thus, agricultural antibiotics produced by microorganisms are now being widely used as fungicides, insecticides, and herbicides. If gibberellin, produced by microorganisms, and well-known as a plant growth regulator, is added to the group, agricultural antibiotics are then being extensively used in every sphere of pesticides, as shown in Table 1 (Ref. 1 & 2).

CHARACTERISTICS OF AGRICULTURAL ANTIBIOTICS

Not only pesticides but all scientific inventions have advantages and disadvantages. The case of agricultural antibiotics is no exception. The favourable and unfavourable points about them may be:

A. Advantages

(1) No environmental pollution problems because of quick degradation
When we evaluate a pesticide only from the standpoint of efficacy and acute toxicity, DDT must be considered the most ideal. What is the reason such a

"non-toxic" chemical as DDT, which did no harm to humans even when it was sprinkled over their heads to exterminate fleas and lice, was prohibited? Because it was learned that the chemical did not decompose easily but that its damaging residue remained in the natural environment posing the threat of chronic toxicity to mammals through its biological concentration in the food chain.

This points out an absolutely indispensable prerequisite for a new pesticide, that is, it must be easily degraded and non-polluting. DDT and BHC were hazardous to the natural environment because they have completely new chemical structures which do not exist in nature and, therefore, cannot be degraded by existing microorganisms. Usually, all living organisms on earth are decomposed by microorganisms after termination of life and resolve in nature. This is why antibiotics, metabolites of microorganisms, are easily decomposable and there is no fear of environmental hazard.

TABLE 1. Pesticidal compounds of microbiological origin

Fungicides	Antifungal antibiotics	Blasticidin S, kasugamycin polyoxin, validamycin
	Antibacterial antibiotics	Streptomycin, etc.
Insecticides	Miticidal antibiotics	Tetranactin
	Bacterial toxins	Bacillus thuringensis
Herbicides	Herbicidal antibiotics	Bialaphos
Growth regulators	Fungal products	Gibberellins

TABLE 2. The concentration of antibiotic for application

(Antibiotic)	Concentration (ppm)
Blasticidin S	10 - 20
Kasugamycin	20 - 40
Validamycin	30 - 50
Tetranactin	100 - 130
Polyoxins	100 - 200
Streptomycin	100 - 200
(Other fungicides)	
Organic phosphorus compounds	500
Organic sulfur compounds	1,000 - 1,500
Inorganic sulfur compounds	2,000
Bordeaux mixture ($CuSO_4$)	4,000

(2) Less amount of application per unit area is sufficient
Because of their stronger effect at lower concentrations, the amount required for plant protection purposes is 1/10 to 1/100 times less than organic synthesized pesticides applied in the field as shown in Table 2. This is not only a great advantage from an environmental point of view but also has merit from an economical standpoint. Low cost is an important condition for a pesticide to be widely used, so the fact that effective spraying can be done

with much less quantity indicates the feasibility of the pesticide. Farmers can use it even when the price is 10 to 100 times higher than that of other synthetic chemicals to spray the equivalent field area.

(3) Selective toxicity to target organisms
If there is any pesticide which can control diseases and insect pests with efficacy and without mammalian toxicity, this is the pesticide we are seeking. The agricultural antibiotics being used in Japan have selective toxicity to target organisms except for blasticidin S, and therefore, are ideal pesticides with low mammalian toxicity.

(4) Advantage in production - no need to change plant facilities for production of different antibiotics
Due to the growing concern about environmental issues, the regulations on industrial wastes have recently been made more rigorous. As a consequence enormous amounts of money are being invested in plant and equipment for the manufacture of new chemicals because waste disposal facilities suited for the chemical synthesis process must be newly established.

In the case of antibiotics varieties of them can be prepared in turn even by using the same tank. Moreover, since there is no great difference in the constituents of culture solution and production process except for the difference in microorganisms to be produced, one set of equipment serves for production of several kinds of antibiotics. Under the present tight financial circumstances, contrary to the past when plant and equipment posed burdens, this will be a great advantage. What is more fascinating about antibiotics is that microorganisms easily produce their complex chemical structure, the synthesis of which involves many sophisticated manufacturing processes.

(5) Materials are inexhaustible
Agricultural antibiotics are produced not from limited resources like those of fossil origin but from crop plants produced by solar energy with the aid of microorganisms living in the soil. The materials are therefore an inexhaustible resource.

B. Limitations

(1) Difficulties in microanalysis
As seen in the case of polyoxins, an antibiotic is generally a mixture of various components. Its analysis depends on bioassay methods, which cannot be expected to give accurate results nor to be duplicated in as simple a manner as in an instrumental analysis. This requires some troublesome effort.

(2) Development of resistance to antibiotics in plant pathogens
Antibiotics generally have selectivity to target organisms and are apt to develop resistance in plant pathogens to them, as has been experienced in the cases of kasugamycin and polyoxin. One countermeasure may be to establish a technology of the combined uses of antibiotics with other chemicals having different mechanisms of action, or by spraying them in rotation.

(3) Misunderstanding from public health aspects
When a medical antibiotic, like streptomycin is to be used for agricultural purposes, sufficient caution must be taken against resistance of pathogens of human diseases. Most of the antibiotics now being used in Japan are not in use for medical purposes and so may be treated in a manner similar to other pesticides. Despite this fact, just because they are called antibiotics, there is a rigid regulation that there must be no residue. This stands in the way not only of research and development but also of attend the world market for these products. To resolve this, a new reasonable residue standard is needed, such as those for other pesticides, to further efforts toward international understanding.

PRESENT SITUATION OF AGRICULTURAL ANTIBIOTICS IN JAPAN

Antibiotics registered as a pesticide in Japan and actually in use are listed in Table 3.

Since antibiotics are used in various forms of formulations like powder, wettable powder or emulsified concentration, the amount consumed is expressed simply as the total. Yet, since antibiotics mixed with other formulations is increasingly applied in the field these days, the figures in the table will be much larger if those used as mixture are added to them.

TABLE 3. Agricultural antibiotics being used in Japan

Antibiotics	Year Registered	Effective against	Consumption (1980) (10^3 Yen)
Streptomycin	1956	Bacterial diseases of fruit trees & vegetables	1,539,510
Blasticidin S	1962	Rice blast	770,639
Kasugamycin	1965	Rice blast	1,194,057
Polyoxins	1968	Fungal diseases of fruit trees & vegetables	1,455,684
		Rice sheath blight	
Validamycin	1972	Rice sheath blight	1,756,168
Tetranactin	1974	Mites of fruit & tea trees	367,354

In accordance with the Agricultural Chemicals Regulation Law amended in 1971, two years of severe safety tests including one on chronic toxicity are required for the registration of a pesticide and must be renewed every three years. These tests involve an enormous amount of money, and as a result, those agricultural antibiotics whose consumption was small, like cycloheximide, griseofluvin, and cellocidin, have disappeared from the market because of the difficulty in preparing sufficient data to satisfy the regulation.

Next, some of the promising agricultural antibiotics now in the developing stage will be introduced briefly. Nikkomycin (Ref. 3) (Fig. 1) is a nucleotide-peptide antibiotic with a chemical structure and bioactivity very similar to that of polyoxin.

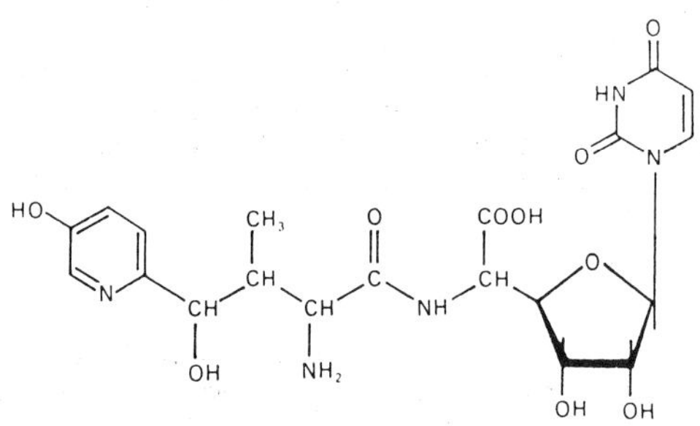

Fig. 1. Structure of nikkomycin

The name is said to originate from the famous Nikko, where during his visit a German scientist happened to collect the soil sample used in the antibiotic research resulting in this great success. After the publication of the report on this discovery, thorough re-examination was conducted on the more than one hundred cultures of microorganisms stored at the Institute of Physical and Chemical Research as producers of polyoxin-like substances. Ten percent of them were found to be nikkomycin-producing organisms. This provides a good lesson for the screening of new antibiotics. Mildiomycin (Ref. 4) (Fig. 2) is a water-soluble and basic antibiotic produced by streptomyces. Its action against powdery mildew of fruit and vegetables.

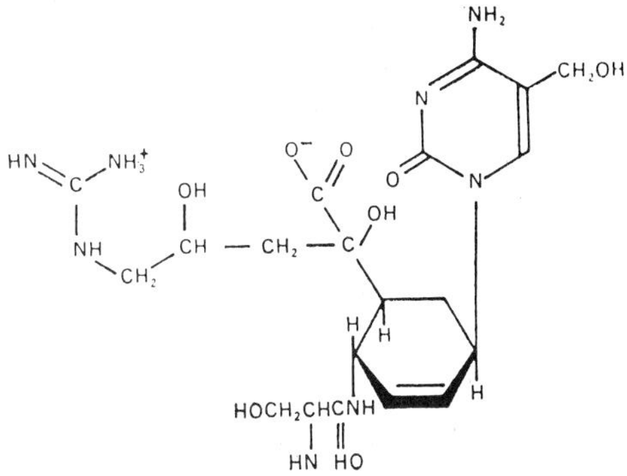

Fig. 2. Structure of mildiomycin

A herbicidal antibiotic, bialaphos (Ref. 5) (Fig. 3), on which the spotlight of attention has focused recently has a chemical structure of (2-amino-4-methylphos-phinoyl-butylyl)-ananylalanine. Its sodium salts is used as a pesticide.

$$CH_3-P(=O)(OH)-CH_2-CH_2-CH(NH_2)-CONH-CH(CH_3)-CONH-CH(CH_3)-COOH$$

Fig. 3. Structure of bialaphos

When sprayed on the leaves and stems of weeds, it is translocated to the roots and kills the plant. Because of this it is applicable to a wide range of plants from annual weeds to perennial plants and shrubs. In comparison with the simmilar type herbicides, gramoxon and glyphosate, it surpasses the former in permeability and translocation ability, and the latter in its fast-acting characteristic. These superior characteristics are expected to make the herbicide internationally popular. The herbicidal effect of bialaphos was discovered in the microbial solution which, because of the phytotoxicity present, did not pass the screening during tests on fungicidal effects. It was then tested on its herbicidal performance, and is truly an example of success as the result of an excellent idea.

CONCLUSION

As mentioned above, the research and development of agricultural antibiotics in Japan are more advanced than in other countries of the world. Their future is bright as non-polluting pesticides with low mammalian toxicity. It is expected that the predictable rapid progress in such aspects of biotechnology as gene manipulation will facilitate mass production of antibiotics of high additional value in the same way as in the case of insulin. In contrast to medical antibiotics which are limited in demand and do not necessarily require mass production, the demand for agricultural antibiotics for pesticidal use are predicted to increase if the price is lowered by mass production. Their production will benefit by the remarkable progress in biotechnology.

With these facts in mind, a research project on the exploitation and utilization of microorganism and plant resources in tropical and subtropical regions was started in 1981 with Science and Technology Agency of the Japanese Government. Under this program collaborative research has been conducted both on medical and agricultural antibiotics between the Shanghai Medicine Research Institute of China and the Institute of Microbial Chemistry of Japan, and between the Shanghai Pesticide Research Institute of China and the Institute of Physical and Chemical Research of Japan, aiming at exploitation of unutilized soil microrganisms in mainland China for medical and agricultural uses. Again, I believe that the field of antibiotic research and development must be explored through collaboration among Asian countries, though countries in other parts of the world have not yet become as enthusiastic about it.

REFERENCES

1. T. Misato, K. Ko and I. Yamaguchi: "Advances in Applied Microbiology", Academic Press, 21, p.53 (1977).
2. T. Misato: "ACS Symposium Series", American Chemical Society, 37, p.170 (1977).
3. U. DÄhn, H. Hagenmaier, H. Höhne, W.A. König, G. Wolf and H. Zähner: Arch. Microbiol. 107, 143 (1976).
4. S. Harada and T. Kishi: J. Antibiot. 31, 519 (1978).
5. H. Sekizawa: (to be presented at this Symposium) (1982).

HOW TO DISCOVER NEW ANTIBIOTICS FOR FUNGICIDAL USE

Keido Ko

Fungicide Laboratory, The Institute of Physical and Chemical Research, Wako, Saitama 351, Japan

Abstract - Many antibiotics were found with various methods including *in vitro* and *in vivo* tests. Many systems of semi-*in vivo* test devised by some researchers for their convenience, are also available for the discovery and the development of new antibiotics. There are some merits and demerits for each method. Therefore, when a screening system is going to be established, several key factors must be considered. They are how to select a pathogenic target, how to treat test compound on test organism, how to make test plant infected, and how to evaluate an efficacy from the experimental results, etc. Recently, some methods, e.g. cell-free system for screening active compound with high-selectivity and semi-*in vivo* tests for purification of non-fungicidal antibiotic, have been devised and tried. Some methods specially used in bioassay of antibacterial and antiviral substances are introduced.

INTRODUCTION

Studies on antibiotics for plant disease protection have been attempted since 1950 by using some medical antibiotics, e.g. streptomycin, chloramphenicol, tetracyclines, etc. and their by-products, e.g. cycloheximides. However, most of the researchers did not believe that an application of antibiotic could be successful in the field of plant disease protection, until the first antibiotic for agricultural use, blasticidin S, was developed in 1958. Since this finding, studies on agricultural antibiotics became active. As for the research process of antibiotics, its principle has not been changed for 30 years as shown in Fig. 1. In this process, all steps are required to be modified usually for finding new active compound. Otherwise, the probability of the finding may be extremely low. Among the steps in this process, how to assay biological activity of test culture broth is most important.

Sample collection (from air, water, soils, etc.)
↓
Isolation
↓
Cultivation ——————→ Clone improvement
↓
Bioassay
↓
Purification ——————→ Toxicity check
↓
Identification
↓
Formulation
↓
Field test

Fig. 1. Outline of research process of antibiotics

METHODS GENERALLY USED FOR SEARCHING NEW ACTIVE COMPOUND

As shown in Table 1, the conventional methods for bioassay of antibiotics are almost the same as that of synthetic compound. They are some *in vitro* tests and *in vivo* tests. Since 1950 s, the spore germination test was rarely used. Because, the inhibition of antibiotic on spore germination is generally not so distinctive. Therefore, the cylinder method has been used mostly. The cylinder method is practical for the assay of not only the antifungal substance but also the antibacterial substance. This method is also useful for the assay of culture broth without pre-sterilization. Later, a similar method, paper disk method was devised and tried almost instead of the cylinder method. A merit of this method is simplicity and convenience. Another method for *in vitro* tests may be the agar streak method. This method can assay many targets in the same assay plate at the same time. Therefore, it has

TABLE 1. Methods usually used to search new active compound

In vitro tests	a. Spore germination test b. Cylinder method c. Paper disk method d. Agar streak method
In vivo tests	a. Pot-test b. Nursery-test c. Field-test

been always used for checking the MIC (Minimum Inhibitory Concentration) of test sample. As for the *in vivo* tests, many methods have been devised and tried (Ref.1). The author intended to introduce a method which was successfully used in developing antiblast compounds including blasticidin S and kasugamycin. As shown in Fig. 2, the 3-4 leaf-stage rice seedlings cultivated in a small pot can be used as test plants. The culture broth is sprayed on the seedlings by foliar treatment before or after conidial inoculation. The inoculum is prepared by cultivating *Pyricularia oryzae*, the causal fungus of rice blast on some media suitable for sporulation. The infected rice seedlings are then incubated in a moisture chamber under 28°C and more than 95% R.H. for 4 days. After the lesion developed, its number is counted and compared with that of the untreated control (Ref.2). As for nursery-test and field-test are rarely used for finding new active substance from culture broth.

Rice seedlings
↓
Foliar treatment with test sample
↓
Conidial inoculation
↓
Incubation under 28°C and more than 95% R.H.
↓
Evaluation

Fig. 2. The process of *in vivo* test for bioassay of anti-blast substance

METHODS USED TO FIND ANTIBIOTICS PRACTICALLY APPLIED IN FIELD

There are several antibiotics practically used in plant disease protection, as shown in Table 2. Among these antibiotics, blasticidin S, kasugamycin, polyoxins and validamycin were developed for agricultural use and are used as agricultural fungicides only, while the others were developed for medical use first and then applied as an agricultural fungicide.

Blasticidin S is the first antibiotic developed for agricultural use by T. Misato and his coworkers in 1958, for preventing rice blast. This antibiotic was found by applying the cylinder method (commonly called cup method in Japan) and the pot-test previously described (Ref.1-3). Also it was only one found by *in vitro* test. Second antibiotic for preventing rice blast is kasugamycin found by T. Ishiyama and his coworkers with the pot-test as previously described (Ref.4). This antibiotic did not show any inhibitory effect under a condition of *in vitro* assay. Essentially, it was hardly purified by the pot-test only. Fortunately, it was found and purified by H. Umezawa and his coworkers already, when they searched some antibiotics against *Pseudomonas aeruginosa* for medical use. Later, it was found that kasugamycin did make an inhibition zone, on agar plate seeded *Pyricularia*

TABLE 2. Some antibiotics practically used and the methods used during their exploitation

Antifungal antibiotics	Disease prevented	Methods
Blasticidin S	Rice blast	Cylinder method
Kasugamycin	Rice blast	Pot test
Polyoxins	Rice sheath blight	Cylinder method
Validamycin	Rice sheath blight	Kosaka's method and reversed layer method
Cycloheximide	Onion downy mildew	Field test
Antibacterial antibiotics		
Streptomycin	Various bacterial diseases	Cylinder method
Tetracyclines	Various bacterial diseases	Cylinder method
Chloramphenicol	Bacterial leaf blight of rice plant	Cylinder method
Novobiocin	Canker of tomato	Cylinder method

oryzae under pH 5. This phenomenon may be a character of this antibiotic. At the same time, S. Suzuki and his coworkers adopted *Rhizoctonia solani* (formerly *Pellicularia sasakii*), the causal fungus of rice sheath blight as a screening target. And they found a group of antibiotics, polyoxins which are excellent antibiotics for preventing several plant diseases, mainly for rice sheath blight and pear black spot (Ref. 5&6). Second antibiotic for preventing rice sheath blight, validamycin, was found in 1970 by using a method with specially devised system and Kosaka's method (Ref. 7-10). As for its detail, K. Matsuura will described it later in this proceeding. The other antibiotics, streptomycin, tetracyclines, chloramphenicol, novobiocin, cycloheximides, etc were all medical antibiotics. And their biological activities were checked by the cylinder method. However, they are less useful in plant disease protection now.

SOME METHODS TRIED TO SEARCH NEW ANTIBIOTIC NOWADAYS

From some knowledges of action mechanisms of antibiotics, some researchers tried to assay biological activities of culture broth with high selectivity. K. Isono and his coworkers attempted to screen some active compounds by using two kinds of cell-free system. One of them is the system of peptidoglycan synthetase reported by K. Izaki et al (Ref. 11). They obtained some new antibiotics, e. g. lipopeptin A which is able to inhibit GDP-[U-^{14}C]mannose and UDP-[U-^{14}C]GlcNAc incorporation into proteo-heteroglycan of *Pyricularia oryzae* (Ref. 12). Another method is the system of chitin synthetase reported by Hori, M. et al (Ref. 13). With this system, they have obtained some new antibiotics, e. g. neopolyoxins which show remarkable inhibitory effect of chitin synthetase and induce mycelium swelling on many plant pathogens as polyoxins did (Ref. 14). Recently, some workers have an experience that there are many active compounds and culture broth effective against some plant diseases show no or less fungicidal activity on some agar plates by usual *in vitro* tests. When such a culture broth is purified with *in vitro* tests, it is impossible to get real active components. Therefore, we must have a method of bioassay, during the purification of active culture broth for tracing the component. However, usual *in vivo* tests required much test sample and test periods. For this reason, the authors attempted to devise a ting activities of test samples, called leaf disk method. This method is one of semi-*in vivo* tests with half-developed leaves of cucumber and conidial suspension of *Botrytis cinerea*. As shown in Fig. 3, the process of the method is described. The leaf disks are prepared by cutting cucumber leaves with cork borer (20 mmin diameter). Then the leaf disks are dipped in test solutions for 1 min. After the treatment of test chemical solutions, the treated leaf disks are set on glass slide in moiture chamber and inoculated by an inoculum paper disk. The inoculum paper disks have been pre-immersed in conidial suspension contained 1-5 X 10^5 spores/ ml, 5% glucose and 1% yeast extract. After 24-36 hr-incubation, the diameter of the lesion is measured and compared with the size of the untreated control (Ref.15). This method could be applied not only to disease caused by Botrytis cinerea, but also on some rotted diseases and some diseases caused by obligate parasites.

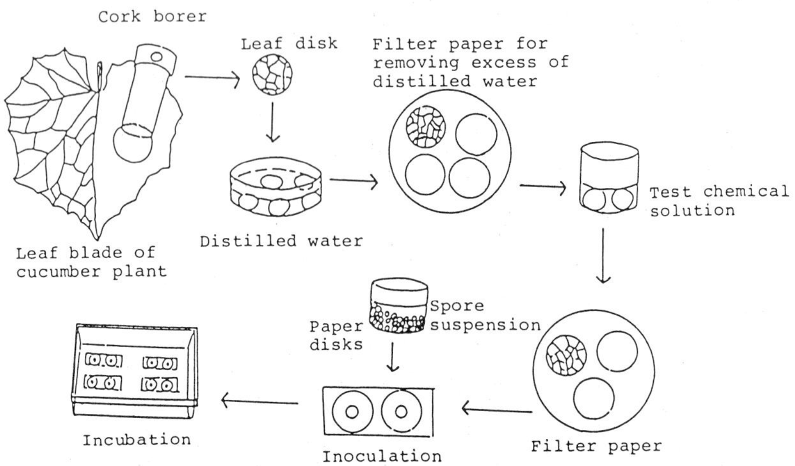

Fig. 3. Procedure of the leaf disk method

METHODS FOR EVALUATING ANTIBACTERIAL AND ANTIVIRAL ACTIVITIES OF TEST CULTURE BROTH

Although, several antibiotics for preventing bacterial diseases are practically used, their efficacy is not so satisfactory. Naturally, many methods for bioassay of antibacterial substances have been devised and tried. I am going to show the most simple one for their representatives. As shown in Fig. 4, a screening method reported by Koike, M. et al (Ref.16). They used radish block and Erwinia aroidea a causal bacterium of soft rot disease to check the activity of the test sample. This is one of the high sensitive

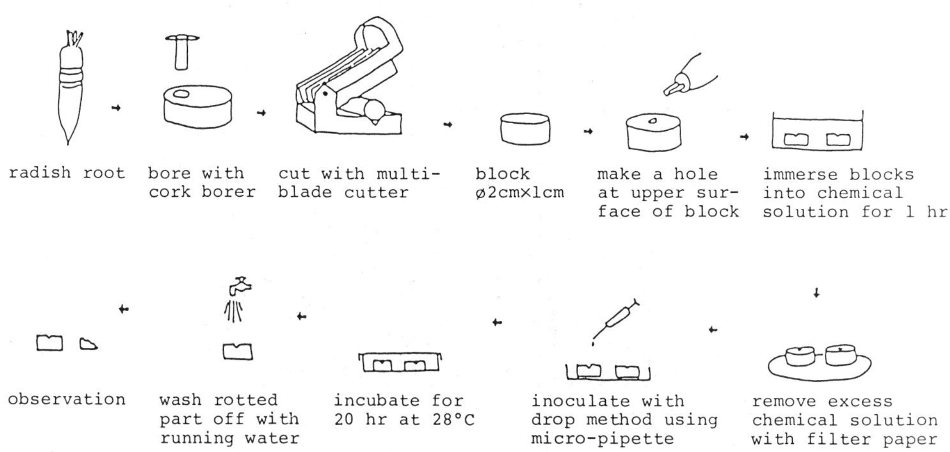

Fig. 4. Procedure of the radish block method (Ref. 16)

method. Using this method and a pot-test of spraying inoculation devised by the authors (Ref.17), we found biological activity of antibiotic, myomycin, which is effective on soft rot disease of vegetables and citrus canker (Ref. 17). As for bioassay of antiviral substance, some methods have been attempted. But there is no effective antiviral agent developed yet. So it can be said that no excellent method is worthy to be recommended. As shown in Table 3, the local lesion assay is the most popular method to detect antiviral substances. The authors used this method to discover a new antibiotic, bihoromycin, also an excellent antiviral antibiotic (Ref.19), and antiviral activity of an antibacterial antibiotic, formycin B (Ref.20). But both are phytotoxic on test plants. Then the authors used systemic host assays of pot-test and leaf disk floating test to discover aabomycin A (Ref.21) which did also show a strong inhibition against *Pyricularia oryzae* on potato dextrose agar plate. The leaf disk floating method is one of the semi-*in vivo* tests for both, local lesion assay and systemic assay. However, virus content should be measured by chemical determination or biological assay, when a systemic host is used. Any method of local lesion assay is generally more convenient than method of systemic assay. Therefore, in many cases, the workers have a tendency to use local lesion assay to evaluate of test substance. However, when a pot-test is always carried out by using local lesion host, some workers may miss to detect some effective multiplication inhibitors. Therefore many workers are now conscious of the importance of *in vivo* test by using systemic host in whole plant. In using such a host however, many difficulties may be considered. For instance, how to inoculate virus as near as possible to natural status, how to control concentration of virus inoculum and various infection conditions etc. still remained to be solved. In order to improve these problems, the authors devised an apparatus for air brush inoculation as shown in Fig. 5. The method was largely improved from a cotton ball rubbing method, a conventional method. With the use of the apparatus, inoculation can be carried out under a certain gauge pressure, exposure period, a certain distance between nozzle and test plant, and a certain concentration of carborundum content. Inoculation under constant conditions would considerably control the diseased ratio of the inoculated plants (Ref.22&23). As for single cell tests, they were generally used to study mode of action of antiviral substances.

TABLE 3. Methods for screening antiviral substance

1. Pot-test	a. Local lesion assay
	b. Systemic host assay
2. Leaf disk floating test	a. Local lesion assay
	b. Systemic host assay
3. Single cell test	a. Leaf hair cell assay
	b. Protoplast of mesophyll assay
	c. Tissue-culture cell assay

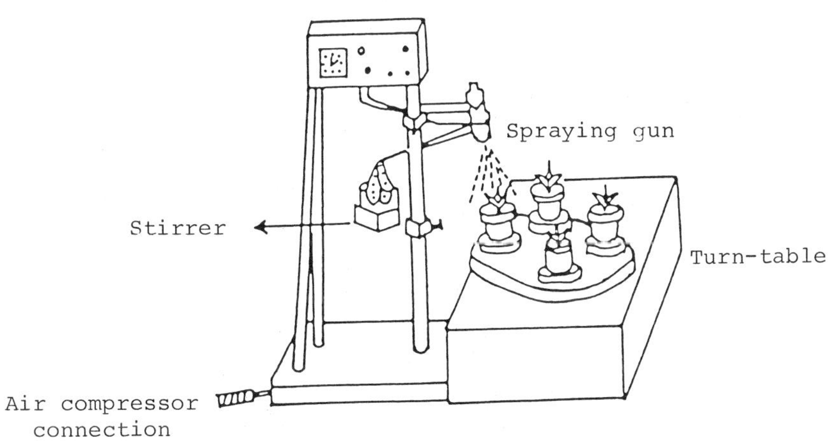

Fig. 5. Automatic sprayer for spraying inoculation

CONCLUSION

From the review as described above, it can be said that a good method can discover a good fungicide. However, there is not so many new fungicides successfully discovered by using the same method without any modification. Another important matter on the discovery of new antibiotic is that one should never overlook a different phenomenon on its biological results, even a slight difference. For instance, the size of an inhibition zone, discoloration or deformity of test organism, etc., they are all important signs of new antibiotics. Therefore, it can be said that a pursuit of new fungicide must be started from pursuiting unusual phenomenon at every step in the whole research process.

REFERENCES

1. K. Fukunaga, T. Misato, I. Ishii and M. Asakawa, Bull. Agric. Chem. Soc. Japan 19, 181-188 (1955).
2. T. Misato, Y. Okimoto, I. Ishii, M. Asakawa and K. Fukunaga, Ann. Phytopathol. Soc. Japan 24, 307-312 (1959).
3. T. Misato, I. Ishii, M. Asakawa and K. Fukunaga, ibid 23, 219-224 (1958).
4. T. Ishiyama, I. Hara, M. Matsuoka, K. Sato, S. Shimada, R. Izawa, T. Hashimoto, M. Hamada, Y. Okami, T. Takeuchi and H. Umezawa, J. Antibiotics Ser. A, 18, 115-119 (1965).
5. K. Isono, J. Nagatsu, Y. Kawashima and S. Suzuki, Agric. Biol. Chem. 29, 848-854 (1965).
6. K. Isono, J. Nagatsu, K. Kobinata and S. Suzuki, Agric. Biol. Chem. 31, 190-199 (1967).
7. T. Kosaka and K. Fukushiro, Shokubutsu Bōeki 10, 331-334 (1956).
8. T. Iwasa, E. Higashide, H. Yamamoto and M. Shibata, J. Antibiotics 24, 107-113 (1971).
9. T. Iwasa, E. Higashide and M. Shibata, J. Antibiotics 24, 114-118 (1971).
10. T. Iwasa, Y. Kameda, M. Asai, S. Horii and K. Mizuno, J. Antibiotics 24, 119-123 (1971).
11. K. Izaki, M. Matsuhashi and J. L. Strominger, J. Biol. Chem. 243, 3180-3192 (1968).
12. K. Tsuda, T. Kihara, M. Nishii, G. Nakamura, K. Isono and S. Suzuki, J. Antibiotics 33, 247 (1980).
13. M. Hori, K. Kakiki and T. Misato, Agric. Biol. Chem. 38, 691 (1974).
14. K. Kobinata, M. Uramoto, M. Nishii, H. Kusakabe, G. Nakamura and K. Isono, Agric. Biol. Chem. 44, 1709 (1980).
15. K. Ko, Y. Kobayashi, K. Akutsu, Y. Matsuzawa and T. Misato, The 6th Annual Meeting of Pesticide Chemical Society held in Nagoya (1981).
16. M. Koike, S. Sekido, K. Yoneyama and T. Misato, J. Pesticide Sci. 3, 433-436 (1978).
17. K. Ko, H. Nagai, Y. Adachi, S. Ohbuchi, Y. Matsuzawa and T. Misato, Proceeding of The Kanto-Tosan Plant Protection Society 21, 79-80 (1974).
18. K. Yoneyama, M. Koike, S. Sekido, K. Ko and T. Misato, J. Pesticide Soc. 3, 359-364 (1978).
19. T. Misato, K.-T. Huang, M. Katagiri, M. Ueda, S. Fukatsu and T. Niida, J. Antibiotics Ser. A, 20, 254-260 (1967).
20. K.-T. Huang, M. Katagiri and T. Misato, J. Antibiotics Ser. A, 16, 75-77 (1966).
21. I. Yamaguchi, R. Taniguchi, K.-T. Huang and T. Misato, J. Antibiotics 22, 463-466 (1969).
22. K.-T. Huang, Y. Matsuzawa and T. Misato, Ann. Phytopathol. Soc. Japan 39, 404-409 (1974).
23. K.-T. Huang, Y. Matsuzawa and T. Misato, Ann. Phytopathol. Soc. Japan 40, 1-5 (1975).

HOW TO DISCOVER NEW ANTIBIOTICS FOR INSECTICIDAL USE

Kunio Ando

Research Laboratories, Chugai Pharmaceutical Co. Ltd., Toshima, Tokyo 171, Japan

Abstract- Our experience on the research and development of miticidal antibiotic, tetranactin, is described. The macrotetrolide antibiotic, tetranactin, has recently been isolated from the fermented broth of Streptomyces aureus S-3466 using Azukibean weevil as a test insect. The antibiotic is, so far as we know, the first pesticidal antibiotic ever commercialized. It has been in use in Japan as an agricultural miticide since 1973. Our screening procedures, chemical and biological properties of tetranactin are summarized in this paper.

INTRODUCTION

Environmental polution is now serious problem all over the world. Especially chemicals such as pesticides sprayed over wide areas are apt to cause ecological changes and subsequent destruction of the environment. The ideal harmless pesticides should have a number of properties, selective toxicity and ready decomposability into small, safe molecules such as water, carbon dioxide and ammonia are most important. Antibiotic pesticides may have such ideal properties because of their selective toxicity and ready decomposability.

More than hundred years ago, when the modern science and technology had not yet developed, mankind had already acquired the wisdom how to control pests using plant extracts. The representatives of active ingredients isolated from the extract are pyrethrin, nicotinoids and rotenone. These facts tell us that living things are capable of producing pesticidal substances. Therefore, we assumed that microorganisms must have also produced varieties of pesticidal antibiotics.

Early in 1960's, Prof. Takemoto of Tohoku Univ., Japan, isolated two insecticidal antibiotics, tricholomic acid (1) and ibotenic acid (2), from mushrooms, which had been empirically known by Japanese as fly-killing mushrooms. For these reasons, research and development of agricultural antibiotics have been actively and extensively pursued in Japan.

Although my assinged task is "HOW TO DISCOVER NEW ANTIBIOTICS FOR INSECTICIDAL USE", my experience is so limited that I am unable to cover all the research activities in this area. Therefore, I will summarize my small experience on the research and development of tetranactin, which is the only antibiotic miticide commercialized in Japan.

ISOLATION OF TETRANACTIN

A screening procedure is the most important for antibiotic research. Our ordinary screening procedure for antibiotic pesticides is shown in Fig. 1. A loopful of microorganism taken from a slant culture is transfered to production medium and the microorganisms are cultured by shaking for several days. Then, the culture broth is filtered and the filter cake is used for the screening source. Because most topically active antibiotic pesticides are water insoluble lipophilic substances and the filter cake contains most of active principles. This procedure is a characteristic point differentiating it from other antibiotic screening. The filter cake is extracted with acetone or methanol at room temperature overnight. Then, the extract is topically applied to Azukibean weevils on filter paper, or a drop of the extract is added to a test tube containing mosquito larvae. The mortality is usually counted 24 h later.

When some extracts showed insecticidal activity, the shake culture was repeated and the reproducibity was confirmed. After confirmation of the reproducibility the active principles were purified from the extract. Our ordinary purification procedures are essentially the same as those for purifying natural products, for example, solvent extraction, concentration in vacuo, fractionation with column chromatography, fractional distillation and recrystalization. For each step of purification, it is essential to determine which fractions the active principles are distributed. Therefore, the test organisms should be readily available and rapidly propagating ones. We used Azukibean weevil as a test insect, because the weevil is readily propagated only with the use of Azukibean and is highly sensitive to pesticides. The wiggler is another suitable insect for screening. The test method is a dipping so that we can detect not only contact poison but also oral poison.

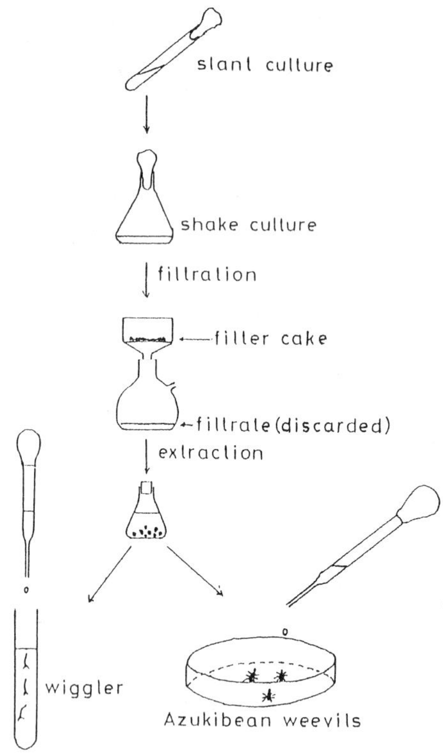

Fig. 1. Our screening procedure for insecticidal antibiotics.

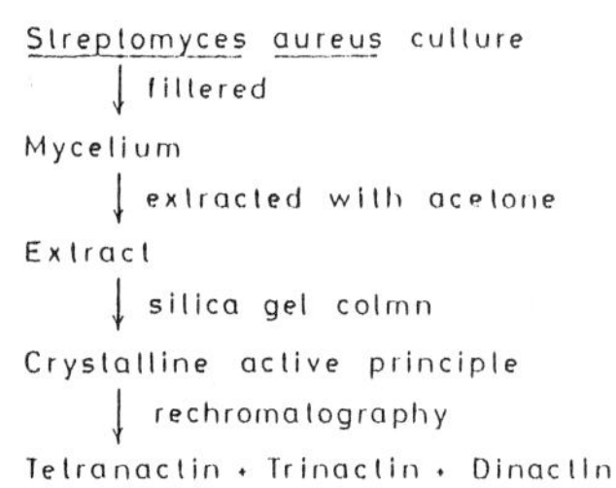

Fig. 2. Isolation procedure for tetranactin.

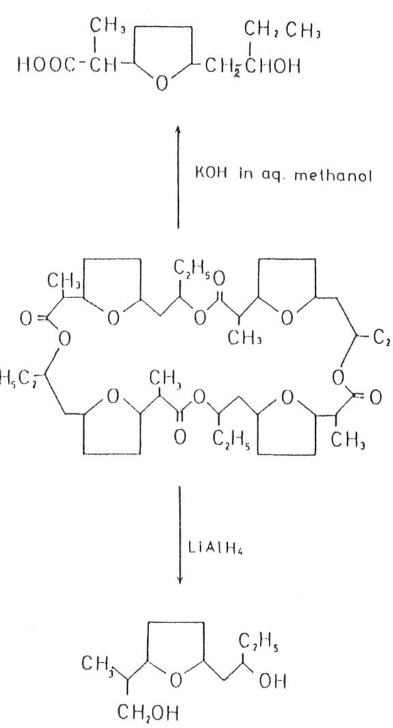

Fig. 3. Structural elucidation of tetranactin.

Using this screening system, we have identified insecticidal activity of some antibiotics. The followings are the examples of such antibiotics. Aureothin is an antimicrobial antibiotic with a nitro group (3). The antibiotic is topically active against certain kinds of insects and mites (4). Antifungal antibiotics, antimycins (5-7) are also active against mites (8). Polyether antibiotics are a large group containing more than 20, and a representative of this group, monensin (9), kills insects and mites when topically applied (unpublished observation). Piericidins were first isolated by Prof. Takahashi of Tokyo Univ (10). The close structural similarity to ubiquinone evoked the interest of biochemists and the effect on electron transport system has been reported (11). Piericidins are highly active against insects and mites.
However, all of these antibiotics are highly toxic to warm-blooded animals. Eighteen years ago, we observed that an unidentified soil streptomycetes

produced potent insecticidal substances in the filter cake of the fermented broth (12). The producing micoorganism was later identified as Streptomyces aureus S-3466 (13). The purification procedure is demonstrated in Fig. 2. The filter cake of the fermented broth was extracted with acetone and the extract was concentrated in vacuo. The residue was applied to silica gel column chromatography yielding crystalline active principle as large prisms. Fig. 3 shows the process of its structural elucidation (14). On alkaline hydrolysis, we obtained homononactic acid as a methyl ester (15). On reduction with lithium aluminum hydride, we isolated a diol with tetrahydrofurane ring as a sole product. Therefore, we could elucidate the structure and designated it tetranactin, because the antibiotic is composed of four equal structural unit called homononactic acid.

MITICIDAL ACTIVITY OF TETRANACTIN

Active spectrum- As shown in Table 1., tetranactin exerts potent pesticidal activity against the carmine spider mite (Tetranychus cinnabarinus) alone. The LC_{50} is 4.8 μg/ml with the spray method. Other pests, for example, the house fly and cockroach are insensitive to it. Azukibean weevil (Callosobruchus chinensis) and larvae of mosquito (Culex pipiens molestus) are moderately sensitive to the antibiotic.

TABLE 1. Active spectrum of tetranactin

organisms	methods	LC_{50} or LD_{50}
Tetranychus cinnabarinus adult	spray	4.8 μg/ml
Aleuroglyphus ovatus adult	film contact	238.8 μg/cm^2
Tyrophagus dimidiatus adult	film contact	80.0 μg/cm^2
Callosobruchus chinensis adult	topical appl.	0.8 μg/weevil
Musca domestica adult	topical appl.	>4.0 μg/fly
Blattella germanica adult	topical application	>4.0 μg/cockroach
Culex pipiens molestus larva	dipping	7.0 μg/ml

Miticidal activity in green house- The LC_{50} 's for four species of mites are shown in Table 2. Concentrations of less than 10ppm are lethal to the adults of the carmine spider, two-spotted spider, kanzawa spider and European red mites. However, tetranactin is only weakly ovocidal against the mites, probably due to the less permeable property of the eggs.

Field test- The miticidal activity was corroborated in field trials by spraying tetranactin suspension on apple trees on whose leaves kanzawa spider mites and European red mites were

TABLE 2. Miticidal activity in green House.

mites tested	LC_{50} (ppm) adult	LC_{50} (ppm) egg
T. cinnabarinus	4.8	59
T. urticae	9.4	80
T. kanzawa	7.2	110
P. ulmi	2.2	50

TABLE 3. Miticidal activity of tetranactin in field test.

agents	mite	concn (ppm)	No. of mite before spray	mite population after spraying (days) 6	24	32
tetranactin	P. ulmi	133	511	1.8 (%)	0.6 (%)	0.6 (%)
		100	403	2.4	0.8	1.6
	T. kanzawa	133	780	1.4	5.5	2.3
		100	430	3.5	9.3	0.0
kelthane	P. ulmi	200	230	0.0	5.0	5.0
	T. kanzawa	"	208	2.4	21.6	11.5
control	P. ulmi		241	408.2	130.0	88.9
	T. kanzawa		114	606.1	42.1	24.6

Numbers of mites/20 leaves collected randomly.
Mite populations were expressed as No. of mites after spray/before spray (%)

naturally parasitic. For comparison kelthane was sprayed on adjacent plots. As the last column of Table 3 shows, on the 32nd day after spraying the mite populations were reduced to 2-3% or less of their pre-spraying numbers where tetranactin was used. Kelthane effectiveness was appreciably less(15).

Acquisition of resistance- It is nearly impossible for mites to acquire resistance to tetranactin. We tried to derive pure strain of resistant carmine spider mites by serial transfers of mites surviving after exposure to sub-lethal concentrations once every three weeks for 6 years. Although LC_{50} of the sensitive strain approximately doubled during the six years (for reason unknown), the resistant strain's LC_{50} was still twice as high as that of sensitive strain (Fig. 4.).

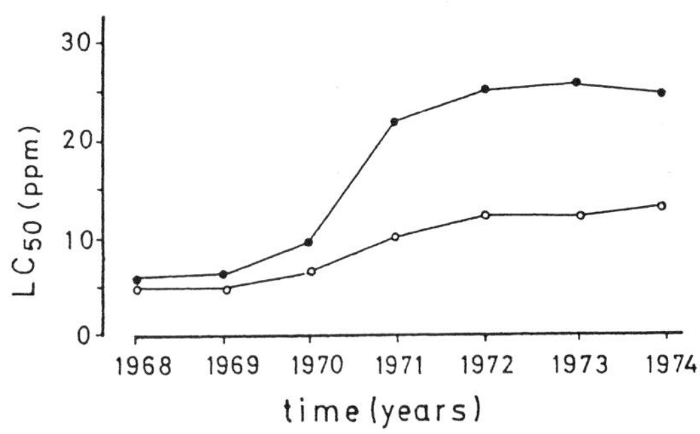

Fig. 4. Acquisition of resistance to tetranactin

The carmine spider mites were used in this study. Filled circles; resistant variants. Open circles; sensitive parent.

Synergistic action with other chemicals- A large number of chemicals were examined to find a synergist for the antibiotic. Consequently, 2-secondary butylphenyl-N-methylcarbamate (BPMC), p-chlorophenyl-p'-chlorobenzenesulfonate (CPCBS) and some organophosphorous insecticides were found potent synergists. Fig. 5 demonstrates synergistic miticidal action of tetranactin with BPMC. As an added bonus the synergistic combinations not only increased the lethal effects on adults but greatly improved the residual ovocidal effect of tetranactin (16,17).

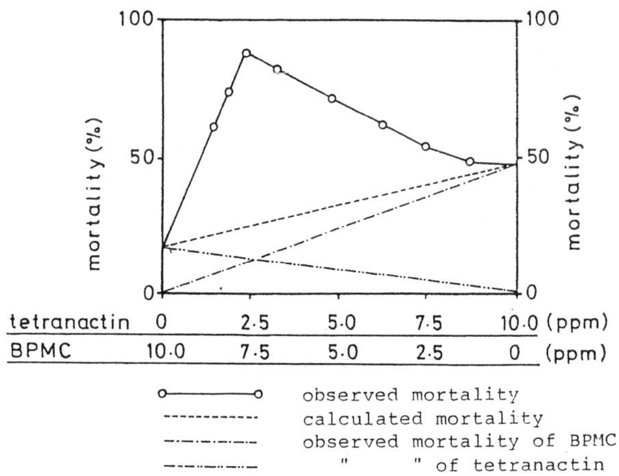

Fig. 5. Synergistic action of tetranactin with BPMC.

The carmine spider mites were used in this study.

FATE OF TETRANACTIN IN SOIL AND PLANTS

Absorption and transfer in plant- Absorption and transfer through the leaf, stem and root of Yabukita strain tea were examined using U-[^{14}C]-tetranactin. It was found that tetranctin is little absorbed through the leaf, stem and root, and it remained intact on the leaf in the dark.

Decay on tea leaf-Tetranactin is highly susceptible to sunlight, although it is resistant to weathering. When U-[^{14}C]-tetranactin was sprayed on tea leaves, it rapidly decomposed on exposure to sunlight. Degradation was more than 50% after 2 days exposure. The degradation products are so complex that they have not been identified yet completely.

Degradation in soil (18)- Degradation of tetranactin seems to be primarily due to soil microorganisms. Soil bacteria such as *Bacillus* species and *Micrococcus* sp. readily hydrolyze the ester bond yielding homononactic acid, although they do not further assimilate the acid (Fig. 6). Soil fungi and other bacteria seem to participate in decomposing homononactic acid into water and carbon dioxide. U-[^{14}C]-tetranactin was degraded to the final products, carbon dioxide and water with a half life of 8-10 days. Thus, by the combined action of soil bacteria and fungi, supplemented by sunlight, the antibiotic rapidly and harmlessly disappears from the environment.

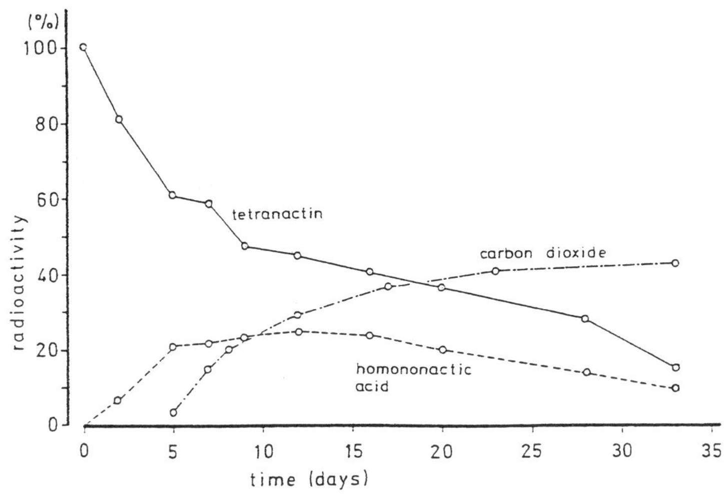

Fig. 6. Degradation of U-[^{14}C]-tetranactin in soil

UTILIZATION OF COMPLEX FORMING PROPERTY

Homononactic acid has four asymetric carbons in its molecule. Therefore, the antibiotic possess 2^{16} stereoisomers. We elucidated the stereochemical structure by x-ray crystallography. Fig. 7 shows the computer drawn structure of tetranactin. The large balls represent oxygens and carbons, the small balls hydrogens. The molecule is rather flat and twisted.

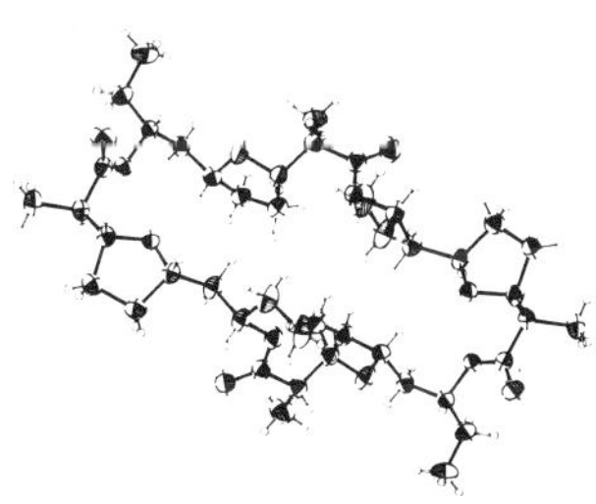

Fig. 7. Stereochemical structure of free tetranactin(19)

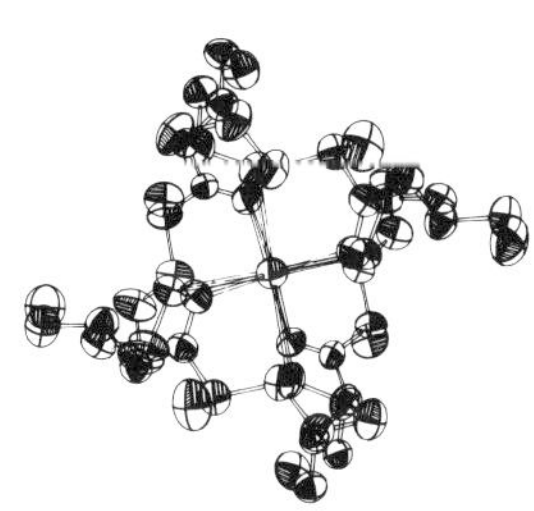

Fig. 8. Structure of tetranactin rubidium complex (20)

The macrotetrolide antibiotic is called an ionophore antibiotic because it specifically forms a complex with alkaline cations. Fig. 8. depicts the crystalline structure of tetranactin-rubidium complex. The molecule is globular in contrast with the free tetranactin. The rubidium ion is located at the center of the globule and is fixed with an ion-dipole of ether and carbonyl oxygens. The surface of the globule is covered with lipophilic moieties such as ethyls, methyls and methylenes. Therefore the complex readily dissolves in most organic solvents, for example, chloroform, dichloromethane and ethylacetate (21,22). This is how the complex works. If an alkaline cation approaches the free tetranactin, the antibiotic envelopes the ion. Both the ether oxygens of tetrahydrofurane and the ester carbonyl oxygens are slightly charged electronegatively due to ion dipole moment, so that they interact with the cation to fix it at the center of the globule. The globule is lipophilic due to its outer covering of lipophilic moieties, so the antibiotic makes the cation lipophilic.

We developed a method for the quantitative determination of tetranactin by utilizing its complex forming property (23). The principle of assay method is based on difference in solubility between the complex and Na salt. The antibiotic and its complex with sodium picrate are readily soluble in dichloromethane but insoluble in water. Sodium picrate is soluble in water but insoluble in dichloromethane. If the antibiotic is present in the lower dichloromethane layer, vigorous shaking with aqueous sodium picrate generates tetranactin-sodium complex. The sodium ion is extracted in association with the picrate ion owing to the interaction between them. Therefore, we can estimate the antibiotic by measuring absorption of the transfered picrate ion. This assay method gives a straight calibration curve from 0 to 40 μg/ml (Fig 9). The method is simple and reproducible. Recently, Prof. Ishibashi of Kyushu Univ., reported a more sensitive assay method. They used a fluorescent compound, 8-aniline-1-naphthalene-sulfonate instead of picrate. His method is approximately 10-100 times more sensitive than ours (23b).

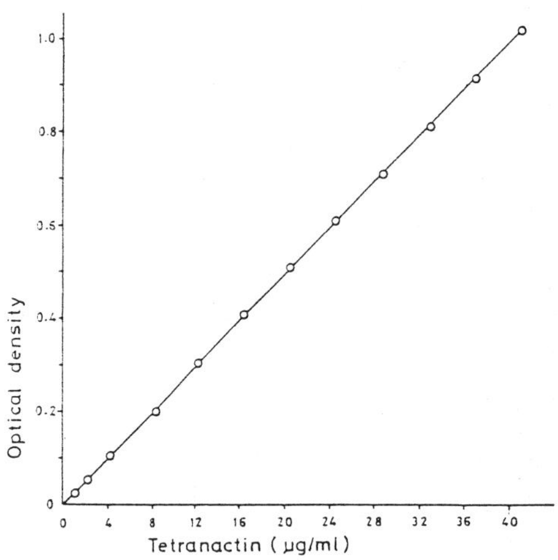

Fig. 9. Standard curve for tetranactin

The upper layer is sodium picrate, 0.4 mg/ml, in distiled water in a total volume of 5ml, and the lower layer dichloromethane (10 ml) containing tetranactin. Optical density of the dehydrated dichloromethane layer is measured at 377 nm.

MODE OF ACTION

Reactivation of tetranactin dry film by water- The macrotetrolide antibiotic acts as an uncoupler in oxydative phosphorylation. We also confirmed that tetranactin causes uncoupling in cockroach mitochondria (unpublished observation). However, when large amounts of powdered tetranactin is applied to the mites they do not die. For example, mites placed on leaves covered with tetranactin dry film were quite safe under various humidity (Table 4). But water was sprayed on these leaves, all of the mites died soon after spraying (17). This activation of the antibiotic dry film is attributable to regeneration of the antibiotic suspension by free water. So water is an essential factor for the miticidal activity.

We can interpret this activation on the basis of the complex formation. All living cells maintain a relatively high potassium content. The intracellular potassium ion is surrounded by water molecules so that it is unable to leak through the biomembrane. However, when the antibiotic aqueous suspension contacts with mites, tetranactin will be incorporated into the biomembrane because of its lipophilic property. Once the antibiotic is incorporated, it makes a hole in the cell membrane which allows the potassium ion to pass out.

TABLE 4. Activation of tetranactin dry film by water

Methods	Mites	Mortality(%) at RH		
		100%	50%	30%
Dry film reactivated by water spraying	P. ulmi	100	100	100
	T. kanzawa	100	100	100
Dry film contact	P. ulmi	10.0	7.5	8.8
	T. kanzawa	12.4	9.5	6.7

Aqueous tetranactin suspension was thoroughly sprayed on the leaves of eggbean planted in pots, and 24 h later the mites were transfered on the leaves with a soft brush. Then, the pots were placed at various humidity with or without spraying water.

In conclusion, the complex forming property is the most important in understanding the biological and chemical properties of tetranactin.
I hope that our limited experience will be useful for those who wish to participate in the research and development of new antibiotics for insecticidal use.

Acknowledgement-This research and development have been carried out in collaboration with my colleagues, Drs. Y.Nawata, H.Oishi, K.Suzuki, H.Sasaki, F.Saitoh, K.Nogaki, T.Sagawa, S. Hirano, T.Ichikawa, M.Hara, M.Yoshimoto, Y.Iwane and K. Togashi. I express my sincere thanks to my colleagues.

REFERENCES

1. T.Takemoto and T.Nakajima, Yakugaku Zashi 84,1230-32(1964)
2. T.Takemoto, T.Nakajima and T.Yokobe, ibid 84, 1232-33(1964)
3. Y.Hirata, H.Nakada and S.Yamada, J.Chem.Soc.Japan 79,390-91(1958)
4. H.Oishi,T.Hosokawa, T.Okutomi, K.Suzukiand K.Ando, Agr.Biol.Chem. 33,1790-91(1969)
5. C.Leben and G.W.Keit, Phytopathology 32,14-18(1947)
6. K.Watanabe, T.Tanaka, K.Fukuhara, N.Miyairi, H.Yonehara and H.Umezawa, J.Antibiot. 10A,39-45(1957)
7. A.J.Birch, D.W.Cameron, Y.Harada and R.W.Richards,J.Chem.Soc.1962,303-5
8. G.S.Kido and E.Spihalski, Science 112,172-3(1950)
9. A.Agtarap, J.W.Chamberlin, M.Pinkerton and L.Steinrauf, J.Am.Chem.Soc. 89,5737-5739(1967)
10. S.Tamura, N.Takahashi, S.Miyamoto, R.Mori, S.Suzuki and J.Nagatsu, Agr.Biol.Chem.27,576-581(1963)
11. S.Yoshida and N.Takahashi, Heterocycles 10,425-467(1978)
12. H.Oishi, T.Sagawa,T.Okutomi, K.Suzuki, H.Okazaki, M.Sawada and K.Ando, J.Antibiot. 23,105-6(1970)
13. K.Ando, H.Oishi, S.Hirano, T.Okutomi, K.Suzuki, H.Okazaki, M.Sawada and K.Ando, J.Antibiot. 24,345-352(1971)
14. K.Ando, Y.Murakami and Y.Nawata, J.Antibiot. 24,418-422(1971)
15. J.Beck, H.Gerlach, V.Prelog and W.Voser, Helv.Chim.Acta 620-30(1962)
16. T.Sagawa, S.Hirano, H.Takahashi, T.Tanaka, H.Oishi, K.Ando and K.Togashi, J.Econ.Entomol. 66,349-51(1973)
17. S.Hirano, T.Sagawa, H.Takahashi,T.Tanaka, H.Oishi, K.Ando and K.Togashi, ibid 65, 372-75(1972)
18. H.Sasaki, K.Suzuki, T.Ichikawa, M.Sawada, Y.Iwane and K.Ando, Appl..Environmental Microbiol. 40,264-68(1980)
19. Y.Iitaka, T.Sakagami and Y.Nawata, Chem. Lett.(Tokyo) 1972,1225-30
19b. Y.Nawata, T.Sakagami and Y.Iitaka, Acta Cryst. B30,1047-68(1974)
20. T.Sakagami, Y.Iitaka and Y.Nawata, Acta Cryst. B32,768-774(1976)
21. T.Sakagami, Y.Iitaka and Y,Nawata, ibid B33,52-59(1977)
22. Y.Kyogoku, M.Ueno, H.Akutsu and Y.Nawata,Biopolymers 14,1049-64(1975)
23. K.Suzuki, Y.Nawata and K.Ando, J.Antibiot. 24,675-79(1971)
23b. K.Kima, K.Shirai and N.Ishibashi, Bunsei Kagaku 27,291-295(1978)

HOW TO DISCOVER NEW ANTIBIOTICS FOR HERBICIDAL USE

Yasuharu Sekizawa and Tetsuo Takematsu*

Laboratory of Agricultural and Veterinary Science, Research Laboratories, Meiji Seika Kaisha Ltd., Kohoku-ku, Yokohama 222, Japan
**Weed Control Research Institute, Faculty of Agriculture, Utsunomiya University, Utsunomiya 320, Japan*

Abstract - The findings of several microbial metabolites having herbicidal activities strongly suggested that microbial metabolites might be a promising source for new herbicidal substances. The current situation of the screening programs operated to find microbial metabolites having herbicidal activities was given.

INTRODUCTION

It has been described that several antibiotics possess the respective herbicidal activities. Those are cycloheximide (1)", anisomycin and toyocamycin (2)" (3)" (4)", herbicidin A and B (5)" (6)", and herbimycin (7)" (8)" (9)" (10)" (11)". Recently, it has been found that bialaphos ; L-2-amino-4-[(hydroxy)(methyl)phosphinoyl]-butyryl-L-alanyl-L-alanine, a streptomyces metabolite (12)" (13)" (14)" (15)" (16)" (17)" (18)" (19)" (20)", has a strong and broad herbicidal activity.

DESCRIPTION ON EACH HERBICIDAL METABOLITE

Cycloheximide

The practical application of cycloheximide antibiotics ; 3-[2-(3,5-dimethyl-2-oxocyclohexyl)-2-hydroxy-ethyl]glutarimide ; MEC (1) as a herbicide was first described by S. Tamura and T. Takematsu (21)". It was observed that MEC could well control perennial shrubs and annual weeds as either the soil-treatment chemicals for upland field or water-treatment chemicals for paddy field. The water-treatment prior to the transplantation of rice seedlings could control the germination and/or emergence of the root system and also completely killed the weeds under the submerged condition. It was confirmed that the dosage of MEC at 50 to 200g/10a of paddy field completely killed barnyard grass (*Echinochloa crus-galli*), broad leaf weeds, needle-upright clubrush (*Eleocharis acicularis*) and pond weed (*Potamogeton distinctus*) without phytotoxicity against rice plant seedlings.

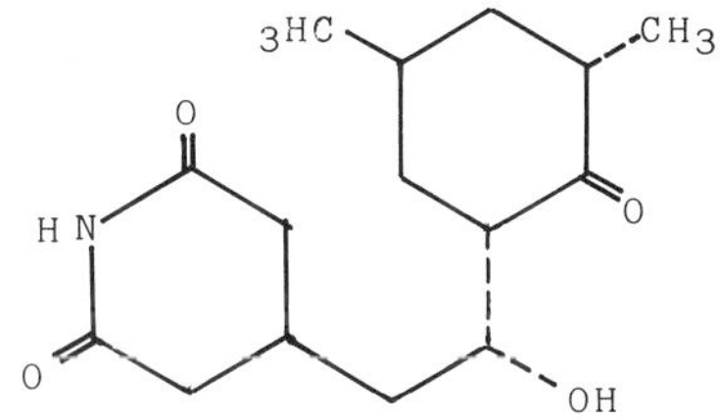

(1)

Anisomycin, toyocamycin and NK-049

O. Yamada, Y. Kaise, F. Futatsuya, S. Ishida, k. Ito, H. Yamamoto and K. Munakata observed that a streptomyces produced plant growth controlling factors which inhibited the growth of root than those did the growth of top of test plants, when the seedlings of rice plant, barnyard grass, crabgrass (Digitaria sanguiralis), lucerne, tomato and turnip were used as test plants (2)". The active substances were identified with the known antibiotics, anisomycin (3)" (2) and toyocamycin (4)" (3).

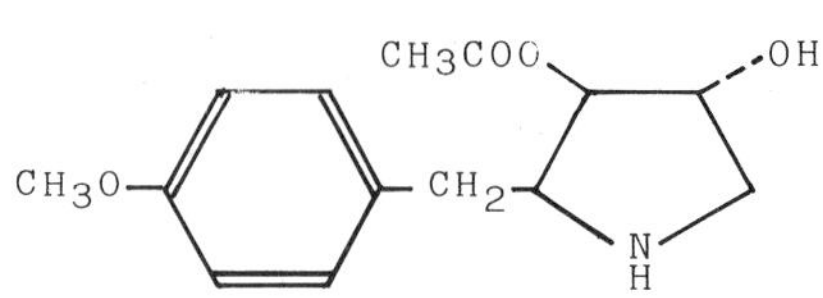

(2)

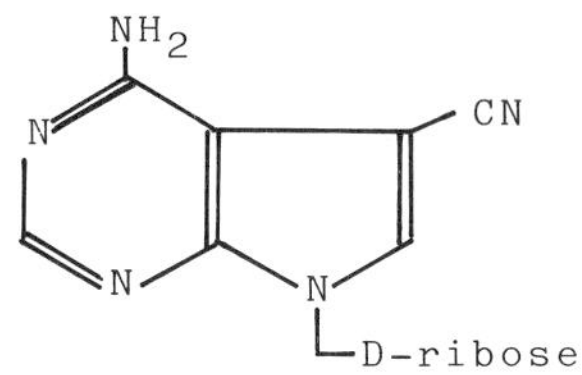

(3)

The N-acetyl-anisomycin derived did not show any of growth controlling activity upon test plants. The extensive synthetic studies on the relatives of anisomycin resulted in the finding of a new type of herbicidal compound, that is, 3,3'-dimethyl-4-methoxy benzophenone ; NK-049 ; methoxyphenone (4). NK-049 showed a high effectiveness against most of annual weed species by the pre-emergence treatment, and it was absorbed mainly via young shoots of weeds at the time of emergence and induced severe chlorosis which led to kill weeds. Thus, NK-049 was succesfully developed and commercialized being found its adaptabilities for an upland and paddy field herbicide (22)" (23)".

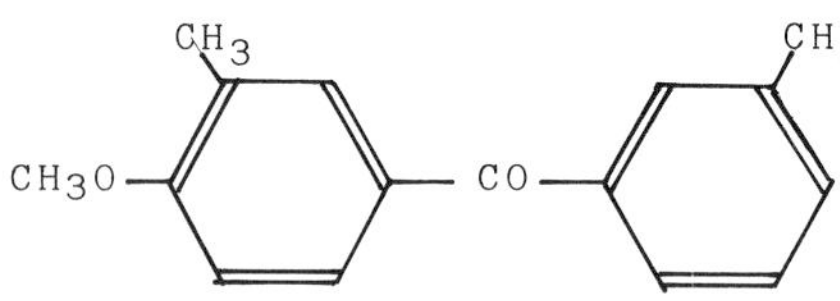

(4)

Herbicidin A and B

M. Arai, T. Haneishi, N. Kitahara, R. Enokita, K. Kawakubo and Y. Kondo described that Streptomyces saganoensis nov. sp. produced two new antibiotics, herbicidin A and B, having selective and contact herbicidal activities and that their characteristic features were brought into relief by their selective and contact killing effect on many dicotyledonous plant as well as their inhibitions upon the germination of plant seeds. Although the final conclusions are not yet given, it is noted that both herbicidin A and B are novel antibiotics of adenine nucleoside analogs having the interrelated chemical structures (5)" (6)".

Herbimycin

S. Omura, Y. Iwai, Y. Takahashi, N. Sadakane, A. Nakagawa, H. Oiwa and Y. Hasegawa found a herbicidal new antibiotic designated as herbimycin (7)" (8)" (9)" (10)" (11)". It was observed that herbimycin exhibited a potent herbicidal activity against most mono- and di-cotyledonous plants, especially against flat-sedge (Cyperus microiria). Rice plant, in turn, showed strong resistance against herbimycin. For most weeds, herbimycin was more active in the pre-emergence use than in the post-emergence use. Extensive studies on the chemical properties of herbimycin revealed that herbimycin was consisted of two active components, A and B, and that herbimycin A and B are two new antibiotics of ansamycin analog (5).

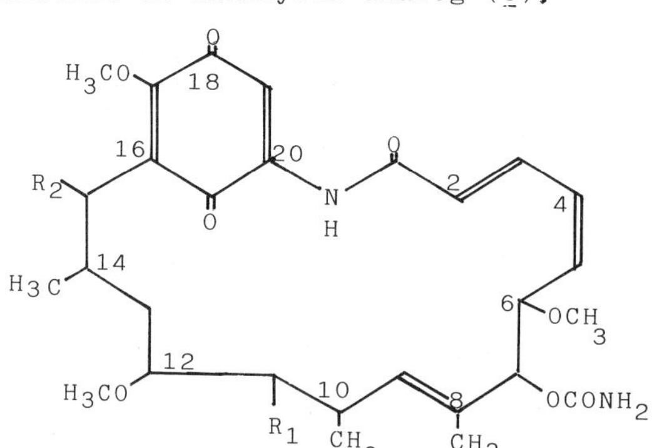

	R_1	R_2
Herbimycin A	OCH_3	OCH_3
Herbimycin B	OH	H

(5)

Bialaphos

Bialaphos ; L-2-amino-4-[(hydroxy)(methyl)phosphinoyl]-butyryl-L-alanyl-L-alanine ; phosphinothricyl-alanylalanine (6)" was an antimicrobial metabolite isolated from culture filtrate of streptomyces by Japanese (12)" (14)" (15)"(16)" (17)" (18)" (19)" (20)" and German (13)" microbial chemists. Afterwards, a strong and broad herbicidal activity of bialaphos was found. Bialaphos controls both dicotyledons and monocotyledons, and is useful for the control of many kinds of weeds of agricultural importance such as barnyard grass, lambs quarter (*Chenopodium album*), purple nutsedge (*Cyperus rotundus*), curly dock (*Rumex crispus*), water hyacinth (*Eichhorma crassiper*).

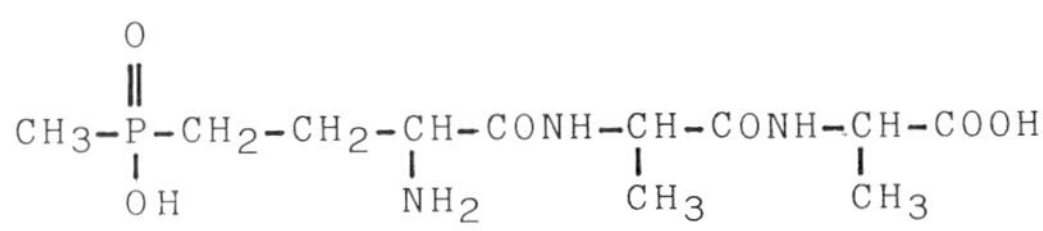

(6)

Merely Japanese cyprus has been found to be tolerant to bialaphos. The standard rate of application of bialaphos is 10 to 30g/a depending on the growth stages of weeds whether or not they are annuals or perennials. Bialaphos is slower acting than paraquat, and significantly faster acting than glyphosate. Bialphos controls the regrowth of perennials longer than paraquat, and has long lasting effect like glyphosate. Bialaphos acts to any growth stage of weeds by foliage treatment, but shows no or very weak activity by soil treatment and shows the possibility of the applications to orchard and mulberry field (19)" (20)". The number of newly formed tubers of purple nutsedge was significantly decreased by the foliage treatment of bialaphos, and L-2-amino-4-[(hydroxy)(methyl)phosphinoyl]-butyric acid ; phosphinothricin ; L-AMPB (16)" (24)" (7), a main active metabolite of bialaphos in the weed, was detected in the tubers of yellow nutsedge (*Cyperus esculentus*).

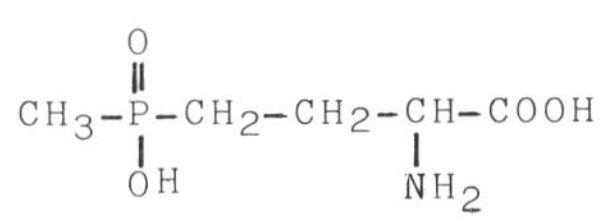

(7)

Further, when 150g/10a of bialaphos was applied upon crabgrass by watering of 100 l/10a, it was observed that bialaphos absorbed into crabgrass at the 4 to 4.5 leaf stage was rapidly metabolized to L-2-amino-4-[(hydroxy)(methyl)-phosphinoyl]-butyryl-L-alanine and the L-AMPB as shown in Fig.1.

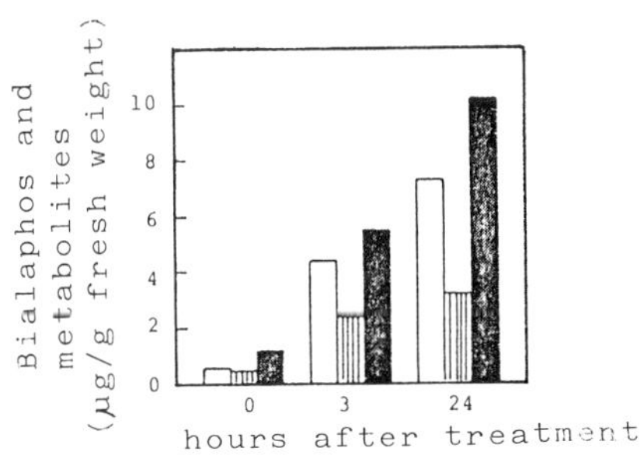

Fig. 1. Absorption of bialaphos into crabgrass and its metabolites in the leaves. Bialaphos and its metabolites were quantitatively analyzed by a Hitachi automatic amino acid analyzer. (open bar); bialaphos, (hatched bar); L-AMPB-ala, (solid bar); L-AMPB.

When 150g/10a to 300g/10a of bialaphos as indicated in Fig. 2 was applied to yellow nutsedge by watering of 100 l/10a, bialaphos killed not simply the terrestrial parts, but also inhibited the regrowth from the underground parts, and L-AMPB was dtermined as shown in Fig. 3 and 4 (25)".

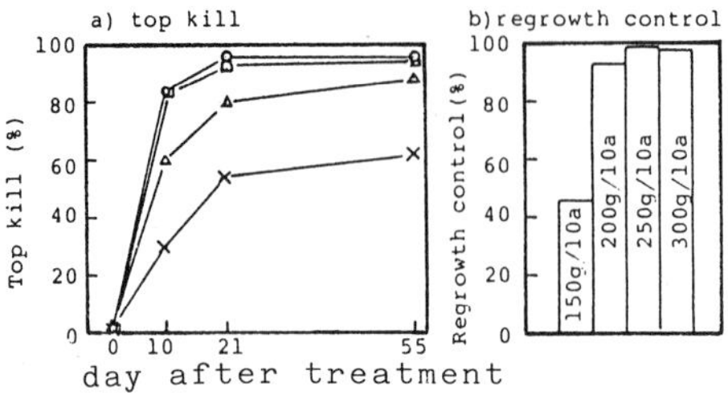

Fig. 2. Herbicidal effect of bialaphos upon yellow nutsedge. —×— ; 150g/10a, —△— ; 200g/10a, —□— ; 250g/10a, —○— ; 300g/10a.

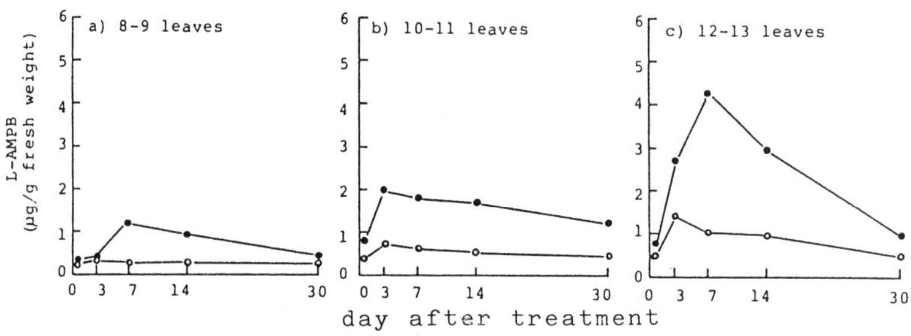

Fig. 3. Translocation of L-AMPB to basal bulb of yellow nutsedge after bialaphos treatment. —○— ; bialaphos 150g/10a, —●— ; bialaphos 300g/10a.

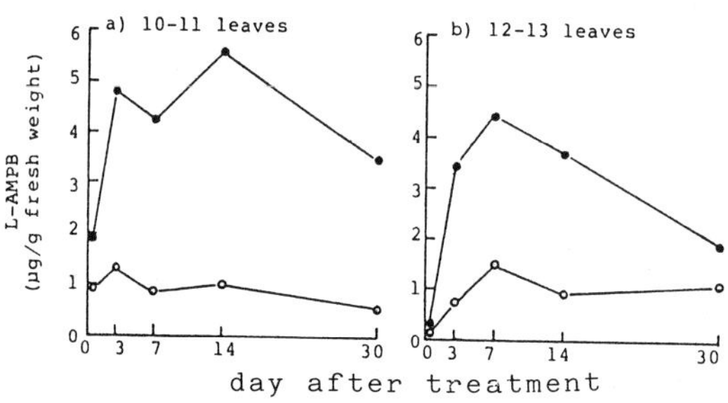

Fig. 4. Translocation of L-AMPB to tubers of yellow nutsedge after bialaphos treatment. —○— ; bialaphos 150g/10a, —●— ; bialaphos 300g/10a.

A new aminotransferase (GOGAT) has been found recently in plants, and is now considered to be functioning for nitrogen assimilation with glutamine synthetase (GS) as GS-GOGAT system (26)". L-AMPB was found to compete with glutamate as a potent inhibitor of plant and microbial GS (13)". As the result of GS inhibition, the accumulation of ammonia was actually observed at 4 to 24 hours after the foliage treatment of bialaphos (27)". Therefore, the inhibition of GS-GOGAT system, which brings about the accumulation of ammonia and the inhibition of nitrogen assimilation, was the main cause of herbicidal activity. It should be reminded that methionine sulfoximine (8) had been proposed for a potent herbicidal compound by B. L. Walworth (28)", although this compound is not a natural product. The compound was also known as an inhibitor upon glutamine synthetase of pea (29)". A surprising event was a recent finding of L-(N^5- phosphono)methionine-S-sulfoximinyl-L-alanyl-L-alanine (9) as an metabolite of unclassified species of streptomyces (30)".

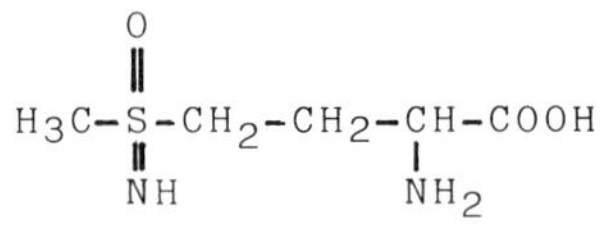

(8)

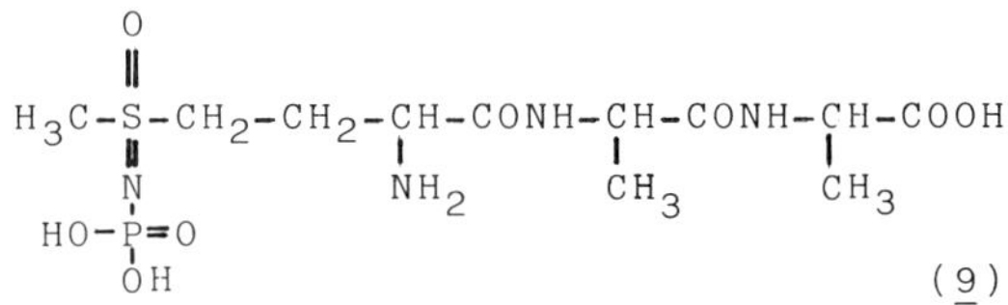

(9)

And L-(N^5-phosphono)methionine-S-sulfoximine moiety (10) was found to be a very potent inhibitor of glutamine synthetase (31)".

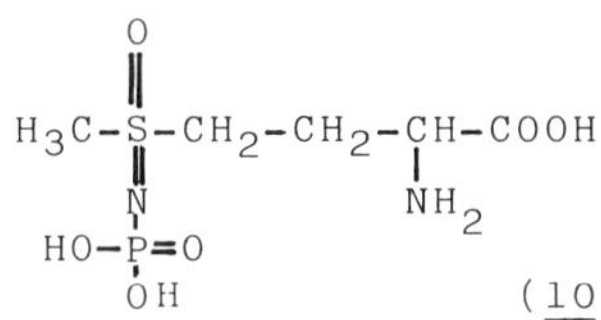

(10)

It should be mentioned relating to those inhibitors upon glutamine synthetase that the tabtoxinine (11) , a moiety of tabtoxin, the wildfire toxin produced by plant pathogen, Pseudomonas tabaci, is also an inhibitor upon glutamine synthetase (29)". The correct chemical structure of tabtoxinine (11) was deceided as following formula by W. W. Stewart (32)". It is remarkable finding that tabtoxinine is a monocyclic-ß-lactum metabolite produced by bacterium.

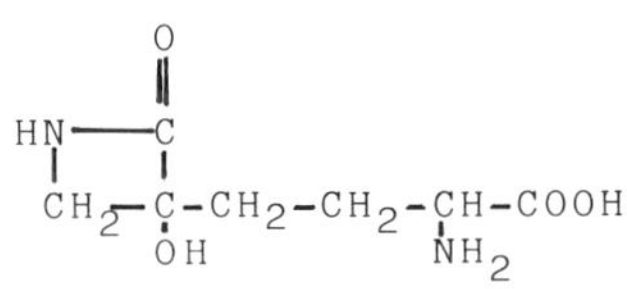

(11)

Regarding optical isomers,that is, D-forms of these glutamine synthetase inhibitors, it is yet unexplored whether these D-forms inhibit the glutamine synthetase activity and whether those possess the individual herbicidal activity. J. Goi, S. Miyado, T. Shomura, A. Suzuki, T. Niwa and Y. Yamada described the optical resolution of racemic AMPB (33)". When N-acyl-D,L-AMPB was fermentatively deacylated using either pseudomonas,streptomyces or aspergillus, merely L-form was deacylated. The resultant solutin of mixture of L-form and N-acylated D-form was subjected to Dowex 50 column to adsorb merely L-form, and the column was eluted with water and concentrated to obtain a pure crystals of L-AMPB. From N-acyl-D-form in the effluent solution, a pure crystals of D-form were prepared. And it was further confirmed that L-AMPB thus obtained exhibited the full herbicidal activity against L-AMPB obtained from bialaphos, in turn, D-AMPB practically did not show the herbicidal activity. As the result, it is concluded that D-AMPB has not the herbicidal activity. The environmental toxicological evaluation of bialaphos is under progress indicating its high feasibility of the practical use in agriculture. The summerized conclusion will be given in near future. From the experiments conducted to analyze the degradation of bialaphos in soil at model conditions, it was indicated as shown in Fig. 5 and 6 that bialaphos was rapidly hydrolyzed to L-AMPB via L-AMPB-alanine and that L-AMPB was further degraded. In the sterilized soil at 120°C for 15 minutes, the degradation of L-AMPB was no more observed as shown in Fig. 7 (34)". These experimental results strongly suggested that the degradation of L-AMPB in soil was operated by microbial actions. Actually,the unclassified soil bacteria isolated catalyzed the deamination of L-AMPB and the subsequent oxidation. At present, a following profile of the degradation pathway is proposed ;

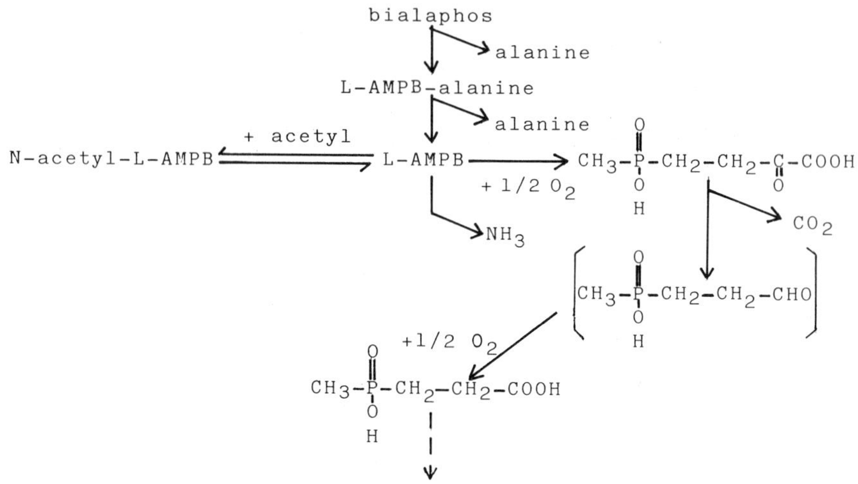

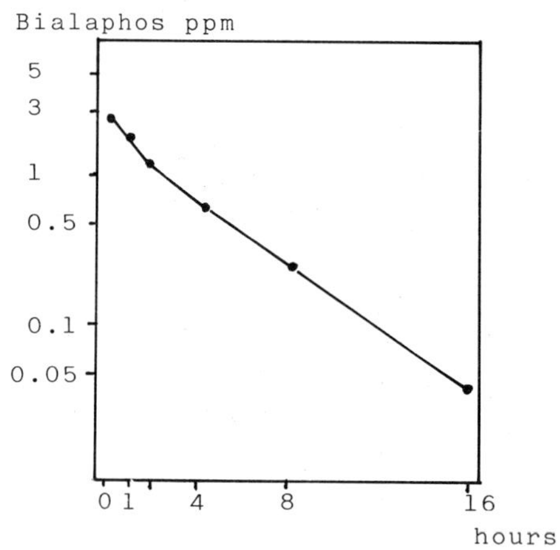

Fig. 5. The decay of bialaphos in soil at a model condition. Bialaphos was determined by a Hitachi automatic amino acid analyzer.

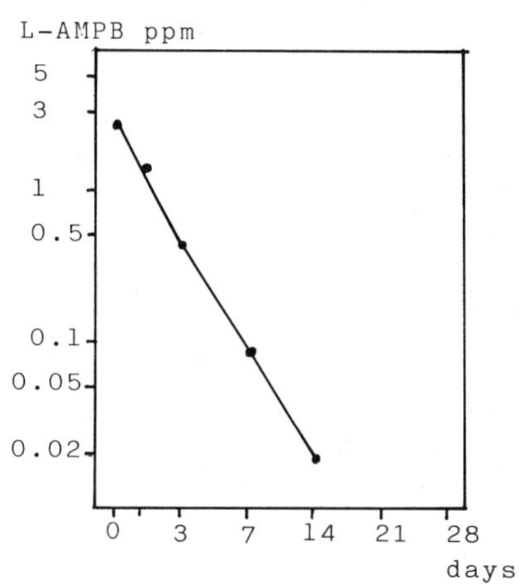

Fig. 6. The decay of L-AMPB in soil at a model condition. L-AMPB was determined by a Hitachi automatic amino acid analyzer.

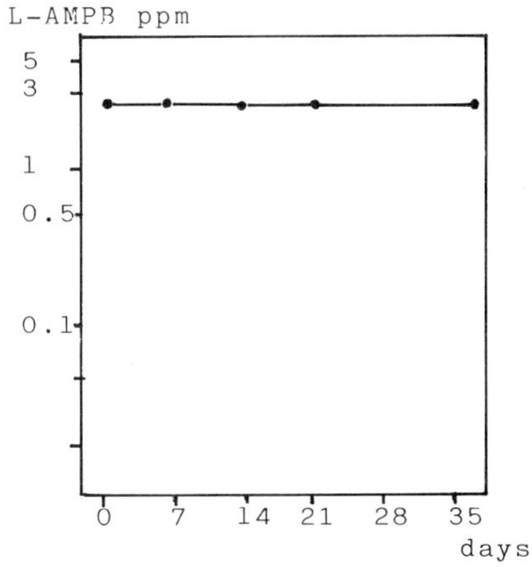

Fig. 7. The decay of L-AMPB in a sterilized soil. The soil was sterilized at 120°C for 15 minutes.

CONCLUDING REMARKS

The knowledges and techniques regarding the screening of bilogically active metabolites from soil microbial source have been extensively accumulated on the basis of soil microbiology since the finding of streptomycin by S. A. Waksman (35)". On the other hand, the chemical control of weeds has been also actively developed depending on the progress of organic synthetic chemistry. The close cooperation between soil microbiology and weed science will bring the novel herbicidal metabolites which have higher adaptabilities in view of their efficacy and the environmental safty.

Acknowledgement - Authors are grateful to Dr. T. Misato, Director, The Institute of Physical and Chemical Research, and Dr. T. Niida, Director, Research Laboratories, Meiji Seika Kaisha, Ltd., for the giving of the opportunity to publish this work.

REFERENCES

1. W.C. Cooper, G.K. Rasmussen, B.J. Rogers, P.C. Peece and W.H. Henry, Plant Physiol., 43 (Pt. B), 1560 - 1576 (1968).
2. O. Yamada, Y. Kaise, F. Futatsuya, S. Ishida, K. Ito, H. Yamamoto and K. Munakata, Agric. Biol. Chem., 36, 2013 - 2015 (1972).
3. B.A. Sobin and F.W. Tanner, Jr., J. Am. Chem. Soc., 76, 4053 (1954).
4. H. Nishimura, K. Katagiri, K. Sato, M. Mayama and N. Shimaoka, J. Antibiotics, 9A, 60 - 62 (1956).
5. M. Arai, T. Haneishi, N. Kitahara, R. Enokita, K. Kawakubo and Y. Kondo, J. Antibiotics, 29, 863 - 869 (1976).
6. T. Haneishi, A. Terahara, H. Kayamori, J. Yabe and M. Arai, J. Antibiotics, 29, 870 - 875 (1976).
7. S. Omura, A. Nakagawa and N. Sadakane, Tetrahedron Lett., 4323 - 4326 (1976).
8. S. Omura, Y. Iwai, Y. Takahashi, N. Sadakane and A. Nakagawa, J. Antibiotics, 32, 255 - 261 (1979).
9. A. Furusaki and T. Matsumoto, A. Nakagawa and S. Omura, J. Antibiotics, 33, 781 - 782 (1980).
10. Y. Iwai, A. Nakagawa, N. Sadakane, S. Omura, H. Oiwa, S. Matsumoto, M. Takahashi, T. Ikai and Y. Ochiai, J. Antibiotics, 33, 1114 - 1119 (1980).
11. A. Nakagawa, N. Sadakane and S. Omura, J. Chem. Soc. Japan ; Chem. & Ind. Chem., 892 - 894 (1981).
12. T. Niida, S. Inouye, T. Tsuruoka, T. Shomura, Y. Kondo, Y. Ogawa, H. Watanabe, Y. Sekizawa, T. Watanabe and H. Igarashi, Japanese Patent, 827,768 (1976).
13. E. Bayer, K.H. Crugel, K. Hägele, H. Hagenmaier, S. Jessipow, W.A. König and H. Zähnen, Hel. Chim. Acta, 55, 224 - 239 (1972).
14. Y. Kondo, T. Shomura, Y. Ogawa, T. Tsuruoka, H. Watanabe, K. Totsukawa, T. Suzuki, C. Moriyama, J. Yoshida, S. Inouye and T. Niida, Sci. Rept. Meiji Seika Kaisha, 13, 34 - 41 (1973).

15. Y. Ogawa, T. Tsuruoka, S. Inouye and T. Niida, Sci. Rept. Meiji Seika Kaisha, 13, 42 - 48 (1973).
16. Y. Ogawa, H. Yoshida, S. Inouye and T. Niida, Sci. Rept. Meiji Seika Kaisha, 13, 49 - 53 (1973).
17. Y. Ogawa, H. Yoshida, S. Inouye and T. Niida, Sci. Rept. Meiji Seika Kaisha, 13, 54 - 59 (1973).
18. N. Ezaki, S. Amano, K. Fukushima, S. Inouye and T. Niida, Sci. Rept. Meiji Seika Kaisha, 13, 60 - 63 (1973).
19. K. Tachibana, Y. Suzuki, T. Watanabe, Y. Sekizawa, M. Konnai and T. Takamatsu, Abstracts of papers, Meeting of The Weed Sci. Soc. Jpn., Tokyo, 133 - 134 (1979).
20. K. Tachibana, Y. Suzuki, T. Watanabe, Y. Sekizawa, H. Kuramochi, M. Konnai and T. Takematsu, Abstracts of papers, Meeting of The Society of Chemical Regulation of Plant, Utsunomiya, 71 (1979).
21. S. Tamura and T. Takematsu, Japanese Patent,45-22,754 (1970).
22. F. Futatsuya, K. Hibi, S. Ishida, O Yamada and K. Munakata, Weed Sci., 10 - 15 (1974).
23. F. Futatsuya, K. Hibi, S. Ishida, O. Yamada and K. Munakata, Weed Sci., 16 - 20 (1974).
24. W. Rupp, M. Finke, H. Bieringer and P. Langelueddeke, Ger. Offen, 2,717,440 (1977).
25. K. Tachibana, H. Izawa, K. Matsumoto, T. Watanabe, Y. Sekizawa and T. Takematsu, Weed Res. Japan, 27 Suppl., 59 - 60 (1982).
26. P.J. Lea and B.J. Miflin, Nature, 251, 614 - 616 (1974).
27. K. Tachibana, T. Watanabe, S. Mase, Y. Sekizawa and T. Takematsu, Abstracts of papers, Meeting of The Pesticide Science Society of Japan, Nagoya, 128 (1981).
28. B.L. Walworth, U. S. Patent, 3,295,949 and 3,323,895 (1967).
29. S.L. Sinden and R.D. Durbin, Nature, 219, 379 - 380 (1968).
30. D.L. Pruess, J.P.Scannell, H.A. Ax, M. Kellet, F. Weiss, T.C. Demny and A. Stempel, J. Antibiotics, 26, 261 - 266 (1973).
31. R.A. Ronzio, W.B. Rowe and A. Meister, Biochemistry, 8, 1066 - 1075 (1969).
32. W.W. Stewart, Nature, 229, 174 - 178 (1971).
33. J. Goi, S. Miyado, T. Shomura, A. Suzuki, T. Niwa and Y. Yamada, Japanese Patent, S-55-47,630 (1980).
34. A. Suzuki, I. Hori, M. Shimura, T. Watanabe and Y. Sekizawa, Abstract submitted to Subtopic Vc, IUPAC, Kyoto (1982).
35. A. Schatz, E. Bugie and S. A. Waksman, Proc. Soc. Exp. Biol. Med., 55, 66 - 69 (1944).

DEVELOPMENT OF RESISTANCE TO AGRICULTURAL ANTIBIOTICS

Johan Dekker

Laboratory of Phytopathology, Agricultural University, Wageningen, The Netherlands

Abstract - Plant pathogenic microorganisms may become resistant to antifungal or antibacterial antibiotics, which are used for plant disease control. In most cases resistance is due to single gene mutation, and as a rule resistant mutants may easily be obtained in laboratory experiments. Most commonly resistance to antibiotics appears to be caused by a change at the site of action, and secondly by a decreased uptake. The mechanisms of resistance will be discussed for a number of antibiotics, and considered in relation to their mechanism of action.

The chance, however, that emergence of antibiotic-resistant cells may lead to disease control failure in the field, varies considerably for different antibiotics. This depends for a large part on the properties of the resistant mutants. When a link exists between resistance and a decrease of fitness, the build-up of a resistant pathogen population will be hampered. The situation with respect to this point, is discussed for the more important agricultural antibiotics.

INTRODUCTION

Many years before the era of systemic fungicides started, antibiotics have been used as model compounds to study selective and systemic action in plant disease control. A prominent example is the systemic antibiotic griseofulvin, detected as early as 1939. In recent years a large arsenal of selective and systemic fungicides has become available. In this way antibiotics have contributed significantly to innovation of chemical control, which until the middle of the 1960's was primarily based on surface protection of plants or seeds by conventional fungicides, such as copper compounds and dithiocarbamates. In addition a few antibiotics themselves have become important plant disease control agents.

Although the use of antibiotics and other selective, systemic fungicides greatly contributes to more efficient control of plant diseases, it also has led to some problems. One of them is the development of resistance to the chemical in plant pathogens, which in several cases has caused failure of disease control. Such problems have not, or only rarely and to a much lesser extent, been encountered with conventional fungicides.

This contribution reviews the mechanisms of action of antibiotics and the mechanisms of resistance to these compounds in plant pathogens. In addition attention will be paid to the hazards that emergence of resistance will lead to failure of disease control in practical agriculture.

MECHANISMS OF RESISTANCE

General

For a proper understanding of the mechanisms of resistance to antibiotics, knowledge of their mechanism of action is important. Many antibiotics appear to be specific-site inhibitors, i.e. they act primarily at specific sites in the fungal or bacterial metabolism, such as protein synthesis, nucleic acid metabolism or nuclear function, chitin synthesis, respiration and functioning of the membranes. In this respect they differ from most conventional fungicides, which act at many sites in the metabolism of the pathogen.

Development of resistance in fungal or bacterial pathogens to specific-site inhibitors may be due to a decreased affinity for the chemical at the reactive site or to compensation for the effects of the inhibition, e.g. by operation of an alternate pathway. Decreased sensitivity may further be caused by changes in the fungal cell that hamper the fungicide to reach the site of action, e.g. increased detoxification or a change in permeability of the protoplast membrane (Dekker, 1977).

Of interest is also naturally occurring resistance in organisms which themselves produce an antibiotic. In such cases compartmentalization, excretion or detoxification are important mechanisms (Vining, 1979).

Resistance to antifungal antibiotics, which are specific-site inhibitors, in most cases appears based on a change at the site of action. Secondly, decreased uptake due to permeability changes may be responsible for resistance. In principle the latter mechanism may apply to specific-site as well as non-specific-site inhibitors.

Protein synthesis

Streptomycin. Streptomycin, discovered in 1944 as a product of *Streptomyces griseus*, has been used primarily for medical purposes. It appeared, however, also active against various plant pathogens, namely bacteria, and some fungi. In studies with *Escherichia coli* it was shown that streptomycin attaches to the 30 S sub-unit of the ribosome, and causes a misreading of the RNA code. In resistant mutants streptomycin does not bind to the 30 S sub-unit because a change in one of the constituting proteins (Ozaki et al., 1969).

Also plant pathogenic bacteria, among which *Erwinia amylovora*, the cause of fire blight, have shown their potential to become resistant to streptomycin. Resistance is caused by chromosomal mutation (Schroth et al., 1979).

Antifungal activity of this antibiotic has been reported for species of Oomycetes, but there is no indication that cytoplasmatic protein synthesis is inhibited in fungi. The probable site of action is mitochondrial protein synthesis (Siegel, 1977). Resistance may be a matter of low permeability, as the sensitive *Pythium* and *Phytophthora* species absorb 2-9 times as much antibiotic as insensitive species and antibiotic-resistant strains (Vörös, 1965).

Cycloheximide. Cycloheximide was discovered in 1946 in a culture filtrate of *Streptomyces griseus*. It shows high antifungal activity against a wide range of fungi and yeasts, but not against bacteria. Originally hailed in the popular press as the 'penicillin in plant disease control' its possibilities for control of plant diseases appeared limited because of phytotoxicity.

Cycloheximide has been shown to be a potent inhibitor of protein synthesis in yeast cells. It affects the transfer of amino acids from aminoacyl-transfer RNA's to the nascent polypeptide chain on the ribosome, and hampers the movement of ribosomes along the messenger RNA. In laboratory experiments cycloheximide-resistant mutants of *Saccharomyces cerevisiae* were easily obtained (Wilkie and Lee, 1965). The incorporation of amino acids into protein was inhibited in a cell free system from wild type cells, but not in that from resistant cells. Combination experiments with ribosomes and supernatant from sensitive and resistant cells learned that it was the ribosome which conferred resistance to the antibiotic (Cooper et al., 1967). It was later shown that the 60 S sub-unit of the ribosome, contains the binding site for the antibiotic, and it has been suggested that resistance involves specific alteration of a single protein component of this sub-unit, due to mutation (Siegel, 1977).

Cycloheximide may also affect RNA synthesis, as was shown in studies with Oomycetes, and a few other metabolic processes (Siegel, 1977).

No development of cycloheximide-resistance has been reported in practical agriculture, but the rather limited use of the antibiotic for control of plant diseases should be taken into consideration.

Blasticidin S. Blasticidin S, discovered in 1958 in the culture broth of *Streptomyces griseochromogenes*, was the first antibiotic, which has been used on a large scale in plant disease control, namely against rice blast, caused by *Pyricularia oryzae*. It has also antibacterial activity. Because of toxic side effects on humans and animals, and a rather small margin between curative and phytotoxic dosage, it has now largely been replaced by kasugamycin and other compounds.

Blasticidin S was reported to inhibit incorporation of amino acids into protein in extracts of *P.oryzae* and *E. coli*, where it binds to the 60 S and 50 S ribosomal subunit, respectively. It inhibits peptidyltransferase activity associated with chain elongation. The antibiotic is rather selective in its action against fungi. It is highly active against *P. oryzae*, but ineffective against *Pellicularia sasakii*, even at high concentrations. Protein synthesis in cell free extracts of the former fungus was inhibited, but not in that of the latter one, so that differences in the ribosome between these fungi might be the cause of selective action (Huang et al., 1964). Strains of *P. oryzae* , resistant to blasticidin S, were obtained on agar medium. Protein synthesis in cell free systems from these strains was, however, equally inhibited as in those from sensitive strains. It was shown that in this case resistance was based on decreased permability of the protoplast membrane for the antibiotic (Huang et al., 1964).

Although resistant strains of *P. oryzae* were easily obtained in the laboratory, no serious problems have been encountered in practice. It is not known whether this might be explained by decreased pathogenicity, as observed in mutants obtained in laboratory experiments (Nakamura and Sakurai, 1962).

Kasugamycin. Kasugamycin, discovered in 1965 in a culture broth of *Streptomyces kasugaensis*, is particularly active against rice blast. It has become the most widely used agricultural antibiotic. Remarkably the antibiotic shows no antifungal activity in vitro at pH 7 and above. Fungitoxicity is only expressed in the plant, or in the presence of plant juice at pH < 6. Inhibition of pathogen development by kasugamycin is observed only after penetration into the plant.

Kasugamycin shows only weak antibacterial activity except for species of *Pseudomonas*, which are relatively sensitive. In a cell free system derived from *E. coli* or from *P. fluorescens* the antibiotic inhibits protein synthesis by reacting with the 30 S ribosomal sub-unit. The ribosomes of a resistant strain, which appeared deficient in the methylation of the 16 S RNA part of the 30 S sub-unit (Helser et al., 1971) did not bind to the antibiotic.

In a cell free system from *P. oryzae* kasugamycin inhibits binding of aminoacyl-tRNA to ribosomes, when ribosomes from the sensitive strain were used, but not with ribosomes from the resistant strain, regardless of the source of tRNA. Thus also with this fungus acquired resistance appears to be due to decreased affinity of the ribosome to the antibiotic (Siegel, 1977).

In 1971 resistant strains of *P. oryzae* were isolated from rice fields, treated with kasugamycin. Genetic analysis of these isolates, which had become possible after the discovery of the perfect stage of this pathogen, *Magnaporthe grisea*, revealed that resistance is due to major gene mutation. So far three loci for kasugamycin resistance have been detected. One of these also controls resistance to blasticidin S (Taga et al., 1979).

Nucleic acid metabolism and nuclear function

Griseofulvin. Griseovulvin, a metabolic product from *Penicillium griseofulvin* and some other *Penicillium* species, is fungistatic for many pathogenic fungi, causing bursting, stunting, excessive branching, abnormal swelling and distortion of hyphae, often at very low concentrations. Fungi, belonging to the class of Oomycetes are insensitive. In the 1980's, more than a dekade after its discovery, it was found that this antibiotic could provide systemic protection of plants against various diseases, especially powdery mildews and *Botrytis* diseases. In the United Kingdom it was released for agricultural use in 1957, but it has, due to high cost and variable performance, not become widely used in plant disease control. In view of the shape of germ tube distortion, it was originally assumed that the antibiotic interferes with chitin synthesis, a theory which now has been abandoned. Studies with *Aspergillus nidulans* showed that spindles were distorted within 30-60 seconds after treatment (Crackower, 1972). In studies with the fungus *Basidiobolus ranarum*, daughter nuclei did not separate during cell division (Gull and Trinci, 1974). It is therefore assumed that griseofulvin inhibits mitosis by interference with formation or functioning of microtubules, but the site of action seems to differ from that of the benzimidazole fungicides.

After its development for agricultural purposes, griseofulvin was found to be useful also in the medical field, namely by oral administration against dermatophytes. Mutagenic treatment of one of these fungi, *Arthroderma simii*, resulted in emergence of strains with a high level of resistance to the antibiotic (Darbord et al., 1974). In all mutants resistance appeared due to mutation in one gene, but the mechanism of resistance has not been studied.

Development of resistance in plant pathogens to griseofulvin has never been reported. The fungistatic rather than fungicidal nature of griseofulvin activity and its limited use in agriculture may have played a role in this respect.

Antibiotics which interfere with nucleic acid metabolism. There are various antibiotics which interfere with steps in nucleic acid metabolism, such as synthesis of nucleotides, replication and transcription of DNA. For more information the reader is referred to a review by Dekker (1977). In this contribution only a few antibiotics will be mentioned, namely those which have shown activity against plant pathogens. Aristeromycin, an adenine analogue produced by *Streptomyces citricolor*, provided control of rice blast, caused by *P. oryzae*, and bacterial leaf blight of rice, caused by *Xanthomonas oryzae*. In studies with the latter pathogen evidence was obtained that the antibiotic interferes with formation of adenylic acid from adenine and adenosine. Bleomycins are a group of basic glycopeptide antibiotics, produced by *Streptomyces verticillus*. One of them, bleomycin B-2, is active against rice sheath blight, caused by *Pellicularia sasakii*. In studies with *E. coli* bleomycins showed binding to DNA and caused scission of the sugar-phosphate backbone of DNA. Phleomycins, polypeptide antibiotics, also produced by *S. verticillus*, are active against various rust diseases. They interfere with DNA synthesis by inhibition of DNA polymerase. Phytoactin, a polypeptide antibiotic produced by an unidentified *Streptomyces* species, gave control of white pine blister rust, caused by *Cronartium ribicola*, and of various other plant diseases. It affects RNA synthesis, possibly by inhibiting DNA dependent RNA polymerase. Cycloheximide, which in most sensitive organisms interferes primarily with protein synthesis, was shown to inhibit RNA polymerase in Oomycetes.

With exception of cycloheximide none of the above mentioned antibiotics have reached the phase of disease control in practice, for various reasons, among which phytotoxicity. Mutational changes resulting in resistance to this type of fungicides do not seem to occur readily, possibly because mutations leading to change in nucleic acid metabolism might be lethal.

Chitin synthesis

Polyoxins. Polyoxins, a group of closely related compounds formed by *Streptomyces cacaoi* var. *asoensis*, have been used for control of plant diseases since 1967. Polyoxin B is very effective against black spot of pear, caused by *Alternaria kikuchiana*, and polyoxin D against rice sheath blight, caused by *Pellicularia sasakii*. Their mechanism of action was elucidated in studies with *Alternaria kikuchiana*. They interfere with the incorporation of uridine diphosphate N-acetylglucosamine into the chitin of the cell wall by competitive inhibition of the enzyme chitin synthetase (Hori et al., 1974). Polyoxins are inactive against bacteria and fungi belonging to the Oomycetes, which lack chitin in their cell wall.

Development of resistance to polyoxin B has been reported, in laboratory experiments as well as in the field. It appeared, however, that chitin synthetase from these resistant strains was unaltered sensitive to the antibiotic, so that emergence of resistance can not be attributed to a change at the site of action. Further studies revealed that polyoxin resistance was closely related with a decrease in uptake (Hori et al., 1976), so that a change in permeability must be held responsible for resistance.

Energy production

Antimycin A. Antimycin A, produced by various *Streptomyces* species, was first discovered in 1947. It inhibits growth of various pathogenic fungi but appeared not suitable for practical application. It interferes with electron transport between cytochrome b and c in the respiratory chain. Leben et al. (1955) obtained strains of *Venturia inaequalis*, the cause of apple scab, by irradiation of conidia. Resistance appeared to be based on single gene mutation, but the mechanism of resistance has not been studied. Natural insensitivity of *Ustilago maydis* to antimycin A has been attributed to the operation of an electron transport pathway, from a site preceding cytochrome b, to an alternate terminal oxidase, thus bypassing the antimycin A blocked site. Elimination of this alternate pathway due to gene mutation leads to sensitivity to antimycin A (Georgopoulos and Sisler, 1970).

Membrane function

Polyene macrolides. Since 1950 a continuously increasing number of antifungal antibiotics, all produced by *Streptomyces* species, have been discovered (Dekker, 1969), and some of these have shown activity against plant diseases, among which pimaricin, rimocidin and nystatin (Dekker, 1963). Fungicidal action is due to complexation with ergosterol, the principal sterol in the fungal membrane, followed by leakage and cell death. Polyene macrolides are inactive against bacteria and Oomycetes, which do not contain ergosterol in the cell membrane. In laboratory experiments strains of various yeasts were obtained, which were resistant to nystatin (Athar and Winner, 1971), and strains of the plant pathogen *Cladosporium cucumerinum*, resistant to pimaricin (Van Tuyl, 1977). It was found that polyene resistance was associated with an altered sterol pattern in fungi. In *Candida albicans* and *C. utilis* the major sterols of successively more nystatin-resistant strains, were successively more primitive biogenetic precursors of ergosterol (Fryberg et al., 1976). The latter possess a lower affinity to polyene antibiotics, and a reduced fitness. A link between resistance and lower fitness was also postulated for pimaricin resistant strains of some plant pathogens (Dekker and Gielink, 1979).

Polyene macrolides can not be used to protect aerial plant parts, since they are readily decomposed in light. Treatment of seeds, tubers and bulbs, however, in principle remains possible. Pimaricin and rimocidin showed activity in internal seed disinfection (Dekker, 1957) and pimaricin has been admitted for control of narcissus bulb rot in the Netherlands (Dekker and Langerak, 1979), but results in practice still appeared erratic. The latter antibiotic is also active as a disinfectant of potato tubers against *Rhizoctonia solani* (unpublished results).

Metabolism associated with pathogenicity

Validamycin. Validamycin, discovered in 1970 in a culture broth of *Streptomyces hygroscopicus* var. *limoneus*, is not fungicidal in vitro. Nevertheless it controls a few fungal diseases, such as sheath blight of rice, caused by *Pellicularia sasakii*, and *Rhizoctonia solani* on potatoes (Wakae and Matsuura, 1975). It seems that the antibiotic interferes with the biosynthesis of myo-inositol, presumed to be indispensable for pathogenic activity. Of much interest is the question, whether the pathogen may overcome the effect of such an antibiotic by a change in its metabolism, after having continuously been exposed to it. No experimental data are yet available.

Unknown mechanism of action

Agrocin 84. The antibiotic agrocin 84, a fraudulent adenine nucleotide, is produced by *Agrobacterium radiobacter* strain 84, an organism used for biological control of crown gall caused by the closely related *Agrobacterium tumefaciens*. The production of this antibiotic is coded for by a plasmid, which also contains the code for insensitivity to agrocin 84. After conjugation, plasmids may be transferred from one bacterium to another. In the laboratory strains of the pathogen *A. tumefaciens* have been obtained which, after plasmid transfer, had become resistant to agrocin 84. If this would occur in nature, the biological control method would become ineffective (Kerr, 1980). The mechanism of action of agrocin 84, and the biochemical resistance mechanism have not been elucidated.

BUILD-UP OF A RESISTANT PATHOGEN POPULATION

General

The preceding paragraphs allow the conclusion that emergence of resistance is a common phenomenon with antibiotics, which are mostly specific-site inhibitors. The fact, however, that in vitro mutants may arise, which are resistant to a particular fungicide, does not necessarily mean that this fungicide will encounter resistance problems in the field. Only after a considerable proportion of the pathogen population has become resistant, failure of disease control has to be expected. Whether this will indeed occur, depends upon a number of factors, among which the comparative fitness in relation to that of the wild type fungus plays a predominant role. In addition, the type of disease, the life cycle of the pathogen, and the management of fungicide application are important.

There is evidence that, at least with some fungicides, resistance of the pathogen is linked to decreased fitness. This may happen when a change in the fungal cell at the site of action, which results in less affinity to the fungicide and consequently in resistance, in itself is unfavourable for the pathogen in absence of the fungicide. This seems to be the case with mutants, resistant to the antibiotic pimaricin. As has been outlined above, ergosterol in the cell membrane of the resistant cells has been replaced by precursors of this compound. These precursors possess lower affinity to the antibiotic, which means resistance, but at the same time they are a less suitable replacement of ergosterol, which means decreased fitness of the resistant cell. This means that resistance is inversely related with fitness, which, of course, will hamper the build-up of a resistant pathogen population.

In the laboratory pimaricin resistant strains of various plant pathogens were obtained, namely of *Cladosporium cucumerinum*, the cause of cucumber scab, and of *Fusarium oxysporum* f.sp. *narcissi*, the cause of narcissus bulb rot. All resistant strains invariably showed decreased pathogenicity (Dekker and Gielink, 1979). Use of pimaricin in disease control has been very limited and it does not allow conclusions with respect to build-up of resistance in practice. This antibiotic, however, has been extensively used to prevent moulding of freshly made cheese without build-up of resistance in the cheese packing houses. Also clinical use of the polyene macrolides pimaricin and pimaricin has never led to a resistant pathogen population (Dekker, 1982).

It would be of interest to know whether also with other compounds resistance is linked to decreased fitness. Such compounds might then be considered as less hazardous with respect to the chance that emergence of resistant cells will lead to failure of disease control. It is not clear whether absence of fungicide-resistance problems with blasticidin S can be explained in this way. In the following paragraphs only those antibiotics will be discussed, which have been used on a large scale, namely kasugamycin, streptomycin and polyoxin.

Kasugamycin

Resistance of *P. oryzae* to kasugamycin was found in 1971 in an important rice-growing district of Japan, where the antibiotic had been used intensely and exclusively for several years. As in that area the major part of the field isolates already had become resistant, application of the antibiotic for control of rice blast was stopped in 1972. In 1975 the proportion of resistant strains appeared to be decreased to 2-20% (Uesugi, 1982), which indicates a lower competitive ability of the resistant strains as compared with that of the original sensitive strains. This was confirmed in a greenhouse test, where plants were inoculated with a 1 : 1 mixture of conidia from resistant and sensitive isolates. In absence of the fungicide the number of lesions caused by the sensitive strain appeared larger than that caused by the resistant isolates. This is assumed to be due to a somewhat slower progress of infection by the resistant isolate (Ito and Yamaguchi, 1979). When, however, the resistant and sensitive isolates were tested separately, no differences in mycelium growth on agar, sporulation or virulence were found (Miura et al., 1976).

Lower fitness of resistant strains means a competitive advantage for the sensitive pathogen, which has escaped the fungicide, or which enters from neighbouring unsprayed fields. In such a case the build-up of a resistant pathogen population may be hampered by interrupting the use of the fungicide, thereby avoiding a continuous selection pressure. Nowadays rice blast can be controlled successfully by a combination product of kasugamycin with tetra-chlorophthalide, named Kasurabcide, used in an alternating sequence with fungicides with a different mode of action, such as probenazole (Sato, personal communication, 1981).

Streptomycin

Streptomycin has been extensively used during many years for control of fire blight in pears, caused by *Erwinia amylovora*. In 1971 disease failure occurred in California, USA, due to development of high level resistance. Laboratory and greenhouse studies revealed that virulence among resistant and sensitive strains varied, but that these were no consistent differences between the two groups. The resistance appeared to be rather persistent. Resistant strains could be isolated from orchards, even six years after termination of streptomycin application (Schroth et al., 1979). It seems that streptomycin resistance is not linked to decreased fitness, which will make it more difficult to avoid resistance problems in practice.

Polyoxins

Four years after introduction of polyoxin B for control of blackspot in pears, in 1971, strains of the pathogen, *Alternaria kikuchiana*, were isolated which had become resistant to the antibiotic. As the season progressed, the resistant strains caused severe losses in pear fruit production. After polyoxin application was stopped, the frequency of resistant strains markably dropped in 1973 (Nishimura et al., 1976). Reduced fitness of resistant strains and dilution of the resistant pathogen population with sensitive strains of neighbouring fields may have played a role. Indications of a somewhat decreased competitiveness of resistant strains were indeed obtained in greenhouse tests. In spite of this, resistant strains did not disappear entirely in the field during several years (Uesugi, 1978). Therefore it has been recommended to avoid a continuous selection pressure by the antibiotic, and to use polyoxin alternatively and in combination with other fungicides. Also occurrence of polyoxin-resistant strains of *Alternaria mali*, which causes apple blotch, have been detected in apple orchards (Nishimura et al., 1976).

DISCUSSION

Antibiotics, as a rule, are specific-site inhibitors. They may affect particular steps in protein-, nucleic acid- or chitin synthesis, or they may interfere with respiration, nuclear function or membrane structure. With such inhibitors emergence of resistant cells appear to be a general phenomenon. It would be of interest to know whether antibiotics exist, which act at such a conservative part of the cell metabolism, that each change in that part by mutation would be lethal. This would preclude the emergence of viable resistant mutants. It seems doubtful, however, whether such compounds would be sufficiently selective for use in plant disease control.

Even when fungicide-resistant cells emerge, this should not necessarily lead to failure of disease control in practice. The latter will only occur after a considerable proportion of the pathogen population has become resistant. This may happen readily with some antibiotics, but slowly or not at all with other antibiotics, depending on the properties of the resistant strains. In view of this we may discern risky and less risky compounds. It would be of interest to know the resistance risks in practice of compounds, which are not fungicidal in vitro, but which interfere with the pathogenicity of the fungus, or which are only fungistatic.

REFERENCES

1. M.A. Athar and H.I. Winner, *J. med. Microbiol. 4*, 505-517 (1971).
2. D. Cooper, D.V. Banthorpe and D. Wilkie, *J. Mol. Biol. 26*, 347-350 (1967).
3. S.H.B. Crackower, *J. Microbiol. 18*, 683-687 (1972).
4. J.C. Darbord, D. Vidon, H. Nguen Van and A. Desvignes, *Ann. Microbiol. 125A*, 17-25 (1974).
5. J. Dekker, *Neth. J. Pl. Path. 63*, 65-144 (1957).
6. J. Dekker, *Ann. rev. Microbiol. 17*, 243-262 (1963).
7. J. Dekker, In: *Fungicides, and Advanced Treatise* (Ed. D.C. Torgeson), vol. 2, 579-635 (1969).

8. J. Dekker, In: *Systemic Fungicides* (Ed. R.W. Marsh), Longman, London and New York, 176-197 (1977).
9. J. Dekker, In: *Antifungal Compounds* (Eds. M.R. Siegel and H.D. Sisler), Marcel Dekker, New York and Basel, vol. 2, 365-398 (1977).
10. J. Dekker, In: *Fungicide Resistance in Crop Protection* (Eds. J. Dekker and S.G. Georgopoulos) Pudoc, Wageningen 128-138 (1982).
11. J. Dekker and A.J. Gielink, *Neth. J. Pl. Path. 85*, 67-73 (1979).
12. J. Dekker and C.J. Langerak, In: *Systemfungizide* (Eds. H. Lyr and C. Polter), Akademie-Verlag, Berlin 63-74 (1979).
13. M. Fryberg, A.C. Oehlschlager and A.M. Unrau, *Arch. Biochem. Biophys. 173*, 171-177 (1976).
14. S.G. Georgopoulos and H.D. Sisler, *J. Bacteriol. 103*, 745-750 (1970).
15. K. Gull and A.J.P. Trinci, *Nature 244*, 292-294 (1973).
16. T.L. Helser, J.E. Davies and J.E. Dahlberg, *Nature (New Biology) 233*, 12-14 (1971).
17. M. Hori, J. Eguchi, K. Kakiki and T. Misato, *J. Antibiotics (Japan) 27, 4*, 260-266 (1974).
18. M. Hori, K. Kakiki and T. Misato, *J. Pestic. Science 1*, 31-40 (1976).
19. K.T. Huang, T. Misato and H. Asuyama, *J. Antibiotics (Tokyo) A 17*, 71-74 (1964).
20. I. Ito and T. Yamaguchi, *Ann. Phytopath. Soc. (Japan) 45* 40-46 (1979).
21. A. Kerr, *Plant Disease 64*, 24-30 (1980).
22. C. Leben, D.M. Boone and G.W. Keitt, *Phytopathology 45*, 467-472 (1955).
23. H. Miura, M. Katagiri, T. Yamaguchi, Y. Uesugi and H. Ito, *Ann. Phytopath. Soc. (Japan) 42*, 117-123 (1976).
24. H. Nakamura and L. Sakurai, *Ann. Phytopath. Soc. (Japan) 27*, 84 (Abstr.) (1962).
25. S. Nishimura, K. Kohomoto and H. Udagawa, *Rev. Pl. Prot. Res. 9*, 47-57 (1976).
26. M. Ozaki, S. Mizushima and M. Nomura, *Nature 222*, 333-341 (1969).
27. M. N. Schroth, S. V. Thomson and W. J. Moller, *Phytopathology 69*, 565-568 (1979).
28. M.R. Siegel, In: *Antifungal Compounds* (Eds. M.R. Siegel and H.D. Sisler). Marcel Dekker, New York and Basel, 399-438 (1977).
29. M. Taga, H. Nakagawa, M. Tsuda and A. Ueyama, *Phytopathology 69*, 463-466 (1979).
30. J.M. van Tuyl, *Mededelingen Landbouwhogeschool, Wageningen, The Netherlands 77-2*, 1-136 (1977).
31. Y. Uesugi, *Japan Pesticide Information 35*, 5-9 (1978).
32. Y. Uesugi, In: *Fungicide Resistance in Crop Protection* (Eds. J. Dekker and S.G. Georgopoulos), Pudoc, Wageningen 207-218 (1982).
33. L.C. Vining, *Adv. appl. Microbiol. 25*, 147-168 (1979).
34. J. Vörös, *Phytopath. Zeitschr. 54*, 249-257 (1965).
35. O. Wakae and K. Matsuura, *Rev. Pl. Prot. Res. 8*, 81-92 (1975).
36. D. Wilkie and B. K. Lee, *Genetic Research 6*, 130-138 (1965)

PERSPECTIVES ON RESEARCH OF ANTIBIOTICS AND LOW MOLECULAR WEIGHT ENZYME INHIBITORS

Hamao Umezawa

Institute of Microbial Chemistry, 3-14-23 Kamiosaki, Shinagawa-ku, Tokyo 141, Japan

Abstract - Blasticidin S, kasugamycin, polyoxin and validamycin have been discovered by screening culture filtrates for antibiotics for agricultural use. Even at the present, the screening of antibacterial antibiotics leads to the discovery of new types of structures, and the derivative studies of β-lactam and aminoglycoside antibiotics have led to the successful developments of derivatives effective against resistant strains.
In the case of antitumor antibiotics, also successful developments are being made in the development of derivatives and analogs of anthracyclines, bleomycin, mitomycin *etc*. Furthermore, antibiotic research has been expanded to low molecular weight enzyme inhibitors and immunomodifiers. Immunomodifiers are contributing to the complete cure of cancer. The study of enzyme inhibitors may contribute to the development of compounds useful in prevention of plant diseases.
I will review our recent studies in my institute on the subjects described above.

The screening for antimicrobial antibiotics is still continuing, and even at the present it is leading to the discovery of compounds with new types of structures to be used for the development of effective agents against infections in humans and animals. It is also leading to the discovery of antibiotics for agricultural use. Research of antitumor antibiotics has also contributed to the development of various cancer chemotherapeutic agents. Moreover, since 1969, antibiotic research has been expanded to the study of low molecular weight enzyme inhibitors. Experience has shown that microorganisms produce an unlimited number of compounds with various structures, and the reason for this is being studied from a genetic perspective.

In this paper, I will review recent studies on antibiotics and low molecular weight enzyme inhibitors.

ANTIBIOTICS FOR PREVENTION OF PLANT DISEASES

About 1950, the possible use of antimycin for the prevention of plant diseases was suggested, but all researchers were pessimistic about producing antibiotics at a low enough cost for agricultural use. At about that time, the late Prof. Sumiki of the Faculty of Agriculture at the University of Tokyo and his coworkers started screening for antimicrobial antibiotics which would prevent rice plant diseases. Blasticidin S (Fig. 1) which was effective in preventing rice blast caused by *Pyricularia oryzae* was thus discovered, and the industrial production of this antibiotic was started in about 1964. At that time, there was an urgent problem in Japan to develop an effective substitute for phenyl mercuric compounds, since an elevated mercury content had been detected in the hair of Japanese people. Therefore, with my colleagues I also undertook a screening for antibiotics effective against rice blast. In this study, a culture filtrate of a streptomyces strain suppressed the rice blast in a pot test. However, the culture filtrate did not inhibit the growth of *Pyricularia oryzae* in media generally used in the screening procedure. But we found that this culture filtrate exhibits a strong effect in inhibiting the growth of this fungus in a rice plant juice medium at a pH of 5.5 or lower than that. Thus, an assay method was established and we were quickly successful in the purification of the active agent. We named it kasugamycin (Ref. 1) and determined its structure (Ref. 2 & 3) (Fig. 1). Moreover, we were successful in the establishment of an industrial fermentation process; and since 1969, more than 90 tons of kasugamycin have been produced yearly. Kasugamycin also inhibits the growth of *Ps. aeruginosa*, and has a low toxicity. Therefore this antibiotic was once clinically studied for its therapeutic effect on urinary infections in humans. Thus, its low toxicity was also proved by this clinical study (Ref. 4). The screening of microbial culture filtrates for activity in inhibiting the growth of *Pellicularia sasakii* led to the discovery of polyoxins (Fig. 1) by Suzuki and others (Ref. 5) and validamycin by Shibata and others (Ref. 6). Polyoxin (Fig. 1) has been used to prevent rice sheath blight, apple leaf spot, *etc*. At present, 100 tons of validamycin are used yearly for the prevention of rice sheath blight.

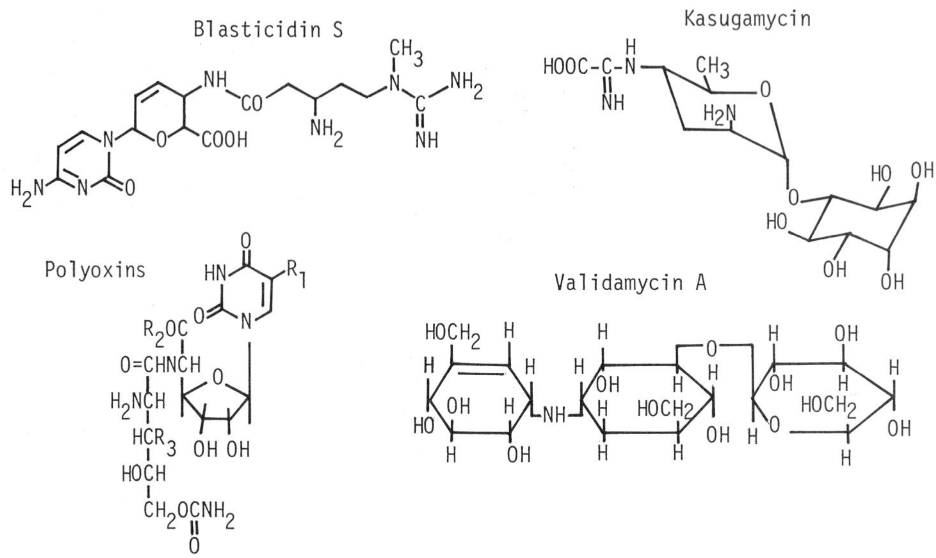

Fig. 1. Antibiotics discovered by the screening for effective agents against rice plant diseases.

Besides the compounds which were discovered by screening culture filtrates for antibiotics for agricultural use, streptomycin and oxytetracycline have been used for the prevention of bacterial leaf spot, _etc_., and novobiocin, for tomato bacterial canker, _etc_. Polynactins have been used as an acaricide to prevent damage to apples caused by the apple-spotted spider mite, _etc_. Also, mildiomycin, botryticidine and nikkomycin are being developed as fungicides; SF1293Na, as a herbicide; and avermectin, as an insecticide.

ANTIMICROBIAL ANTIBIOTICS AND THEIR DERIVATIVES USEFUL IN THE TREATMENT OF INFECTIONS IN HUMANS

In the case of antibiotics for agricultural use, it seems to be very difficult to effectively produce their derivatives at a low enough cost for practical use. However, in the case of antibiotics for medical use, new chemotherapeutic agents have been developed in the last 10 years by preparing their derivatives and analogs.

During the decade of the 1970's, the following 16 β-lactams were introduced for clinical use in Japan with the year of introduction shown in parenthesis: penicillin analogs: phenethicillin (1960), propicillin (1963), methicillin (1961), oxacillin (1962), cloxacillin (1964), dicloxacillin (1968), flucloxacillin (1970), ampicillin (1963), hetacillin (1970), talampicillin (1977), amoxycillin (1975), pivmecillinam (1979), cyclacillin (1974), carbenicillin (1970), carindacillin (1976), carfecillin (1977), sulbenicillin (1973); cephalosporin analogs: cephaloridine (1965), cephalothin (1966), cephaloglycin (1969), cephalexin (1970), cefazolin (1971), ceftezol (1978), cefapirin (1977), cefradine (1977), cephacetrile (1978).

Thereafter, there was a further rapid progress in the synthesis of new effective β-lactam compounds, and during the 27-month period from January, 1980 to April, 1982, the following 17 new β-lactams were introduced for clinical use in Japan: penicillin analogs: ticarcillin (1980), piperacillin (1980), bacampicillin (1981), mezlocillin (1982); cephalosporin analogs: cefatrizine (1980), cefotium (1981), cefsulodin (1981), cefotaxime (1981), cefoperazone (1981), cefroxadine (1982), cefuroxime (1982), cefaclor (1982), cetizoxime (1982), cefadroxil (1982); cephamycin analogs: cefoxitin (1980), cefmetazole (1980); oxadethiocephamycin analog: latamoxef (1982).

Although the development of these useful β-lactam compounds is due to advances in chemistry, all new types of structures from which useful derivatives and analogs originated have been discovered by screening for β-lactam antibiotics.

In 1981, N-sulfonyl single β-lactam antibiotics (Fig. 2) were discovered in bacteria by Imada, _et al_. (Ref. 7) and by Sykes, _et al_. (Ref. 8), and the name, "monobactam" was proposed for these β-lactams produced by bacteria. Based on this new type of structure, an effective analog with a potential usefulness, SQ26,776 has already been synthesized (Fig. 2).

In addition to β-lactam antibiotics, great progress has been made in aminoglycoside antibiotics in the last 15 years. I was able to elucidate the enzymatic mechanism of resistance to

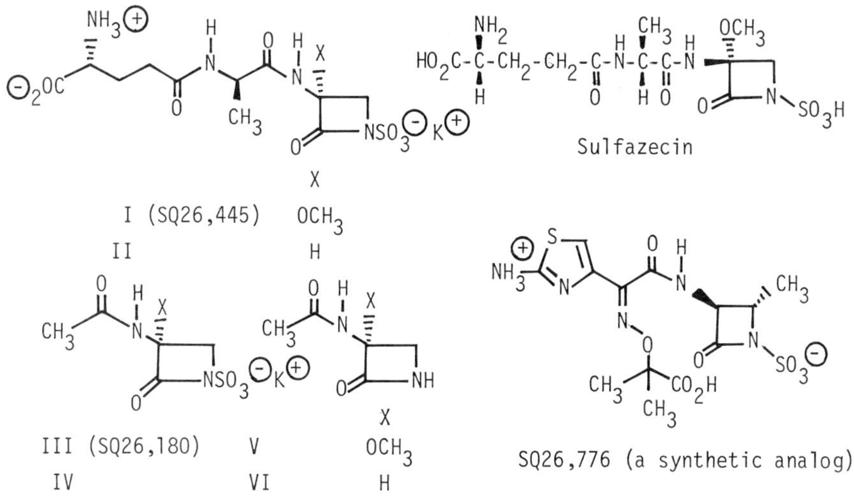

Fig. 2. β-Lactam antibiotics produced by bacteria and synthetic analog.

aminoglycoside antibiotics in 1967 (Ref. 9): most strains resistant to kanamycins A, B and C produced 3'-O-phosphotransferases which transferred the terminal phosphate of ATP to the 3'-hydroxyl group (Fig. 3) of kanamycin A, B and C; and the involvement of these enzymes in the mechanism of resistance was proved by the chemical synthesis of 3'-deoxykanamycin A (Ref. 10) and 3',4'-dideoxykanamycin B (Ref. 11) which inhibited the growth of resistant strains. Thus, on the basis of the enzymatic mechanism of resistance, it became possible to predict the structures of aminoglycosides which would inhibit the growth of resistant strains, and such derivatives have indeed been synthesized (Ref. 12).

At the present, 3'- and 2"-O-phosphotransferases or 4'- and 2"-O-adenylyltransferases and 3-, 2'-, and 6'-N-acetyltransferases shown in Fig. 3 are known to be involved in the enzymatic mechanism of resistance to deoxystreptamine-containing antibiotics (Ref. 12 & 13). Resistant strains forming other O-phospho or O-adenylyltransferases may appear in the future. Therefore, I was interested in antibacterially active structures which had the least number of hydroxyl groups. We synthesized deoxy derivatives of kanamycin B and found that the derivatives, shown in Fig. 4, which contain only one hydroxyl group have a strong antibacterial activity (Ref. 14). This indicates that amino groups have a predominant role in the antibacterial action of aminoglycosides.

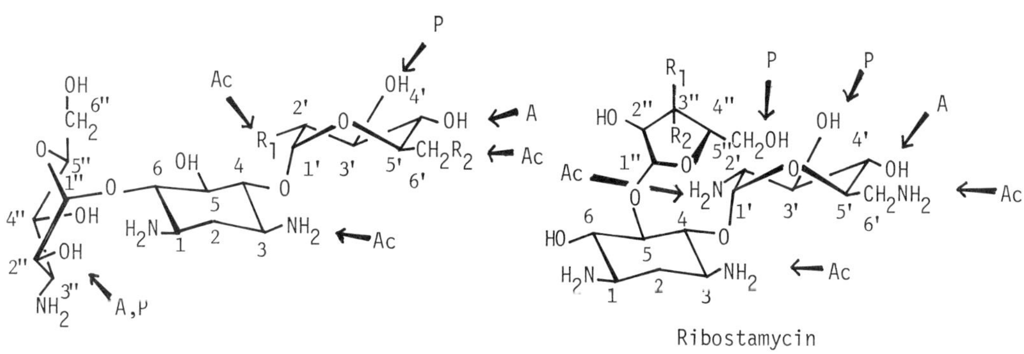

Kanamycin A: R_1=OH, R_2=NH_2
Kanamycin B: R_1=NH_2, R_2=NH_2
Kanamycin C: R_1=NH_2, R_2=OH

Fig. 3. O-Phosphotransferases (P), O-adenylyltransferases (A) and N-acetyltransferases (Ac) involved in resistance mechanism.

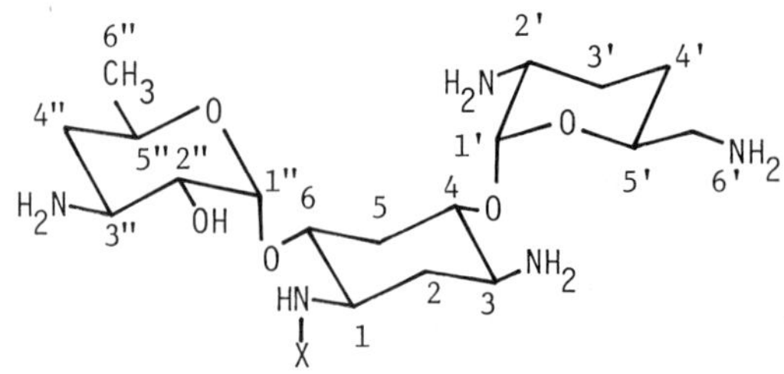

Fig. 4. Active kanamycin derivatives which have the least number of OH groups.

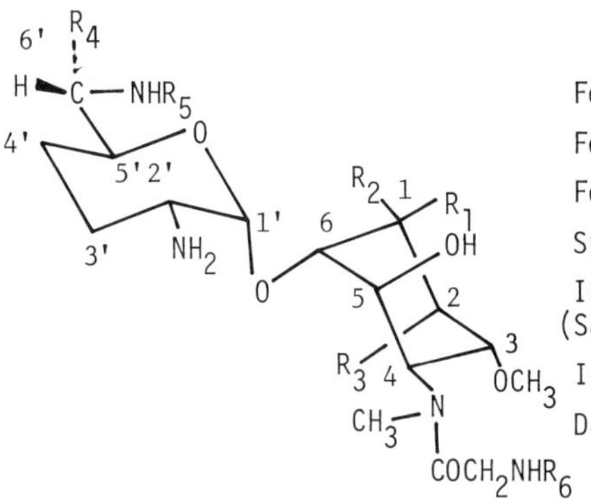

	R_1	R_2	R_3	R_4	R_5	R_6
Fortimicin A	NH_2	H	OH	CH_3	H	H
Fortimicin C	NH_2	H	OH	CH_3	H	$CONH_2$
Fortimicin D	NH_2	H	OH	H	H	H
Sporaricin A	H	NH_2	H	CH_3	H	H
Istamycin A (Sannamycin A)	NH_2	H	H	H	CH_3	H
Istamycin B	H	NH_2	H	H	CH_3	H
Dactimicin	NH_2	H	OH	CH_3	H	CH=NH

Fig. 5. Fortimicin group antibiotics.

Also by screening, aminoglycoside antibiotics which contain only one hydroxyl group have been found in actinomycetes. Among the fortimicin group of antibiotics shown in Fig. 5 (Ref. 13), sporaricins and istamycins contain only one hydroxyl group. Members of the fortimicin group are useful in the treatment of infections; and moreover, their derivatives with improved activity are being synthesized (Ref. 15).

Besides β-lactam and aminoglycoside antibiotics, studies are going on tylosin and other macrolides and leading to the development of derivatives effective against resistant strains.

ANTITUMOR ANTIBIOTICS

Also in the case of antitumor antibiotics, since our first successful report in 1953 (Ref. 16), the screening study has been continued, and moreover, in the last 10 years a great deal of effort has been made to develop derivatives and analogs more effective than their parent antitumor antibiotics.

In the first step of cancer treatment, tumors should be macroscopically eliminated by surgery, radiation, chemotherapy, or their combination. The effectiveness of adriamycin (Fig. 6), discovered by Arcamone, stimulated the study of anthracyclines. 4'-epi-Adriamycin (Fig. 6), developed by Arcamone, has lower toxicity than adriamycin and is becoming a useful therapeutic agent. Very recently, the same investigators suggested that 4-demethoxyadriamycin would be more effective than adriamycin (Ref. 17). The group of compounds which include adriamycin are called anthracyclines and their aglycone parts, anthracyclinones. These terms were proposed in about 1964 by Brockmann who first studied the chemistry of this group of antibiotics. Besides Arcamone's group, anthracyclines have been studied by many other researchers. It is said that the National Cancer Institute of the U.S.A. has tested over 600 anthracyclines up to 1980. As examples, I will report here on our studies of anthracyclines. Aclacinomycin A (Fig. 6) (Ref. 18), which we had discovered, has been confirmed to exhibit a therapeutic effect against leukemia and lymphoma, even against those cases resistant to adriamycin treatment. We have studied the biosynthetic pathways of anthracyclines and have prepared many mutants of aclacinomycin-producing strains. One of the mutants produced a new anthracyclinone which was elucidated to be 2-hydroxyaklavinone; aklavinone is the name of the aglycone of aclacinomycin. The 2-hydroxyaklavinone was converted by a non-pigmented mutant of the aclacinomycin-producing strain to 2-hydroxyaclacinomycins A and B which have significantly higher therapeutic indices than aclacinomycins against L1210 mouse leukemia (Ref. 19). They may be

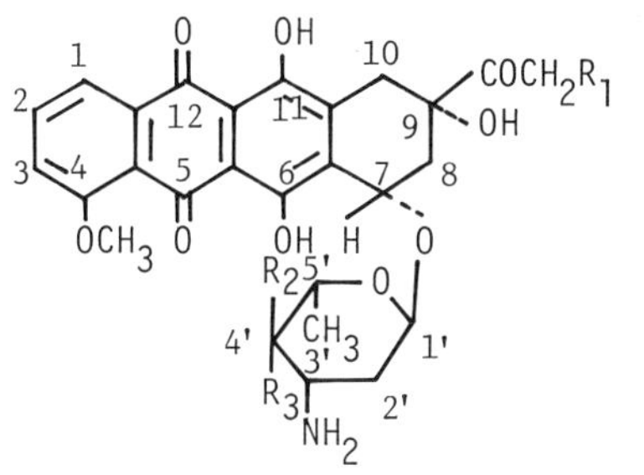

Daunomycin: R_1, R_2=H, R_3=OH
Adriamycin: R_1=OH, R_2=H, R_3=OH
4'-*epi*-Adriamycin: R_1, R_2=OH, R_3=H

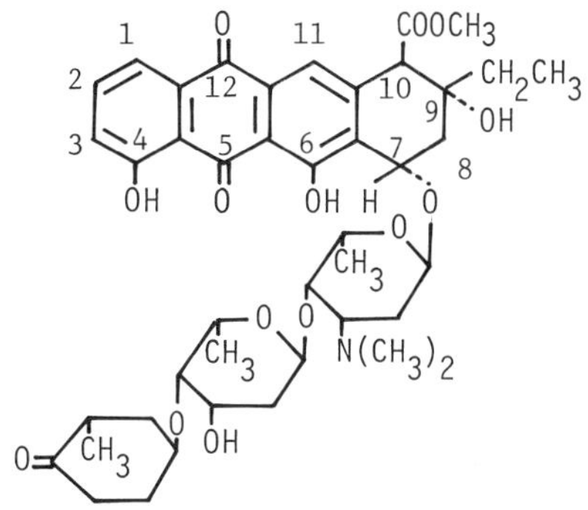

Aclacinomycin A (R=H)

Fig. 6. Anthracyclines.

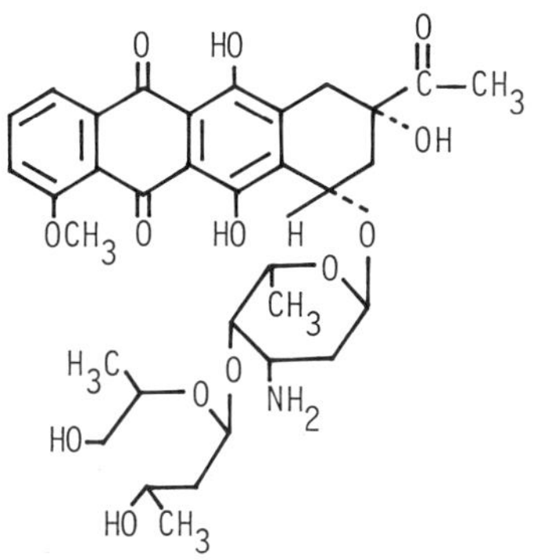

Baumycin A1

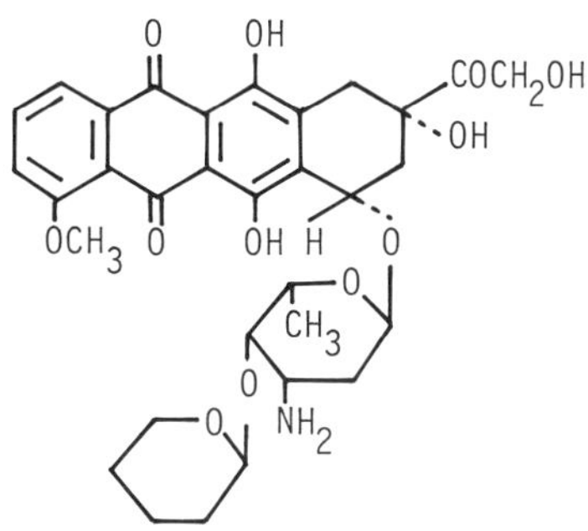

4'-O-Tetrahydropyranyladriamycin

Fig. 7. Baumycin A1 and 4'-O-tetrahydropyranyladriamycin.

worthy of further study. We also discovered baumycin A1, A2, B1, and B2 (Fig. 7) (Ref. 20) which are 4'-glycosides of daunomycin. A1 showed good inhibitory activity against L1210. Therefore, we synthesized the 4'-O-glycosidic derivatives of daunomycin and adriamycin and discovered that 4'-O-tetrahydropyranyladriamycin (Fig. 7) (Ref. 21) has a stronger activity than adriamycin against mouse tumors. This derivative was found by Mathé and others (Ref. 22) to have significantly lower cardiac and skin toxicity in hamsters than adriamycin and has been clinically studied. Practically, it does not cause nausea, vomiting, or hair loss and is effective; thus, this derivative will become a useful anthracycline for cancer treatment. 4-Demethoxy-11-deoxyadriamycin (Ref. 23) which we synthesized also has a strong antitumor activity against L1210 and may be worthy of further study.

In 1956, I discovered phleomycin (Ref. 24), an antibiotic which forms a complex with copper. This antibiotic is very effective in preventing bean and wheat rust. Soon thereafter, we found that this antibiotic has a strong therapeutic effect against Ehrlich carcinoma and sarcoma 180. But it unfortunately produced strong renal damage in dogs. Therefore, I continued screening for antibiotics of this type. By 1966 I had discovered new antibiotics which could be differentiated from phleomycin by paper chromatography and which did not have renal toxicity. I named this group of antibiotics bleomycin.

Bleomycin (Fig. 8) has been used in the treatment of Hodgkin's lymphoma, tumors of the testis, and carcinomas of the skin, head, and neck. We determined the complicated structure of bleomycin (Ref. 25) and very recently were successful in its total chemical synthesis (Ref. 26). Bleomycin binds strongly to cupric ion, producing an equimolar complex. We also determined the structure of the bleomycin-Cu(II) complex (Fig. 9) (Ref. 27). Bleomycin and its metal complex bind to DNA (Ref. 28): the bithiazole moiety intercalates into double-stranded DNA (Ref. 29) and the terminal amine is also involved in the binding (Ref. 28). We also determined the structure of phleomycin (Ref. 26): one of double bonds of the bithiazole ring

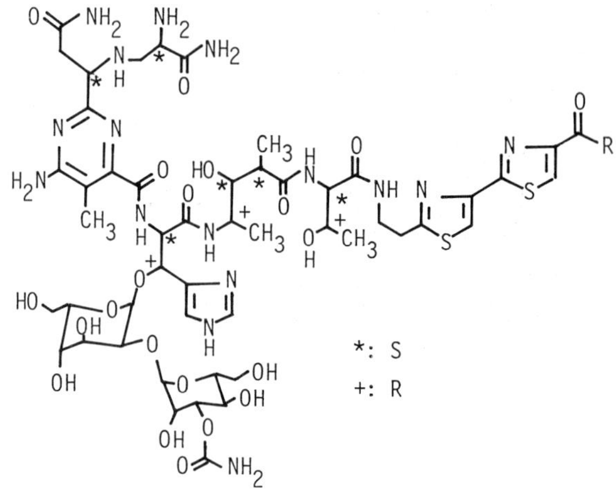

A1: R = $NH-(CH_2)_3-SO-CH_3$

Demethyl-A2: R = $NH-(CH_2)_3-S-CH_3$

A2: R = $NH-(CH_2)_3-\overset{+}{S}(CH_3)_2$

A2'-a: R = $NH-(CH_2)_4-NH_2$

A2'-b: R = $NH-(CH_2)_3-NH_2$

A2'-c: R = $NH-(CH_2)_2$- 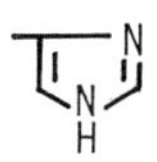

A5: R = $NH-(CH_2)_3-NH-(CH_2)_4-NH_2$

A6: R = $NH-(CH_2)_3-NH-(CH_2)_4-NH-(CH_2)_3-NH_2$

B1': R = NH_2

B2: R = $NH-(CH_2)_4-NH-C(=NH)-NH_2$

B4: R = $NH-(CH_2)_4-NH-C(=NH)-NH-(CH_2)_4-NH-C(=NH)-NH_2$

Bleomycinic acid: R = OH

PEP: R = $NH-(CH_2)_3-NH-CH(CH_3)$- 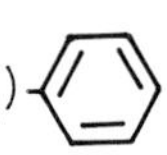
(PEP=Peplomycin)

BAPP: $NH-(CH_2)_3-NH-(CH_2)_3-NH-(CH_2)_3-CH_3$

Fig. 8. Natural bleomycins, peplomycin, BAPP, and bleomycinic acid.

in the bleomycin molecule is saturated in phleomycin. In this connection, it is interesting that phleomycin does not intercalate into double-stranded DNA (Ref. 30). Phleomycin causes more single-strand than double-strand scission (Ref. 31). We have proposed a structure for the bleomycin-Fe(II)-O_2 complex (Ref. 27, 32 & 33). Although the structure of bleomycin-Fe(II)-O_2 complex proposed by us has not yet been conclusively proved, there are no conflicting experimental data. The bleomycin-Fe(II)-O_2 complex binds to double-stranded DNA and causes double-strand scission. The active species of this complex has been suggested to be bleomycin-Fe(III)-$^{-}O_2H$ (Ref. 34 & 35). The reaction products of the bleomycin-iron-O_2 complex with DNA have been isolated (Ref. 36). Thus, the reaction sequences involved in DNA strand scission are suggested as shown in Fig. 10.

One of the amino acid moieties of bleomycin has a pyrimidine ring, and we thus named this amino acid "pyrimidoblamic acid". A bleomycin analog which lacks the methyl group in the pyrimidoblamic acid moiety has also been found in culture filtrates of actinomycetes (Ref.

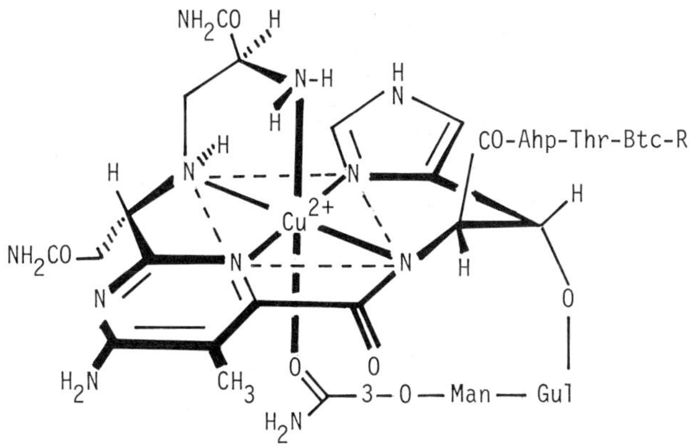

Ahp = 4-amino-3-hydroxy-2-methylpentanoyl

Thr = threonyl

Btc = 2'-(2-aminoethyl)-2,4'-bithiazole-4-carboxyl

R = terminal amine

Man-Glu = 2-O-(α-D-mannopyranosyl)-α-L-gulopyranosyl

Fig. 9. Bleomycin-copper complex.

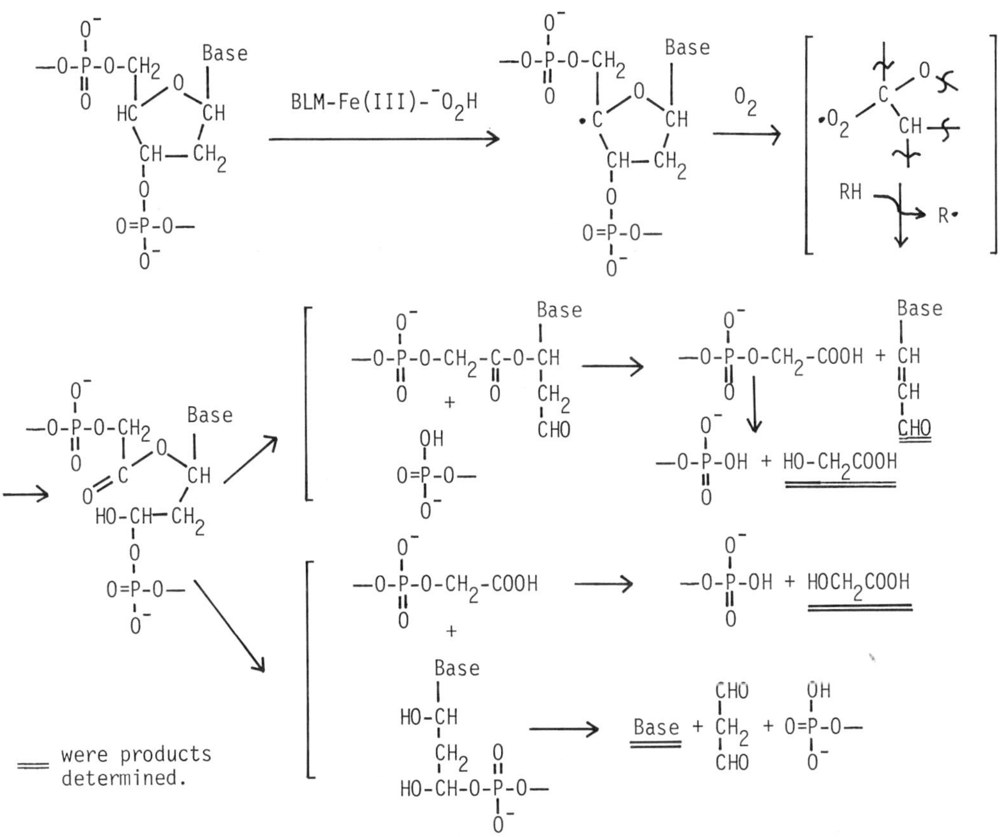

Fig. 10. Reaction of bleomycin (BLM) with DNA, resulting in DNA strand scission.

37). Testing incorporation of labeled amino acids into the pyrimidoblamyl and bithiazole acid moieties, and isolating biosynthetic intermediates, we have almost completely elucidated the biosynthetic pathway to the peptide part of bleomycin (Ref. 38). On the basis of this biosynthesis study, various bleomycin analogs are being prepared.

New bleomycins containing various terminal amines can be prepared by the addition of amines to fermentation media (Ref. 39 & 40). They can also be synthesized from bleomycinic acid which is obtained by hydrolysis of bleomycin B2 by agmatine amidohydrolase of Fusarium sp (Ref. 41) or by the CNBr reaction with bleomycin demethyl A2 (Ref. 42). Thus, more than 400 bleomycins have been prepared. Peplomycin shown in Fig. 11 is one of them; it had a lower pulmonary toxicity than bleomycin and was clinically effective not only against bleomycin-sensitive tumors but also against prostatic carcinoma.

All kinds of human and animal cells contain bleomycin hydrolase which hydrolyzes the α-aminocarboxamide bond (Fig. 8) of the pyrimidoblamyl moiety of bleomycin (Ref. 40). Using the product of this hydrolysis, the α-aminocarboxamide moiety of bleomycin can be chemically modified. Such bleomycin derivatives are resistant to bleomycin hydrolase. In this paper, I will report two examples, PEP-PEP and DBP-PEP, shown in Fig. 11. Both were resistant to bleomycin hydrolase, and have good antitumor activity as well as bleomycin. Thus, derivatives which have a wider anticancer spectrum than bleomycin are being developed.

As described above, derivatives and analog studies are in progress for the modification of anthracycline, bleomycin, mitomycin (Ref. 43), etc. Clinical study is also under way for other types of antibiotics such as neothramycin (Ref. 44), etc. Among pyrrolo-(1,4)benzo-diazepine antibiotics (Fig. 12) (Ref. 45), neothramycin (Fig. 12) has the lowest toxicity; it exhibits a strong inhibition against Yoshida rat sarcoma and Novikoff hepatoma and has a very low cumulative toxicity. Bactobolin (Ref. 46) (Fig. 13), which was discovered by 3 Japanese research groups, inhibits protein synthesis in the mammalian ribosome system and is being subjected to study using a human stem cell assay.

Even at present, successful results are being obtained by screening for new types of antitumor antibiotics. Spergualin (Fig. 13) (Ref. 47 & 48), very recently discovered by us, is one example. It has an interesting activity against L1210 mouse leukemia, but it does not inhibit the synthesis of DNA, RNA, or protein. Also, it does not cause differentiation of malignant cells.

As already discussed, the first step in curing a cancer should be the macroscopic elimination of the tumors. In this case, inhibition of the action or generation of suppressor cells should enhance the effect of radiation and chemotherapy. It is reasonable to assume that there would be cytotoxic antibiotics which inhibit the action or generation of suppressor cells more strongly than that of effector cells. In fact, cyclophosphamide, aclacinomycin

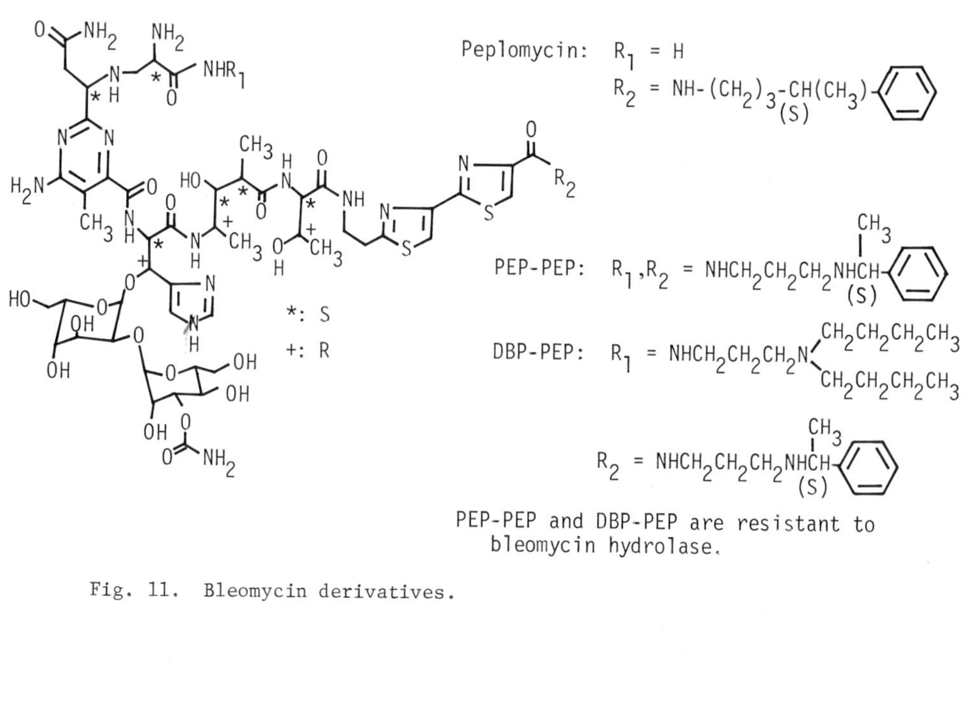

Fig. 11. Bleomycin derivatives.

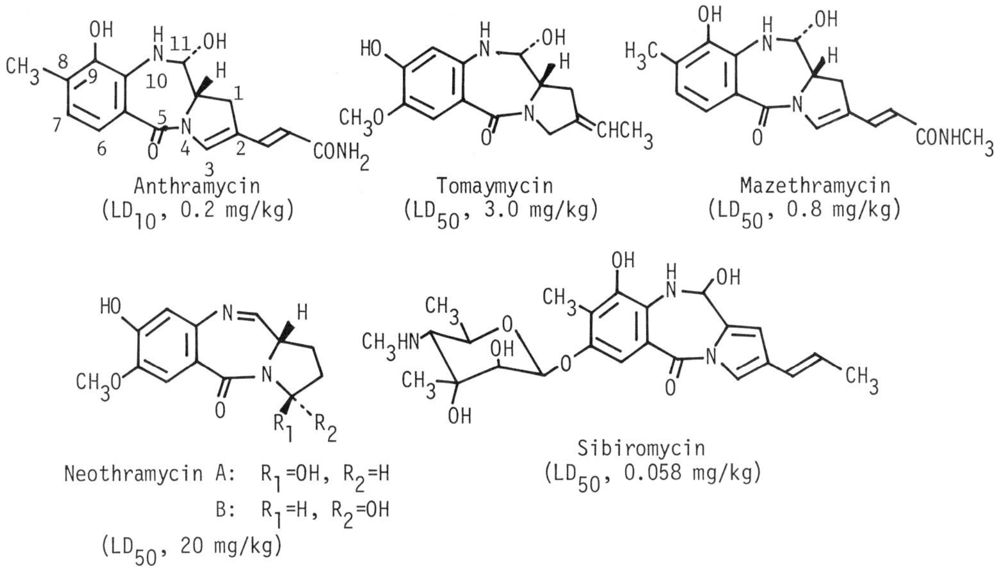

Fig. 12. Anthramycin group antibiotics.

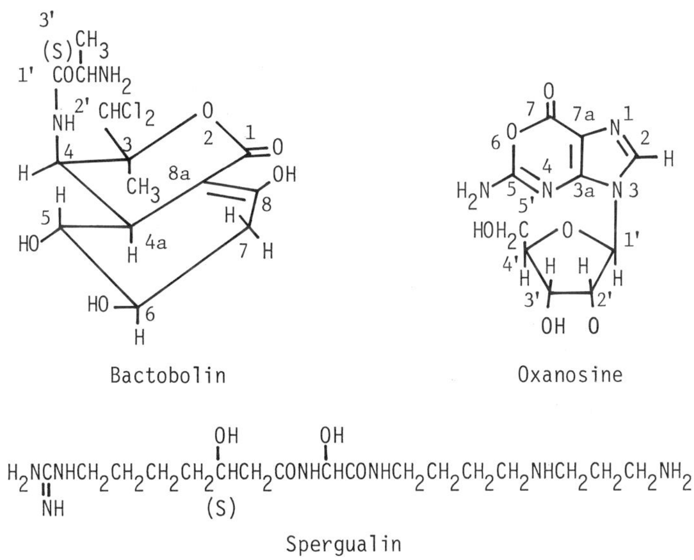

Fig. 13. New antitumor antibiotics.

(Ref. 49), adriamycin, etc. have been observed to inhibit the action or generation of suppressor cells in mice. Oxanosine (Ref. 50 & 51) (Fig. 13), a nucleoside antitumor antibiotic which we discovered recently has been suggested to inhibit the generation of suppressor cells. Research on antitumor antibiotics is now being extended to those compounds which inhibit the action, growth, or generation of suppressor cells.

LOW MOLECULAR WEIGHT IMMUNO-MODIFIERS

In order to cure cancer, minimal residual tumors after macroscopic elimination should be completely eliminated by the action of the host defense system or additional chemotherapy. Therefore, I undertook a study to find microbial products which would enhance immune responses and restore the reduced immune-resistance commonly found in cancer patients.

As described later, I initiated the screening for low molecular weight enzyme inhibitors, reporting the first work in 1969 (Ref. 52). We then expanded the study of enzyme inhibitors to the study of low molecular weight immuno-modifiers.

In 1972, we found that a very low dose of coriolin, antitumor antibiotics produced by *Coriolus consor* and its derivative, diketocoriolin B (Fig. 14), increased the number of mouse spleen cells producing antibody to sheep red blood cells (Ref. 53). We also found that diketocoriolin B inhibits Na^+-K^+-ATPase (Ref. 54). Therefore, I thought that the binding of coriolin and diketocoriolin B to ATPase in cell membranes caused the blastogenesis of lymphocytes producing antibody. Later, we confirmed that the action of diketocoriolin B in increasing the number of antibody-forming cells is due to its interaction with B lymphocytes producing antibody to sheep red blood cells (Ref. 55).

I assumed that the screening of compounds which bind to cell membranes or surfaces would result in the finding of immuno-modifiers; so, with my colleagues, I began a search for inhibitors of enzymes located on cell surfaces or membranes. We first found that all aminopeptidases are not only in cells but also located on their surfaces (Ref. 56). These enzymes are not released extracellularly. Alkaline phosphatase and esterase were also found to be located on cell surfaces. Searching for inhibitors of these enzymes, we found bestatin (Ref. 57 & 58), inhibiting aminopeptidase B (Ki=6 x 10^{-8}M) and leucine aminopeptidase (Ki=2 x 10^{-8}M); amastatin (Ref. 58 & 59), inhibiting aminopeptidase A (Ki=1.5 x 10^{-7}M) and leucine aminopeptidase (Ki=1.5 x 10^{-6}M); forphenicine (Ref. 58 & 60), inhibiting chicken intestine alkaline phosphatase; and esterastin (Ref. 58 & 61) (Ki=2 x 10^{-10}M) and ebelactones A and B (Ref. 58 & 62), inhibiting esterase (Ki=9.2 x 10^{-8}M for A; Ki=5 x 10^{-10}M for B). Their structures are shown in Fig. 15. All these inhibitors, except for esterastin, enhanced immune responses (Ref. 58).

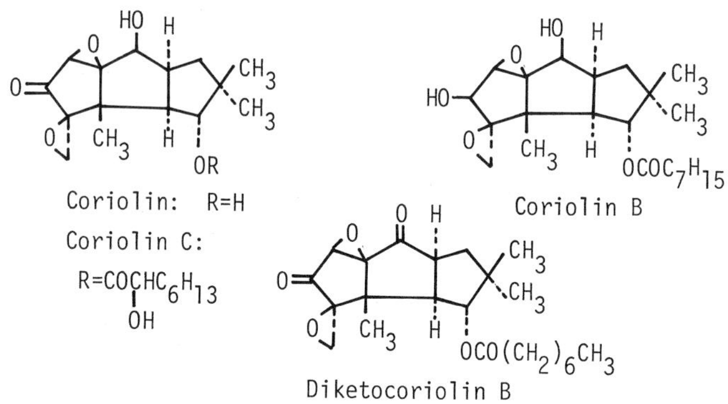

Fig. 14. Coriolins, products of *Coriolus consor*, and their derivatives.

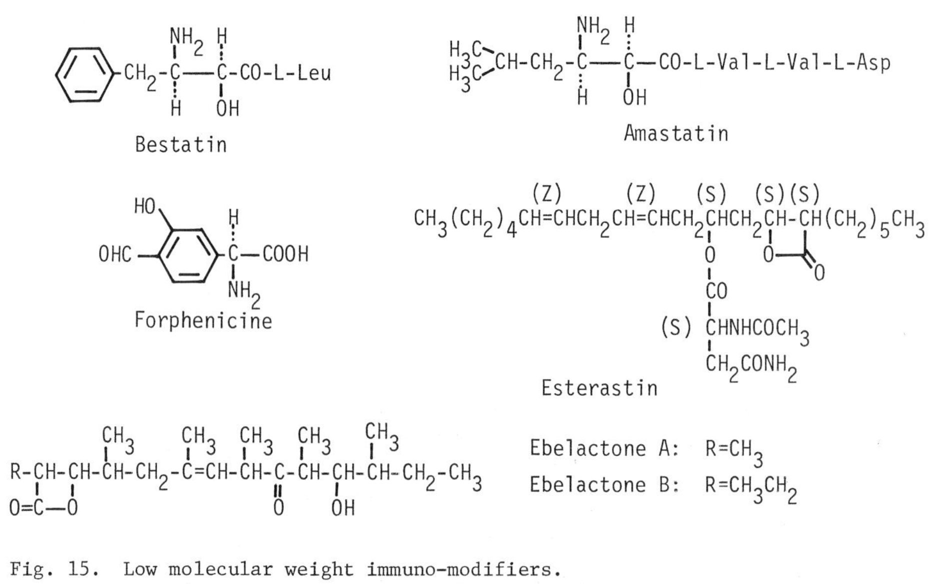

Fig. 15. Low molecular weight immuno-modifiers.

A low dose (1-100 μg/mouse) of bestatin enhanced delayed-type hypersensitivity (DTH) to sheep red blood cells, and, at higher doses (1 mg/mouse), it increased the number of antibody-forming cells in spleen. Amastatin increased the number of antibody-forming cells. Forphenicine (1-100 μg/mouse) enhanced DTH and also increased the number of antibody-forming cells (10-1,000 μg/mouse). Ebelactone enhanced DTH. But esterastin suppressed DTH and reduced the number of antibody-forming cells.

We have synthesized all stereoisomers of bestatin (Ref. 58). Those isomers which have the S-configuration at the 2-C of the 3-amino-2-hydroxy-4-phenylbutyryl moiety showed similar activity as bestatin in inhibiting aminopeptidase B and enhancing DTH, but the other isomers having the R-configuration at this carbon atom had no activity.

Very recently, we have found an inhibitor which is completely specific for aminopeptidase B. We elucidated its structure (Fig. 16) and named it "arphamenine". This was isolated from culture filtrates of a bacterial strain classified as Chromobacterium violaceum. Arphamenines A and B (Fig. 16) inhibit aminopeptidase B very strongly (50% inhibit concentrations were 0.006 μg/ml for A (Ki=2.5 x 10^{-9}M) and 0.002 μg/ml for B (Ki=8 x 10^{-10}M); however, they do not inhibit aminopeptidase A or leucine aminopeptidase. Arphamenines enhanced delayed-type hypersensitivity.

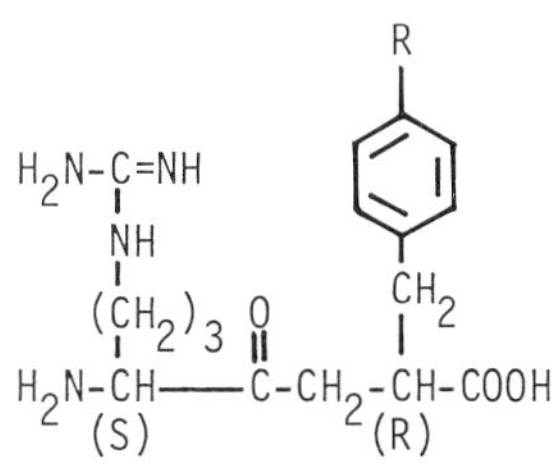

Arphamenine A: R=H
Arphamenine B: R=OH

Fig. 16. Arphamenine.

Among low molecular weight immuno-modifiers described above, bestatin, forphenicine, forphenicinol and arphamenine A have been tested for antitumor effects. All showed antitumor action against mouse tumors *in vivo*. Among them, bestatin has been studied in most detail (Ref. 58). It enhanced immune responses in mice and humans and stimulated the production of both interleukin 1 and 2. Bestatin has been clinically studied and studies using randomized schedules are indicating its effect in suppressing relapse after elimination of macroscopic tumors.

LOW MOLECULAR WEIGHT ENZYME INHIBITORS

One of the reasons why antibiotic research is still being continued is due to the expansion of its research area. By 1965, NMR and X-ray crystallography had already been introduced into natural product chemistry, and it became possible to elucidate the structures of low molecular weight microbial products very quickly. Moreover, at about that same time, an understanding of the biochemistry of various diseases began to make rapid progress. Therefore, I initiated the screening of culture filtrates for low molecular weight enzyme inhibitors (Ref. 52). In this study with my colleagues, I have discovered about 50 new compounds which have various pharmacological activities.

Testing for the activities of streptomyces culture filtrates in inhibiting various proteases, the following protease inhibitors (Fig. 17) have been discovered (Ref. 63): leupeptin (Fig. 17), inhibiting plasmin, trypsin, papain, and cathepsin B; antipain (Fig. 17), inhibiting papain, trypsin, and cathepsin B; chymostatin (Fig. 17), inhibiting chymotrypsin; elastatinal (Fig. 17), inhibiting pancreatic elastase; phosphoramidon (Fig. 18), inhibiting metalloproteinases such as thermolysin, *etc.*; and pepstatin (Fig. 19), inhibiting carboxylproteinases such as pepsin, cathepsin D, renin, *etc.*

Trypsin, chymotrypsin or elastase hydrolyze peptide bonds at the carboxyl side of arginine, phenylalanine or alanine moiety in peptides, and leupeptin, chymostatin, and elastatinal contain the argininal, phenylalaninal or alaninal moiety. This aldehyde structure for inhibition of serine and thiole proteinases was first found in these inhibitors. β-MAPI recently reported by Murao, *et al.* (Ref. 64) inhibits chymotrypsin and thiol proteinases and also has the phenylalaninal moiety. The L-leucyl-L-tryptophan N-phosphate is the active structural moiety of phosphoramidon. Talopeptin (Fig. 18) recently reported by Murao, *et al.* (Ref. 65) also has this active structural moiety.

The protease inhibitors described above have been widely used for the identification of proteases and analysis of their roles in normal biological and disease processes. Pepstatin was used as the functional group for affinity chromatography of renin, and this enzyme was first purified by such chromatography. Leupeptin exhibits an effect in preventing genetic mouse muscular dystrophy. The medicinal application of protease inhibitors are being studied from various aspects for treatment of thrombosis, muscular dystrophy, cancer, etc.

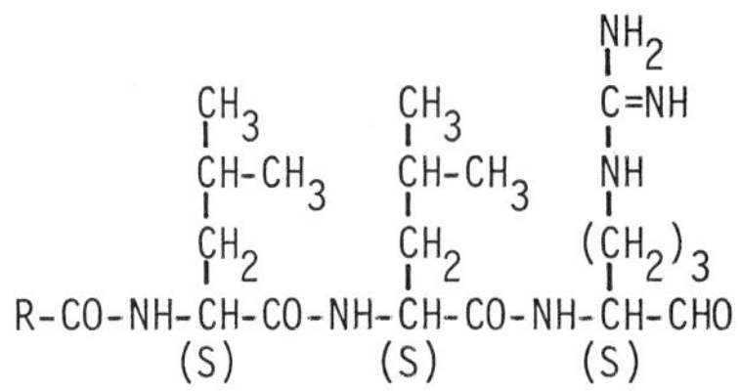

Leupeptin

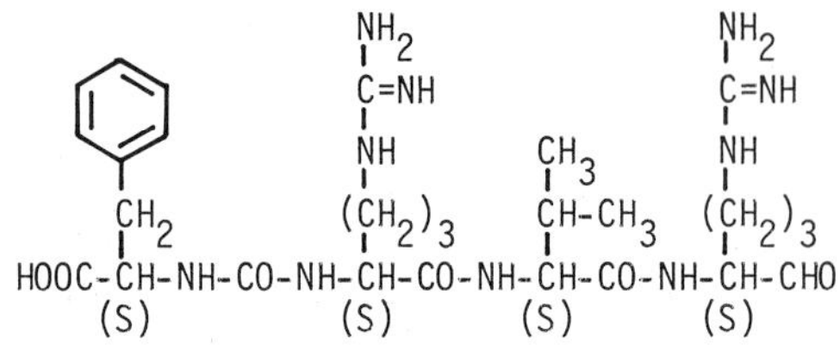

Antipain

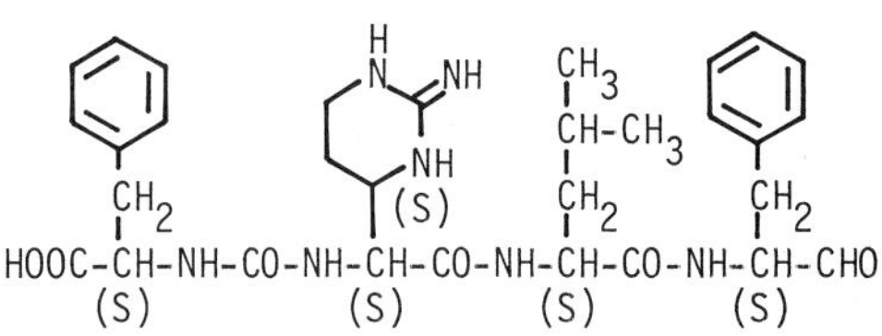

Chymostatin

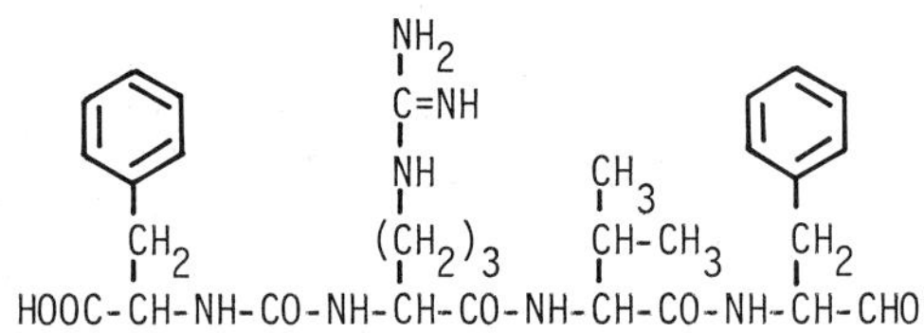

β-MAPI

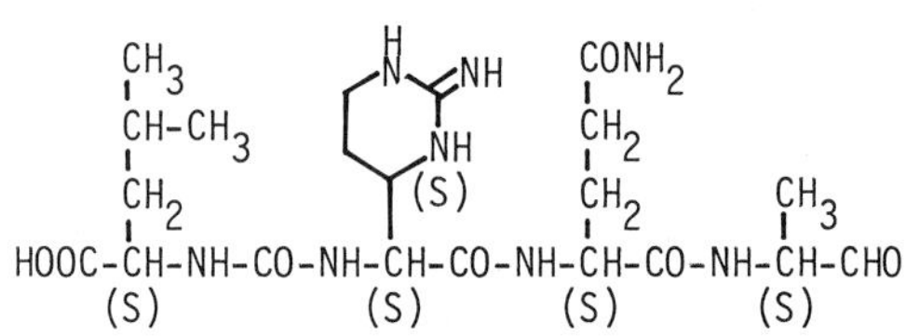

Elastatinal

Fig. 17. Inhibitors of serine and thiol proteinases.

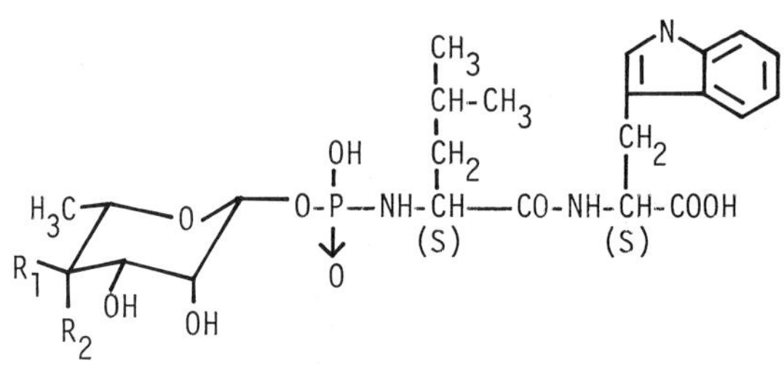

Phosphoramidon: R_1=OH, R_2=H

Talopeptin (MK-I): R_1=H, R_2=OH

Fig. 18. Inhibitors of metalloproteinases.

We have also found inhibitors of enzymes involved in the biosynthesis of noradrenaline (Ref. 52 & 66); that is, oudenone (Fig. 20) inhibits tyrosine hydroxylase; various isoflavone compounds (Fig. 20) inhibit dopa decarboxylase; dopastin (Fig. 20) inhibits dopamine β-hydroxylase. During the screening studies, we also found that fusaric (fusarinic) acid (Fig. 20) has a strong effect in inhibiting dopamine β-hydroxylase. All of these inhibitors show a hypotensive effect against hypertension of spontaneously hypertensive rats. A clinical study has also confirmed the hypotensive effect of fusaric acid against essential hypertension.

RCO-L-Val-L-Val-STA-L-Ala-STA

Pepstatin

RCO-L-Val-L-Val-STA-L-Ser-STA

Hydroxypepstatin

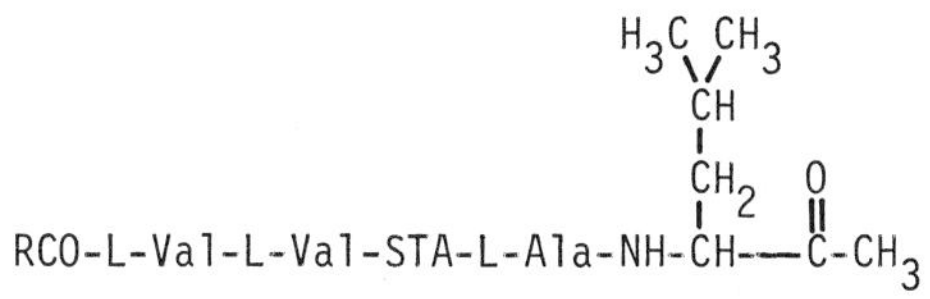

Pepstanone

$R = (CH_3)_2CH\text{-}(CH_2)_n\text{-}, \quad CH_3\text{-}(CH_2)_n\text{-} \quad (n=0,\ 1\text{-}20)$

$STA\ (statin) = (CH_3)_2CH\text{-}CH_2\text{-}\underset{(S)}{CH}(NH_2)\text{-}\underset{(S)}{CH}(OH)\text{-}CH_2COOH$

Fig. 19. Inhibitors of carboxyl proteinases:

R of pepstatin widely used is $(H_3C)_2CHCH_2$-

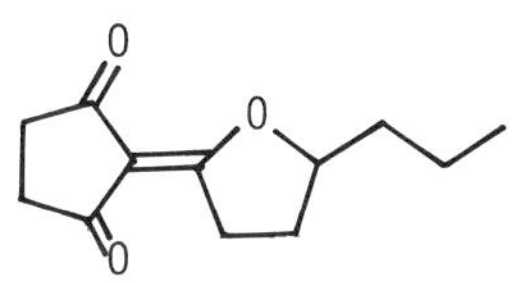

Oudenone (TH)

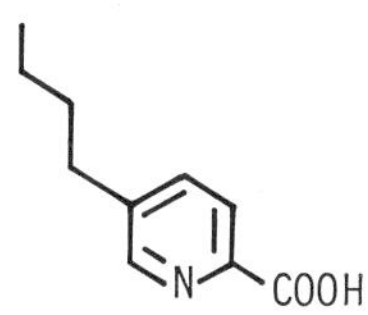

Fusaric acid (DβH)

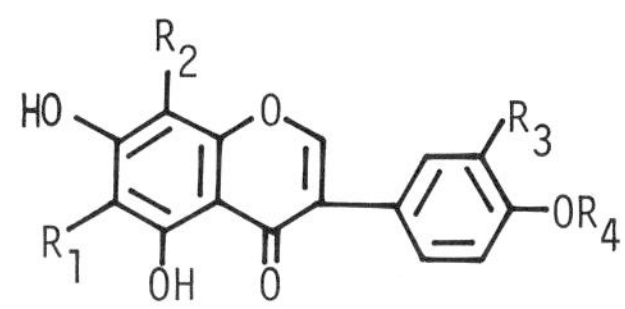

(DpdC)

Compound	R_1	R_2	R_3	R_4
I	H	H	OH	H
II	H	OCH_3	OH	H
III	H	OCH_3	H	H
IV	H	OH	H	H
V	OCH_3	H	OH	CH_3
VI	H	OCH_3	OH	CH_3

(I=Orobol)

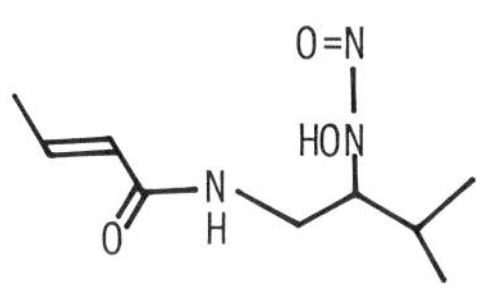

Dopastin (DβH)

Fig. 20. Inhibitors of enzymes involved in noradrenaline synthesis:

Tylosine $\xrightarrow[\text{TH}]{}$ DOPA $\xrightarrow[\text{DpdC}]{}$ Dopamine $\xrightarrow[\text{D}\beta\text{H}]{}$ Noradrenaline;

( ) means the enzyme inhibited.

Up to the present, we have found about 50 enzyme inhibitors and have elucidated all of their structures (Ref. 66 & 67). All of them have no significant activity in inhibiting the growth of microorganisms. The study of enzyme inhibitors is now under way in the laboratories of pharmaceutical companies. For example, inhibitors (ML-236B and mevinolin, Fig. 21) (Ref. 68 & 69) of 3-hydroxy-3-methylglutaryl-CoA reductase involved in mevalonate synthesis have been reported to be useful in the treatment of cholesteremia (Ref. 70).

As described above, the study of enzyme inhibitors is leading to the discovery of various compounds which have therapeutic effects on various diseases in humans and animals. For instance, bestatin and forphenicinol which bind to cell surfaces or membranes described in a

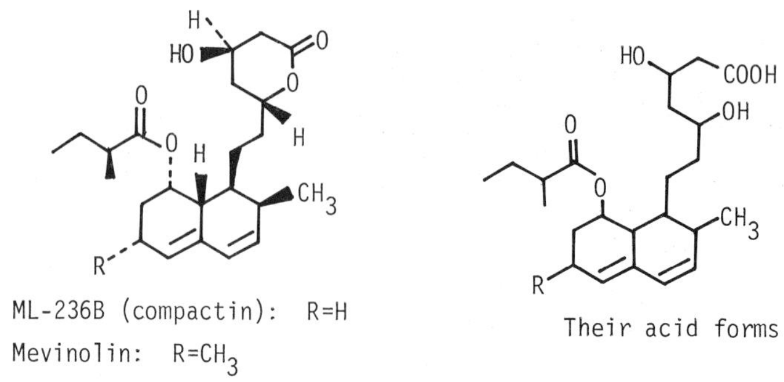

Fig. 21. Compactin and mevinolin.

previous paragraph were recently found by Matsushita *et al*. at the Wakayama Medical School to exhibit a therapeutic effect on genetic mouse muscular dystrophy.

The study of low molecular weight enzyme inhibitors may lead to the discovery of microbial products useful as pesticides.

CONCLUSION

Studies of antibiotics and low molecular weight enzyme inhibitors have indicated that microorganisms produce compounds which have various structures and biological activities. The reason why microorganisms produce an almost unlimited number of compounds is being studied from its genetic aspect. Therefore, parallel to progress in the analysis of plant disease processes, screening methods will be established and new compounds useful in preventing plant diseases will be found among microbial products.

Moreover, although up to now, our search for new microbial products has been dependent on microorganisms collected from nature, in the future we may be able to utilize recent technology to make new genes for the production of new useful compounds.

REFERENCES

1. H. Umezawa, Y. Okami, T. Hashimoto, Y. Suhara, M. Hamada and T. Takeuchi, *J. Antibiotics* *18A*, 101-103 (1965).
2. T. Ikekawa, H. Umezawa and Y. Iitaka, *J. Antibiotics* *19A*, 49-50 (1965).
3. Y. Suhara, F. Sasaki, K. Maeda, H. Umezawa and M. Ohno, *J. Am. Chem. Soc*. *90*, 6559 (1968).
4. Symposium on Kasugamycin-Fundamental and Clinical Studies Published by Microbial Chemistry Research Foundation, 3-14-23 Kamiosaki, Shinagawa-ku, Tokyo (1966).
5. K. Isono, J. Nagatsu, Y. Kawashima and S. Suzuki, *Agric. Biol. Chem*. *29*, 848-854 (1965).
6. T. Iwasa, H. Yamamoto and M. Shibata, *J. Antibiotics* *23*, 595-602 (1970).
7. A. Imada, K. Kitano, K. Kintaka, M. Muroi and M. Asai, *Nature* *289*, 590-591 (1981).
8. R.B. Sykes, C.M. Cimarusti, D.P. Bonner, K. Bush, D.M. Floyd, N.H. Georgopapadokou, W.H. Koster, W.C. Lin, W.L. Parker, P.A. Principe, M.L. Rathnum, W.A. Slusarchyk, W.H. Trejo and J.S. Wells, *Nature* *291*, 489-491 (1981).
9. H. Umezawa, M. Okanishi, S. Kondo, K. Hamana, R. Utahara, K. Maeda and S. Mitsuhashi, *Science* *157*, 1559-1561 (1967).
10. S. Umezawa, T. Tsuchiya, R. Muto, Y. Nishimura and H. Umezawa, *J. Antibiotics* *24*, 274-275 (1971).
11. H. Umezawa, S. Umezawa, T. Tsuchiya and Y. Okazaki, *J. Antibiotics* *24*, 485-487 (1971).
12. H. Umezawa, *Advances in Carbohydrate Chemistry and Biochemistry*, Vol. 30, p. 183, Academic Press, New York (1974).
13. H. Umezawa, *Jap. J. Antibiotics* *32* (Suppl.), S1-S14 (1979).
14. H. Umezawa, *Microbial Drug Resistance*, Vol. 3, Japan Sci. Soc. Press, Tokyo (1982, in press).
15. Y. Horiuchi, D. Ikeda, S. Kondo and H. Umezawa, *J. Antibiotics* *33*, 1577-1580 (1980).
16. H. Umezawa, T. Takeuchi, K. Nitta, T. Yamamoto and S. Yamaoka, *J. Antibiotics* *6A*, 101 (1953).
17. A.D. Marco, A.M. Casazza, F. Giuliani, G. Pratesi, F. Arcamone, L. Bernardi, G. Franchi, P. Giardino, B. Patelli and S. Penco, *Cancer Treatment Reports* *62*, 375-380 (1978).
18. T. Oki, Y. Matsuzawa, A. Yoshimoto, K. Numata, I. Kitamura, S. Hori, A. Takamatsu, H. Umezawa, M. Ishizuka, H. Naganawa, H. Suda, M. Hamada and T. Takeuchi, *J. Antibiotics* *28*, 830-834 (1975).

19. T. Oki, A. Yoshimoto, Y. Matsuzawa, T. Takeuchi and H. Umezawa, J. Antibiotics 34, 916-918 (1981).
20. Y. Takahashi, H. Naganawa, T. Takeuchi and H. Umezawa, J. Antibiotics 30, 622-624 (1977).
21. H. Umezawa, T. Takahashi, M. Kinoshita, H. Naganawa, T. Masuda, M. Ishizuka, K. Tatsuta and T. Takeuchi, J. Antibiotics 32, 1082-1084 (1979).
22. D. Dantchev, M. Paintrand, M. Hayat, C. Bourut and G. Mathe, J. Antibiotics 32, 1085-1086 (1979).
23. H. Umezawa, Y. Takahashi, M. Kinoshita, H. Naganawa, K. Tatsuta and T. Takeuchi, J. Antibiotics 33, 1581-1585 (1980).
24. K. Maeda, H. Kosaka, K. Yagishita and H. Umezawa, J. Antibiotics 9A, 82-85 (1956).
25. T. Takita, Y. Muraoka, T. Nakatani, A. Fujii, Y. Umezawa, H. Naganawa and H. Umezawa, J. Antibiotics 31, 801-804 (1978).
26. T. Takita, Y. Umezawa, S. Saito, H. Morishima, T. Tsuchiya, T. Miyake, H. Umezawa, Y. Muraoka, M. Suzuki, M. Otsuka and M. Ohno, Tetrahedron Lett. 23, 521-524 (1982).
27. T. Takita, Y. Muraoka, T. Nakatani, A. Fujii, Y. Iitaka and H. Umezawa, J. Antibiotics 31, 1073-1077 (1978).
28. H. Kasai, H. Naganawa, T. Takita and H. Umezawa, J. Antibiotics 31, 1316-1320 (1978).
29. L.F. Povirk, M. Hogan and N. Dattagupta, Biochem. 18, 96-101 (1979).
30. L.F. Povirk, Biochem. 20, 665-670 (1981).
31. H. Okubo, Y. Abe, M. Hori, H. Asakura and H. Umezawa, J. Antibiotics 34, 1213-1215 (1981).
32. N.J. Oppenheimer, L.O. Rodriguez and S.M. Hecht, Biochem. 18, 3439-3445 (1979).
33. N.J. Oppenheimer, C. Chang, L.-H. Chang, G. Ehrenfeld, L.O. Rodriguez and S.M. Hecht, J. Biol. Chem. 257, 1606-1609 (1982).
34. H. Kuramochi, K. Takahashi, T. Takita and H. Umezawa, J. Antibiotics 34, 576-582 (1981).
35. R.M. Burger, J. Peisach and S.B. Horwitz, J. Biol. Chem. 256, 11636-11644 (1981).
36. L. Giloni, M. Takeshita, F. Johnson, C. Iden and P. Grollman, J. Biol. Chem. 256, 8608-8615 (1981).
37. T. Shomura, S. Omoto, K. Ohba, H. Ogino, M. Kojima and S. Inouye, J. Antibiotics 33, 1243-1248 (1980).
38. A. Fujii, Bleomycin: Chemical, Biochemical and Biological Aspects, Springer-Verlag, Heidelberg (1979).
39. H. Umezawa, Pure Appl. Chem. 28, 665-680 (1971).
40. H. Umezawa, GANN Monograph on Cancer Research, No. 19, p. 3, Univ. Tokyo Press, Tokyo (1976).
41. H. Umezawa, Y. Takahashi, A. Fujii, T. Saino, T. Shirai and T. Takita, J. Antibiotics 26, 117-119 (1973).
42. T. Takita, T. Fukuoka and H. Umezawa, J. Antibiotics 26, 252-254 (1973).
43. C. Urakawa, K. Nakano and R. Imai, J. Antibiotics 33, 804-809 (1980).
44. T. Takeuchi, M. Miyamoto, M. Ishizuka, H. Naganawa, S. Kondo, M. Hamada and H. Umezawa, J. Antibiotics 29, 93-96 (1976).
45. L.H. Hurley, J. Antibiotics 30, 349-370 (1977).
46. S. Kondo, Y. Horiuchi, M. Hamada, T. Takeuchi and H. Umezawa, J. Antibiotics 32, 1069-1071 (1979).
47. H. Umezawa, S. Kondo, H. Iinuma, S. Kunimoto, Y. Ikeda, H. Iwasawa, D. Ikeda and T. Takeuchi, J. Antibiotics 34, 1622-1624 (1981).
48. S. Kondo, H. Iwasawa, D. Ikeda, Y. Umeda, Y. Ikeda, H. Iinuma and H. Umezawa, J. Antibiotics 34, 1625-1627 (1981).
49. M. Ishizuka, T. Takeuchi, T. Masuda, S. Fukasawa and H. Umezawa, J. Antibiotics 34, 331-340 (1981).
50. N. Shimada, N. Yagisawa, H. Naganawa, T. Takita, M. Hamada, T. Takeuchi and H. Umezawa, J. Antibiotics 34, 1216-1218 (1981).
51. N. Yagisawa, N. Shimada, H. Naganawa, T. Takita, M. Hamada, T. Takeuchi, H. Umezawa, H. Nakamura and Y. Iitaka, Nucleic Acid Research, Symposium Series 10, 55-58 (1982).
52. H. Umezawa, Enzyme Inhibitors of Microbial Origin, Univ. Tokyo Press, Tokyo (1972).
53. M. Ishizuka, H. Iinuma, T. Takeuchi and H. Umezawa, J. Antibiotics 25, 320-321 (1972).
54. T. Kunimoto, M. Hori and H. Umezawa, Biochim. Biophys. Acta 298, 513-525 (1973).
55. M. Ishizuka, T. Takeuchi and H. Umezawa, J. Antibiotics 34, 95-102 (1981).
56. T. Aoyagi, H. Suda, M. Nagai, K. Ogawa, J. Suzuki, T. Takeuchi and H. Umezawa, Biochim. Biophys. Acta 452, 131-143 (1976).
57. H. Umezawa, T. Aoyagi, H. Suda, M. Hamada and T. Takeuchi, J. Antibiotics 29, 97-99 (1976).
58. H. Umezawa (Ed.), Small Molecular Immunomodifiers of Microbial Origin - Fundamental and Clinical Studies of Bestatin, Japan Sci. Soc. Press, Tokyo, Pergamon Press, Oxford (1981).
59. T. Aoyagi, H. Tobe, F. Kojima, M. Hamada, T. Takeuchi and H. Umezawa, J. Antibiotics 31, 636-638 (1978).
60. T. Aoyagi, T. Yamamoto, K. Kojiri, F. Kojima, M. Hamada, T. Takeuchi and H. Umezawa, J. Antibiotics 31, 244-246 (1978).
61. H. Umezawa, T. Aoyagi, T. Hazato, K. Uotani, F. Kojima, M. Hamada and T. Takeuchi, J. Antibiotics 31, 639-641 (1978).

62. H. Umezawa, T. Aoyagi, K. Uotani, M. Hamada, T. Takeuchi and S. Takahashi, J. Antibiotics 33, 1594-1596 (1980).
63. H. Umezawa, Methods in Enzymology, Vol. 45, p. 678, Academic Press, New York (1976).
64. T. Watanabe, K. Fukuhara and S. Murano, Tetrahedron 38 (1982, in press).
65. K. Fukuhara, S. Murano, T. Nozawa and M. Hatano, Tetrahedron 38 (1982, in press).
66. H. Umezawa, Jap. J. Antibiotics 30 (Suppl.), S138-S163 (1977).
67. K. Maeda and M. Ohno, Heterocycles 13, 49-85 (1979).
68. I. Kaneko, Y. Hazama-Shimada and A. Endo, Eur. J. Biochem. 87, 313-321 (1978).
69. A.W. Alberts, J. Chen, G. Kurou, V. Hunt, J. Huff, C. Hoffman, J. Rothrock, M. Lopez, H. Joshua, E. Harris, A. Pachett, R. Monaghan, S. Currie, E. Stapeley, G. Albers-Schonberg, O. Hensens, J. Hirshfield, K. Hoogsteen, J. Liesch and J. Springer, Proc. Natl. Acad. Sci. U.S.A. 77, 3957-3961 (1980).
70. A. Yamamoto, H. Sudo and A. Endo, Atherosclerosis 35, 259-266 (1980).

BIOLOGICAL PROPERTIES OF KASUGAMYCIN

Kiyoshi Sato

Central Research Laboratories, Hokko Chemical Industry Co. Ltd., Toda 2165, Atsugi, Kanagawa 243, Japan

Abstract - Kasugamycin (KSM) is one of the main fungicides for rice blast control. Recently, it is also employed as a single and mixture formulation with copper oxychloride for control of many bacterial plant diseases. KSM resistant strains of rice blast fungus was found in Shonai district of Yamagata Prefecture in 1971. However, the density of resistant strains decreased after ceasing from KSM application, and practically disappeared 3 years later in this district. This fact suggests that the competitive ability and survival ability of the resistant strain are inferior to that of sensitive one. KSM resistant plant pathogenic bacteria have not been found yet in field. It was recognized that KSM resistant strains of plant pathogenic bacteria isolated in *in vitro* selection were sensitive to several antibiotics including Streptomycin. Resistant bacteria to clinical-use antibiotics, having the inactivation enzyme, did not have cross-resistance to KSM.

INTRODUCTION

Kasugamycin (KSM) is produced by *Streptomyces kasugaensis* isolated from soil sample collected around Kasuga shrine in Nara city (Ref. 1). Its chemical structure, physico-chemical properties and toxicity were studied by research group of Institute of Microbial Chemistry (Ref. 2 & 3). On the other hand, its antifungal activity to rice blast fungus (*Pyricularia oryzae*) was studied in Hokko Chem. Co. (Ref. 4). KSM was proved to be highly safe to human and animals and excellently effective to rice blast, and has been widely used in commercial name "Kasumin" since 1965. This paper introduces recent information about KSM.

CONTROL OF BACTERIAL PLANT DISEASES

Recently, it was found that KSM has good activities against plant bacterial diseases. Table 1 shows that KSM is very effective for the control of bacterial seedling rot, severe disease of rice seedling caused by *Pseudomonas glumae* with soil treatment in nursery box (Ref. 5).

TABLE 1. Effect of KSM granule against rice bacterial seedling rot with soil treatment in seedling nursery box

Chemical	Rate g(a.i.)/box*	Percent of Rotten	Percent of Browning	Percent of Symptomless
KSM 1 % granule	0.05	9.7	3.6	86.7
	0.1	2.6	5.8	91.6
	0.2	1.0	5.7	93.3
	0.3	0	0.9	99.1
None	0	63.8	8.2	28.0

*Box size: 60x30x3 cm

The antibiotic has sufficiently preventive and curative effect for cucumber angular leaf spot (*Ps. syringae* pv. *lachrymans*) with foliar application (Ref. 6). It was found that the mixture of KSM and copper oxychloride shows marvelous effect against citrus canker (*Xanthomonas campestris* pv. *citri*), one of the major diseases of citrus fruit. Although single application of KSM is not effective to the disease, KSM combined with copper oxychloride has higher effect than copper oxychloride alone (Table 2). It is assumed that KSM works as a synergist and plays an important role in the control of this disease. On the other bacterial diseases, KSM performed well in laboratory and greenhouse tests against vegetable soft rot (*Erwinia carotovora* subsp. *carotovora*), bean haloblight (*Ps. syringae* pv. *phaseolicola*), cucumber marginal blight (*Ps. marginalis* pv. *marginalis*) and rice sheath brown rot (*Ps. fuscovaginae*). Practical usefulness of KSM against these diseases is evaluating under field conditions.

TABLE 2. Effect of mixture of KSM and copper oxychloride on control of citrus canker caused by *Xanthomonas campestris* pv. *citri* in greenhouse (1981)

Chemical	Concentration ppm(a.i.)	Disease severity[a)]
Mixture of KSM and copper oxychloride	50 + 450	29.0
KSM	50	100
Copper oxychloride	450	52.4
Unsprayed		100

a) Disease severity $= \dfrac{\text{Sum of individual ratings}}{7 \times \text{Number of leaves assessed}} \times 100$

Disease rated 0 to 7 with 0 = no lesion, 7 = more than 21 lesions on a leaf.

RESISTANCE TO RICE BALST FUNGUS

KSM resistant strains of rice blast fungus could be easily selected *in vitro* without any inductive treatment, and control effect of the antibiotic on rice plant infection by these strains was found to be very low (Ref. 7). Frequency of the resistant clones among conidia from culture strains did not vary with the various concentration of the antibiotic, but varied with strains and culture conditions (Ref. 8). These results would indicate that KSM does not participate in induction of mutation, but it selects the spontaneous KSM mutant during reproduction of the fungus. A decline in the control of rice blast by KSM was recognized in fields of Shonai district of Yamagata Prefecture in 1971 (Ref. 9 & 10). In this district, the antibiotic was used exclusively almost 90%, spraying 4 to 5 times a year over 3 years (Table 3). The intensive use of the antibiotic increased the density of KSM resistant strains in field, that resulted in decreased control effect of the antibiotic to rice blast. A similar phenomenon was found in Niigata Prefecture in 1974 (Ref. 13). The density of resistant strains decreased year by year after ceasing from KSM application, and practically disappeared 3 years later in Shonai district (Fig. 1). Thus, the resistant strains might disappear under the field condition free from selection pressure of the antibiotic. This tendency was reproducible in inoculation pot test with a mixture of equal numbers of sensitive and resistant spores, and it is recognized that the competitive ability of resistant strains would generally be more inferior to that of sensitive ones (Ref. 14).

In general, a relation between efficacy and resistance has been discussed only comparison with each proportion but not population of sensitive and resistant strains. According to the results of field experiments in the problem area, though the ratio of KSM resistant population in Phthalide and the mixed product of KSM and Phthalide was not decreased as much as unsprayed control, but each fungicide fairly controlled the rice ear blast (Fig. 2).

TABLE 3. Usage of KSM to control rice blast and development of KSM resistance problem in Yamagata Prefecture (1975)[a]

Year	Shonai district with the problem		The other districts free from the problem	
	% Coverage area with KSM	Spray times of KSM	% Coverate area with KSM	Spray times of KSM
1967	36	2.7	28	1.3
1968	54	3.5	46	1.9
1969	94	4.6	66	2.7
1970	90	4.2	57	2.0
1971	87	5.0	60	2.4

a: Adapted from Yamaguchi (Ref. 11) and Miura *et al*. (Ref. 12).

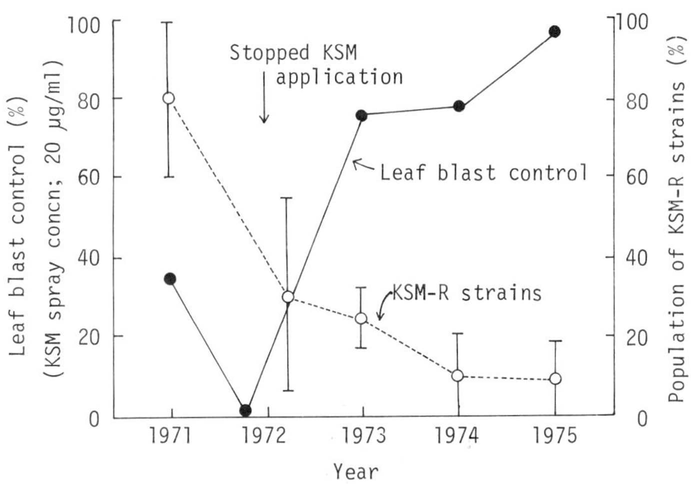

Fig. 1. Fluctuation of KSM-R population and effect of KSM to rice blast after stopped KSM application at Shonai district in Yamagata Prefecture (Ref. 12).

The percentage of ear blast in Phthalide or KSM plus Phthalide is significantly low, and the population of KSM resistant strains in the ear blast is obviously less than that in KSM or untreated check plot. To evaluate the effect of fungicides, relative survival inoculum population of resistant strains is more important rather than the ratio of resistant ones in the field. The only practical approach to cope with fungicide resistance is to avoid consecutive use of single fungicide. The best method is to use several groups of fungicides having different mode of action. The mixed product of KSM and Phthalide (Kasurabcide) is now being used with appropriate regulation in the previous KSM resistance problem areas.

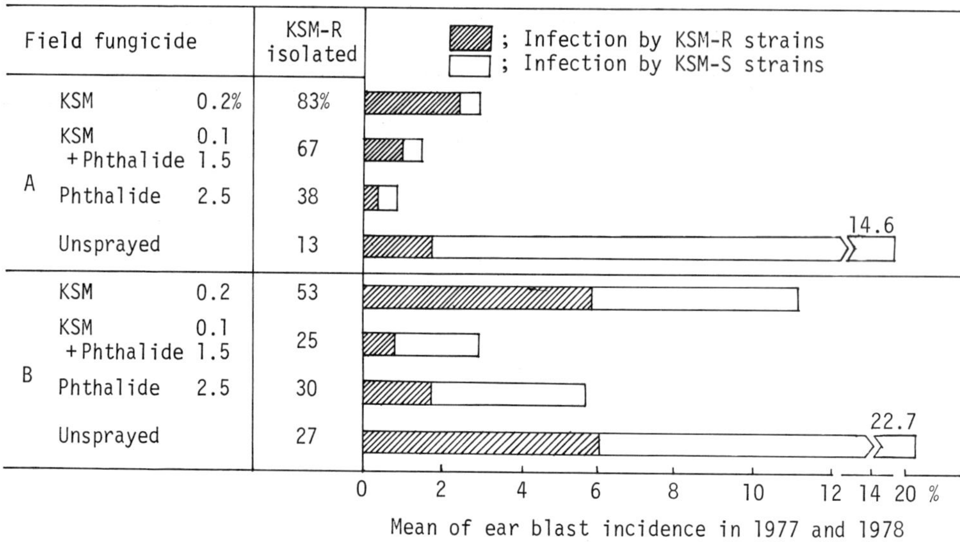

Fig. 2. Population of KSM-R strains in the ear blast after each fungicide spray (Ref. 15). Field, A: at Kubiki district in Niigata Pref.; B: at Yamato district in Niigata Pref.

MODE OF ACTION

KSM inhibits the protein synthesis by affecting the ribosomes in bacteria and fungal cells (Ref. 16). In the ribosome system of *Ps. aeruginosa*, *Ps. fluorescens* and *Escherichia coli* KSM inhibits the incorporation of amino acids. For example, the synthesis of poly phenylalanine on poly-U in *E. coli* is inhibited by 54% at 40 µg/ml of KSM (Ref. 17). KSM shows almost no inhibition against the protein synthesis in the ribosomes of rat liver cells. Eight hundred µg/ml of KSM showed only about 16% inhibition of protein synthesis by the liver cells (Ref. 18). These results indicate that KSM should have an antibacterial effect, but low toxicity to animals. Comparative studies of the inhibition of protein synthesis of bacteria by KSM, Streptomycin and Kanamycin have shown that KSM does not cause misreading of code, but Streptomycin and Kanamycin cause misreading. On the site of action of KSM in *E. coli*, Sparling, Davies and Tanaka pointed out that KSM was a specific inhibitor of the binding of fMet-tRNA to ribosome (Table 4 & 5).

TABLE 4. Effect of KSM(100 µg/ml) on *in vitro* polypeptide synthesis by hybrid ribosomes.

Ribosomes		% Inhibition	
30S	50S	Poly U-directed[a] ^{14}C-phenylalanine incorporation	Poly UG-directed[b] ^{14}C-valine incorporation
KSM^s	KSM^s	42	71
KSM^s	KSM^r	39	68
KSM^r	KSM^s	8	38
KSM^r	KSM^r	11	28

a: Data from Sparling (Ref. 19). b: Data from Helser and Davies (Ref. 20)

KSM^r: resistant strain

KSM^s: sensitive strain

TABLE 5. Effect of antibiotics on binding of fMet-tRNA to ribosomes

Ribosome	Messenger	Antibiotic	Concentration	% Inhibition
a. 70S	f2 RNA	KSM	2×10^{-4} M	98
	+ GTP	SM	2×10^{-5}	100
70S	f2 RNA	KSM	2×10^{-4}	100
	+ GMPPCP	SM	2×10^{-5}	8
70S	AUG	KSM	2×10^{-4}	100
30S	poly AUG*	KSM	2×10^{-4}	62
		SM	2×10^{-5}	1
b. 70S	f2 RNA	KSM	100 μg/ml	75
	+ GTP	TC	100	106
	f2 RNA	KSM	100	78
	+ GMPPCP	TC	100	23
30S(KSM^s)	poly AUG	KSM	100	55
30S(KSM^r)	poly AUG	KSM	100	3

a: Data from Okuyama *et al.* (Ref. 21). b: Data from Helser and Davies (Ref. 20). poly AUG*: Random copolymer of uridine, guanosine and adenosine. KSM: Kasugamycin SM: Streptomycin TC: Tetracycline.

CROSS RESISTANCE OT OTHER ANTIBIOTICS

KSM-resistance of rice blast fungus obtained from *in vitro* and *in vivo* selection seemed to be controled by major chromosomal genes (Ref. 22). On the resistance mechanism of KSM, *in vitro* selected KSM resistant mutant seemed to have the decreased affinity of ribosome to KSM (Table 6). On the other hand, there is no report that KSM resistant bacteria were isolated *in vivo*. And R factor-mediated drug resistance to KSM has not been obtained. Our studies revealed that KSM resistant phytopathogenic bacteria obtained by *in vitro* selection did not show to have any cross-resistance to the following antibiotics (Table 7). The resistant bacteria, having the inactivation enzyme to clinical-use aminoglycoside and macrolide antibiotics, did not have cross-resistance to KSM. It seems that these facts are attributed to the very unique structure of KSM, consisting of *d*-inositol and amidine carboxylic acid moiety and its different mode of action from other antibiotics.

TABLE 6. Effect of KSM on binding of aminoacyl-tRNA to ribosome of *Pyricularia oryzae*.

sRNA	Ribosome	Without KSM 15min**	30min	With KSM 20ppm 15min	30min
S	S	288*	452	147	249
S	R	60	109	59	120
R	R	53	129	47	128
R	S	255	556	168	338

* = c.p.m./0.1 OD_{280nm}
**= incubation periods

TABLE 7. Minimum inhibitory concentration of antibiotics to KSM resistant and sensitive phytopathogenic bacteria

(μg/ml)

Test organism		KSM	Strepto-mycin	Kana-mycin	Chloram-phenicol
Ps. syringae pv. *mori*	S*	25	3.13	12.5	50
	R**	200	6.25	12.5	100
Ps. syringae pv. *lachrymans*	S	50	1.56	25	6.25
	R	800	0.78	25	12.5
Ps. syringae pv. *syringae*	S	50	25	25	6.25
	R	3200	6.25	12.5	6.25
X. campestris pv. *campestris*	S	200	6.25	6.25	<0.39
	R	1600	6.25	6.25	<0.39
X. campestris pv. *oryzae*	S	200	25	25	<0.39
	R	1600	25	50	<0.39
X. campestris pv. *citri*	S	100	12.5	6.25	<0.39
	R	800	12.5	12.5	<0.39
X. campestris pv. *pruni*	S	100	3.13	0.78	<0.39
	R	1600	6.25	0.78	<0.39

Tested by agar dilution streak method.
Medium: Na-glutamate 0.2%, Sucrose 2.0%, K_2HPO_4 0.2%, Peptone 0.5%, Yeast extract 0.2%, $MgCl_2$ 0.1%, $FeSO_4$ 0.01%, pH 7.0
Incubated at 24°C for 48hrs.
* = KSM sensitive strain.
**= KSM resistant isolate selected from sensitive strain.

TABLE 8-1. Minimum inhibitory concentration of clinically used aminoglycoside antibiotics

(μg/ml)

Test organism	DSM	NM	PM	KM	GM	KSM
E. coli K-12	1.56	0.78	1.56	0.78	0.20	100
E. coli K-12 R5[a)]	>100	12.5	12.5	>100	3.13	100
E. coli K-12 J5R11-2[b)]	12.5	>100	>100	>100	1.56	200
E. coli K-12 ML1410 R81[b)]	>100	>100	>100	>100	0.78	200
E. coli K-12 LA290 R55[c)]	3.13	3.13	3.13	50	12.5	100
E. coli JR66/W677[c),d)]	>100	>100	>100	>100	25	200
E. coli K-12 C600 R135[e)]	50	1.56	3.13	1.56	50	100
Ps. aeruginosa A3	1.56	1.56	12.5	12.5	0.39	100
Ps. aeruginosa TI-13[b)]	>100	12.5	>100	50	3.13	200
Ps. aeruginosa GN315[a)]	50	25	>100	>100	6.25	200
Ps. aeruginosa 99[e)]	>100	100	>100	>100	>100	200
Ps. aeruginosa 21-75[f)]	>100	>100	>100	>100	>100	200
Ps. aeruginosa K-Ps102[g)]	>100	>100	>100	>100	6.25	200

Resistance mechanism: a) AAC(6') b) APH(3')-I c) AAD(2") d) APH(3')-II e) AAC(3) f) APH(3')-III g) permeability
Antibiotic DSM: Dihydrostreptomycin NM : Neomycin
PM : Paromomycin KM : Kanamycin
GM : Gentamicin KSM: Kasugamycin
Tested by agar dilution streak method using Mueller-Hinton medium.
Incubated at 37°C for 18hrs.
Adapted from Institute of Microbial Chemistry (I.M.C.) Data.

TABLE 8-2. Minimum inhibitory concentration macrolide antibiotics and KSM

(μg/ml)

Antibiotic	E.coli K-12	E.coli ML1629	E.coli LA290R55	Sal.enteritidis 1891	Sal.typhi T-63
MT[a]	25	100	25	1.56	50
JM[b]	>100	>100	12.5	12.5	>100
KSM[b]	100	50	100	50	50

Tested by agar dilution method.
a: Data adapted from Tanaka (Ref. 24); Nutrient agar medium.
b: Data adapted from I.M.C.; Mueller-Hinton medium.
MT: Mycaminosyl tylonolide JM: Josamycin

REFERENCES

1. H. Umezawa, Y. Okami, T. Hashimoto, Y. Suhara, M. Hamada and T. Takeuchi, J. Antibiot. 18, 101-108 (1965).
2. H. Umezawa, M. Hamada, Y. Suhara, T. Hashimoto, T. Ikekawa, N. Tanaka, K. Maeda, Y. Okami and T. Takeuchi, Antimicrob. Agents and Chemother. 753-757 (1965).
3. Y. Suhara, K. Maeda, H. Umezawa and M. Ohno, Advances in Chemistry Series 74, 15-40 (1968).
4. T. Ishiyama, T. Hashimoto, M. Hamada, Y. Okami, T. Takeuchi and H. Umezawa, J. Antibiot. 18, 115-119 (1965).
5. K. Tsujimoto, H. Yamamura and K. Sato, Ann. Phytopath. Soc. Japan 47, 402 (1981).
6. K. Sato, M. Kanda and H. Yamamura, ibid. 42, 61 (1976).
7. K. Ohmori, J. Antibiot. 20, 109 (1976).
8. H. Miura, M. Katagiri, T. Yamaguchi, Y. Uesugi and H. Ito, Ann. Phytopath. Soc. Japan 42, 117-123 (1976).
9. H. Miura, H. Kimura and S. Takahashi, ibid. 39, 230-240 (1973).
10. H. Miura, H. Ito and S. Takahashi, ibid. 41, 415-417 (1975).
11. T. Yamaguchi, Plant Protection 33, 471-476 (1979).
12. H. Miura and S. Takahashi, Ann. Phytopath. Soc. Japan 42,372 (1976).
13. N. Goh, T. Yaoita, K. Aoyagi, U. Ikeda and H. Sakurai, Proc. Assoc. Pl. Prot. Hokuriku 25, 58-60 (1977).
14. I. Ito and T. Yamaguchi, Ann. Phytopath. Soc. Japan 45, 40-46 (1979).
15. N. Ono, N. Goh and A. Enami, Proc. Assoc. Pl. Prot. Hokuriku 27, 34-36 (1979).
16. H. Masukawa, N. Tanaka and H. Umezawa, J. Antibiot. 21, 73-74 (1968).
17. N. Tanaka, Y. Yoshida, K. Sashikata, H. Yamaguchi and H. Umezawa, J. Antibiot. 19, 65-68 (1966).
18. N. Tanaka, T. Nishimura, H. Yamaguchi, C. Yamamoto, Y. Yoshida, K. Sashikata and H. Umezawa, J. Antibiot. 18, 139-144 (1965).
19. R.F. Sparling, Science 167, 56-57 (1970).
20. T.L. Helser and T.E. Davies, Bact. Proc. 137 (1971).
21. A. Okuyama, N. Machiyama, T. Kinoshita and N. Tanaka, Biochem. Biophys. Res. Commun. 43, 196-199 (1971).
22. M. Taga, M. Tsuda and A. Ueyama, Plant Protection 33, 471-476 (1979).
23. K. Ko, Y. Hoshino and T. Misato, Ann. Phytopath. Soc. Japan 35, 134 (1969).
24. A. Tanaka, T. Tsuchiya, Y. Okada and S. Umezawa, J. Antibiot. 35, 113-116 (1982).

CHARACTERISTICS OF VALIDAMYCIN A IN CONTROLLING *RHIZOCTONIA* DISEASES

Kazuho Matsuura

Research Laboratories, Agricultural Chemicals Division, Takeda Chemical Industries Ltd., Sakyo, Kyoto 606, Japan

Abstract - Validamycin A (VMA) is a kind of aminocyclitol antibiotic produced by *Streptomyces hygroscopicus* var. *limoneus*. This antibiotic is widely used for the control of sheath blight on rice, black scurf on potatoes, bottom rot on lettuce, and damping-off on tobacco and vegetable seedlings caused by *Rhizoctonia solani*. VMA caused retardation of mycelial growth, inhibited formation of infection cushion and suppressed the pathogenisity of *R. solani*. VMA did not inhibit growth of more than 2,100 strains of fungi and 760 strains of bacteria. The contents of protein and RNA in mycelia and those of glucose and glucosamine in the cell wall of *R. solani* were not affected by VMA-treatment. Production of inositol in culture broth of *R. solani* was inhibited by VMA. Recovery from growth retardation and suppression of the pathogenisity by VMA-treatment was observed by addition of inositol. In 1976 - 1978, sheath blight lesions were collected from more than 650 paddy fields throughout Japan, and no resistant strains of *R. solani* to VMA were detected. Resistant strains have not been obtained in a laboratory yet. The acute oral LD50 of VMA for mice and rats is more than 2g/kg. Skin and eye application caused no irritation to rabbits. In 24-month feeding test, no effects were produced on mice fed 10,000ppm nor on rats fed 1,000ppm. Carcinogenic, teratogenic and mutagenic effects were not observed. Residue in rice and straw after 6-time application was below the limit of detection. VMA was non-toxic to chicken, quail, honeybees, carp, killifish and 147 species of plants. No effect of VMA was observed on the sensitivity of *Staphylococcus aureus*, *Escherichia coli* and *Mycobacterium smegmatis* to the other aminocyclitol antibiotics.

INTRODUCTION

Recent remarkable changes in methods of rice cultivation in Japan, such as early transplantation, introduction of early maturing cultivars, high plant populations and high fertilization, have resulted in increase of the sheath blight occurence. This disease has come to be one of the most common and destructive diseases. Up to the middle of 1960s, organoarsenic compounds were solely used for the control of this disease. Application of those compounds often caused phytotoxicity to rice plants(1).

In 1966, *Streptomyces* sp., strain No. T-7545, was found to produce antibiotic substances showing curative effect on sheath blight(2,3,4,5,6). As a result of isolation, purification and characterization of the active substances, they were found to be new antibiotics and the major product was named validamycin A(5,7). This paper describes the chemical, biological and toxicological properties of validamycin A.

CHEMICAL AND PHYSIOLOGICAL PROPERTIES

Structural formula of VMA is presented in Fig. 1 and its chemical name is N-[(1*S*)-(1,4,6/5)-3-Hydroxymethyl-4,5,6-trihydroxy-2-cyclohexenyl][O-β-D-glucopyranosyl-(1→4)-(1*S*)-(1,2,4/3,5)-2,3,4-trihydroxy-5-hydroxymethylcyclohexyl]amine(8,9).

It was isolated from the culture broth of *Streptomyces hygroscopicus* var. *limoneus*. The culture broth was treated with Amberlite IR-120(H) and IR-45(OH) and then applied to a column of Dowex-50X-2. The antibiotic was adsorbed on the resin and then eluted with aqueous ammonia. The eluate concentrate was chromatographed on Dowex-50X-2 with pyridine-acetic acid, pH 7.5, and the eluate was concentrated to give pure validamycin A(5).
VMA is a colorless hygroscopic powder, its melting point is 135°C, $[\ ]_D^{24}$ 110° ± 15°(*c* 1,H_2O),

110° ± 15°(c 1, pyridine) and pKa 6.0. It is soluble in water, methylalcohol, dimethylformamide and methylsulfoxide, slightly soluble in ethylalcohol and acetone, and insoluble in ethylacetate and diethylether. Validamycin A is stable in sunlight or water(5).

Analysis The formulated sample and residues of VMA are extracted with solvents and evaporated under reduced pressure after interfering substances are removed by cleanup procedure. The dry samples are analyzed by gas chromatography using a flame ionization detector after the preparation of VMA trimethylsilyl derivative(10).

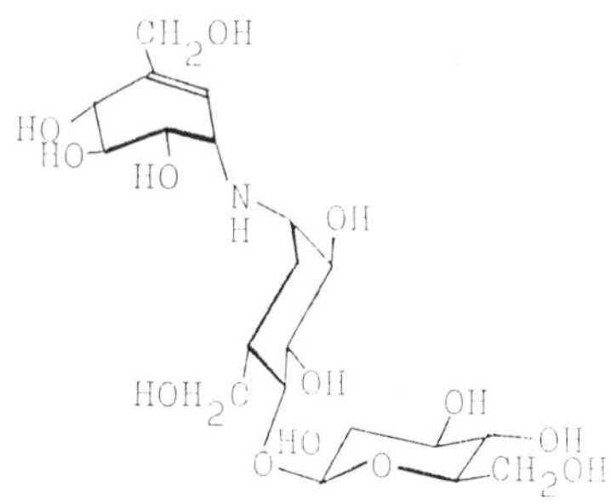

Fig. 1. Structural formula of validamycin A.

BIOLOGICAL PROPERTIES

Disease cycle of sheath blight Wintered sclerotia of *Rhizoctonia solani* are dug out by tillering in spring, spread out by floating on irrigated water and attach to lower parts of sheaths. Sclerotia are masses of fungus mycelia. The outer layer of sclerotium consists of mycelial cells without cytoplasm, but the inside consists of those with cytoplasm(Fig. 2). This structure makes the sclerotia easy to float. Initial infections in the seedling stage originate from mycelial growth from these sclerotia and expand to higher sheaths. One of the typical characteristics of *R. solani* penetrating into host tissues is the formation of infection cushions(Fig.5). Penetration hyphae grow from the infection cushion through the inner surface of the sheath and into the interior of the sheath. From that site, the hyphae penetrate adjacent cells, kill plant tissues and form visible symptoms. Severely diseased plants often snap at the upper diseased parts or lodge on the ground. The greatest loss results when the plants are infected up to the uppermost leaf and sheath.

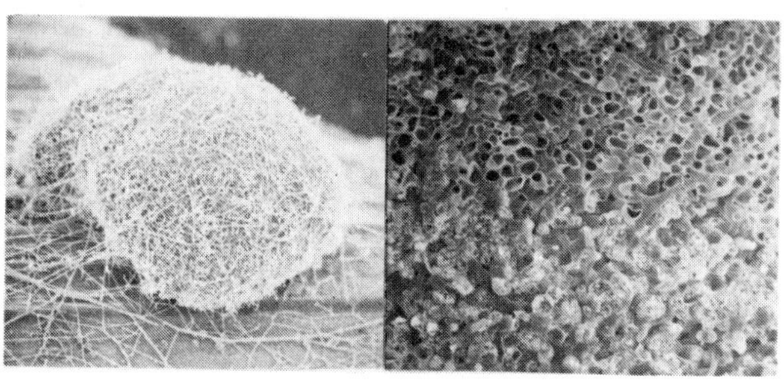

Fig. 2. A SEM image of sclerotium of *Rhizoctonia solani* (left, x130) and its cross section(right, x31).

Effect of VMA on mycelial growth of R. solani *R. solani*, strain No. TKF-44, was incubated on a potato sucrose agar for 2 days at 28°C. Mycelial disks, 9mm in diameter, were dipped in a test solution for a few seconds, inoculated on Czapek and plain agar plate in a 9cm petri dish and incubated at 28°C.

Growth of R. solani was retarded and the margin of the mycelial mat became dense. Retardation of growth was more remarkable on plain agar than on Czapek agar medium(Fig. 3). Microscopic observation of the tip part of the VMA-treated mycelia was illustrated in Fig. 4. The cell length of the trunk and branching hyphae was shorter(TABLE 1) and the angle of branching was wider in VMA-treated than in non-treated group(TABLE 2)(11,12,13).

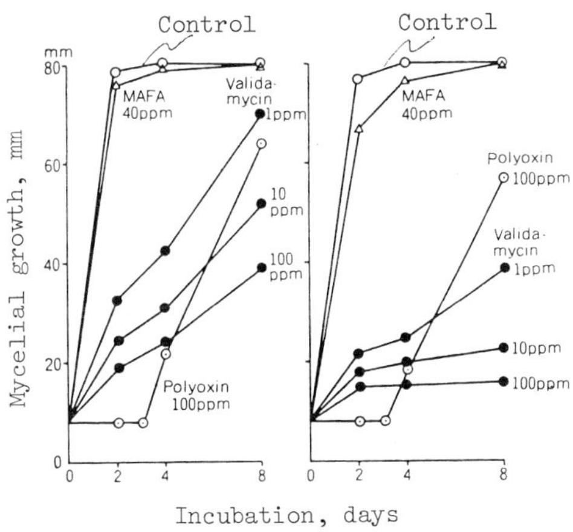

Fig. 3. Effect of validamycin A on growth of Rhizoctonia solani on Czapek(left) and plain agar(right).

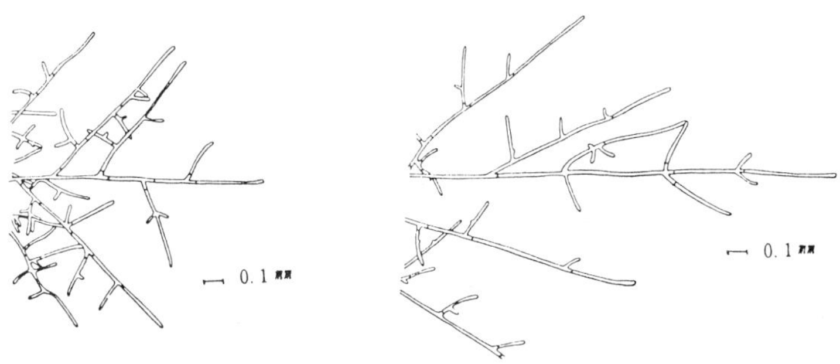

Fig. 4. Tip part of hyphae of Rhizoctonia solani grown in the presence(left) and absence(right) of validamycin A.

TABLE 1. Effect of validamycin A on the length of mycelial cell in Rhizoctonia solani

Treatment	Cell length (μm)			
	Trunk		Branch	
	Tip	Basal	Tip	Basal
Control (a)	381	292	242	168
Validamycin A 10μg/ml (b)	247	156	210	135
Ratio (b/a, %)	64.8	53.4	86.8	80.3

TABLE 2. Effect of validamycin A on the angle of hyphal branching in Rhizoctonia solani

Treatment	Angle of branching
Control	42.7°
Validamycin A 10 μg/ml	56.8°

Effect of VMA on infection cushion formation The leaf samples were cut into pieces, 5mm square, dipped in 2% glutaraldehyde for 3 hours. After washed with deionized water, the samples were dehydrated in a graded ethylalcohol series, then in a graded ethylalcohol-iso-amyl acetate series and finally placed into 100% iso-amyl acetate. They were then dried in a criticalpoint dryer, coated with an ion coater and observed in a scanning electron microscope(SEM) Hitachi S-430.

VMA caused remarkable inhibition of infection cushion formation at the concentration of 1ppm(TABLE 3, Fig.5)(13,14).

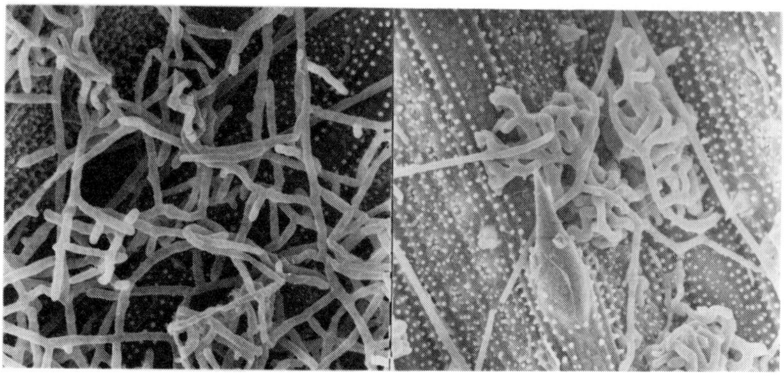

Fig. 5. A SEM image of mycelia and infection cushions on non-treated leaf (right, x300) and validamycin A-treated leaf(left, x300)(Photo by O. Wakae).

TABLE 3. Effect of validamycin A on infection cushion formation in Rhizoctonia solani

Treatment		Infection cushion formation[a)] on	
		Rice sheath	Broad bean leaf
Control		++	++
Validamycin A	0.1 ug/ml	+	+
	1.0	±	-
	10.0	-	-
	100.0	-	-

a) ++: abundant, +: poor, -: none

Effect of VMA on cellular constituents In order to determine the effect of VMA on the net increase in cellular constituents, Nioh and Mizushima(16) compared the increase in protein and RNA contents during growth with and without VMA.
The increase in the amount of protein and RNA was not affected significantly by the addition of VMA(TABLE 4).

Nioh and Mizushima determined the cell wall components of R. solani grown in the presence and absence of VMA, since the results reported by Mahadevan and Tatum(17) suggested a close relationship between the morphological changes and the components of its cell wall in Neurospora crassa.
Three neutral sugars(glucose, mannose and xylose) and glucosamine were found in the wall hydrolysate with or without VMA. There was no difference in the content of glucose and glucosamine in the cell wall of the fungus(TABLE 5)(16).

TABLE 4. Amounts of RNA and protein in mycelia of Rhizoctonia solani

Validamycin A (ug/ml)	RNA (ug/plate)	Protein (^{35}S) (cpm/plate)
0	13.1	3860
0.1	13.2	3220

TABLE 5. Contents of glucose and glucosamine in cell wall of Rhizoctonia solani

Validamycin A (ug/ml)	Cell wall (%)	Glucose (mg/10mg cell wall)	Glucosamine (mg/10mg cell wall)
0	16.5	3.15	1.03
0.1	17.2	3.07	1.01

Effect of VMA on inositol production The amount of inositol in the culture broth of R. solani grown in the presence and absence of VMA was checked by the bioassay method(18). Neurospora crassa, ATCC-9683 inositol-less mutant, was incubated on the Fries minimal medium containing inositol. One part of the 4-fold concentrated Fries medium and 3 parts of the culture broth of R. solani were mixed together with agar, autoclaved and solidified in a petri dish. Mycelial disk of N. crassa prepared above was inoculated to the center of the petri dish and incubated for 5 days at 25°C. Diameter of the mycelia was measured.
The amount of inositol in the culture broth of R. solani was markedly inhibited by VMA at concentrations of 0.75, 7.5 and 75 µg/ml(TABLE 6)(13).

VMA-treatment reduces the pathogenisity of R. solani. As inhibition of inositol production byVMA was observed, effect of inositol on the pathogenisity of R. solani grown in the presence and absence of VMA was examined by the following method. R. solani was incubated on PSA with or without VMA and/or inositol for 2 days at 28°C in a petri dish, and the surface sterilized seeds of cucumber, Cucumis sativus, cultivar Suyo, were placed on the margin of the mycelial mat at 10 seeds/plate. Inhibition of germination was examined 4 days after seeding.
As shown in Table 7, addition of inositol,at the concentration of 0.1µg/ml, to the medium containing VMA at the concentrations of 2.5 and 5.0µg/ml increased the pathogenisity of R. solani.

TABLE 6. Detection of inositol in the broth of Rhizoctonia solani with or without addition of validamycin A by inositol-less mutant of Neurospora crassa ATCC-9683

Medium	Diameter of mycelia[a] (mm)
Fries minimal medium (MM)	5
MM + Inositol 4 µg/ml	>85
MM + Inositol 4 µg/ml + VMA 7.5 µg/ml	>85
MM + Inositol 4 µg/ml + VMA 75 µg/ml	>85
MM + R. solani broth (VMA 0 µg/ml[b])	>85
MM + R. solani broth (VMA 0.75 µg/ml)	31
MM + R. solani broth (VMA 7.5 µg/ml)	24
MM + R. solani broth (VMA 75 µg/ml)	17

a) Diameter of inoculum disk: 5 mm

b) Three parts of broth of Rhizoctonia solani were mixed with one part of the minimal medium with 4 fold concentration.

TABLE 7. Recovery from pathogenisity of validamycin A-treated mycelia of Rhizoctonia solani by addition of inositol

Inositol, ug/ml	Infected cucumber seeds (%)[a]			
	Concentration of validamycin A, ug/ml			
	0	2.5	5.0	10.0
0	100	33	10	3
0.1	100	67	30	7

a) Thirty seeds in each treatment were examined.

Greenhouse and field studies to detect resistant strains Rice plants were inoculated with mycelia of R. solani and kept in a moist chamber at 28°C and 95%r.h. with an illuminance of 6000lx for 2 days. Validamycin A solution was sprayed at the rates of 50 µg/ml, then the plants were dried and kept in the moist chamber for another 2 days. The mycelia isolated from the treated lesions were used again as the next inoculum. This procedure was repeated 16 times. The sensitivity of the isolates to VMA was checked by the dendroyed method(4).

In 1976, 1977 and 1978, sheath blight lesions were collected from more than 650 fields throughout Japan. The lesions were washed with water, dipped in 80% ethylalcohol for a few seconds, placed on a PSA plate in a petri dish and incubated for 2 days at 25°C. Sensitivity of these isolates to VMA was assayed with the dendroyed method in Saga University(19).

As a result, no resistant strain has been obtained in a greenhouse(Fig. 6) and field.

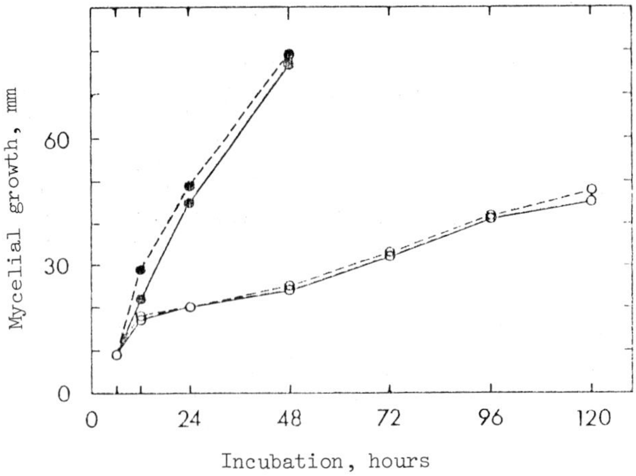

Fig. 6. Growth of *Rhizoctonia solani* on plain agar with (o) or without (•) addition of validamycin A.
——— Sixteen-generation pretreatment strain and
------ Mother strain.

TABLE 8. Summary of toxicological studies

Toxicity	Organism	Route	Duration	No effect level
Acute	Rat	Oral		LD50>20g/kg
	Mouse	"		LD50>20g/kg
	Rat	Dermal		LD50>5g/kg
	Mouse	"		LD50>5g/kg
	Rabbit	Ocular irritation		>10mg/eye
	"	Skin irritation		>10mg/cm^2 skin
	Rat	Inhalation		>12.5mg/liter air
Subclonic	Rat	Diet	3 months	10,000ppm
	Mouse	"	"	10,000ppm
Clonic	Rat	"	2 years	1,000ppm
	Mouse	"	"	10,000ppm
Environmental	Chicken	Oral	23 days	>12.5g/kg
	"	Diet	60 days	>2,000ppm
	Quail	Oral	23 days	>12.5g/kg
	"	Diet	28 days	>2,000ppm
	Carp		72 hours	>40ppm
	Killifish		"	>10,000ppm
	Water flea		24 hours	>40ppm
	Silkworm			No hazard at practical spray rate
	Honeybee			
	D. tenera[a)]			
	P. malinus[b)]			

a) *Dyschiriognatha tenera*

b) *Pseudoaphycus malinum*

TOXICOLOGICAL PROPERTIES

Toxicological studies Data from toxicological studies are summarized in Table 8. VMA has low toxicity to mammals(20) and is nonhazardous to livestock, poultry and wild life such as arthropods and fish(21). It showed no phytotoxicity to 147 species of plants in various stage.

Metabolism of VMA VMA seems to be rapidly degraded biologically(Fig. 8). Rats, rice plants and Pseudomonas denitrificans hydrolyzed VMA to D-glucose and validoxylamine A. The further decomposition of validoxylamine A proceeded via valienamine and validamine in P. denitrificans(22).

Residue in crop and in soil Residue of VMA on brown rice and straw after 6-time repeated application of VMA at a rate of 60ga.i./ha was less than the limit of detection(TABLE 9). When VMA was added to alluvial and volcanic ash soil, the amount decreased to half by a few hours. In sterilized soil, little degradation of VMA occurred(23).

TABLE 9. Residue of validamycin A in rice

Dosage g/ha (ai)	Sampling (Location)	No. of spray	Harvest(Days after last spray)	Analyzed portion	Limit of detection	Residue (ppm)
60	Hokkaido	6	0	Brown rice	0.007	<0.007
"	"	6	0	Straw	0.02	<0.02
60	Chiba	6	1	brown rice	0.007	<0.007
"	"	6	1	Straw	0.02	<0.02

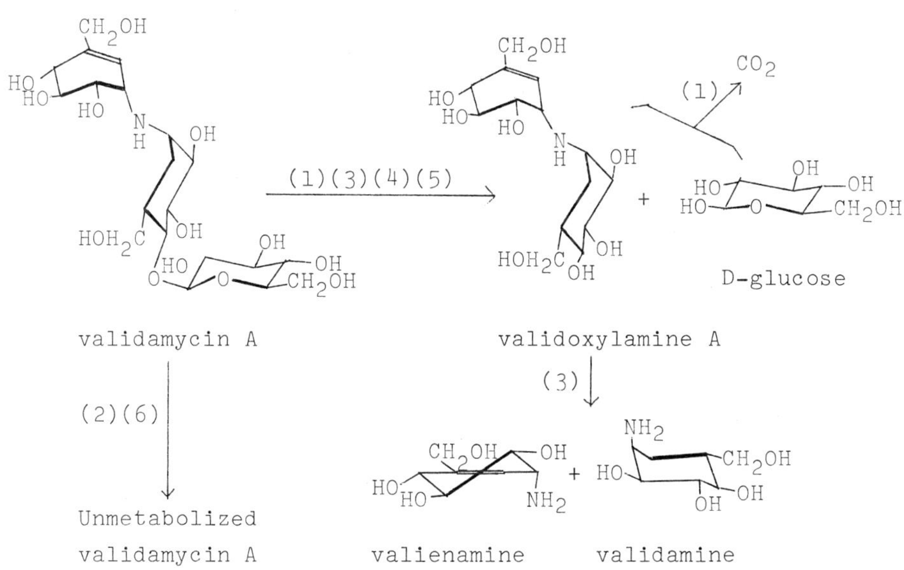

Fig. 8. Metabolism of validamycin A.
(1) Rat(oral), (2) Rat(intravenous), (3) Bacteria, (4) Rice plant, (5) Soil(unsterilized), (6) Soil(sterilized).

Cross resistnace with the other aminocyclitol antibiotics Antibiotics tested were kanamycin A, dextromycin, dihydrostreptomycin, zygomycin A2 and validamycin A. *Staphylococcus aureus* 209 P, *Escherichia coli* IFO12734, *Mycobacterium smegmatis* IFO3083 were successively cultured on a medium containing 1000μg/ml of VMA for 20 generations(transplantations), and minimum inhibitory concentration of those antibiotics were checked.
No change of the sensitivity of those bacteria to any of the four antibiotics was detected (TABLE 10).

TABLE 10. Cross resistance between validamycin A with some other aminocyclitol antibiotics

Antibiotic	Minimal inhibitory concentration (μg/ml)					
	Staphylococcus aureus		*Escherichia coli*		*Mycobacterium smegmatis*	
	+VMA*	-VMA	+VMA*	-VMA	+VMA*	-VMA
Kanamycin A	0.7	0.7	1.0	1.0	1.0	1.0
Dextromycin	0.1	0.1	1.0	1.0	0.3	0.3
Dihydrostreptomycin	1-3	1-3	1-3	1-3	0.5	0.5
Zygomycin A2	0.5	0.5	7.0	7.0	1.0	1.0

* Twenty generations preincubation in the medium with or without addition of validamycin A, at the concentration of 1000 ug/ml.

CONCLUSION

Validamycin A is a non-fungicidal antibiotic with a low mammalian toxicity and has little or no effect on nontarget organisms. Even to the target organism, *Rhizoctonia solani*, validamycin A only reduced mycelial growth and formation of infection cushion on rice plants, i.e. validamycin A controls *Rhizoctonia solani* on rice plants by lowering the infection potency of the pathogen.

REFERENCES

1. T. Kozaka, Rev. Plant Protec. Res. 8,69-80 (1975)
2. T. Iwasa, H. Yamamoto and M. Shibata, J. Antibiotics 23, 595-602 (1970)
3. T. Iwasa, E. Higashide, H. Yamamoto and M. Shibata, J. Antibiotics 24, 107-113 (1971)
4. T. Iwasa, E. Higashide and M. Shibata, J. Antibiotics 24, 114-118 (1971)
5. T. Iwasa, Y. Kameda, M. Asai, S. Horii and K. Mizuno, J. Antibiotics 24, 119-123 (1971)
6. O. Wakae and K. Fujimori, Ann. Phytopath. Soc. Japan 36, 355 (1970)
7. S. Horii, T. Iwasa and Y. Kameda, J. Antibiotics 24, 57-58 (1971)
8. S. Horii and Y. Kameda, J.C.S. Chem. Comm. 747-748 (1972)
9. T. Suami, S. Ogawa and N. Chida, J. Antibiotics 33, 98-99 (1980)
10. K. Nishi and K. Konishi, Analytical Methods for Pesticides and Plant Growth Regulators viii, 309-318, Academic Press , New York (1976)
11. K. Matsuura, E. Oniki and O. Wakae, Ann. Phytopath. Soc. Japan 37, 192 (1971)
12. O. Wakae and K. Matsuura, Ann. Phytopath. Soc. Japan 40, 224 (1974)
13. O. Wakae and K. Matsuura, Rev. Plant Protec. Res. 8, 81-92 (1975)
14. H. Ishizaki, M. Fujino, M. Kohno and H. Kunoh, Bullet. Fac. Agr. Mie Univ. 59, 1-32 (1979)
15. O. Wakae and K. Fujimori, Ann. Phytopath. Soc. Japan 37, 389 (1971)
16. T. Nioh and S. Mizushima, J. gen. appl. Microbiol.20, 373-383 (1974)
17. P. R. Mahadevan and E. L. Tatum, J. Bacteriol. 90, 1073 (1965)
18. G. Tamura, Biseibutsu jikkenho (Methods in Microbiology) 135-155, Kyoritsu Shuppan, Tokyo (1956)
19. F. Nonaka, Unpublished data
20. Y. Shirasu, Abstructs, 5th Int. Cong. Pestic. Chem., Kyoto, Xs-10 (1982)
21. A. Asaka and M. Sakai, J. Takeda Res. Lab. 40, 83-89 (1981)
22. Y. Kameda, S. Horii and T. Yamano, J. Antibiotics 28, 298-306 (1975)
23. K. Nishi, A. Takabatake, M. Hattori, O. Wakae and K. Matsuura, Ann. Phytopath. Soc. Japan 39, 169 (1973)

RESIDUE ANALYSIS OF POLYOXINS B, D AND BLASTICIDIN S IN CROPS AND SOILS

Eiichi Ebata

Kaken Chemical Co. Ltd., Honkomagome, Bunkyo-ku, Tokyo 113, Japan

Abstract - Quantitative bioassay methods for blasticidin S, and polyoxins B and D were established by using sensitive fungal strains. Before the quantitation to know residue levels of these antibiotics in crops and soils after application to control various diseases, extraction and clean-up were carried out by general ways, except that blasticidin S was extractable from soils under considerably severe conditions. The recoveries of polyoxins were 65-87 % in crops and 59-86 % in soils, and those of blasticidin S were 70-82 % and 53-69 %, respectively. The detection limit in both crops and soils is found to be 0.05 ppm, except for that of polyoxins B in melon and D in rice straw at 0.1 ppm. The actual residue levels of these antibiotics in crops became generally undetectable 3 days after application. While polyoxin B in grape and blasticidin S in rice straw were detectable during the first 21 and 7 days, respectively. The half life periods of the antibiotics in soils were 2 to 3 days after application.

INTRODUCTION

In 1958, blasticidin S has been found in the culture broth of Streptomyces griseochromogenes, showing both anti-bacterial and anti-fungal activities (Ref. 1). Interestingly, blasticidin S was exclusively developed to prevent rice blast disease, and a success in large scale production led this antibiotic to use practically in Japan and other countries as an excellent anti-blast agent. As well known, this first success stimulated attempts to find and develop agricultural use antibiotics against various plant diseases. Then, in 1965, polyoxins, which consist of thirteen componenets having very close structures, have been discovered in the culture broth of Streptomyces cacaoi (Ref. 2). Polyoxins are active against various phytopathogenic fungi, but have no anti-bacterial activity. Furthermore, since these antibiotics only affect on cell wall chitin synthesis, they are quite harmless to plant and mammals (Ref. 3). Anyway, polyoxin B has been practically used to control various diseases of fruits, vegetables and tobacco (Ref. 4). And also polyoxin D has been widely used to control rice sheath blight (Ref. 5). Kaken Chemical has exclusively produced these antibiotics and distributed manufacturing use or formulated products. During the registration process of these antibiotics according to the guideline standardized by the Agricultural Chemicals Regulation Law, the data of crop and soil residues were absolutely required to be submitted to the Ministry of Agriculture, Forestry and Fisheries. To determined their residue levels, bioassay methods were established using sensitive fungal strains. In general, antibiotic residues in crops or soils are very low level, though a large amount of interfering substances are present. Therefore, prior to the antibiotic quantitation, extraction and cleanup became necessary under considerably mild condition in order to avoid antibiotic decomposition during the procedures.

Presented at the Vth International Congress of Pesticide Chemistry (IUPAC), Kyoto, 1982.

EXTRACTION AND CLEANUP OF POLYOXINS B AND D IN CROPS

A chopped sample (100 g) is homogenized in a blender, then first extracted with 150 ml of absolute methanol. Although polyoxins are almost insoluble in methanol, water retained in crops is enough to make each antibiotic extractable into the solvent. Use of methanol for the first extraction is advantageous to leave certain high molecular impurities, such as proteins and polysaccharides, as insoluble residue, and to facilitate filtration. The residue is re-extracted once with 200 ml of 80 % aqueous methanol and the combined extracts are concentrated under a reduced pressure below 40 °C to a small volume (ca. 50 ml). After adjusting pH to 2.0 with 6N hydrochloric acid the extract is allowed to stand overnight in a refrigerator and then filtered to remove precipitate. The resulting filtrate is passed through the column packed with 20 ml of ion exchange resin, Dowex 50W-X4. This strong acidic resin with lower cross linking degree is quite available for purification of polyoxins. The resin buffered at pH 2.1 is effective to prevent the adsorption of pigmented impurities. While polyoxins are amphoteric substances and charged positively at the given pH, thus being adsorbed by the resin. A large portion of unionized compounds retained in the resin are then washed out with 1000 ml of 50 % aqueous acetone. The antibiotics still present in the column are eluted with 200 ml of 0.3N hydrochloric acid, of which concentration is optimal to obtain a good polyoxin yield and also to prevent elution of strongly adsorbed impurities. The acid eluate from resin column is adjusted to pH 6.0 with 5N sodium hydroxide, then subjected to carbon (0.8 g) chromatography to remove sodium chloride caused by neutralization and also to put forward the cleanup. As shown in Table 1, even though by 60 % aqueous acetone, the yield of each antibiotic is around 50 %. However, the recovery of polyoxins with this solvent is increased satisfactorily by pretreatment of carbon with 2 % aqueous aniline solution.

TABLE 1. Effect of aniline pretreatment of active carbon on recovery of polyoxins eluting with 60 % aqueous acetone

Aniline conc. (%)	Recovery (%) Polyoxin B	Polyoxin D
0	49	53
0.5	76	81
1	81	79
2	82	84

So that the aniline pretreatment is used and the column adsorbing polyoxin B is washed with 100 ml of 5 % aqueous ethanol. However, in the case of polyoxin D, the aqueous ethanol washing is cut down because it leads to a loss of the adsorbing antibiotic. The same extraction and cleanup procedures are available for these polyoxins except only this washing process of carbon column. Each 60 % aqueous acetone eluate (200 ml) is evaporated under a reduced pressure to dryness and the resulting residue is dissolved in a definite volume (20 ml) of sterile distilled water to prepare the assay solution.

EXTRACTION AND CLEANUP OF BLASTICIDIN S IN CROPS

Extraction and cleanup procedures are similar to those for polyoxins. One hundred grams of rice straw or soiling rice is cut to small pieces less than 2 cm and extracted twice with 1000 ml of 80 % aqueous methanol. After concentration under a reduced pressure the extract (ca. 100 ml) is adjusted to pH 2.0 and applied to the Dowex 50W-X4 (H, 20 ml) column. The column is washed with 1000 ml of 50 % aqueous acetone. As compared to polyoxins, adsorption of blasticidin S through its guanidine group is quite strong, therefore 0.5N ammonium hydroxide solution (300 ml) is used to complete elution instead of 0.3N hydrochloric acid. The alkaline eluate is neutralized and subjected again to an active carbon (1 g) column. As similar to polyoxins, pretreatment of carbon is needed for a good recovery of blasticidin S. After investigation of various conditions shown in Table 2, 1 % aqueous p-toluenesulfonic acid solution is found to be available for the purpose.

TABLE 2. Effects of pretreatment of active carbon on recovery of blasticidin S eluting with 50 % acetone in 0.1N hydrochloric acid

Pretreatment	Recovery (%)
None	45
2 % Aniline	43
0.1 % Stearic acid	49
1 % p-Toluenesulfonic acid	83
2 % p-Toluenesulfonic acid	75

The column adsorbed blasticidin S is washed with 50 % aqueous acetone to remove colored impurities, then elution of the antibiotic is performed effectively with 200 ml of 50 % acetone in 0.1N hydrochloric acid. After neutralization and evaporation of the eluate to dryness, the residue is dissolved in a definite volume (20 ml) of sterile distilled water and submitted to bioassay.

EXTRACTION AND CLEANUP OF POLYOXINS B AND D IN SOILS

In the case of soil residue analysis, a largely differed extraction procedure is employed as compared to that for crops. Table 3 shows per cent values of recovery rate of polyoxins B and D when various solvents are used to extract soils fortified with each antibiotic. Among the extractants investigated, phosphate solutions, specially 1M aqueous dibasic potassium phosphate solution shows a good efficacy.

TABLE 3. Effects of various extractants on recovery of polyoxins from soil

Extractant	Recovery (%)	
	Polyoxin B	Polyoxin D
0.1N HCl	14	12
1N HCl	0	0
Acetone • 0.2N HCl (1:1)	22	19
Acetone • H_2O (1:1)	0	0
1M KH_2PO_4	44	51
0.5M K_2HPO_4	81	79
1M K_2HPO_4	85	83
2M K_2HPO_4	84	80
1M Na_2HPO_4	69	63
1M $(NH_4)_2HPO_4$	38	58
1M CH_3COONH_4	0	0

Actually 400 ml of this solution is used to extract twice a sample of 40 g dried weight of soil. The combined extracts are adjusted to pH 6.0 with hydrochloric acid and left overnight in a refrigerator to filter off resulting precipitates. The filtrate is subjected to active carbon (2 g) column pretreated with 0.01 % aniline aqueous solution. The antibiotics are eluted with 400 ml of 60 % aqueous acetone. After evaporation of the eluate to dryness, the residue is dissolved in a definite volume (10 ml) of sterile distilled water and submitted to bioassay.

EXTRACTION AND CLEANUP OF BLASTICIDIN S IN SOILS

In the case of blasticidin S extraction from soil, severer conditions are needed because of its strong adsorption (Ref. 6). As shown in Table 4, one factor to increase yield of this antibiotic is a strength of hydrochloric acid using for extraction. Also addition of acetone to acid solution and heating during the extraction are important.

TABLE 4. Conditions affected on blasticidin S recovery from soil

Condition	Recovery (%)
1N HCl	0
2N HCl	0
5N HCl	45
8N HCl	45
Acetone · 6.6N HCl (1:3)	50
Acetone · 6.6N HCl (1:3), 60 °C	62
Acetone · 10N HCl (1:1)	51
Acetone · 10N HCl (1:1), 60°C	63
5N H_2SO_4	0
5N H_3PO_4	0
1M K_2HPO_4	12

Therefore, extraction of blasticidin S from soil (40 g) has been performed by using 400 ml of 50 % acetone in 12N hydrochloric acid at 60°C for a short period (e.g. 5 minutes) with agitation. After addition of citric acid (80 g) as a masking agent preventing colloidal precipitation, the extract is adjusted to pH 6.0 and evaporated to dryness. The dried residue is dissolved in 1000 ml of water and the solution is allowed to stand overnight in a refrigerator to filter off resulting precipitates. The filtrate is passed through the carbon (1 g) column, and the column is washed with 100 ml of 10 % aqueous acetone. Blasticidin S is eluted from carbon with 200 ml of 50 % acetone in 0.2 N hydrochloric acid. After neutralization, the eluate is evaporated to dryness. The residue is dissolved in 10 ml of sterile distilled water and subjected to the following bioassay.

BIOASSAY

An agar-plate diffusion method using stainless steel cylinders is employed for the antibiotic quantitation. Organisms using in the assay are all plantpathogenic fungi. Those are *Alternaria mali* AKI-3 strain and *Rhizoctonia solani* ACI 1134 strain for polyoxins B and D, respectively, and *Cladosporium fulvum* ACI 1164 strain for blasticidin S (Ref. 7 & 8). Agar mediums to prepare plates vary in composition with organisms. For inoculation to agar medium, spore suspension of *Alternaria* and *Cladosporium*, and mycelial suspension of *Rhizoctonia* are used. The spore or mycelial suspension is inoculated to a melted assay medium when its temperature is around 47 °C. After mixing well, a portion of 5 ml of the inoculated medium is spread onto each Petri dish to prepare agar plate. Four empty cylinders are placed on a plate at equal intervals and two of them are filled with standard solutions containing each antibiotic at 1 or 0.5 u/ml. The other two cylinders are filled with sample solutions at original or twice diluted concentrations. Five plates are used for each sample. To enhance assay sensitivity, prediffusion of antibiotic into agar plates is carried out at a low temperature, such as 5°C, regulating the growth of test organism to slow rate. Table 5 shows conditions of prediffusion and succeeding incubation of assay plates. When inhibition zones are formed around the cylinders, their diameters are measured.

TABLE 5. Conditions for prediffusion of antibiotic and incubation of test organisms

Antibiotic	Prediffusion period at 5°C (hrs)	Incubation Temp. (°C)	Incubation Period (hrs)
Polyoxin B	5	31	40
Polyoxin D	5	31	20
Blasticidin S	18	27	24

From the results obtained by measuring standard inhibition zones a linear relation between the logarithmic potencies and the diameters is observed. For an example, dose-response relationship for polyoxin B is shown in Fig. 1.

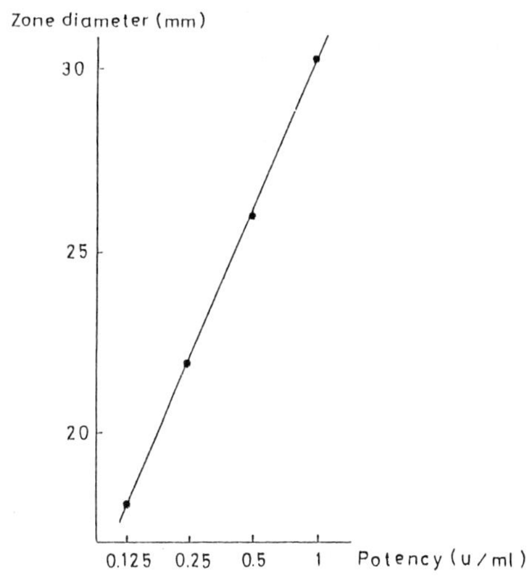

Fig. 1. Dose-response relationship for polyoxin B

After confirming linear relationships the following formulas can be used to calculate antibiotic potency in sample solution.

$$\log \theta = \frac{(\Sigma UH + \Sigma UL) - (\Sigma SH + \Sigma SL)}{(\Sigma UH + \Sigma SH) - (\Sigma UL + \Sigma SL)} \times \log 2$$

$$\theta = \frac{Pu}{Ps}$$

In which θ is ratio of sample potency, Pu, to standard potency, Ps, and SH and SL are diameters of inhibition zone caused with standards at concentration of 1 u/ml and 0.5 u/ml, respectively. Similarly UH or UL is a zone diameter caused with a respective sample solution. Based on antibiotic contents thus obtained from these formulas, the residue levles in crops or soils are estimated.

DETECTION LIMITS

Detection limits of these antibiotics in samples are determined by the following method. For example, appropriate amounts of polyoxin B are fortified to a sample of grape, onion or soil and the values of measured inhibitory zones on agar plate are shown in Table 6.

TABLE 6. Detection limit of polyoxin B

Sample	Fortification level (ppm)	Zone diameter (mm)
Grape	0.02	N.D.
	0.05	17.9
	0.1	23.2
Onion	0.02	N.D.
	0.05	18.3
	0.1	23.6
Soil	0.02	N.D.
	0.05	18.2
	0.1	22.4

From the results obtained, the lowest residue level of these antibiotics detectable by the proposed procedures is at 0.05 ppm, except for that at 0.1 ppm of polyoxin B in melon or D in rice straw.

RECOVERY TEST

Table 7 indicates that the mean recovery rates of each antibiotic from fortified crops are above ca. 70 %, of which relative standard deviations are less than 10 %.

TABLE 7. Recoveries from crops

Antibiotic	Crop	Fortification level (ppm)	Recovery (%)	S.D./$\bar{X}$ (%)
Polyoxin B	Tomato	0.2 0.5	74.6 79.0	6.0
	Melon	0.2 0.5	82.8 84.4	5.0
	Grape	0.5 1	75.1 79.0	4.5
	Onion	0.5 1	79.8 82.9	2.7
Polyoxin D	Unpolished rice	0.5 1	69.9 72.2	2.2
	Rice straw	0.5 1	69.4 74.6	6.4
	Apple	0.2 0.5	76.9 84.8	5.7
Blasticidin S	Soiling rice	0.5 1	74.4 78.8	4.4
	Rice straw	0.5 1	74.2 77.2	4.4
	Unpolished rice	0.1	74.0	5.0

While, as shown in Table 8, the antibiotic recoveries from soils are varied considerably. Specially, as mentioned before, blasticidin S yields are somewhat low due to the tight adsorption. These are in the range of 56.1 to 81.4 %.

TABLE 8. Recoveries from soils

Antibiotic	Soil	Fortification level (ppm)	Recovery (%)	S.D./$\bar{X}$ (%)
Polyoxin B	Volcanic ash (Ibaraki)	0.1 0.5	77.9 78.7	5.7
	Alluvial (Saitama)	0.1 0.5	78.6 81.4	
Polyoxin D	Volcanic ash (Tochigi)	0.5 1	71.1 75.3	8.6
	Alluvial (Mie)	0.5 1	63.1 65.8	
Blasticidin S	Volcanic ash (Tochigi)	0.32 0.96	56.1 58.3	9.7
	Alluvial (Mie)	0.32 0.96	60.1 69.2	

ANTIBIOTIC RESIDUES IN CROPS

Table 9 shows the results of periodical residue analysis in various crops treated with the antibiotic in field. These crops were sampled at the Prefectural Agricultural Experiment Stations indicated.

TABLE 9. Antibiotic residues in various crops (ppm)

Antibiotic	Crop	Sampling place	Days after application to harvest 1	3	7	14	21	30	45
Polyoxin B	Tomato	Tochigi	<0.05	<0.05	<0.05	<0.05			
		Kanagawa	0.06	<0.05	<0.05	<0.05			
	Melon	Ibaraki	<0.1	<0.1					
		Nagano	<0.1	<0.1					
	Grape	Yamanashi			0.28	0.20	0.10	<0.05	<0.05
		Ōsaka			0.16	0.06	<0.05	<0.05	<0.05
	Onion	Ibaraki		<0.05	<0.05	<0.05	<0.05		
		Hokkaidō		<0.05	<0.05	<0.05	<0.05		
Polyoxin D	Unpolished rice	Fukushima	<0.05		<0.05				
		Ehime	<0.05		<0.05				
	Rice straw	Fukushima	<0.1		<0.1				
		Ehime	0.49		<0.1				
	Apple	Iwate	<0.05				<0.05		
		Aomori	<0.05				<0.05		
Blasticidin S	Soiling rice	Tochigi	0.08	<0.05	<0.05	<0.05	<0.05		
		Gifu	0.10	<0.05	<0.05	<0.05	<0.05		
	Rice straw	Tochigi			0.06	<0.05	<0.05		
		Gifu			<0.05	<0.05	<0.05		
	Unpolished rice	Niigata			<0.05 (25 days)				
		Shizuoka			<0.05 (41 days)				

The data are means of duplicate determinations. Residue levels of these compounds were found to become undectable at 3rd day after application except that polyoxin B in grape and blasticidin S in rice straw needed 30 and 14 days after application to decrease under the detection limit, respectively.

IN VITRO TEST ON DEGRADATION OF ANTIBIOTICS IN SOIL

Degradation of these antibiotics in soils was examined under flooded or upland conditions. For flooded condition water was added up to 1 cm deep from the soil surface, while for upland condition, soil was moistened with water to 60 % of its maximum water capacity. After preincubation at 25°C for 1 week the antibiotic was added to soil at the concentrations designed on a dried soil weight basis. The antibiotics were extracted and determined periodically by the methods described above. Degradation profiles in soils under these conditions are shown in Fig. 2.

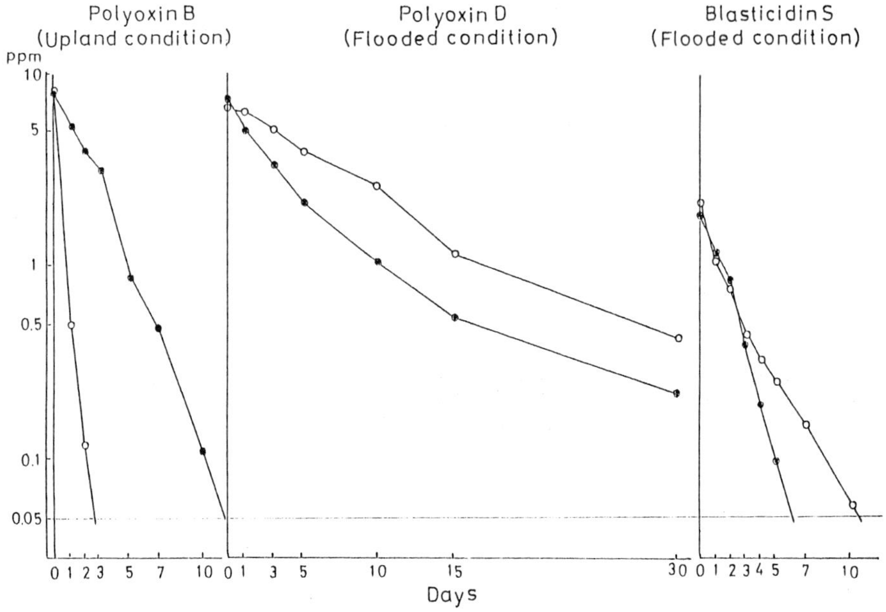

Fig. 2. In vitro test on degradation of polyoxins and blasticidin S in soil (•:volcanic ash; o:alluvial)

Although the degradation curves are varied to some extent with each antibiotic and soil, the half life periods of polyoxins and blasticidin S are estimated to be 2 or 3 days.

CONCLUSION

From the results, it is evident that, when blasticidin S, and polyoxins B and D are used practically in fields to control various plant diseases, the residue levels in crops and soils become undetectable during a short period after application because of their quick decomposition. Therefore, it can be said that each antibiotic is less liable to cause environmental pollution. Also the bioassay methods used here for these antibiotics are quite sensitive and accurate as compared to other physico-chemical assays investigated for them elsewhere.

Acknowledgement - I wish to thank Dr. Masahiro Hori of Kaken Chemical Co., Ltd., for a critical reading of the manuscript.

REFERENCES

1. S. Takeuchi, K. Hirayama, K. Ueda, H. Sakai and H. Yonehara, J. Antibiotics Ser. A9, 1-5 (1958).
2. K. Isono, J. Nagatsu, Y. Kawashima and S. Suzuki, Agric. Biol. Chem. 29, 848-854 (1965).
3. M. Hori, K. Kakki, S. Suzuki and T. Misato, Agric. Biol. Chem. 35, 1280-1291 (1971).
4. J. Eguchi, S. Sasaki, N. Ota, T. Akashiba, T. Tsuchiyama and S. Suzuki, Ann. Phytopath. Soc. Japan 34, 280-288 (1968).
5. S. Sasaki, N. Ota, J. Eguchi, Y. Furukawa, T. Akashiba, T. Tsuchiyama and S. Suzuki, Ann. Phytopath. Soc. Japan 34, 272-279 (1968).
6. I. Yamaguchi, K. Takagi and T. Misato, Agric. Biol. Chem. 36, 1719-1727 (1972).
7. H. Sakurai, T. Morita, H. Suzuki and K. Yoshida, Bull. Agr. Chem. Inspect. Stn. No.9, 30-36 (1969).
8. H. S. Baba, H. Sakurai and H. Nakamura, Bull. Agr. Chem. Inspect. Stn. No.10, 79-82 (1970).

HERBICIDES AND PLANT GROWTH REGULATORS FOR RICE CULTURE

WEED SUCCESSION BY LONG-TERM APPLICATION OF HERBICIDES IN JAPAN

Kunikazu Ueki

Weed Science Laboratory, Faculty of Agriculture, Kyoto University, Kyoto 606, Japan

Abstract - In an attempt to determine weed floral changes affected by the long-term application of herbicides in transplanted rice in Japan, a survey was made of weed specialists in 53 prefectural agricultural experiment stations throughout the country. Ninety percent of the questionnaires were returned. The majority of prefectures began herbicide application with 2, 4-D or MCPA in the period between 1950 and 1959. From then until 1975, PCP, nitrofen, thiobencarb and many other herbicides were introduced on rice. Sixty-one percent of the respondents indicated a trend of weed shift to perennials in their prefectures during this period. *Scirpus juncoides* (probably subs. *juncoides*) and *Sagittaria pygmaea* are the perennials indicated to have been most dominant by 44 and 27% of the respondents, respectively. This weed floral change has resulted not only from the long-term application of herbicides, but also from the changes of paddy management for rice, such as abandonment of intercultivation and hand-weeding, pre-plant soil preparation with rotary tillage, and shallower flooding level of the water. Many rice growers do not cultivate fields after harvesting, and the rest do so with rotary tillage.

INTRODUCTION

Paddy weeds were formerly controlled in Japan by physical means such as hand-weeding, coal-trimming rake, paddy tiller and later by rotary weeders. However, 2,4-D introduction as a rice herbicide remarkably changed the weeding schedule. Since then many herbicides have been introduced for the crop, and herbicides have generally become widely used. The total acreage of herbicide application has steadily increased: 57 thousand hectares in 1950, 1,058 in 1960, 4,560 in 1970 and 5,735 in 1980. Rice was produced on a total of 2,500 thousand hectares in 1980, and at present there are few paddy fields remaining on which herbicides are not used.

Among their advantages, herbicides can provide early-season weed control, and some can be applied even during the puddling period. They can control weeds around the crop stands where intercultivation is not possible. These advantages largely minimize the competition between rice and weeds during the early stage of crop growth. But herbicides are more or less selective among weed species, and have a residual efficacy in the soil. Although some herbicides can kill perennial propagules located below the soil surface, most rice herbicides cannot do so. Therefore, it is reasonable to anticipate a spectrum shift of weeds by repeated application of herbicides. Matsunaka et al. (2) reported a spectrum shift of paddy weeds in non-weeded plots of herbicide evaluation fields located at 34 prefectural agricultural experiment stations, and Sakamoto et al. (3) revealed a shift to perennial weeds by 5-years of repeated application of an herbicide in Miyazaki Prefectural Agricultural Experiment Station. The research reported herein is the result of our survey undertaken in 1981 on changes in the weed flora and paddy management during the past 30 years.

METHOD OF SURVEY

In the fall of 1981 a survey was made by sending a questionnaire to weed specialists of 53 prefectural agricultural experiment stations throughout Japan. Subjects in question covered a broad range of the aspects relating to changes in weed species and weeding schedules in transplanted rice from 1950 to 1981. Information on changes in paddy management such as cultivation methods and flooding level were also sought. The period from 1950 to 1981 was divided into four terms: I; 1950 to 1959, II; 1960 to 1969, III; 1970 to 1975, IV; 1976 to 1981. We asked weed specialists of all prefectures to list the five leading species of annual and perennial weeds during each term. Degree of dominance of a weed was estimated for the districts by giving the first leading species 5 points, the second 4, the third 3, the fourth 2 and the fifth 1, and by calculating the mean value of points for each species as shown in

PC 2 - K*

Figure 1.

RESULT OF SURVEY AND DISCUSSION

Forty-eight of the 53 experiment stations answered the questionnaire, a recovery rate of 91%. Answers from throughout the country, grouped into six districts, were closely examined. It was found that the majority of prefectures, 81% of all respondents, began herbicide application with 2,4-D of MCPA between 1950 and 1959. In this decade, paddy fields with a relatively small acreage were thoroughly prepared by ploughing prior to planting, and rice growers weeded mostly by frequent hand-weedings and intercultivations (Figure 1). The broadleaved weeds, which had eluded physical control and had grown at the midseason drainage, were applied with phenoxy herbicides. Major weed species composing the paddy weed community in this decade were *Echinochloa* spp., *Monochoria vaginalis, Cyperus* spp., *Rotala indica, Lindernia pyxidaria, Dopatrium junceum, Eleocharis acicularis, Sagittaria pygmaea, Potamogeton distinctus* and a few others (Table 1). Kasahara (1) surveyed paddy weed species in 1959 throughout Japan and indicated that the total number of species was 191 of 43 families. Though the quantity of emergence varied from prefecture to prefecture, leading species of the dominant weeds did not greatly differ, probably because a paddy field in a waterlogged condition is relatively stable for those weeds resistant to water stress.

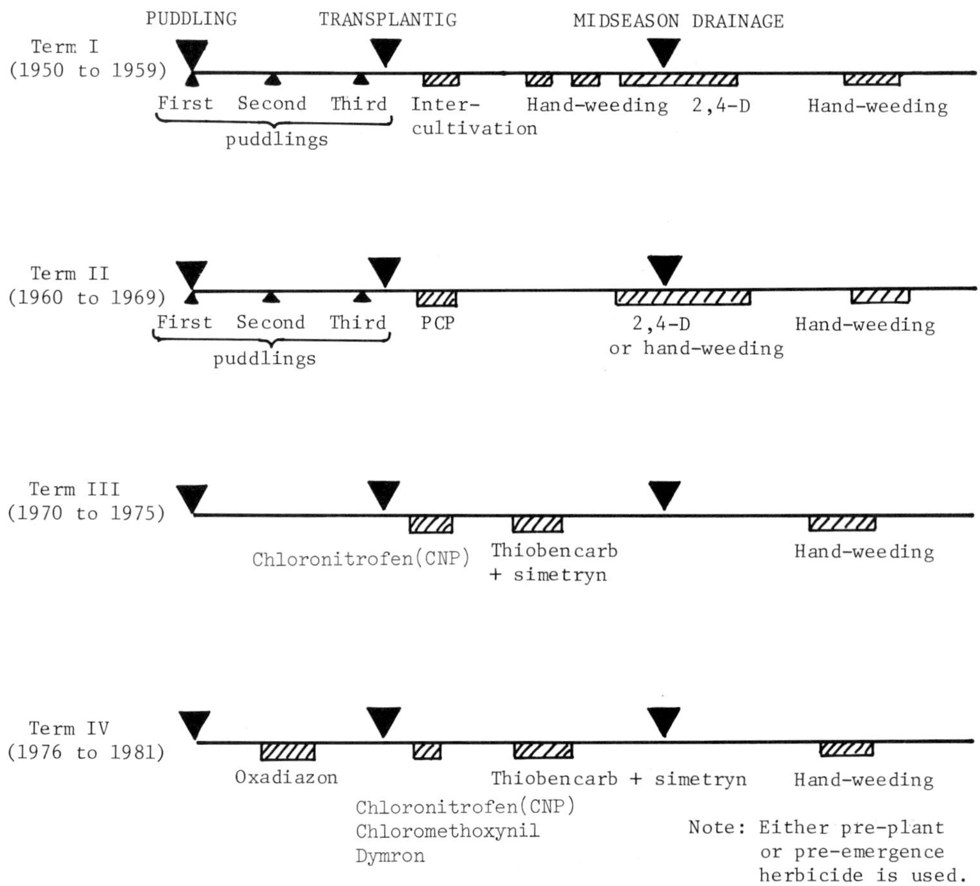

Figure 1. Change in weeding schedule for transplanted rice between 1950 and 1981. Data for this figure was obtained from the Saitama Prefectural Agricultural Experiment Station. The herbicides listed herein are not exclusive for each stage; many other herbicides could be substituted depending on a grower's choice.

Table 1. Estimated degrees of dominance of weeds for Term 1 (1950 to 1959) and lV (1976 to 1981).

	Districts[a]													
	A		B		C		D		E		F		Total	
Annual weeds	I	IV	I	IV	I	IV	I	IV	I	IV	I	IV	I	IV
Echinochloa spp.	5.0	5.0	5.0	5.0	5.0	5.0	4.6	4.8	4.7	4.8	5.0	4.6	4.9	4.9
Monochoria vaginalis		0.8	3.3	1.2	3.3	3.7	3.3	3.6	4.1	3.3	3.9	3.3	3.0	2.7
Rotala indica	2.3		1.0	0.6	3.0	3.0	1.3	1.3	1.2	0.8	2.4	2.6	1.9	1.4
Cyperus spp.			1.6		0.7		2.3	2.2	1.9	2.1	1.9	1.9	1.4	1.0
Dopatrium junceum					0.7		1.4	0.1	0.7	0.2	0.1		0.5	0.1
Lindernia pyxidaria	2.3	1.0		0.4	1.3	1.0	0.3	0.9	0.3	0.1	0.9	0.6	0.9	0.7
Aneilema keisak							0.4						0.1	
Elatine triandra	1.3	1.0				0.7							0.2	0.3
Eclipta prostrata								0.3		0.9	0.3		0.2	0.1
Ammannia multiflora								0.1		0.2				0.1
Gratiola japonica		0.8		0.8										0.3
Ludwigia prostrata										0.2				
Polygonum spp.								0.1						
Aeschynomene indica										0.2				
Leptochloa chinensis												0.3		0.1
Lythrum anceps										0.1				
Monochoria korsakowii		1.0												0.2
Bidens tripartita		0.5												0.1
Leersia oryzoides		1.0												0.2
Eriocaulon robustius			1.0	0.6										0.3
Lindernia dubia				0.2										
Perennial weeds														
Eleocharis acicularis	4.7	1.5	4.5		3.3	1.6	4.5	2.5	4.0	1.9	4.3	1.7	4.2	1.5
Sagittaria pygmaea		1.3		2.2	1.0	4.0	0.5	3.6	3.5	4.4	1.2	4.3	1.0	3.3
Sagittaria trifolia		1.8	0.5	1.6		0.7	0.4	0.9	0.2	0.3	0.3	0.4	0.2	1.0
Cyperus serotinus			3.0	3.4	3.0	4.0	0.6	2.6	0.7	2.0	1.4	2.1	1.5	2.4
Eleocharis kuroguwai					0.7	0.7	1.3	0.6	0.8	0.3	0.6	0.7	0.6	0.4
Scirpus juncoides	0.7	0.5		2.8	1.3	2.3	0.2	3.3		3.6		2.1	0.4	2.4
Alisma canaliculatum	1.0	4.0		1.0				0.4		0.3			0.2	1.0
Potamogeton distinctus	3.0		3.8	1.0			0.4	0.2	0.8	0.3	1.0	0.3	1.5	0.3
Oenanthe javanica							0.7	0.4	0.7	1.4	0.6	0.4	0.3	0.4
Scirpus maritimus											0.6	0.7	0.1	0.1
Paspalum distichum										0.2		0.9		0.2
Sagittaria aginashi							0.2							
Scirpus wallichii				0.8										0.1

[a] A: Hokkaido, B: Tohoku, C: Hokuriku, D: Kanto and Tokai, E: Kinki, Chugoku and Shikoku, F: Kyushu, Total: Countrywide. The values shown are mean figures. Refer to the text.

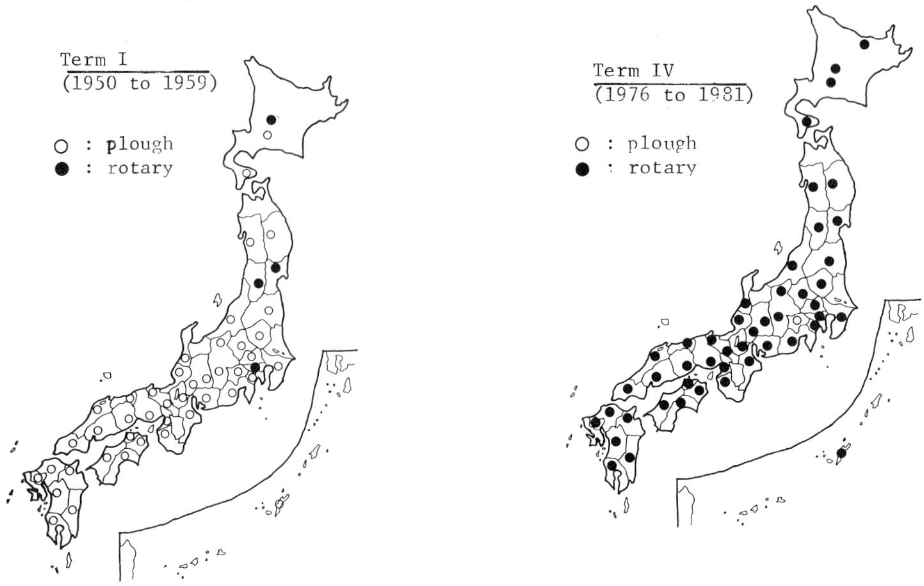

Figure 2. Change in method of pre-plant cultivation from Term 1 (1950 to 1956) to Term 1V (1976 to 1981).

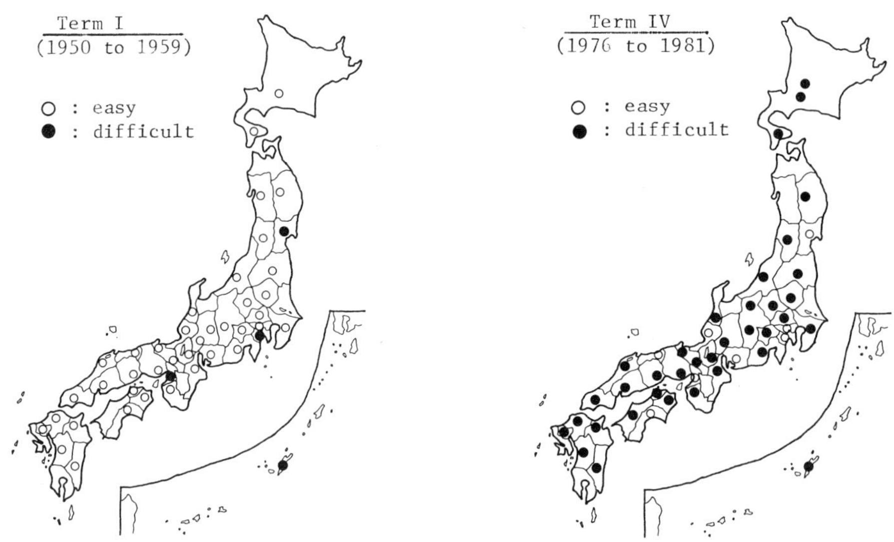

Figure 3. Paddy maintenance of flooding level of water in Term 1 (1950 to 1959) and in Term 1V (1976 to 1981).

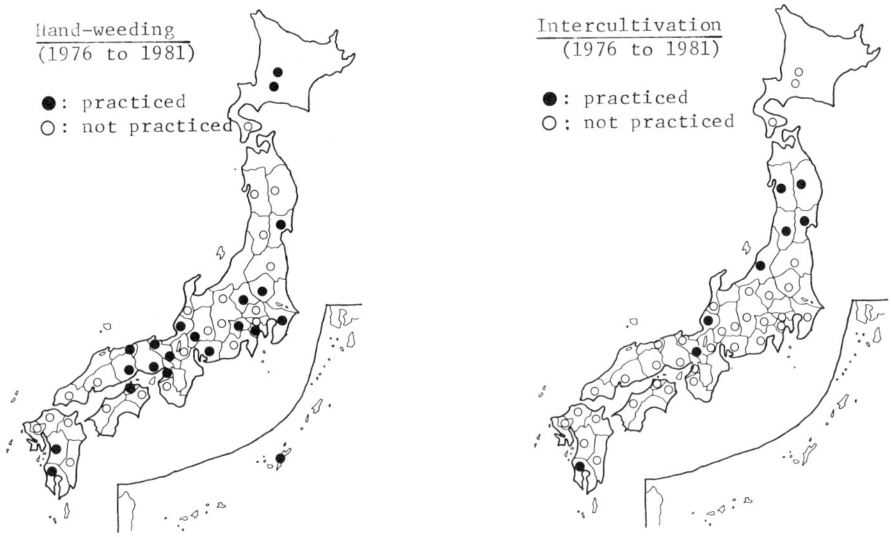

Figure 4. Practice of hand-weeding and intercultivation in Term lV (1976 to 1981).

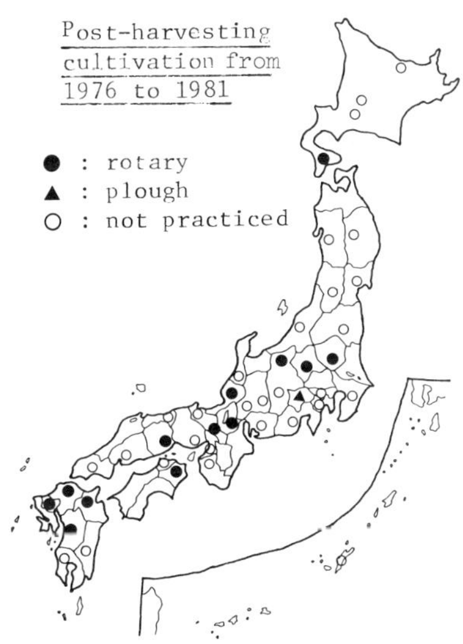

Figure 5. Methods of post-harvesting cultivation in Term lV (1976 to 1981).

From 1950 until 1975, PCP, nitrofen, thiobencarb and many other herbicides were introduced for rice, and these herbicides became widely used. Sixty-one percent of the questionnaire respondents indicated a trend in weed spectrum shift to perennials in their prefectures during this period. Among these, 90% observed the trend between 1970 and 1975. During these years, total acreage of herbicide application to rice exceeded that of rice cultivation. Most of the fields were treated with a post-transplanting herbicide 3 to 4 days after the transplanting operation and again 10 to 15 days later with a post-emergence herbicide,though this schedule depended on area, weed population and dominant species. Rice growers abandoned both intercultivation and hand-weeding before the midseason drainage. In the decade from 1950 to 1959, *Eleocharis acicularis* was the perennial weed which 65% of the respondents ranked as the most dominant, while 10% did so between 1976 and 1981. The species composing the weed flora in rice changed little from 1950 to 1981. However, *Scirpus juncoides* (probably subs. *juncoides*) and *Sagittaria pygmaea* are the perennials which were indicated to have the largest trend of dominance by 44 and 27% of the respondents, respectively. The other perennial weeds showing this trend are *Potamogeton distinctus, Cyperus serotinus, Alisma canaliculatum, Eleocharis kuroguwai, Oenanthe javanica,* and *Sagittaria trifolia* (Table 1). Although *Echinochloa* spp. is the most dominant annual at present, 83% of all respondents reported a reduction in its quantity of emergence. Results of our previous survey (2) showed a similar trend of the spectrum shift to perennial. That survey studied the weed community changes in population and dominant species in non-weeded plots of herbicide evaluation fields located at 34 prefectural agricultural experiment stations from 1968 to 1978, and showed that there was a remarkable increase of perennial weeds such as *Cyperus serotinus, Scirps juncoides, Alisma canaliculatum, Sagittaria pygamaea, Sagittaria trifolia,* with an exceptional reduction of *Eleocharis acicularis.* In the experiment by Sakamoto et al. (3), the original weed population was compared with 5-years of repeated application of an herbicide and an increased population of perennial weeds such as *Cyperus serotinus* and *Scirpus juncoides* was also found.

This weed floral change has resulted not only from the long-term application of herbicides, but also from the changes in rice paddy management. In the decade of 1950 to 1959, the majority of prefectures (92% of the respondents) had conducted pre-plant soil preparation by ploughing, but between 1976 and 1981, 98% began to do it with rotary tillage (Figure 2). In the latter period the flooding level of water became shallower and more difficult to maintain because of the increase in acreage of strips of fields (Figure 3). At present most of the rice growers depend for weeding solely on preplanting herbicides plus early postplanting and/ or late postplanting herbicides (Figure 1). But half of the prefectures (46%) reported hand-weeding of *Echinochloa* spp. by their rice growers after the midseason drainage (Figure 4). Only 31% of all respondents indicated that in their prefectures the fields were cultivated in autumn after rice harvesting, but with rotary tillage (Figure 5).

Yamagishi (5) indicated in his review on a spectrum shift of paddy weeds to perennial in Japan, two causal factors: change in agricultural technologies and situational changes in agriculture. The former includes changes in the cultivation system, the form of paddy utilization, cultural and soil preparation and in weeding technology. The situational changes in agriculture include a labor shortage owing to the outflow of labor to other industries and an increase of fallow paddy fields for the production adjustment of rice. These factors are thought to create, directly and indirectly, conditions suitable for perennial weeds to propagate and dominate. Herbicides play an important role in rice production in Japan. As Shaw and Jansen (4) indicated in the paper relating to problems and risks in chemical weed control, massive use or repeated application of the chemicals may bring about crop injury, environmental contamination, spectrum shift and resistance development of weed species. To avoid these problems and risks, we need to have sufficient knowledge on the physiology and ecology of weeds, populational dynamics of the weed community, competition mechanisms between crop and weeds and also on herbicidal behavior in the environment. Integrated control of weeds in rice can be accomplished on the basis of such knowledge by rationally combining cultural (ecological), mechanical and biological control measures with chemical measures.

Acknowledgements - The author expresses his sincere appreciation to weed specialists of prefectural agricultural expériment stations throughout this country for their cooperation in answering the questionnaire for this survey.

REFERENCES

1. Y. Kasahara, *Nōgaku Kenkyū 14*, 123 (1959)
2. S. Matsunaka, K. Ueki and N. Ichizen, *Weed Research (Japan) 24*, 33 (1979)
3. S. Sakamoto, H. Eto, A. Kajimoto and Y. Umeki, *Weed Research (Japan) 24*, 39 (1979)
4. W.C. Shaw and L.L. Jansen, *Pest Control Strategies for the Future*, p.197, NAS (1972)
5. J. Yamagishi, *Nōgyō-oyobi-Engei 50(1)*, 1118 (1975)

ESSENTIAL CHARACTERISTICS OF HERBICIDES FOR RICE CULTURE

Shooichi Matsunaka

Department of Plant Protection, Faculty of Agriculture, Kobe University, Nada-ku, Kobe 657, Japan

Abstract - Rice cultivation, especially under flooded conditions, has been done by a particular type of management. The weeding methods in rice culture are also rather special. The essential characteristics which the rice herbicides should possess are somewhat different from those for other crop plants. The following items may be proposed as such characteristics: (1) Herbicidal properties: Herbicides should of course have stable activities to noxious weeds in paddy fields. In upland rice culture, the weeds belonging to C_4-plants are important targets of herbicides because of their keen competition with rice, a C_3-plant. (2) Selectivity or rice safety: The injury of rice by herbicides should be minimal or none at all. The detoxification activity of rice plants such as aryl acylamidase I may be utilized in the design of new selective herbicides. (3) Physico-chemical properties: Under flooded conditions, considerations of water solubility and adsorption activity to clays and organic matter are more important than in upland conditions. (4) Formulation: Granular formulations may be profitable to rice culture on a small scale, especially when transplanting is done, because of the safety factor to rice and the fact that no application equipment is necessary. (5) Environmental problems: Low toxicity to fish or shellfish and no flow-out from paddy fields is essential. Both reductive degradations of herbicides in paddy soils and their co-distillatory properties from flooded water should be considered. (6) Economic factor: The cost of herbicide application should be in economic balance with the hand-weeding wage.

INTRODUCTION

Rice cultivation is often done under flooded conditions. Although the cultivation of lotus roots or rush for *tatami* mats is practiced under flooded farm conditions, almost all agricultural production is performed under non-flooded upland conditions. Flooded rice culture is thus a special case and requires a particular type of management. Even in upland rice culture in the hot summer season, the severe competition of the crop with vigorous C_4-weeds should be considered. Here we should give special attention to the weeding methods in rice culture. The essential characteristics needed in rice herbicides are rather special. In this paper, these characteristics will be compiled and accompanying problems described.

HERBICIDAL ACTIVITIES

Herbicides should control all the noxious weeds in paddy fields. As described in Ueki's paper, after long term application of herbicides, changes in the target weeds should be considered. In Japan, the succession from annual to perennial weeds has been clearly observed. These problems are being solved by two practices: one is a two or three times application of herbicides, and the other is the development and use of combined herbicides.

The first application of herbicides just before or after transplantation is intended to control the annual weeds, especially barnyardgrass. The second is applied 10-20 days after transplantation to kill perennial weeds and broadleaves.

A single herbicide has a limited spectrum of weed control, so that if we want to control several species of weeds, two or three herbicides should be combined to widen this spectrum. In Japan, 42% of all herbicides applied to paddy fields are combined herbicides, while the amount used on upland crops is less than 3%. For this difference, Miyahara (1) gave the following explanation: in upland cultivation, herbicidal activity is unstable because of various environmental conditions, and mechanical weeding measures which are effective to all weed species are those primarily used. The improvement of the activity thus is of first importance and widening of the weeding spectrum becomes secondary. In the flooded rice culture, the efficacy of herbicides is very stable and can control almost all noxious weeds; they are therefore used almost exclusively in these conditions. Thus in Japan many combined herbicides were developed to broaden the weeding spectrum. Table 1 shows the typical combination of herbicides for rice culture.

TABLE 1. Typical combined herbicides for rice culture in Japan

Component herbicides (content in %)	Trade name
Thiobencarb (7) + simetryn (1.5)	Saturn S Granule
Thiobencarb(10) + simetryn (1.5) + MCPB (0.8)	Kumilead SM Granule
Thiobencarb (7) + simetryn (1.5) + bentazon (7)	Esgran Granule
Thiobencarb (7) + chlornitrofen (6)	Saturn M Granula
Thiobencarb(10) + bentazon (10)	Satagran Granule
Thiobencarb(10) + bentazon (7) + MCPB (0.8)	Gra-M Granule
Thiobencarb (7) + propanil (17)	Saturn-DP Granule
Thiobencarb (7) + simetryn (1.5) + methoxyphenone (2)	K-Saturn S Granule
Thiobencarb(10) + simetryn (1.5) + MCPB (0.8) + methoxyphenone (3)	K-Kumilead SM Granule
Thiobencarb (7) + chloronitrofen (6) + methoxyphenone (2)	K-Saturn M Granule
Molinate (6) + simetryn (1.5)	Mamet Granule
Molinate (8) + simetryn (1.5) + MCPB (0.8)	Mamet SM Granule
Chloronitrofen (9) + dymron (7)	Shōron M Granule
Chloronitrofen (8) + molinate (6)	Ordram M. Granule
Butachlor (2.5) + pyrazolate (6)	Kusakarin Granule 25
Butachlor (3.5) + pyrazolate (6)	Kusakarin Granule 35
Butachlor (7) + naproanilide (3.5)	Ohza Granule
Butachlor (12) + oxadiazon (8)	Delcut E.C.
Piperophos (4.4) + dimethametryn (1.1)	Avirosan Granule
Swep (20) + MCPA (0.7)	Swep M Granule 20
Simetryn (2.5) + MCPB ethyl (1)	Pawnax M Granule 3.5
Simetryn (2.5) + MCPA thioethyl (0.7)	Grakill Granule 2.5
Bentazon (10) + MCPA (1.5)	Grassdin M Granule

In these combinations, we can hope to get not only an enlargement of the weeding spectrum, but also a synergistic action on the weeds. This means that we may use combined herbicides having lower contents of single component herbicides. Chisaka (2) proposed a method of estimating the joint action of herbicides, when mixed, using isobole line analysis. He found that in each combination of thiobencarb + simetryn, propanil + thiobencarb, and simetryn + butachlor, respective herbicides acted synergistically with each other to two leaf stage barnyardgrass, while the combination of thiobencarb + butachlor was additive and that of simetryn + chloronitrofen antagonistic.

In the development of new herbicides, the prediction of the future flora of noxious weeds in the target area becomes most important. A short history of such succession in Japan reported by Ueki in the previous paper becomes a valuable reference.

In upland rice culture, special attention should be paid to C_4-weeds which are more dominant than rice plant, a C_3-plant. Flooding of the paddy field is done for two reasons: one is to decrease the total amount of weeds and the other is selective depression of C_4-weeds. Arai and others (3) surveyed weed species and their amounts under three conditions of soil humidity. Recently Tanaka (4) rearranged their results from the standpoint of C_3- and C_4-plant classification and found that in flooded conditions only C_3-weeds dominate as shown in Table 2.

On the other hand, a compiled result of herbicide evaluation tests in upland cultivation in Philippines showed not only lower grain yield in hand-weeded plots but also very severe weed damage in non-weeded plots compared with flooded conditions, as shown in Table 3 (5,6). This information shows us that in upland rice cultivation the herbicides effective on C_4-weeds are the best to use.

TABLE 2. Changes in the distributions of weeds with different photosynthetic pathways as affected by soil moisture (Tanaka, 1976)(4)

Photosynthetic pathway	Flooded	Water saturated	Upland
C_3-Type	8.65*(89)	1.70 (6)	3.85 (7)
C_4-Type	1.05 (11)	29.10 (94)	54.0 (93)
Total (C_3 + C_4)	9.70(100)	30.80 (100)	57.85(100)

*Figures represent total weight of weeds in gram/0.81 m^2 (%).

TABLE 3. Comparison of loss in grain yield by weeds between flooded and upland rice plants

	Grain yield (kg/ha)	Yield loss by weed (%)	No. of experiments
Flooded culture *	4,891	36	8
Upland culture **	2,049	84	5

Figures represent the average of two series of experiments by Vega and others - *(5), **(6).

SELECTIVITY OR RICE SAFETY

In rice culture, there are several methods of cultivation. Direct seeding methods may be roughly divided into two: one is seeding into dry soil followed by flooding at the several leaf-age of rice plants, and the other is seeding under flooded conditions, which is widely recommended in the United States. Transplantation is practiced by hand with relatively taller seedlings or by transplanting machine with shorter seedlings. Currently in Japan machines suitable for two to three leaf-age seedlings are utilized, but those for larger seedlings are also being developed. Regarding rice safety using herbicides, we should consider various problems attendant with each cultivation method.

In direct seeding methods, the rice plant has no advantage of stage difference so that in the earlier application an absolute selectivity is necessary for the herbicides. Weed infestation is more severe than in the transplanting method, and higher herbicidal activity and selectivity are required. Biochemical or absolute selectivity should be utilized in this case, and propanil can be recommended.

Rice plants can hydrolyze and detoxify propanil by their own special propanil hydrolyzing enzyme (aryl acylamidase I) (7). In the co-existence of organophosphorus or carbamate insecticides which inhibit the hydrolyzing enzyme, the application of propanil may also cause injury in rice plants. Rice aryl acylamidase I has the following substrate specificity as shown in Table 4 (8); therefore this enzyme activity may be utilized in the design of new selective pesticides.

TABLE 4. Substrate specificity of aryl acylamidase I in the presence of 0.02% Triton X-100 (Akatsuka, 1979) (8)

Substrate	R.A.*	Substrate	R.A.
3,4-DCPA**	100	3,4-DCAA***	62
2,3-DCPA	151	2,3-DCAA	117
2,4-DCPA	145	2,4-DCAA	107
2,6-DCPA	0	2,6-DCAA	0
2,5-DCPA	107	2,5-DCAA	39
Swep	5		

* Relative activity, ** DCPA: dichloropropionanilide, *** DCAA: dichloroacetanilide

In the transplanting system, the differences in growth stage and position of growth points between rice plants and weeds can be utilized for safety. During the 30 year history of herbicide utilization, the most delightful development in this field is the utilization of granular formulation of herbicides. Over 20 years ago, 2,4-D acid applied to paddy fields after draining sometimes reached mulberry tree fields and others, causing severe damage. Then esters, i.e. ethyl esters, of 2,4-D or MCPA which were granulated and could be applied under flooded conditions without any drainage, were introduced. As a result of such improvements almost no problem was found in the susceptible crops around paddy fields.

The next step was the development of PCP (pentachlorophenol) granules. If we apply PCP-Na solution to transplanted rice fields, the rice leaves show severe injury. However, PCP granules, not being adhesive to the foliage of the plants, cause no injury to the crop but sink to the mud of the paddy fields and form a firm and thin herbicide layer in or on the soil surface. They thus have proved reasonably effective in killing weeds, mainly barnyardgrass, whose growing points are halted at the level of the herbicide layer, and in preventing crop injury through the roots (9).

Following the PCP granules, almost all herbicides for rice culture in Japan have been of granular formulation even though it has the disadvantages of somewhat higher cost of preparation, storage, and transportation; these are compensated by the advantages in the above-described safety for the plants and by ease of application.

Simetryn is utilized safely in transplanted rice culture except in extremely high temperatures. However, some rice varieties, especially those crossed with the indica type, are susceptible to this herbicide as shown by Ichizen (10).

Not only the herbicides themselves, but also derivatives or metabolites from original herbicides sometimes show injury to rice plants or other crops.

PHYSICO-CHEMICAL PROPERTIES

TABLE 5. Correlation coefficients between soil factors and phytotoxic activities of oxadiazon in 26 paddy soils (Hirai and Kawamura, 1975)

Soil factors	Phytotoxicities	
	ED_{90} to barnyardgrass	Length of brown spots on rice leaves
Concentration in water	-0.5986**	0.8074**
Clay content	0.3203	-0.5073*
Bulk density of soil	-0.3808	0.5525**
Carbon total	0.7589**	-0.5160**
Cathion Exchange Capacity	0.516-**	-0.4553*
pH	-0.4194*	0.0872

Leaching of an herbicide with water through soil layers may cause both a decrease in herbicidal activity on weeds and an increase in the toxicity to the plants through root absorption. Thus, herbicides for flooded rice culture should be absorbed slightly at the soil surface. Just-emerged weeds can then receive herbicide molecules bound to the soil as they pass through the treated soil zone. To such fundamental characteristics, both the content of clay and organic matter is contributing. One example is the case of oxadiazon shown in Table 5, reported by Hirai and Kawamura (11).

Co-distillatory activity of herbicides with paddy field water is also one of the important characteristics. Some thiocarbamate herbicides can be easily co-distillated with water in hot summer months and may cause sometimes severe damage on neighboring vegetable crops. Yukimoto et al. (12) showed that the herbicides with higher vapor pressures and lower solubilities in water showed higher volatility. Among those tested the evaporating amount of dichlobenil was the largest, successively followed by monilate, thiobencarb, nitrofen, and butachlor. Simetryn showed almost no evaporation.

FORMULATIONS

As shown in the section on rice safety, granular formulation contributed to selectivity, especially in the transplanted rice culture. However, as stated above, this has the disadvantage of higher cost of manufacture, transportation and storage. On the other hand, no application equipment is needed and a high selectivity may be realized. For the purpose of lower cost, sands coated with some kinds of herbicides may be utilized. In Japan, a large share of the herbicides is directed to rice culture and granules play a very important role, as shown in Table 6 (12).

One exceptional formulation of herbicide is the emulsifiable concentrate of oxadiazon. This concentrate is applied by hand directly from special holes of a container like a Coca-cola bottle onto the muddy water surface without any dilution. The floating soil particles adsorb the herbicide, then precipitate and form a firm soil-herbicide layer on the water bottom. Oxadiazon E.C. can easily disperse into the water and adsorb to the soil particles. These two properties have made the formulation applicable as described above (14).

ENVIRONMENTAL PROBLEMS

As shown in a following paper, the toxicity of rice herbicides to environmental organisms, especially aquatic animals which may be an important protein source for residents, should be extremely low. Flooded paddy fields are connected with lakes or seas through water channels, and herbicides applied in paddy fields may thus be easily transferred to such aquatic areas. PCP granules had been found to be a very nice herbicide as described above, however, when heavy rain came, small particles of soil adsorbed with PCP flowed out from the fields to the lake or shallow sea where the herbicide killed many fish or shellfish. PCP cannot therefore

Table 6 Formulation type of pesticide in Japan (1980)

Formulation	Insecticide	Fungicide	Herbicide	Others	Total
Dust	28,707 *	24,914	107	371	54,103
Granule	20,926	11,986	50,401	74	83,388
E.C. & Liquid	45,599	8,087	27,795	3,162	84,642
Wettable powder	27,147	50,258	12,597	1,849	91,851
Dust-granule	1,239	384	614	-	2,237
Others	14,946	3,183	420	2,190	20,740
Total	138,563	98,817	91,934	7,648	336,962

* Sales in thousand Yen

be practically used in the flooded paddy fields in Japan because of its mode of action which inhibits oxidative phosphorylation. Although transplanted rice plants are safe after PCP application as described above, aerobic organisms having the same susceptible site as weeds will be damaged. In general, herbicides having a mode of action which inhibits oxidative phorphorylation may not be suitable to flooded rice culture.

Under flooded conditions, especially with raw organic materials, where soils can easily be reduced we should pay attention to the reduction of herbicides to prevent unfavorable compounds. One such example is the dechlorination (15, 16) of thiobencarb to produce *N,N*-diethyl benzylthiocarbamate which has already no selectivity to rice plants. Fortunately this process could be inhibited and the problem was solved by the co-existence of another herbicide methoxyphenone (3,3'-dimethyl-4-methoxybenzophenone) or other compounds. Reduction of nitro-diphenylether herbicides, chloronitrofen and others, to their amino derivatives lengthened their residual periods (18). Another example in this field is the reductive dechlorination of pentachlorobenzoic acid produced from a rice blast fungicide pentachlorobenzylalchol (PCBA). Partially dechlorinated benzoic acids became auxin-type herbicides to broadleaved vegetables through the application of manure made from rice straw containing PCBA.

ECONOMIC PROBLEMS

Economic assessment of weed control in rice culture will also be discussed in a following paper. The labor cost is very low in most rice producing countries, so the price of the herbicides themselves and the application cost should also be low. The cost of herbicides and their application should be much less than hand-weeding if we want to utilize herbicides for rice culture. In this case governmental regulation costs such as monitoring or residue analysis of herbicides should be considered (19).

REFERENCES

1. M. Miyahara, Nōyaku (Pesticide Design - Strategy and Tactics), 1,005-1,012, Soft Science, Tokyo (1979).
2. H. Chisaka, Weed Res. (Japan) 14, 12-18 (1972), 15, 16-20 (1973), 19, 72-77 (1975).
3. M. Arai, M.Miyahara and H. Yokomori, J. Kanto-Tosan Agric. exp. Stn.8, 56-62 (1955).
4. I. Tanaka, Proc. Symposium on Climate and Rice, 223-247, International Rice Research Institute, Los Banos (1976).
5. M.R. Vega, J.D. Ona and E.C. Paller, Jr., Proc. 1st Asian-Pacific Weed Control Interchange 63-66 (1969).
6. M.R. Vega, J.D. Ona and F.L. Punzalan, Proc. 1st Asian-Pacific Weed Control Interchange, 59-62 (1969).
7. S. Matsunaka, Pesticide Terminal Residues, 343-365, Butterworth, London (1971).
8. T. Akatsuka, Weed Res. (Japan), 24, 55-63 (1979).
9. S. Matsunaka, Proc. 1st Asian-Pacific Weed Control Interchange, 41-44 (1969).
10. N. Ichizen, Weed Res. (Japan), 21, 80-83 (1976).
11. K. Hirai and Y. Kawamura, Weed Res. (Japan), 20, 61-66 (1975).
12. M. Yukimoto, T. Kawahara and T. Nakahara, J.Pesticide Sci., 4, 447-451 (1979).
13. Anonymous, Nōyaku-yōran 1981, 38, Japan Plant Protection Ass., Tokyo (1981).
14. Y. Kawamura, Proc. 3rd. Conf. Asian-Pacific Weed Sci, Soc., 176-179 (1971).
15. T. Yamada, H. Chisaka, Y. Koyama and Y. Takeichi, Weed Res. (Japan), 24, 272-280 (1979).
16. K. Ishikawa, R. Shinohara, A. Yagi, S. Shigematsu and I. Kimura, J. Pesticide Sci., 5, 107-109 (1980).
17. S. Shigematsu, Y. Yamada, Y. Fukai, H. Abe, I. Kimura, K. Ozawa and T. Nakano, Weed Res. (Japan), 26 (Suppl.) 159-160 (1981).

18. T. Yamada, Weed Res. (Japan), 14, (Suppl.) 117-119 (1975).
19. S. Matsunaka, Rice in Asia, 438-457, Univ. Tokyo Press, Tokyo (1975).

USE OF PLANT GROWTH REGULATORS IN RICE CULTIVATION

Yasuo Ota

Department of Physiology and Genetics, National Institute of Agricultural Sciences, 1-1, Kannondai-3, Yatabe-machi, Tsukuba-gun, Ibaraki 305, Japan

Absracts - This paper reports on three main plant growth regulators presently used or shortly to be used in rice cultivation in Japan.

Since 1961, mechanical transplanting methods for rice cultivation, which require nursery boxes for producing the seedlings, have been widely developed in Japan. Rice seedlings grown in nursery boxes are apt to be susceptible to soil-borne diseases and physiological damping-off (Murenae), because of the special and densely populated cultivation. The application of hymexazol (3-hydroxy-5-methylisoxazole) to the nursery boxes has a remarkable effect on the control of these harmful phenomena.

Meanwhile, anti-lodging agents are needed to adopt to mechanical harvesting as well as to obtain a high yield and a good quality of rice in Japan. Although many anti-lodging agents have been tested, none of them has given satisfactory results except IBP (*O*,*O*-diisopropyl-*S*-benzyl thiophosphate), a rice blast fungicide. IBP has preventive effects for lodging of rice by shortening internodes without decreasing yields.

In the direct sowing method of rice cultivation in sumberged fields, other problems must be recognized such as low germination, possible floating of seedlings and of lodging due to poor roots. For coated seeds the use of calcium peroxide, which release oxygen slowly in submerged soil, was found to be very effective in promoting emergence and establishment of rice seedlings by direct sowing in submerged field conditions.

INTRODUCTION

The use of plant growth regulators in rice cultivation has become prevalent throughout Japan from a labor saving point of view. In particular, the modification of rice seedlings which are used ina mechanical transplantting method has been successfully achieved with a growth regulator, hymexazol. This has not only shown high fungicidal effects against soil-borne plant pathogenic organisms (such as *Aphanomyces*, *Phthium*, *Fusarium sp.*) of rice and sugar beet but has also encouraged the physiological characteristics of the respective seedlings.

The harvesting method using combines is becoming more popular, and the anti-lodging agent is increasing more requested by farmers. IBP is a systemic fungicide which has excellent effects on *Pyricularia oryzae*, *Pellicularia sasakii*, and *Helminthosporium sigmoideum*, and acts as an effective plant growth regulator. It is effectively preventing lodging by shortening rice internodes.

Although with the direct sowing culture of paddy rice in submerged fields it is difficult to get stands of seedlings as uniform as with a transplanted culture, direct sowing is expected to become more popular if a technique for stabilizing the emergence and establishment of seed-is found. This will then help to save labor. To promote the germination of rice seeds sown in submerged conditions, therefore, many studies have been carried out but no trial had been made on improving seedling emergence and establishment by supplying oxygen to the seeds. The method presented in this paper is to supply oxygen to sown seeds treated with calcium peroxide, which releases oxygen slowly in submerged soil. The emergence and establishment of seedlings directly sown in submerged paddy fields is thereby improved.

The conventional method of direct sowing of rice has several defects: low germination rate and poor root growth due to lack of oxygen, uneven growth of seedlings due to staggered germination, lianility to lodge (direct-sown rice formd advantitious roots on the soil surface which do not have sufficient strength to support a mature plant), and difficulty of weed control as compared with transplanted rice. The use of calcium peroxide for coating seeds was found very effective in promoting emergence and establishment of rice seedlings in direct sowing in submerged conditions.

In addition, it was also found that, when seeds were coated with the mixture of calcium peroxide and hymexazol (3-hydroxy-5-methylisoxazole), a growth regulator effective in promoting growth and physiological activity of roots, the emergence and early growth of seedlings were further improved.

EXPERIMENTAL

Plant growth-promoting activities of hymexazol (3-hydroxy-5-methylisoxazole, trade name; Tachigaren)

The chemical structure of hymexazol is similar to those of tricholomic acid and ibotenic acid found in mushrooms.

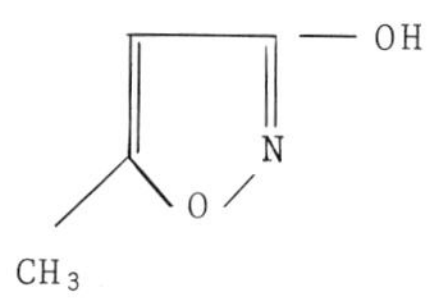

The effect of hymexazol on the growth of rice (*Oryza sativa* L. c.v. *Nihonbare*) seedlings was examined in nursery boxes using non-sterilized or sterilized soil. In both soils, the weight of shoot and root increased in soil treated with hymexazol as compared with the untreated soil as shown in Table 1. The increase in weight due to hymexazol treatment was greater for roots than for shoots. Therefore these results indicate that hymexazol has a growth-promoting effect on the rice seedlings.

Table 1. Effect of hymexazol (3-hydroxy-5-methylisoxazole) on growth of rice seedlings in non-sterilized and sterilized soils

Treatment	Plant height (cm)	Root length (cm)	Fresh weight (mg)	
			Shoot	Root
Non-sterilized soil				
control	12.4	5.7	86	21
treated	15.4	6.7	99	29
Sterilized soil				
control	14.7	6.8	89	25
treated	15.2	6.8	95	34

Note: About 7,500 rice seedlings were grown densely at 13-18°C in a nursery box (30x60x3cm). Five hundred ml of solution containing 0.15g of hymexazol per nursery box was applied to the soil immediately after sowing in the treated plot. Measurements were made at 20 days after sowing. Figures are average of 20 individuals.

The effect of hymexazol on the growth of roots was also observed in other plant species such as sweet potato, taro, shallot, lotus, carrot, strawberry, onion, tea, tomato, eggplant, cucumber and chrysanthemum, when it was applied to the soil after sowing or planting. In general, the application of hymexazol at about $0.9g/m^2$ promoted the development of branched roots and root hairs as well as the growth of roots.

Fig. 1 shows a comparison of α-naphtylamine-oxidizing activity in roots between hymexazol treated and control plots. It is evident from these figures that the oxidizing activity of roots of the hymexazol-treated plot was higher than that of the control when expressed on a per plant basis or per gram fresh weight of roots.

It is known that the occurrence of Murenae (physiological damping-off) is closely related to the physiological activity of roots. Roots from Murenae-affected plants show low α-naphthylamine-oxidizing activity. The results mentioned above indicate that hymexazol stimulates the physiological activity of roots while preventing their infection by the damping-off organisms. This increased physiological activity may also prevent the occurrence of Murenae in seedlings.

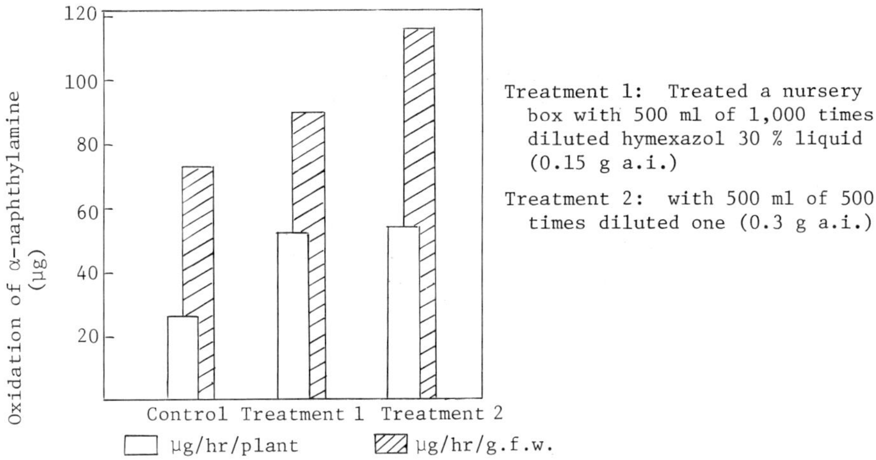

Fig. 1. Effect of 3-hydroxy-5-methylisoxazole on α-naphthylamine oxidizing activity in rice roots 20 days after sowing

Hymexazol is absorbed by plants and translocated acropetally to the shoots of plants. In plants, hymexazol is readily converted to its *N*-β-glucoside and *O*-β-glucoside derivatives, shown in Fig. 2. The two metabolites were examined about their effect on the growth of rice seedlings. The growth effects of the metabolites were similar to those observed when rice seedlings were treated with hymexazol. The metabolites promoted root growth and development of root hairs, and increased the oxidizing activity of roots.

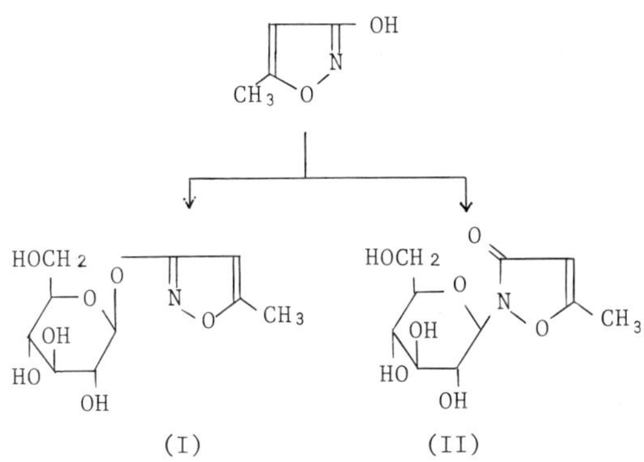

(I) 3-(β-D-glucopyramosyloxy)-5-methylisoxazole (*O*-β-glucoside)
(II) 2-(β-D-glucopyramosyl)-5-methyl-4-isoxazolin-3-one (*N*-β-glucoside)

Fig. 2. Metabolism of 3-hydroxy-5-methylisoxazole in higher plants

As shown in Fig. 3, *N*-β-glucoside and *O*-β-glucoside gave marked elongation of roots for a short (6-day) period after germination in water culture.

The results strongly suggest that the growth-promoting effect of hymexazol is possibly due to the conversion of the compound to two kinds of glucosides, especially to *N*-β-glucoside. It is known that *O*-β-glucoside is antifungal, but *N*-β-glucoside is not. Both metabolites, however, seem to be successful in promoting the growth of roots. The hymexazol-treated seedlings had a high geotropic curvature response. Hymexazol showed no auxin activity in the rice lamina joint test. However, the auxin activity of indoleacetic acid was increased in the presence of hymexazol, as shown in Fig. 4. Therefore, the increased geotropic curvature response of rice seedlings may be due to a synergistic effect of hymexazol on endogenous auxin. It is considered that the increased response of rice seedlings caused by hymexazol is a very important factor in mechanical transplanting of rice seedlings.

It was observed that the pre-treatment of rice seedlings with hymexazol increases cold resistance, and a drastic reduction in overhead flooding damage in rice. Hymexazol also reduced the phytotoxic action of herbicides such as simetryn, swep-MCPA, nitrofen, chloronitrofen and propanil. These phenomena may be attributed to increased seedling vigor induced by hymexazol.

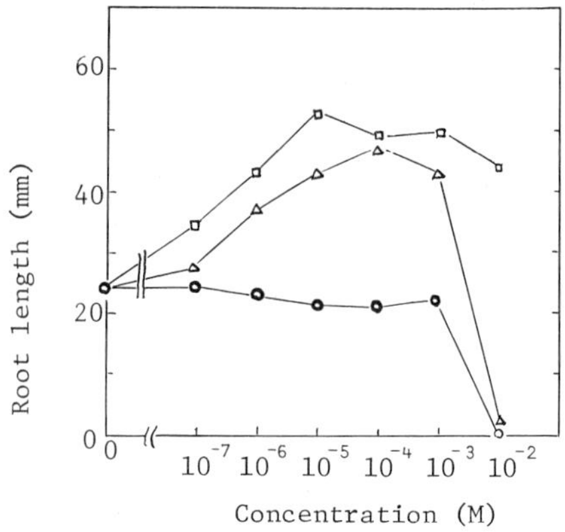

Fig. 3. Effect of hymexazol (3-hydroxy-5-methylisoxazole) and its two metabolites on root growth of rice seedlings

Note: Rice seeds were germinated and five seeds each were transferred to a small test tube (2.5x6.0 cm) containing 2ml of hymexazol or its metabolites. The test tubes were kept at 30°C under constant light (4,000 lux). Measurements were made 6 days after sowing.

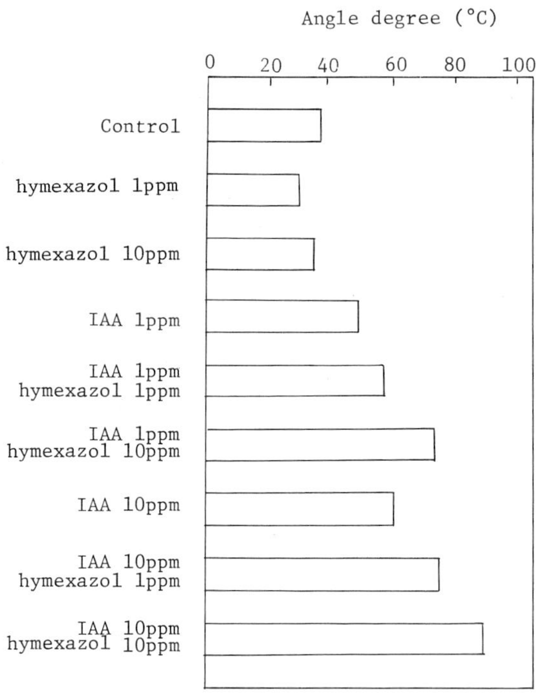

Fig. 4. Effect of hymexazol (3-hydroxy-5-methylisoxazole) on the auxin-induced inclination of lamina in etiolated 2nd leaves of rice

Note: Segments consisting of laminal joint with intact lamina and 2 cm of sheath were treated in various solutions of IAA and hymexazol after pre-treatment for 24 hours by deionized water, and the inclination of lamina was measured at 48 hours after treatment.

Anti-lodging activities of IBP (*O,O*-diisopropyl-*S*-benzyl thiophosphate, trade name:Kitazin P)
Although many chemicals have been tested for preventing the lodging od paddy rice, none of them have given satisfactory results. For example, some hormonal compounds such as 2,4-D, and MCPA are known to depress the growth of culm and make rice plants more resistant to lodging. The depression made by these compounds, however, may affect the length and weight of panivles which leads to poor yield of crops, while IBP shortens the culm length without decreasing the yield. Usually an increase of the yield is observed. Fig. 5 shows the shortening effect of IBP on the length of culms and panicles.

It is found that the length of culms is shortened by 5 to 10 % at the dose of 40-60 kg(17 % of a.i. granule)/ha, and the most effective time for application for this purpose is 18-29 days before heading.

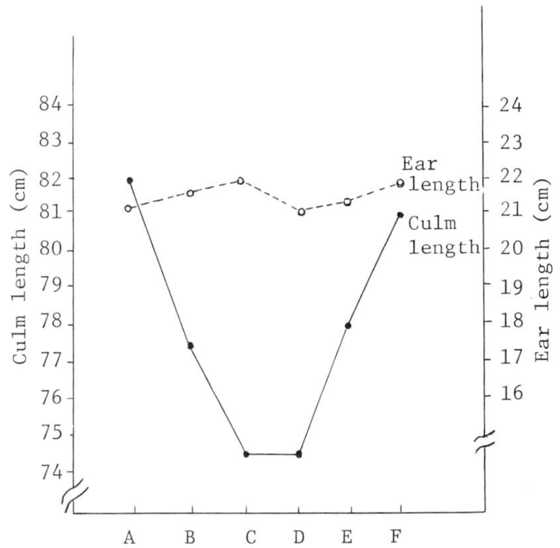

Date of the application

A: No treatment
B: July 14 (39 days before heading)
C: July 24 (29 days before heading)
D: Aug. 4 (18 days before heading)
E: Aug. 13 (9 days before heading)
F: Aug. 23 (Heading)

Fig. 5. Length of the culm and ear as influenced by the application time of IBP

Generally, when growth retardants are applied, the length of culms is shortened and the length of ears is also shortened simultaneously. However, IBP has no influence on the length of ears but has a good effect on the shortening of culms.

It is also observed that the strength of the culms is incresed because the culm walls of the lower internodes (N_4, N_5) become thicker (Table 2).

Table 2. Influence of IBP on lodging
(Kyushu Agr. Expt. Stn., 1969)

Treatment	Breaking strength of the 4th internode (kg)	Moment	Lodging index
Control	0.578 (100)	1,108 (100)	192
Treatment 31 days before heading	0.728 (126)	1,018 (92)	131
Treatment 20 days before heading	0.717 (124)	998 (90)	139
Treatment 10 days before heading	0.674 (117)	969 (87)	144

Note: IBP granules (a.i. 17 %) applied at the rate of 50 kg/ha.

Furthermore, when IBP is applied, the flag leaves become erect at the ripening stage, the physilogical activity of roots can be well maintained and the silica content is particularly increased. Therefore, IBP makes it possible to apply a large quantity of fertilizers because of its anti-lodging effect, which results in higher rice yield.

Promotion of emergence and establishment of rice seedling using calcium peroxide-coated seeds

Calcium peroxide (CaO_2) is itself stable at room temperature. However, it decomposes slowly in humid soil and generate oxygen in the reaction to form calcium hydroxide. In the soil, calcium hydroxide may eventually combined with atmospheric carbon dioxide to form calcium cabonate.

$$CaO_2 + H_2O = Ca(OH)_2 + (O)$$
$$Ca(OH)_2 + CO_2 = CaCO_3 + H_2O$$

This method paved the way for the commercial use of calcium peroxide known in the market as Calper G dust. Calper G dust is composed of:

CaO_2	more than 35 %
$CaSO_4$ 1/2 H_2O(gypsum)	more than 25 %
Other materials	less than 40 %

In practice, wet seeds are placed in the rotary pan of a coating machine. An equal amount of Calper G dust is gradually mixed with the rice seeds to coat them uniformly.

Rice seeds can germinate in submerged paddy soil where the oxygen supply is limited. Subsequent growth, however, may be highly impaired unless the oxygen supply is adequate. The oxygen concentration required for organ development is 2 ppm for appearance of radicle, 4 ppm for root elongation, more than 5 ppm for active root elongation and 5-6 ppm for growth of the first leaf. Effect of different coating ratios of Calper G dust on seedling emergence was determined with the treated seeds covered with 2 cm soil and 2 cm water depth at 25°C (Table 3). It was clearly shown that Calper G dust coating is very effective in promoting seedling emergence, and the coating ratio of 100 % gave the greatest effect.

Table 3. Coating ratio of Calper G dust and seedling growth

Seedling growth	Coating ratio (%)				
	0	25	50	75	100
Shoot emergence (%)	36	57	74	76	77
First leaf emergence (%)	7	26	41	59	73
Plant height (cm)	2.0	3.9	7.8	10.1	11.4
Dry weight (mg/plant)	10	20	40	50	60

Note: Measurement was made 11 days after sowing.

$$\text{Coating ratio} = \frac{\text{Weight of Calper G dust}}{\text{Weight of dry seeds}} \times 100\ (\%)$$

Even though the seedling emergence is improved by the use of Calper G dust in direct sowing at low temperature, the growth of young leaves and roots is often retarded by low temperature, sometimes causing seedling rot infection. In such cases the use of the mixture of Calper G dust and hymexazol was found to be very effective in promoting the early growth of seedlings (Table 4). This effect of the combined use of hymexazol with Calper G dust has been proved useful not only at a low temperature but also at high temperatures.

For the direct sowing on a submerged paddy field, the sowing has to be done at the time when the mean temperature of 5 consecutive days has reached 14-15°C or higher, and at a sowing rate of 40 to 60 kg of seeds per 1 ha. The sowing depth is critical for seedling emergence of Calper G coated seeds: 1-2 cm is ideal and should not exceed 3 cm. The application of a highly selective herbicide, pyrazolate granule (trade name, Sanbird) from soon after sowing to 5 days after sowing is the most preferable for weed control.

Table 5 shows the result of a field trial conducted at the Central Agricultural Experiment Station, Konosu, Saitama in 1979. Yields of c.v. "Koshihikari" (*japonica car.*) and "Milyang 23" (*japonica* x *indica var.*) were fairly high, compared with mechanical transplanting culture.

Table 4. Effect of seed coating with a mixture of hymexazol dust and Calper G dust on growth of rice seedlings

(Growth in mg of fresh weight, % in parentheses)

Temperature	Plant part	Untreated	Calper G dust	Mixture of Calper G dust with hymexazol dust***
Low temperature*	Top	53 (100)	76 (143)	82 (153)
	Root	30 (100)	43 (146)	59 (199)
Medium temperature**	Top	60 (100)	83 (138)	93 (155)
	Root	28 (100)	53 (189)	66 (239)

Note: * Temperature was adjusted to 18°C in daytime and 13°C in nighttime. Measurement was taken 30 days after sowing.
** Temperature was kept at 32 - 34°C for 3 days after sowing, then lowered gradually to 16 - 25°C at nighttime from the 4th to 7th day, and kept at 18°C in daytime and 13°C in nighttime after 8th day. Measurement was made 20 days after sowing.
*** Hymexazol dust (4 % a.i.) was used at the rate of 3 % of dry seed weight.

Table 5. Grain yields and their components

Variety	No. of panicles/m^2	No. of spikelets/ panicle	Percentage of ripened grains	Weight of 1,000 grains (g)	Kernel yield (ton/ha)
"Koshihikari"	312	76.9	89.4	21.2	4.51
"Milyang 23"	324	132.0	73.6	22.6	7.12

Note: Seeds were coated with mixture of Calper G and hymexazol. Date of sowing: 23, May 1979. Sowing rate: 50kg/ha. Application of fertilizer for "Koshihikari": 50kg N/ha as basal, 70kg N/ha as top dressing splitted three times. For "Milyang 23": 100kg N/ha as basal, 100kg/ha as top dressing splitted twice. Weeds were controlled by pyrazolate granule applied one day after sowing.

REFERENCES

1. Ogawa, M. & Ota, Y.: Plant growth-regulating activities of 3-hydroxy-5-methylisoxazole. I. Effects of 3-hydroxy-5-methylisoxazole and metabolities in plants on growth of rice seedlings. *Proc. Crop Sci. Soc. Japan,* 42, 499-505 (1973).
2. Ogawa, M. & Ota, Y.: II. Effect of 3-hydroxy-5-methylisoxazole on the geotropic response of rice seedlings. ibid. 43, 278-282 (1974).
3. Ota, Y. & Ogawa, M.: Plant growth regulating activities of 3-hydroxy-5-methylisoxazole in rice seedlings. *Plant Grwoth Substances* 1973, 494-503. (1973)
4. Takeichi, Y. & Yamagishi, A.: Inhibition of non-parasitic damping-off ("Murenae") of young rice seedlings in nursery boxes. I. Effect of 3-hydroxy-5-methylisoxazole on damping-off and growth of rice seedlings. *Proc. Crop Sci. Soc. Japan,* 43, 24-30 (1974).
5. Ogawa, M. & Ota, Y.: Combined use of Calper and Tachigaren to improve seedling emergence under submerged condition. *Agr. & Hort.,* 48, 1297-1304 (1973) [In Japanese].
6. Ota, Y. & Nakayama, M.: Effect of seed coating with calcium peroxide on germination under submerged condition in rice plant. *Proc. Crop Sci. Soc. Japan,* 39, 535-536 (1970) [In Japanese with English summary].
7. Ota, Y., Nakamura, Y. & Imamura, S.: The utilization of oxygen generating agent calcium peroxide in direct sown paddy rice. *Proc. 7th Asian-Pacific Weed Sci. Soc. Conf.,* 267-270 (1979).
8. Mitsuishi, S.: Study on the direct underground sowing in the submerging field of rice. *Special Bull. Ishikawa Pref. College Agr.,* 4, 1-59 (1975) [In Japanese with English summary].
9. Mitsuishi, S. & Nakamura, Y.: Studies on direct sowing into flooded soils. I. Method of calcium peroxide coating. *Proc. Crop Sci. Soc. Japan,* 46 (Suppl. No.1), 35-36 (1977) [In Japanese].
10. Yamada, N.: Calcium peroxide as an oxygen supplier for crop plants. *Proc. Crop Sci. Soc. Japan,* 21, 65-66 (1951) [In Japanese with English summary].
11. Yoshida, S. & Rivera, C.T.: Effect of calcium peroxide on seedling emergence of IR 36 from puddled soil at different temperatures. *Int. Rice Res. Newsl.,* 3, 17-18 (1978).

THE FATE OF HERBICIDES IN CALIFORNIA RICE CULTURE

Donald G. Crosby

Department of Environmental Toxicology, University of California, Davis, California 95616, USA

Abstract - Rice has become a major crop in California. Weeds remain a severe problem, and over one million kg of herbicides are applied annually for control. The rice field represents a chemical reactor containing active reagents into which the herbicidal compound is introduced and subsequently moved and degraded. Of particular importance are volatilization (as illustrated by molinate), photonucleophilic substitution reactions (propanil), photooxidation (thiobencarb), and loss in spray drift (MCPA). Investigation and application of these principles may permit prediction of the ricefield fate of other pesticides and adjustment of their properties to produce improvements important to efficacy, environmental safety, and public health.

The United States of America ranks rather low among the rice-producing nations of the world. Despite geographical size, its 1.2 million hectares of rice land represent less than 1% of the world's rice-producing area, and the 6.4 million metric tons it produces is less than 2% of the world total (1). California, now the principal rice-growing state, produces only about 1.6 million metric tons on some 220,000 hectares (less than 0.5% of its land area).

However, the impact of California rice production is disproportionately large. At present, the California yield of 7.3 metric tons/ha (6500 lbs/acre) is almost three times the world average, a major proportion is exported to other nations, and California cultivars, production methods, and research have attracted worldwide interest. The rice comes from the Great Central Valley fed by the Sacramento and San Joaquin rivers; the fields are levelled accurately--generally under laser-beam control---flooded to 6-15 cm depth, and fertilizer, seed, and pesticides applied by aircraft during the growing season (April-September). During much of this period, there is no rain, water temperature lies between 25° and 30°C, and atmospheric humidity is low.

Fortunately, California rice suffers few insect and disease pests. However, weeds remain a major problem (Table I). In addition to flooding and other cultural methods of weed-control, over 1 million kg of chemical herbicides now are applied annually, most by aircraft (Table II) (2). About 10 herbicidal compounds are used regularly, and several others are used occasionally or are under investigation. What happens to this large amount of biologically-active chemicals? The answer is important to economical rice production, to environmental quality and safety, and to human comfort and health. In this paper, I will review some basic principles, describe our experience with the fate of several of the herbicides most widely used in California rice culture, and try to draw at least tentative conclusions.

Table I. Principal California Rice Weeds

Barnyard grass	*Echinochloa crus-galli*
Sprangletop	*Leptochloa fascicularis*
Naiad	*Najas guadalupensis*
Roughseed bulrush	*Scirpus mucronatus*
Umbrella plant	*Cyperus difformis*
Purple ammania	*Ammania coccinea*
Arrowhead	*Sagittaria* spp
Cattail	*Typha latifolia*
Chara	*Chara* spp
Waterhyssop	*Bacopa eisenii*

Table II. Herbicides applied to California rice, 1981 (2)

Common Name	Trade Name	Structure	Amount applied Kg	ha
Molinate	Ordram	IX	766,077	173,899
MCPA (salts)	MCP-Amine	VI	203,789	160,327
Thiobencarb	Bolero	V	130,356	29,409
Bentazon (No Salt)	Basagran		58,475	64,972
Propanil	STAM	II	51,630	12,340
2,4-D (PGBE ester)	Esteron		3,388	1,108
2,4-D (salts)	2,4-D	I	2,752	2,059
Silvex (PGBE ester)	Kuron, Weedone 2,4,5-TP		2,697	1,288

RICE FIELDS AS REACTORS

The rice field may be viewed as a chemical reactor. It contains, in aqueous solution, reactive nucleophiles such as hydroxide ion (pH 8-10), ammonia and amines, and sulfide; dissolved oxygen and other oxidants (3); organic and inorganic reducing agents; and the biochemical agents produced by microorganisms. Heat and light provide energy. The herbicide released into this reactor will be subjected to the physical forces of dissolution, adsorption, and volatilization as well as to biotic and abiotic breakdown.

A uniform application of one pound/acre (1.1 kg/ha) of herbicide represents a concentration of about 1 mg/L in a typical rice field. The pure rice herbicides all are soluble at that level although their distribution in water may be affected by application as immiscible formulations. Adsorption is inversely related to aqueous solubility (polarity), and so most rice herbicides are not considered to be highly adsorbed although some may become chemically bound. However, volatilization proves to be an especially important dissipative force. Mackay (4) has investigated the volatilization of pesticides and other chemicals from water and shown that the rate is influenced by solubility, vapor pressure, and water depth; it is apparent that vapor loss from the warm, shallow rice fields generally will be significant.

The high pH of the water results in the hydrolysis of carboxylic esters even in the dark. However, other dark reactions are slow; sunlight is the important driving force (5). Most California rice herbicides absorb ultraviolet (UV) radiation in the 290-350 nm range from sunlight, and the light-energized molecules undergo reactions with surrounding environmental reagents resulting primarily in oxidation (oxygenation), reduction (hydrogenation), and photonucleophilic replacement of substituents by hydroxyl derived from water. These reactions are illustrated by 2,4-D (I, Fig. 1) (6). Simultaneously, oxidation occurs on the side-chain (Eq. 1), the chlorines are replaced by H (reduction, Eq. 2) and by hydroxyl (Eq. 3), and these photolysis products subsequently are further degraded. Similarly, pentachlorophenol (PCP), at one time

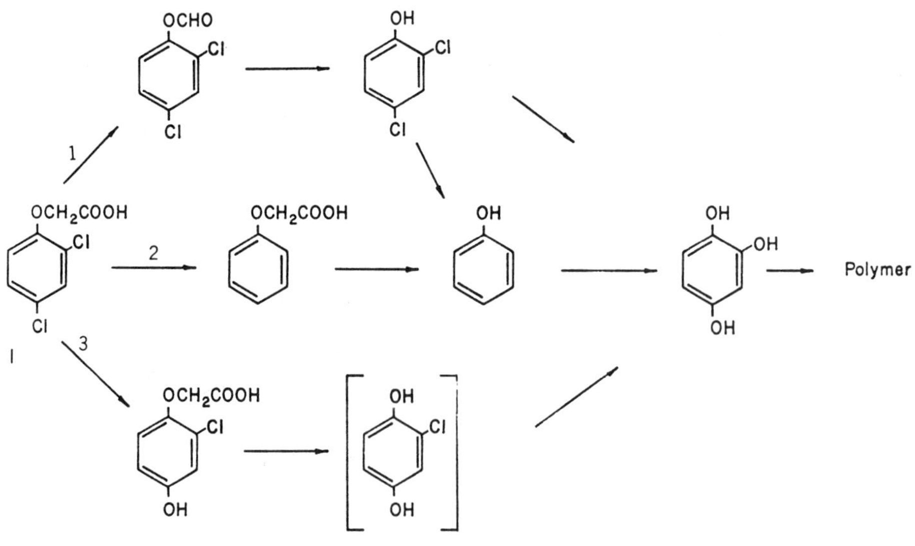

Fig. 1. Photodegradation of 2,4-D in aqueous solution (6).

extensively used in rice culture, initially undergoes photoreduction and photonucleophilic loss of Cl, and the resulting products then become oxidized or otherwise photolyzed, eventually to small fragments (7).

Being acids, 2,4-D and PCP volatilize only very slowly from rice field water, and atmospheric photochemistry may be relatively unimportant to their fate. However, most neutral substances--herbicides and their photoproducts alike--are more volatile, and vapor-phase photo-oxidation may become a significant factor (8). While microbial degradation in water often is slow compared to other routes of loss, it becomes important for those (largely neutral) herbicides which are applied pre-emergence to the soil. Likewise, metabolism by rice plants, weeds, and algae always takes some part in herbicide fate, and these biological aspects have been reviewed for many rice herbicides (9). Unfortunately, they still have received little attention under California conditions, and the present article must be concerned primarily with physical movement and chemical degradation.

THE ENVIRONMENTAL FATE OF RICE HERBICIDES

The results from environmental fate investigations of several herbicides underscore a number of important principles. Among these are the interesting and general phenomenon of photonucleophilic reactions (propanil), the photochemical generation and reactions of oxidants in field water (thiobencarb and molinate), degradation in spray droplets (MCPA), and the often-significant of volatilization from water (molinate).

Propanil. Propanil (II, mp 93°C, water soly 225 mg/L, vp 9 x 10^{-5} torr/60°C) usually is applied at 4-5 kg/ha from an EC formulation (STAM^R). It was found to be stable in water in the dark, but its aqueous solutions were slowly degraded by sunlight (Fig. 2) (10). Three major pathways were evident. In one, ring-chlorines were replaced by hydroxyl, and the resulting destabilized molecule became oxidized to the quinone imide which underwent rapid hydrolysis. In another, chlorines were replaced by H. Both propanil and its dichlorinated products also underwent light-energized hydrolysis to the corresponding anilines; dichloroaniline (III) was photodegraded as rapidly as it formed ($t_{1/2}$=0.5 day) (11), a small proportion forming 3,3',4,4'-tetrachloroazobenzene (IV)(10, 11).

The replacement of ring-chlorines by OH represents photonucleophilic reactions. For 3,4-dichloroaniline, Miller et al. (12) have provided evidence that formation of 2-chloro-5-aminophenol is a photosolvolysis in which water itself is the reagent; other evidence (13) suggests that replacement of the para-Cl is a photonucleophilic displacement. These reactions appear to be general for many types of pesticides and other substances in water (13), involving halogen, nitro, and even methoxyl as leaving groups; photonucleophilic substitution reactions may be expected to provide a major aquatic degradation pathway for many present and future rice herbicides.

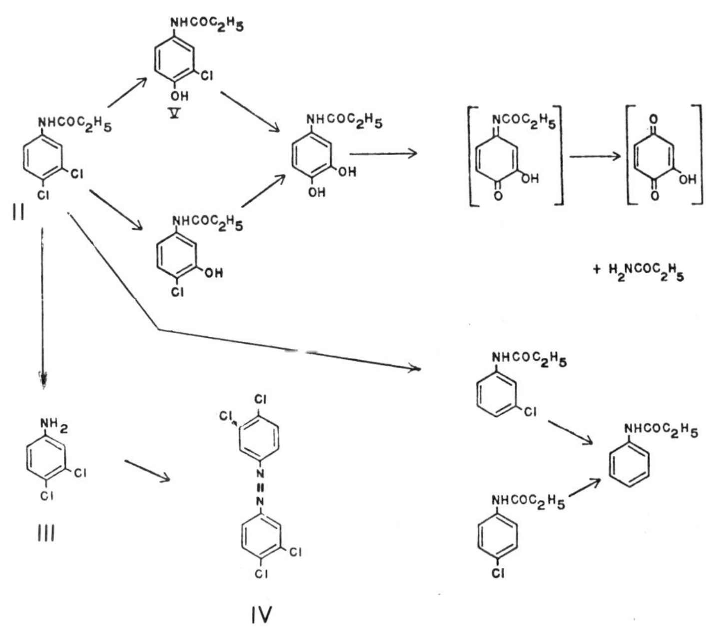

Fig. 2. Photodegradation of propanil in water (10)

Surprisingly, propanil appeared to be lost slowly, if at all, by volatilization from water (10). It is known to be degraded rapidly by plants and microorganisms (14), initially by hydrolysis to dichloroaniline which then may become bound to soil, but investigation of this route has not been reported for California field conditions. A survey of California rice soils (15) did not reveal any residual propanil, but one of 19 samples contained 0.01 ppm tetrachloroazobenzene. Thus, it seems reasonable that while only a small proportion of the applied propanil will be degraded directly by light or higher plants, and some will be adsorbed from solution by soil, most may be rapidly metabolized by microorganisms and any water-borne dichloroaniline subsequently photolyzed.

Thiobencarb. This compound (V), sold as Bolero[R] or Saturn[R] (bp 126-29°C/0.008 torr, soly 30 mg/L, vp 1.48×10^{-6} torr/20°C) is applied at 3-6 kg/ha from an EC or WP formulation to control grassy weeds. In aqueous solution, it does not absorb sunlight UV and also was is relatively stable in the dark. However, in rice field water, it was rapidly photodegraded ($t_{1/2}$=6 hrs) (16). Photolysis products included p-chlorobenzaldehyde, p-chlorobenzyl alcohol, p-chlorobenzoic acid, and hydroxylated benthiocarb (16,17) (Fig. 3).

Our earlier work (3) had demonstrated the presence of oxidants generated by photochemical action in field water. Pesticides were shown to be oxidized at rates which increased during the day but which then dropped off to zero after nightfall. Eventually, hydrogen peroxide was isolated from sunlit field water and shown to reproduce in vitro the photooxidation observed in the rice fields (18), including that of thiobencarb.

The herbicide proved to be quite volatile (19); at 30°C, pure thiobencarb was lost from aqueous solution with a half-life of about 2 days, although $t_{1/2}$=8 days at 25°C. In commercial-scale field tests, $t_{1/2}$ from maximum concentration was 5-7 days due, perhaps, to differences in water temperatures, and p-chlorobenzaldehyde and p-chlorobenzoic acid were detected in field water.

Both photochemical and microbial degradation have been reported by others (20). The picture of thiobencarb fate which emerges is one of rapid breakdown in the field accompanied by equally rapid loss to the atmosphere. However, the surprising "photodecomposition" in water of a pesticide which does not absorb sunlight UV--that is, degradation by photochemical oxidant--seems to be a general phenomenon and one which must alter our methods of laboratory prediction of pesticide environmental fate.

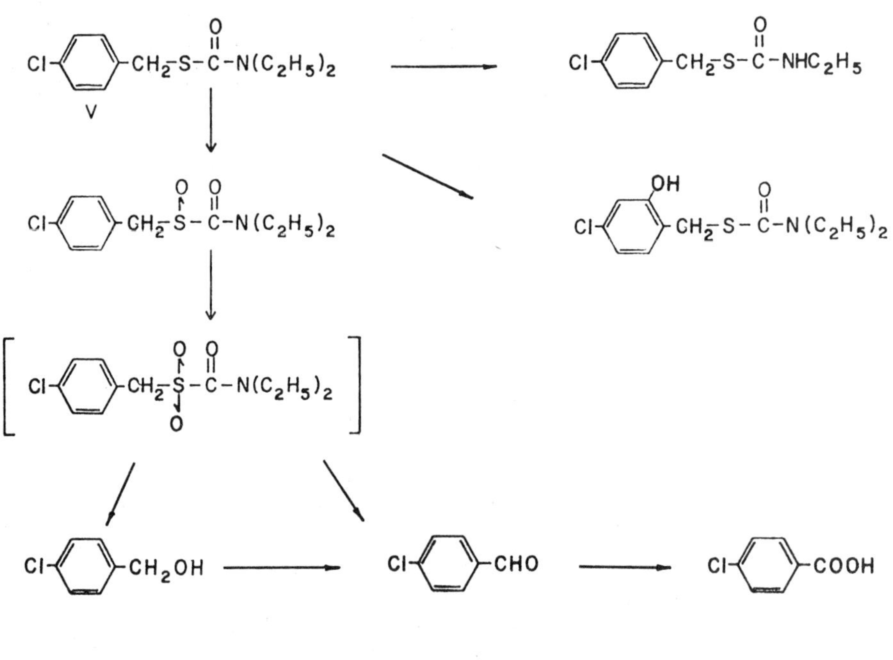

Fig. 3. Photodegradation of thiobencarb in water (16,17).

MCPA. MCPA (VI) most often is applied for broadleaf weed control as a 15 g/L (0.06 M) aqueous solution of its dimethylamine (DMA) salt to provide about 1 kg/ha as MCPA. That which reaches the water (pH 8) remains largely in anionic form, and there is little if any volatilization (except perhaps from soild surfaces). Although relatively stable in the dark, dilute MCPA solutions undergo moderately rapid photodegradation (21) ($t_{½}$=17 days) characterized by oxidation of the acetate and methyl groups and eventual replacement of Cl by OH (Fig. 4A). However, microbial action is observed even in the dark in field water, and sterilized field water in sunlight produces a $t_{½}$ of only 5 days.

At the high concentrations found in evaporating spray droplets, the environmental situation is quite different. As the airborne droplets evaporate, the contained chemicals become increasingly concentrated rather than more dilute, and volatile photoproducts are more rapidly evaporated from their surface. Photolysis is quite rapid ($t_{½}$=3 days), and, while major photoproducts remain the same, others such as the amide VII are observed which are not present after irradiation of dilute solutions (Fig. 4B) (22). As photolysis proceeds, the droplets become more acidic, and MCPA, 4-chloro-2-methylphenol (chlorocresol, VIII), and other products are lost and can be detected in the atmosphere over rice fields (23).

The application efficiency of MCPA was only about 50% in our experiments , meaning that perhaps as much as half of the spray becomes airborne (21,23). The fraction which reaches the flooded field is degraded with a half-life of about 3 days by photochemical and microbial action; the principal intermediate is 4-chlorocresol (21). That which remains airborne for any significant length of time is photolyzed increasingly to a mixture of unidentified acids or salts. The atmospheric fate of MCPA vapor still is unknown.

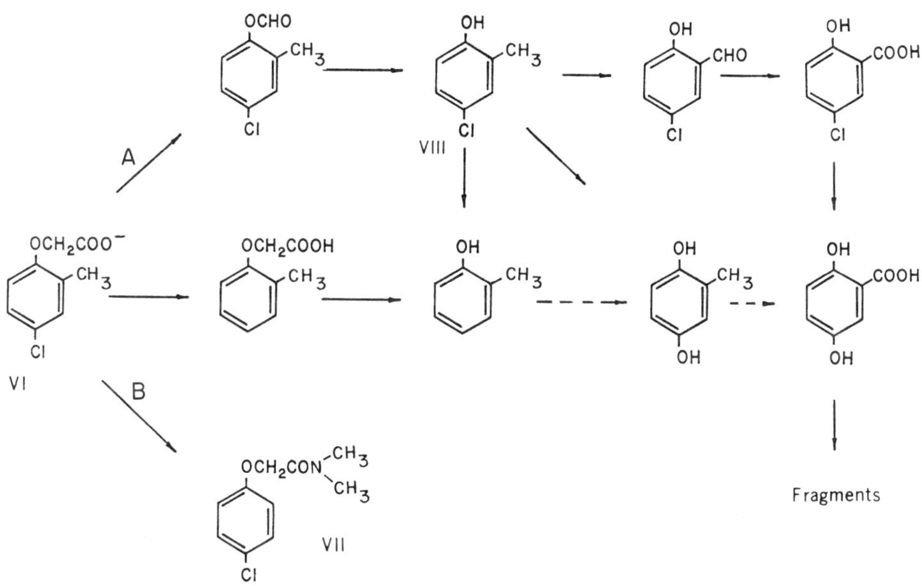

Fig. 4. Photodegradation of MCPA (DMA salt) in water and spray droplets (21,22).

Molinate. This thiol ester (IX, bp 202°C/10 torr, water soly at 20°C 800 mg/L, vp 5.6×10^{-3} torr/25°) generally is applied for water-grass control at 3-4 kg/ha as granular Ordram[R]. It does not absorb UV radiation at sunlight wavelengths and is relatively stable in the dark (24). However, like thiobencarb, it is rapidly photooxidized by hydrogen peroxide, and a number of photolysis products have been identified in laboratory experiments (Fig. 5) and detected in field tests.

Microorganisms, too, have been shown to degrade molinate in vitro (25), but neither light nor microbes usually have much time to take effect due to the rapid volatilization of the herbicide (24). The volatilization rate increases with temperature; on a typical application date in late May, with an average water temperature of 28°C, a $t_{½}$ of 2.5 days may be attributed to volatility alone (24).

Once in the atmosphere, molinate can be degraded by ozone and other photooxidants without itself absorbing ultraviolet radiation (26). The oxidation process eventually leads to adipimide (X) and then on to smaller fragments (Fig. 5). Thus, molinate applications lead to small (and diminishing) amounts in water and increasing movement into air; plant uptake, too, leads primarily to release into the atmosphere (27).

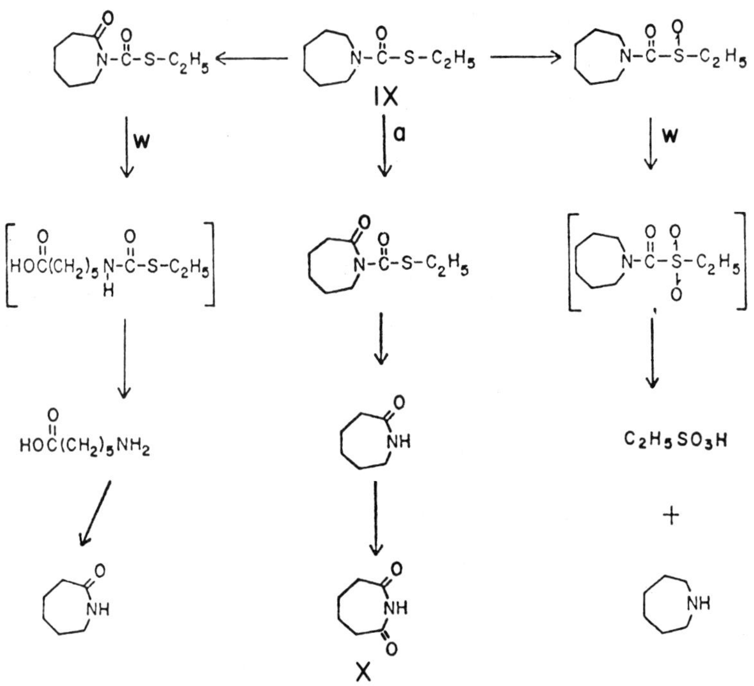

Fig. 5. Photodegradation of molinate in water (W) and air (a).

CONCLUSIONS

The fate of herbicides in California rice culture obviously is a complex issue, involving, as it does, both movement and degradation in air, water, soil, and plants. However, the California rice field environment can be characterized, and differentiated from many others, by the continual presence of warm, alkaline water, aerial application of seed and chemicals, and intense sunlight. These factors lend special emphasis to the importance of photonucleophilic reactions, photooxidation in aqueous solution, volatilization from water, and atmospheric reactions as vapor and particulates.

Dissipation of the herbicides ordinarily is quite rapid. Using molinate as an example, a 3.36 kg/ha application as a 10% granular formulation results in an initial surge of chemical in the field water as it is released from the granules, followed by a 50% decline within 2.5 days (Fig. 6). An estimate of the relative importance of each dissipation route (Table III) demonstrates the significance of volatility; the rate of molinates eventual atmospheric degradation is moderate, and depends upon airborne oxidant levels, but it is not known with accuracy.

Table III. Field distribution of applied molinate

Process	Estimated Loss (%)
Soil adsorption and metabolism	<10
Plant uptake and metabolism	< 5
Aqueous microbial metabolism	< 1
Hydrolysis	< 1
Photolysis	5 - 10
Volatilization to atmosphere	75 - 85

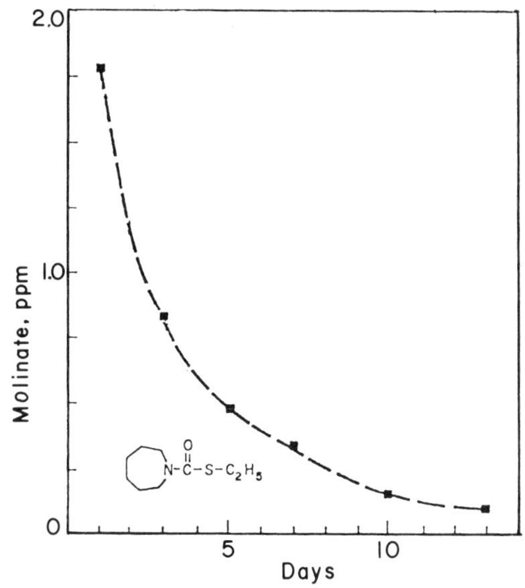

Fig. 6. Dissipation of molinate from rice-field water (24).

The environmental distribution and dissipation of rice herbicides is becoming a major public and political as well as scientific issue in Northern California. The problem associated with propanil primarily concerns its now well-known interaction with cholinesterase-inhibiting insecticides (the organophosphates and carbamates). While satisfactorily nonvolatile and degradable in water and soil, it is found to drift for several km during and after application; where it impacts the leaves of fruit trees which have been sprayed with the insecticides, it can cause damage because of the tree's altered ability to detoxify it. Neither photonucleophilic nor microbial degradation operates to reduce the hazard under these conditions.

MPCA also can present a drift problem, again in relation to particularly sensitive orchard crops such as pistachio (*Pistacia vera*) close to the sites of application. While the herbicide eventually disappears from water and air, the odor of its degradation product, chlorocresol, permeates sprayed areas for some time, and residents have expressed concern over possible effects of the vapor on their health. Molinate presently is being implicated in fish-kills on Northern California agricultural drainage canals and has caused controversy and investigation as the possible source of off-flavor in drinking water of the State Capitol, Sacramento; thiobencarb also will come under scrutiny.

The fate of herbicides in California rice culture can be seen to reflect our climate, application methods and formulations, and the physical and chemical characteristics of each substance. This suggests several possible approaches to manipulation of herbicide dissipation and alleviation of our perceived problems. It often may be possible to hold the water on a treated field long enough to allow volatilization or degradation to take place; changes in formulation or time of application may be useful in gaining longer or shorter persistence and reducing release of spray particles to the atmosphere; intentional stimulation of aquatic oxidation processes may not be out of the question.

Control of rice weeds satisfactory to both grower and public is not likely to come either from use of just *more* herbicides and different cultural practices on the one hand or from oppressive government regulation on the other, but rather from rational understanding and then control of the environmental dissipation and fate of our limited supply of useful chemical tools.

ACKNOWLEDGEMENT

It is a pleasure to acknowledge the continued support of the California Rice Research Foundation and USDA Regional Research Project W-45.

REFERENCES

1. J.N. Rutger and D.M. Brandon, Scientific American **244** (2), 42 (1981).
2. California Department of Food and Agriculture, Pesticide Use Report 1981, Sacramento, Calif., 1982.
3. R.D. Ross and D.G. Crosby, Chemosphere **5**, 277 (1975).
4. D. Mackay and P.J. Leinonen, Environ. Sci. Technol. **4**, 420 (1970).
5. D.G. Crosby, Advances in Chem. Ser. **111** , 173 (1972).
6. D.G. Crosby and H.O. Tutass, J. Agr. Food Chem. **14**, 596 (1966).
7. A.S. Wong and D.G. Crosby, J. Agr. Food Chem. **29**, 125 (1981).
8. D.G. Crosby, Proc. Fifth Intern. Congress Pestic. Chem., Kyoto, 1982.
9. S. Matsunaka and S. Kuwatsuka, Environ. Qual. Safety **4**, 149 (1975).
10. K.W. Moilanen and D.G. Crosby, J. Agr. Food Chem. **20**, 950 (1972).
11. G.C. Miller, R. Zisook, and R. Zepp, J. Agr. Food Chem. **28**, 1053 (1980).
12. G.C. Miller, M.J. Miille, D.G. Crosby, S. Sontum, R.G. Zepp, Tetrahedron **35**, 7797 (1979).
13. D.G. Crosby, K.W. Moilanen, M. Nakagawa, and A.S. Wong, in Environmental Toxicology of Pesticides (F. Matsumura, G. Boush, and T. Misato, eds.), Academic, New York, 1972, p. 423.
14. G.G. Still, Science 159, 992 (1968); L.E. Deuel, K.W. Brown, F.C. Turner, D.G. Westfall, and J.D. Price, J. Environ. Qual. **6**, 127 (1977).
15. A.E. Carey, H.S.C. Yang, G.B. Wiersma, H. Tai, R.A. Maxey, and A.E. Dupuy, Pestic. Monit. J. **14**, 23 (1980).
16. R.D. Ross, Ph.D. Thesis, University of California, Davis, Calif. 1975; W.M. Draper, Ph.D. Thesis, Univ. of Calif., Davis, Calif. 1979.
17. K. Ishikawa, Y. Nakamura, Y. Niki, and S. Kuwatsuka, J. Pestic. Sci. **2**, 17 (1977).
18. W.M. Draper and D.G. Crosby, J. Agr. Food Chem **29**, 699 (1981).
19. K. Ishikawa, Y. Nakamura, and S. Kuwatsuka, J. Pestic. Sci. **2**, 127 (1977).
20. Y. Nakamura, K. Ishikawa, and S. Kuwatsuka, J. Pestic. Sci **2**, 7 (1977).
21. C.J. Soderquist and D.G. Crosby, Pestic. Sci. **6**, 17 (1975).
22. D.G. Crosby, J.B. Bowers, and K.P. Downes, Abstr. 179th National Meeting, Amer. Chem. Soc., Las Vegas, Nev., 1980 PEST 9.
23. D.G. Crosby, M.Y. Li, J.N. Seiber, and W.L. Winterlin, Environmental Monitoring of MCPA in Relation to Orchard Contamination, Univ. of Calif., Davis, Calif., 1981.
24. C.J. Soderquist, J.B. Bowers, and D.G. Crosby, J. Agr. Food Chem **25**, 940 (1977).
25. L.E. Deuel. F.T. Turner, K.W. Brown, and J.D. Price, J. Environ. Qual. **7**, 373 (1978).
26. D.G. Crosby, K.W. Moilanen, and J.N. Seiber, Abstr. Fourth Internat. Congress Pestic. Chem., Zurich, 1978.
27. G.A.L. Ferreira and J.N. Seiber, J. Agr. Food Chem. **29**, 93 (1981).

FATE OF HERBICIDES IN FLOODED PADDY SOILS

Shozo Kuwatsuka

Faculty of Agriculture, Nagoya University, Chikusa, Nagoya 464, Japan

Abstract - The soil environment of paddy fields differs largely from that of upland fields in respects of soil properties, aquatic conditions and organisms including weeds. These factors define the properties of herbicides applied in paddy fields and largely influence the fate and behavior of the herbicides. Major pathways of disappearance of herbicides in paddy fields are photodegradation in flooding water, wolatilization and run-off from flooding water, and degradation in soil. In general, degradation in the soil, especially microbial degradation, is the major route of disappearance of many herbicides in the fields. In many cases, the degradation rates and major degradation pathways of herbicides in paddy soil differ greatly from that in upland soil. The fate of the principal paddy herbicides such as benthiocarb, molinate, chlornitrofen, chlomethoxynil, MCPA, butachlor and other herbicides in paddy soils is discussed.

INTRODUCTION

Rice is one of the most important crops in the world. It is cultivated in an area of some 145,100,000ha, mostly in flooded paddy fields. Although a large portion of this area is still not applied with pesticides, their application is important for greater food output and to save labor. The herbicide application in paddy fields is increasing rapidly even in developing countries. Many studies have been reported on the fate and behavior of herbicides in the soil environment in past two decades, and many detailed reviews and books on these studies have been published. These studies, however, are mostly for herbicides used in upland fields, and reports on paddy herbicides are quite few compared with upland herbicides. The soil environment of paddy fields largely differs from that of upland fields in respects of physical, chemical, and biological properties of soil as well as the aquatic conditions and the kinds and ecology of animals and plants including weeds (1). These factors largely influence the fate and behavior of these herbicides, and many herbicides used in paddy fields differ from those used in upland fields. For controlling weeds in paddy fields, thiocarbamate herbicides such as benthiocarb (thiobencarb) and molinate, anilide herbicides such as butachlor and propanil, diphenylether herbicides such as chlornitrofen (CNP), chlomethoxynil and bifenox, phenoxy herbicides such as 2,4-D and MCPA and their esters, and other miscellaneous herbicides including simetryn, oxadiazon, pyrazolate and dymuron are consumed in large quantities in Japan and other East Asian countries. PCP, nitrofen, and swep have also been used to a large extent in the past.

FATE OF HERBICIDES IN PADDY FIELDS

The herbicides used for weed control in paddy fields are generally applied to flooding water. In such cases, their photochemical decomposition and microbial degradation in the water and the evaporation from the water should occur. The analysis of this behavior, however, is difficult, and therefore, investigations and established results in this area are still inadequate. The leaching of herbicides with water occurs more extensively in paddy than upland fields because herbicides in soil are always washed away with leaching water. However, many kinds of paddy herbicides are strongly adsorbed by the soil particles and are retained mostly in the surface soil. Run-off of herbicides with irrigation drainage and by overflooding in some cases is also one of the main factors of loss for many paddy herbicides.

In general, the degradation of pesticides in soil is the most important pathway of their disappearance in the environment. This degradation is largely affected by physical and chemical properties of soil and soil conditions. Soils in paddy fields are quite different from upland soil in respects of aerobic and redox conditions and soil pH. According to this difference, not only degradation rates but also major degradation products sometimes differ between flooded and upland conditions of soil.

1. Photodegradation

Photodegradation is one of the important factors affecting the fate of paddy herbicides in the environment. Until herbicides are adsorbed into the soil layer, they stay in flooding water as a diluted solution or suspension. For example, benthiocarb takes about 5 days to disappear in flooding water after application (2). During this period pesticides are irradiated by strong sunlight, because paddy herbicides in general are applied under the strongest sunshine in May to July not only tropical areas but even in temperate areas, Soderquist et al. (3) reported that a large portion of molinate applied in paddy fields disappear by photodegradation and volatilization. Benthiocarb in aqueous solution was also rapidly decomposed under sunlight to produce 4-chlorobenzylalchohol and 4-chlorobenzyl aldehyde as major degradation products and more than 20 minor products (4).

2. Volatilization

Volatilization of herbicide chemicals from flooding water to the atmosphere is also one of the major manners of dissipation for some paddy herbicides. Molinate is volatilized off quite easily from the aqueous solution (3, 5). Benthiocarb is less volatile than molinate, but it is still easily volatilized from the aqueous solution (6). Volatilization occurred in proportion to the evaporation of water. The rate of volatilization, however, decreased when a soil layer was placed at the bottom of the solution due to the rapid adsorption of benthiocarb to soil particles prior to volatilization. When benthiocarb was applied to the surface of unflooded soil, volatilization was less than 1/5 of that from aqueous solution. These results indicate that the volatilization of herbicides from flooding water in paddy fields may be much larger than that from the soil surface of upland fields, and that the volatilization is decreased by rapid adsorption of herbicides into the soil surface. Many pesticides, not only volatile chemicals but also those which are hardly volatile ones, may be easily evaporated by co-distillation with water. Not only molinate, benthiocarb, and other thiolcarbamate herbicides but also many other pesticides were evaporated by steam distillation, but chloronitrofen and simazine were not (7). The volatilization of benthiocarb from the aqueous solution was largely affected by temperature as well as by the strength of the wind (8). The loss of butachlor by volatilization from 0.05 M $CaCl_2$ was 4.5% at 21.5°, and it increased 30% at 40°C (9).

3. Leaching

The leaching of herbicides in flooded paddy fields should be greater than in upland fields because in submerged soil they always washed with leaching water. However, large portions of many kinds of paddy herbicides are retained in the surface soil layer even several months after application. Benthiocarb, which is a moderately adsorbed herbicide among the pesticides examined, was still retained mostly in the surface 2 cm layer and partly in 2-5 cm layer of soil in paddy fields one month after its application (2). Many kinds of herbicides are strongly adsorbed on soil components, especially humic substances. This retention in the soil surface for a certain period of time is necessary for a paddy herbicide to keep the residual activity for controlling weed seedlings, and these retaining herbicides are selected for development. Many results of ricemeter or soil column experiments have shown that the amount of herbicides leached into the subsoil layer is negligible or very low. Acid herbicides such as 2,4-D and MCPA are not strongly adsorbed on soil, but are degraded before leaching down into the ground water.

4. Run-off

The run-off of paddy herbicides from rice fields to river and sea mainly through irrigation drain and partly by overflow is an important factor in their fate in the environment. This pollution by herbicides has occasionally caused fish kill in river and ponds or the accumulation in fish and shellfish in lakes and seas. In Japan, the use of fish-toxic pesticides are limmited by law. The paddy field use of PCP, which was the most important herbicide until 1971, was prohibited because of its strong fish-toxicity.

Yusa and Ishikawa (10) reported changes in the benthiocarb concentration of water in creeks and a river in Saga Plain in Southwest Japan. The benthiocarb concentration in creek water was closely related to the amount and term of the herbicide applied. The concentration began to increase together with its application in June, and reached the maximum concentration (8 to 40 ppb at 8 monitoring sites), and then decreased rapidly to the starting level (<0.2 ppb) by September. In the river, benthiocarb was not detected in water sampled from upper streams in the forest area through the year, in lower streams, the seasonal changes in the benthiocarb concentration were very similar to those in creek water, and the concentration was greater at lower reaches. The maximum concentration of benthiocarb was about 10 ppb, which was apploximately the same level as that found in other rivers in Japan (11, 12).

Kato and Maru (12) also investigated changes in the concentration of benthiocarb, molinate, and chlornitrofen (CNP) in creeks and a river in an area of central Japan. The concentration of these herbicides in the water changed with their application. The concentration of both herbicides in the river was approximately half of those in the creeks. In addition, the concentration of molinate was more than twice that of benthiocarb, although both herbicide chemicals were applied at about same quantity in this area. Chloronitrofen was also applied in this area, but the concentration in the river and creek was negligibe. The rates of loss of herbicides by run-off was etimated to be 20 to 30% for molinate, about 10% for benthiocarb, and 2 to 3% for chlornitrofen. This fact may indicate that water solubility of herbicides are largely related to the run-off of herbicides or the pollution of river and sea by pesticides.

5. Degradation in soil

Degradation in the soil is the largest fate of many herbicides in the paddy fields. Paddy herbicides are usually applied to flooded water, and a large portion of the applied amount enters into the soil layer with leaching water. Many herbicides are retained in the surface layer of soil for a relatively long term and are degraded there mostly by soil microorganisms.

The degradation rates or persistence of herbicide chemicals vary largely according to the properties of the pesticides. Table 1 shows the half life periods of various paddy herbicides in flooded soils under laboratory conditions and in paddy fields. The degradation rates of many herbicide chemicals in soil also vary greatly according to the properties and conditions of the soils (see Table 1). For example, the degradation rates of PCP in several soils differed considerably, and the half life period ranged from 12 to 70 days under flooded conditions, and from 18 to 120 days under upland conditions (13). A large variation in degradation rates according to the kind and condition of soil have also been observed in many paddy herbicides such as chloronitrofen, nitrofen, chlomethoxynil (14), bifenox (15), molinate (16, 17) benthiocarb (18), and 2,4-D (19). The degradation of chemicals in soil is affected by physicochemical soil properties such as the content of organic matter, kind of clay minerals, clay content, CEC, pH, redox potential, moisture content, soil structure, and soil texture. These properties affect each particular herbicide in different ways. For example, the degradation rate of PCP was approximately proportional to the organic content of soil and was also affected by the kinds of clay (13). Disappearance of diphenylether herbicides, such as chloronitrofen, nitrofen, chlomethoxyl, and bifenox was much faster in soils under anaerobic (reduced) conditions than under aerobic (oxidative) conditions (14, 15, 20), while thiolcarbamate herbicides such as benthiocarb and molinate were degraded more rapidly under oxidative soil conditions (16, 17, 18). The residual periods of some herbicides such as molinate, butachlor and others in paddy fields are sometimes considerably shorter than that in soil under laboratory conditions (Table 1).

TABLE 1. Half life time (days) of paddy herbicides in flooded soils[1)]

Herbicide	In laboratory experiments[2)]	In paddy fields[3)]
2,4-D	30-40	35, 48
2,4-D ethyl	<1 hr	
MCPA	3, 4, 7, 7, 15, 20	7, 7
MCPA ethyl	7-14	
Phenothiol	<1	<5
Darapon	3-5, 14-21	10-15, 20-31
PCP	5, 10-17, 12-70 (mean 30), 60	3-4, 6-7, 10-17
Benthiocarb	7-100 (mean 40)	3-8, 7, 8, 14, 62
Molinate	7, 15, 18, 30	<1, <5, <5, <5, <9, 11
Swep	2-9, 10-11, 7-14	<10
Propanil	<1-1, 1, <5	<1-1
Naproanilide	5, 6	2, <4, 4
Napropamide	49, 56	<20, 20
Butachlor	9-30	6, 8
Credazine	90-150	22, 45
Trifluralin	9, 10, 22, 45	10, 45
Nitrofen	3-35 (mean 11)	ca.14
Chlornitrofen	7-35 (mean 15), 17, 35	7, 9, 12, 13, ca.14
Chlomethoxynil	7-35 (mean 15), 30	7-8
Bifenox	4, 4	4, 4
Oxadiazon	75, 93-98	
Bentazone	5, 33, 45	15, 15
Simetryn	<37, 63	
Prometryne	100, 120	
Paraquat	>180	>180
Diquat	>150	

1) Data were collected from various sources.
2) Each chemical was mixed with soil and incubated at 25-30°C in dark.
3) Persistence in soils in paddy rice fields in Japan. Most herbicides were applied in May or June.

This may be because many factors such as photodegradation, volatilization, leaching, and run-off affect the dissipation of herbicides in fields.

When soil is submerged, soil microorganisms exhaust oxygen in the soil, and the soil becomes in a reductive state, except that uppermost 0.5 to 1 cm of the surface soil layer is kept in an oxidative state. This is because a limmited ammount of air can only enter to the surface soil by diffusion through flooded water. Thus, flooded soil except the surface layer is made reductive where Eh is below -100 mV, iron is reduced to ferrous ion, soil pH reaches to 6-7, aerobes are inactive and anaerobes are abundant (1, 21). These phenomena may result in the activity of the soil microbes responsible for the degradation of chemicals, and in widely different degradation rates and mechanisms for upland and flooded soils and, furthermore, for the oxidative and reductive layers of flooded soil. Benthiocarb is degraded to carbon dioxide more rapidly in upland soil than in flooded soil and more rapidly under aerobic conditions than anaerobic conditions (18) (Fig. 2). Chlornitrofen (CNP) is transformed to its amino derivative with ferrous ion more rapidly in the reductive sublayer than in the oxidative surface layer of flooded soil (20). Diphenylether herbicides such as chloronitrofen, nitrofen, and chlomethoxynil are persistent in soil under upland conditions (15). Chlorine atoms of PCP were replaced with hydrogen more rapidly in flooded soil (13). These observations can be explained by the differences in soil conditions and in degrading microbes between upland and flooded soils.

The degradation rates of herbicides in soil are largely affected by the soil temperature. The temperature effect is larger than expected because many herbicides in soil are degraded by microorganisms. The degradation of many herbicides is largely limitted to below 10°C. In paddy fields in northern Japan, it was found that considerable residues of chlornitrofen (CNP) and its amino derivative remained at harvest time, while these residues were only negligible in the warmer southwest of Japan (22). The same results were found for benthiocarb residues in three different districts of the country. (23).

FATE OF PRINCIPAL PADDY HERBICIDES IN SOIL

1. Benthiocarb

Of the thiolcarbamate herbicides, benthiocarb (thiobencarb, Saturn®, Bolero®, *S-p*-chlorobenzyl *N,N*-diethylthiocarbamate) is consumed in the largest amount of all pesticides used in Japan. This herbicide is used mainly for controlling paddy weeds in combination with simetryne, chlornitrofen, or other herbicide chemicals as in granular formulation. In recent years, molinate (Ordram®) has also been used to a large extent in paddy fields. The other thiolcarbamates such as EPTC (Eptam®), vernolate (Vernam®), and orthobencarb are used mainly in upland fields.

The fate and behavior of benthiocarb in the environment have been studied in detail and were reviewed recently by Ishikawa (24). Ishikawa et al. (2) reported that the residual amount of benthiocarb in soil and flooding water of paddy fields decreased rapidly within one week after application in central Japan. The half life period was 3 to 8 days in the soil and the degradation slowed after the 10th day of application. Most of the residue was retained in the surface 2 cm layer of soil, and only a small amount was detected in the 2 to 5 cm layer. Yamada et al. (23) reported that the benthiocarb residues in soil after rice harvest were 18 to 48% in one cold district of Japan, 10 to 19% in central Japan, and 3 to 4% in a warmer district. In tropical areas, benthiocarb as well as other herbicides should disappear in shorter periods than in temperate areas.

The photodegradation rate of benthiocarb is relatively high, as compared with 6 other pesticide chemicals tested (4). The photodegradation process of benthiocarb in aqueous solution and as thin film on glass and silica gel plates was studied by Ishikawa et al. (4, 25) and Chen et al. (26). They identified benthiocarb sulfoxide, desethyl benthiocarb, 4-chlorobenzyl alcohol, 4-chlorobenzaldehyde, 4-chlorobenzoic acid, the 4-hydroxy analogue of benthiocarb, 2-hydroxybenthiocarb, 4-chlorobenzyl mono- and di-sulfide as the photodegradation products of benthiocarb. A part of these products evaporated into the atomsphere (4, 6). Another large portion of them enters to the soil layer in paddy fields, together with parent benthiocarb. As discussed already, the volatilization and run-off of benthiocarb from flooding water are also important factors of the dissipation of benthiocarb in paddy fields. The leaching of benthiocarb in soil is not great because of the strong adsorption on soil particles (2, 27).

The degradation rates of benthiocarb in soil differ largely according to the soil conditions. Phenyl-^{14}C-benthiocarb was readily degraded in soils under aerobic upland conditions, less readily in flooded soils under aerobic conditions, and most slowly in flooded soil under anaerobic conditions (18, 28). In this case, $^{14}CO_2$ was evolved from phenyl-^{14}C-benthiocarb according to the degradation rates in the soil under different conditions. Little degradation of benthiocarb and no evolution of $^{14}CO_2$ occurred in sterile soil. Radioactive materials extracted with organic solvents consisted mainly of benthiocarb itself. More than 20 degradation products were detected, but none of them exceeded 3% of the applied radioactivity. Bound residues unextractable with organic soilvents were relatively small in amount. As degradation products in the soil, benthiocarb sulfoxide, 2-hydroxybenthiocarb, desethyl benthiocarb, 4-chlorbenzyl alcohol, 4-chlorobenzoic acid, 4-chlorobenzyl sulfoxide and its sulfone were identified (25, 28).

Recently, a new degradation product of benthiocarb was found from a soil where dwarfing of rice plants had occurred and identified as dechlorinated benthiocarb (29, 30). This dwarfing of rice plants or the dechlorination of benthiocarb occurred only in some particular soils under some specific conditions such as excessive application of benthiocarb and organic materials to the soils (31). The dechlorination of benthiocarb was inhibited by the herbicide methoxyphenone (32). This dechlorinated benthiocarb is also rapidly degraded in flooded soil especially under aerobic conditions to produce the sulfoxide, desethyl and 2-hydroxy derivatives, and benzyl methyl sulfoxide and its sulfone, and finally CO_2 (33).

In soil perfusion with benthiocarb, the chemical was degraded after a lag period. By the successive addition of benthiocarb into the perfusion system, the lag period was shortened and the degradation rate was increased (34). This enrichment effect was just like the cases of 2,4-D and MCPA in Audus's experiment (35). Benthiocarb-degrading microbes seemed to proliferate during the lag period.

A strain of Coryneform bacteria which decompose benthiocarb was isolated from a soil perfusate enriched with benthiocarb. This strain was not able to degrade dechlorinated benthiocarb (34). On the other hand, another strain of Coryneform bacteria, which decomposed dechlorinated benthiocarb but not benthiocarb, was also isolated from a perfusate enriched with dechlorinated benthiocarb (36). Microbiological characteristics of the two strains were quite similar, but the modes of degradation pathways were quite different. The former strain decomposed benthiocarb through dealkylation and sulfoxidation to *p*-chlorobenzoic acid and finally CO_2, while the latter strain decomposed only the benzene ring of *S*-benzyl *N,N*-dialkyl thiolcarbamates without any degradation of other portions of the molecule to accumulate *N,N*-dialkyl thiocarbamoylacetic acid (37). This compound, however, was not detected in soil which was incubated with the parent compounds, probably because it was degraded further by other microorganisms (33).

The dechlorination of benthiocarb in the soil is quite a special reaction in the light of difficulty in the dechlorination of monochlorophenyl compound. In laboratory experiments, the dechlorination of benthiocarb occurred after a lag period only when benthiocarb was incubated in some particular soils containing organic materials such as rice straw or sugars. The repeated application of benthiocarb into the soil resulted in shortening of the lag period and increase of the reaction rate. The dechlorination activity, however, rapidly decreased after benthiocarb in the soil was exhausted. In a suspension of the activated soil, the dechlorination occurred only at narrow ranges of temperature, pH, Eh, and with certain content and kind of organic additives. Sugars promoted the reaction but amino acids did not. Ascorbic acid promoted but cysteine and ferrous ions did not. $NADPH_2$ increased the reaction rate greatly but the reaction occurred after a lag time of several days as with the control. The isolation of this "special" microorganism, however, has not yet been successful (31, 38, 39).

Fate of benthiocarb in a rice paddy model ecosystem using ^{14}C-benthiocarb was studied recently by Chen et al. (40), and they concluded that benthiocarb in the environment seemed to be pretty safe according to the ecological magnification and the biodegradability. S. Duah-Yentumi and Kuwatsuka reported that the amendments of rice straw, compost, and chemical fertilizers of N, P, and K, especially P, promoted the degradation of benthiocarb in the soil in laboratory experiments (41).

2. Molinate

Molinate (Ordram®, *S*-ethyl *N,N*-hexamethylenethiocarbamate) has also been applied to a large extent in paddy fields in recent years. Unlike benthiocarb, however the fate and behavior of molinate in the environment have not yet been broadly studied enough.

In paddy fields, molinate dissipates rapidly by photodegradation and volatilization (3, 5) as already described. The period of molinate persistence in field soil is remarkably shorter than that in the laboratory experiment in which molinate is mixed with soil (see Table 1). The loss of molinate by run-off is also higher than that of benthiocarb (12).

In soil, molinate is degraded more rapidly under aerobic conditions than under anaerobic conditions (16, 17). The degradation rates in different soils differ largely depending on the soil properties (16). Thomas et al. (17) reported that the degradation products of molinate in soil were sulfoxide and sulfone of molinate, azepin-ring-4-hydroxy and 4-oxo derivatives, *S*-carboxy methyl derivative, and hexamethyleneimine. Recently, Imai and Kuwatsuka (16) further recognized azepine-ring-2-oxo derivative, *S*-2-hydroxyethyl derivative, and ethane sulfonate in addition to the products reported by Thomas et al. The latter, however, detected *N*-acetyl hexamethyleneimine, hexamethyleneimine thiocarbamate and its methyl ester, although the former had not detected these products.

Golovleva et al. (42) reported the degradation of molinate by *Mycrococcus* sp., and Skyabin et al. (43) reported that by *Mycrococcus* ap. and *Bacillus.* sp. Imai and Kuwatsuka (44) also isolated about 20 strains of molinate degrading microbes and identified the highly active ones as *Mycobacterium* sp. and *Flavobacterium* sp. of bacteria, *Streptomyces* sp. of actynomycetes, and *Fusarium* sp. of fungi. The degradation pathways of molinate by these isolates differed largely according to the strain. Only the fungi and the actynomycetes decomposed ^{14}C-azepin ring of molinate completely to $^{14}CO_2$, but the bacterial isolates only oxidized *S*-ethyl and 2- and 4-positions of the azepin ring without cleavage (44).

In soil which was not applied with molinate, the population of molinate-degrading microbes counted by the MPN-method was 20 to 35% of total aerobic microbial population by plate dilution method. The ratio of numbers of molinate-degrading microbes to total microbial population did not change through soil perfusion with molinate, nor did the molinate-degrading activity increase during soil perfusion which had no lag period (44). These phenomena differ largely from the case of benthiocarb degradation in the soil perfusion. These things indicate that there are many molinate-degrading microbes originally in soil and that they are not increased by molinate application. This differs greatly from the case of the other thiocarbamate herbicide benthiocarb, in which there are initially few benthiocarb-degrading microorganisms in soil and these proliferate by repeated application of benthiocarb (34).

3. Butachlor and other anilide herbicides

Butachlor (Machete®) and alachlor (Lasso®) of the chloroacetamides and propanil (DCPA in Japan, Stam®) of the acylamides are used in paddy fields. *N*-butoxymethyl-2-chloro-2',6'-diethylacetanilide, is the most important paddy in Korea and Taiwan, and is also consumed to a large extent in other countries.

The fate and behavior of butachlor in the environment have been studied mainly by Y.L. Chen and his co-workers (9, 45, 46, 47). Butachol in aqueous solution was readily degraded under UV or sunlight, and produced at least 24 compounds including 15 identified compounds, such as 2-chloro-2',6'-diethyl-*N*-(butoxymethyl)acetanilide, 1-chloroacetyl-2,3-dihydro-7-ethylindole and *N*-2',6'-diethylphenyl-2,5-dihydrooxazol-4-one (45). The photodegradation of butachlor in aqueous solution is more rapid and more complicated than that of thin film on glass and silica gel plates (46). Its volatilization from aqueous solution and the adsorption in the soil were also studied by Chen and Chen (9). These were found to be significantly influenced by temperature.

The degradation of butachlor by several microbial isolates in a medium and a soil was studied by Chen and Wu (47). Seven species of fungi and Bacillus sp. had butachlor-degrading activity. The most active, Mucor sufui NTU-358 produced at least 8 to 12 metabolites including 2-chloro-2',6'-diethylacetanilide, 2-hydroxy-2',6'-diethylacetanilide, 2,6-diethylaniline, *N*-chloroacetyl-7-ethyl-2,3-dihydroindole, 2,6-diethylacetanilide, and *N*-methyl-2-chloro-2',6'-diethylacetanilide. Lee (48) also studied the degradation of butachlor by a strain of soil fungi *Chaetomium globosum*. More than 10 metabolites were isolated, and some of them were characterized.

Alachlor (Lasso®, 2-chloro-2',6'-diethyl-*N*-methoxymethylacetanilide) is also applied in paddy fields. This herbicide chemical is decomposed in soil mainly by soil microorganisms to produce 2,4-diethylaniline as the main product and the other several intermediates. The metabolism of alchlor by a soil fungus *Chaetomium globosum* produced *N*-chloroacetyl-7-ethyl-2,3-dihydroindole in addition to the degradation products in soil (49). Photodegradation of alachlor was studied by Fang (50).

Propanil (DCPA in Japan, Stam®, 3',4'-dichloropropionanilide) was once used in substantial quantities for controlling barnyard grass in rice fields because of its wonderful herbicidal selectivity. At present, however, this herbicide is not much used in Japan. The degradation of propanil in soil and the microbial metabolism as well as the plant metabolism have been studied in detail, and many reviews on these have been published. Propanil is readily degraded in soil and produces 3,4-dichloroaniline (DCA), 3,3',4,4'-tetrachloroazobenzene (TCAB), and other minor polimers. DCA is strongly adsorbed on soil particles resulting in its long persistence in soil. The formation of TCAB in flooded soil is less than in upland soil and the quantities produced are negligible in flooded soil.

Naproanilide (Uribest®, 2-(2-naphthyloxy)propionanilide) is a newly developed anilide herbicide applied in paddy fields. This herbicide was rapidly degraded in flooded soils under both oxidative and reductive conditions to produce 1-(2-naphthoxy)propionic acid as the major product and other minor degradation products identified (51).

4. Diphenylether herbicides (Chlornitrofen, nitrofen, chlomethoxynil, bifenox)

Diphenylether herbicides such as chlornitrofen (CNP, MO®, 2,4,6-trichlorophenyl 4-nitrophenyl ether), nitrofen (NIP, TOK®), 2,4-dichlorophenyl 4-nitrophenyl ether), chlomethoxynil (X-52, 2,4-dichlorophenyl 3-methoxy-4-nitrophenyl ether) and bifenox (MOWDOWN®, methyl 5-(2,4-dichlorophenoxy)-2-nitrobenzoate) are pre-emergene herbicides, mainly used in paddy fields. Chlornitrofen has been consumed in the largest amount in the past in Japan. Chlomethoxynil is also used to a large extent. Nitrofen has largely used in the past but is not largely at present.

Kuwatsuka and his co-workers (14,15,20,52,53,55-58) have studied the fate and behavior of diphenylether herbicide mainly chlornitrofen, chlomethoxynil, nitrofen and bifenox in soils in the laboratory using ^{14}C-labeled compounds. These herbicide chemicals were rapidly degraded in flooded soils to produce their amino derivatives, but very slow under upland conditions, where amino derivatives were hardly detected (14). The degradation rates of CNP in flooded soils under anaerobic (reductive) conditions were 3-4 times faster than under aerobic (oxidative) conditions. The compounds produced in flooded soil were 4-amino, 4-acetylamino, and 4-hydroxy derivatives replaced at 4-amino group, and p-nitrophenol, p-aminophenol, 2,4,6-trichlorophenol, and unidentified minor compounds (20). In soil, the reduction of the nitro group of chlornitrofen was attributed to a chemical reduction with ferrous ion which was metabolically produced by iron reducing bacteria in flooded soil, although many strains of bacterial isolates could reduce the nitro group of chlornitrofen (14, 52). The amino derivative of CNP is strongly adsorbed to soil components, especially humic substances, to make complexes, initially by ionic adsorption and later by covalent bonding probably with benzoquinone moieties of humic substances (53). The amino compound has rather long-term persistence in soils both in the laboratory (14) and in the field (54).

Nitrofen was degraded in soil to produce the same analogues as the degradation products of chlornitrofen and the hydroxy analogues at each of the nitro, 2-chloro, 4-chloro and 6-hydrogen positions (55). Chlomethoxynil produced the compounds analogues to the degradation products of nitrofen with methoxy group, and additionally their demethylated compounds (56). Bifenox, which has a methoxycarbonyl group adjacent to the nitrogroup of nitrofen, was rapidly degraded in soils under both upland and flooded conditions. The main products were the free acid of molinate derived by hydrolysis in soil under upland conditions and were the free acid and the amino analogues of bifenox and its free acid under flooded conditions (57). The amino derivatives of bifenox as well as chlomethoxynil were not strongly adsorbed on soil particles unlike the aminoderivative of chlornitrofen. The strength of adsorption was largely related to pK a values of the amino derivatives (58).

5. Phenoxy herbicides

One of the major groups of paddy herbicides is phenoxy herbicides such as 2,4-D (2,4-dichloroactic acid), MCPA (4-chloro-2-methylphenoxyacetic acid), MCPB (4-(4-chloro-2-methyl) butyric acid), and their esters. In paddy fields, the esters of 2,4-D and MCPA are mainly used as water-treating agents. The ethyl esters are hydrolyzed chemically and also microbiologically to the free acids within one day, but phenothiol (ethylthioester of MCPA) was hydrolyzed mainly microbiologically to MCPA in soil (59). MCPB was also degraded rapidly in flooded soils. MCPA as the degradation product, however, was only detected in usually prepared flooded soil but not in strongly reduced soil (60). The degradation of 2,4-D and MCPA in soils and by isolated microorganisms, especially the latter, has been reported in a numbers of papers and reviewed in many books. However, the fate and behavior of 2,4-D and MCPA in soils have not yet been well clarified. MCPB was degraded to produce MCPA in usual flood soil, but MCPA was not detected in the soil under strongly reduced conditions, although MCPB was degraded at approximately same rates under both conditions (61).

REFERENCES

1. F.N. Ponnamperuma, *advances in agronomy 24,* 29 (1972)
2. K. Ishikawa, Y. Asano, Y. Nakamura and K. Akasaki, *Weed Research, Japan 21,* 16 (1976)
3. C.J. Soderquist, J.B. Bowers and D.G. Crosby. *J. Agric. Food Chem. 25,* 940 (1977)
4. K. Ishikawa, Y. Nakamura, Y. Niki and S. Kuwatsuka, *J. Pesticide Sci. 2,* 17 (1977)
5. L.E. Devel, F.T. Turner, K.W. Brown and J.D. Price, *J. Environ. Qual. 7,* 373 (1977)
6. K. Ishikawa, Y. Nakamura and S. Kuwatsuka, *J. Pesticide Sci. 2,* 127 (1977)
7. Y.H. Moon and S. Kuwatsuka, *Abstr. Annual Meeting of Soc. Sci. Soil and Manure, Japan 27,* p.177 (1981)
8. S. Matsunaka: *Annual Report of Special Research Project of Envir. Sci.,* Ministry of Education Science and Culture, Japan *B8-R12-6,* p.65 (1980)
9. Y.L. Chen and J.S. Chen, *J. Pesticide Sci. 4,*432 (1979)
10. Y. Yusa and K. Ishikawa, *Proc. 6th Asian-Pacific Weed Sci. Soc. Confer.,* Jakarta, *1977,* p.596 (1979)
11. M. Suzuki, Y. Yamato and T. Akiyama, *Water Research 11,* 257 (1977)
12. M. Kato and S. Maru, *Bull. Chiba-ken Agric. Exp. Station No.19,* 127 (1978)
13. S. Kuwatsuka and M. Igarashi, *Soil Sci. Plant Nutr. 21,* 405 (1975)
14. Y. Niki and S. Kuwatsuka, *Soil Sci. Plant Nutr. 22,* 223 (1976)
15. H. Ohyama and S. Kuwatsuka, *J. Pesticide Sci. 3,* 401 (1978)
16. Y. Imai and S. Kuwatsuka, *J. Pesticide Sci.* in press
17. V.H. Thomas, G.L. Holt and J.R. DeBaun, *J. Environ, Sci. Health B15,* 475 (1980)
18. Y. Nakamura, K. Ishikawa and S. Kuwatsuka, *J. Pesticide Sci. 2,* 7 (1977)
19. T. Yoshida and T.F. Castro, *Soil Sci. Plant Nutr. 21,* 397 (1975)
20. M. Oyamada and S. Kuwatsuka, *J. Pesticide Sci. 4,* 157 (1979)
21. S. Ishizawa and H. Toyoda, *Bull. National Institute of Agric. Sci. B14,* 203 (1964)

22. T. Yamada, *Abstr. 14th Meeting of Weed Sci. Soc. Japan* p.117 (1975)
23. T. Yamada, H. Nakamura, S. Sakamoto and S. Matsunaka, *Weed Research, Japan 24,* 18 (1979)
24. K. Ishikawa, *Rev. Plant Protec. Res. 14,* 149 (1981)
25. K. Ishikawa, Y. Nakamura and S. Kuwatsuka, *J. Pesticide Sci. 5,* 603 (1980)
26. Y.L. Chen, C.H. Fang, L.J. Chen and Y.S. Wang, *Proc. 5th Asian-Pacific Weed Sci. Soc. Congr.,* Tokyo p.236 (1975); *J. Chinese Agric. Chem. Soc. 14,* 59 (1976)
27. Y. Nakamura and S. Kuwatsuka, *Abstr. 1st Annual Meeting Pesticide Sci. Soc. Japan* p.224 (1976)
28. K. Ishikawa, Y. Nakamura and S. Kuwatsuka, *J. Pesticide Sci. 1,* 49 (1976)
29. K. Ishikawa, R. Shinohara, A. Yagi, S. Shigematsu and I. Kimura, *J. Pesticide Sci. 5,* 107 (1980)
30. T. Yamada, H. Chisaka, Y. Koyama and Y. Takeichi, *Weed Research, Japan 24,* 272 (1979)
31. H. Abe, K. Anma, T. Oishi and S. Kuwatsuka, *Abstr. 5th Annual Meeting Pesticide Sci. Soc. Japan* p.129 (1980)
32. S. Shigematsu, Y. Yamada and I. Kimura, *Weed Research, Japan 25, suppl.* 27 (1980)
33. H. Abe and S. Kuwatsuka, *Abstr. 6th Annual Meeting of Pesticide Sci. Soc. Japan* p.245 (1981)
34. H. Abe and S. Kuwatsuka, *Abstr. 4th Annual Meeting Pesticide Sci. Soc. Japan* p.204 (1979)
35. L.J. Audus, *Plant Soil 3,* 170 (1951)
36. H. Abe, Y. Nakamura and S. Kuwatsuka, *Abstr. 5th Annual Meeting Pesticide Sci. Soc.* p.128 (1980)
37. H. Abe and S. Kuwatsuka, *Abstr. 5th International Congress of Pesticide Chem.* Vf-11 (1982)
38. Y.H. Moon and S. Kuwatsuka, *Abstr. 6th Annual Meeting of Pesticide Sci. Soc. Japan* p.305 (1981)
39. Y.H. Moon and S. Kuwatsuka, *5th International Congress of Pesticide Chem.* Vc-15 (1982)
40. S.J. Chen, E.L. Hsu and Y.L. Chen, *J. Pesticide Sci. 7,* 335 (1982)
41. S. Duah-Yentumi and S. Kuwatsuka, *Soil Sci. Plant Nutr. 26,* 541 (1980)
42. L.A. Golovleva, E.L. Golovlev, A.M. Zyakum, Yu. V. Shurukhin and Z.I. Finrelstein, *Izv. Akd. Nauk SSSR, Ser. Biol. 1,* 44 (1978)
43. G.K. Skryabin, L.A. Golovleva, A.M. Zyakum, V.G. Sakharovsky, A.L. Klysheva, Yu.V. Shurukhin and M.Iu. Nefedova, *Dokladwi Akad. Nauk SSSR 239,* 717 (1978)
44. Y. Imai and S. Kuwatsuka, *Abstr. 5th International Congress of Pesticide Chem.* Vc-14 (1982)
45. Y.L. Chen, C.C. Lo and Y.S. Wang, *J. Pesticide Sci. 7,* 41 (1982)
46. Y.L. Chen, and C.C. Chen, *J. Pesticide Sci. 3,* 143 (1978)
47. Y.L. Chen and T.C. Wu, *J. Pesticide Sci. 3,* 411 (1978)
48. J.K. Lee, *J. Korean Agric. Chem. Soc. 21,* 1 (1978)
49. J.M. Tiedje and M.L. Hagedorn, *J. Agric. Food Chem. 23.,* 77 (1975)
50. C.H. Fang, *J. Chinese Agric. Chem. Soc. 15,* 14, 53 (1977)
51. M. Oyamada and S. Kuwatsuka, *J. Pesticide Sci. 5,* 495 (1980)
52. M. Oyamada and S. Kuwatsuka, *Abstr. Annual Meeting of Soc. Sci. Soil Manure, Japan* p.8 (1974)
53. H. Shimotori and S. Kuwatsuka, *1st Ann. Meeting of pesticide Sci. Soc. Japan* p.222 (1976)
54. T. Yamada, *Abstr. 14th Meeting of Weed Soc. Japan* p.117 (1975)
55. H. Ohyama and S. Kuwatsuka, *Abstr. 1st Annual Meeting of Pesticide Sci. Soc. Japan* p.220 (1976), *J. Pesticide Sci.* in preparation
56. Y. Niki and S. Kuwatsuka, *Soil Sci. Plant Nutr. 22,* 233 (1976)
57. H. Ohyama and S. Kuwatsuka, *J. Pesticide Sci. 3,* 401 (1978)
58. H. Ohyama and S. Kuwatsuka, *J. Pesticide Sci.* in press
59. H. Ohyama, J. Tamura and S. Kuwatsuka, *Weed Research, Japan 22* suppl. 37 (1977)
60. T. Izawa and S. Asaka, *J. Pesticide Sci. 4,* 61 (1979)
61. A. Kurozumi, T. Kurokawa, I. Yamaguchi and T. Misato, *J. Pesticide Sci. 5,* 37 (1980)

EFFECTS OF HERBICIDES ON AQUATIC ANIMALS

Yasushi Hashimoto and Yasuhiro Nishiuchi

Tokai Regional Fisheries Research Laboratory, Ueda, Nagano 386, Japan and Agricultural Chemicals Inspection Station, Kodaira, Tokyo 187, Japan

Abstract - Although most of the herbicides now used in paddies have practically no adverse effects on aquatic animals, pentachlorophenol-sodium (PCP) and molinate caused a series of massive fish kills in the past and a possibility that they cause hazards is suggested for some other herbicides by experimental findings. Acute toxicity of PCP is high in a variety of aquatic animals. It is not greatly influenced by water temperature and developmental stage in carp. Water and surface soil in paddies treated with the recommended rate of PCP remain toxic for about 10 days, and are required to be kept there during the period. Acute toxicity of molinate is very low in all the aquatic animals tested. However, hemorrhagic anemia, which frequently leads to death, was induced in carp exposed to 10 ppb or higher concentrations of molinate for more than one week in both the laboratory and the field. This anemia is specific for carp. In addition, experiments reveal that trifluralin and benthiocarb induce vertebral deformity in certain kinds of fish.

INTRODUCTION

Application of herbicides in paddies before or after the transplanting of rice seedlings is now one of the agricultural practices essential to rice culture. However, since the application is made mostly during or before the wet season when the water and surface soil containing the residual herbicides overflow into the aquatic environment including fishery nurseries, potential herbicidal toxicity to aquatic organisms is of great concern.

At present, more than 30 kinds of herbicides are registered for paddy use in Japan. In this paper, the toxicity data for these herbicides, especially PCP and molinate, are presented, and some discussion is made on the kinds of herbicides dangerous to aquatic animals.

TOXICITY OF REGISTERED HERBICIDES TO FOUR REPRESENTATIVE AQUATIC ANIMALS

The herbicides registered for paddy use are listed in Table 1 with their chemical class, postulated phytotoxicological mechanism (target in killing plant) and acute toxicity measured as LC-50 values to four representative aquatic aminals, that is, the teleost fish: carp, *Cyprinus carpio*, Crustacea: *Daphnia pulex*, Molluscaean univalve: *Physa acuta*, and tadpole of Amphibian frog: *Bufo bufo japonicus*.

HISTORY OF PCP USE

PCP was first registered as a fungicide for orchard use in 1956. Its herbicidal effect and high toxicity to fish had already been recognized and it was not until 1959 that PCP was permitted to be used as an herbicide in paddies under the condition that every precaution be taken against aquatic hazards.

Since it could control at a reasonable price graminaceous weeds including barnyard grass *Echinochloa crus-galli*, against which 2,4-D was ineffective, PCP was used throughout the country within a few years. However, with its increased use, fish or shellfish kills suspected to be caused by the herbicide occurred more frequently. The major reason was its high toxicity.

TABLE 1. Common name, chemical class, target in plant and acute toxicity to aquatic animals of the herbicides registered for paddy use

Herbicide Name and chemical class	Target	Toxicity (48-hour LC-50: ppm) Carp	Daphnia	Physa	Tadpole
(Phenoxy acid)					
2,4-D dimethylamine	H	>40	>40	>40	>40
2,4-D sodium	H	>40	>40	>40	>40
2,4-D ethylester	H	1.0	10	10	>20
MCPA sodium	H	>40	>40	>40	>40
MCPA ethylester	H	14	30	1.3	>10
MCPB ethylester	H	5.6	3.3	14	>10
MCPA thioethyl	H	2.5	>40	10	28
Naproanilide	H	3.2	>40		
(Phenol)					
Pentachlorophenol	R	0.12	3.6	0.32	0.25
(Diphenylether)					
Nitrofen	-	2.1	>40	2.2	3.8
Chlornitrofen	-	>40	>40	16	14
Chloromethoxynil	-	1.2	>40	3.0	>40
Befenox	-	3.1	>40		
(Carbamate)					
Swep	P	3.5	>10	>10	2.5
Benthiocarb	B	1.5	0.75	5.2	3.5
Molinate	B	34	>40	24	34
(Acidic amide)					
Propanil	P	13	>40	8.8	2.5
Butachlor	B	0.81	21	2.3	1.8
(Urea)					
Linuron	P	7.0	>10	>40	>10
Dymron	P	>40	>40	>40	>40
(Triazine)					
Simazine	P	>40	>40	>40	>40
Simetryn	P	>10	>40	>40	>40
Prometryn	P	5.2	>40	>10	20
Dimethametryn	P	3.5	>40	>40	13
(Diazine)					
Oxadiazon	-	32	>40	8.7	2.5
Pyrazolate	P	0.75	>40		
Bentazone	P	>40	>40	>40	>40
(Bipyridium)					
Paraquat	P	>40	>40	17	14
(Dinitroaniline)					
Trifluralin	B	1.0	>40	30	14
(Nitril)					
Dichlobenil	B	>10	>10	>10	7.5
Chlorthiamid	B	>40	>40	>40	>40
(Benzoic acid)					
2,3,6-TBA	H	>40	>40		
(Naphtoquinon)					
Aminochloronaphtoquinone	R	0.65	8.0	2.0	0.85
(Benzophenon)					
Methoxyphenon	P	3.0	2.0	3.8	6.5
(Organophosphate)					
Pyperophos	B	3.5	0.04		

1). 3-hour LC-50 values are shown for *Daphnia pulex*.
2). H, R, P and B mean phytohormone, respiration, photosynthesis and biosynthesis, respectively.

In addition to the data given in Table 1, the following LC-50 values of PCP have been obtained:

Goldfish, *Carassius auratus*	0.12 (48 h)
Medaka, *Oryzias latipes*	0.082 (48 h)
Dojo (Pond loach), *Misgurnus anguillicaudatus*	0.12 (48 h)
Guppy, *Poecilia reticulata*	0.42 (48 h)
Rainbow trout, *Salmo gairdneri*	0.056 (48 h)
Water flea, *Moina macrocopa*	3.0 (3 h)
Mayfly, *Cloëon dipterum*	16 (48 h)
Crayfish, *Procambarus clarki*	28 (72 h)
Red snail, *Indoplanorbis exustus*	0.62 (48 h)
Tanishi (Marsh snail), *Semisulcospira libertina*	0.77 (48 h)
Asari (Short-necked clam), *Tapes philippinarum*	0.24 (96 h)

These figures show that PCP is highly toxic to a broad spectrum of aquatic animals except the arthropodan. It is almost equally toxic to carp in a wide range of water temperatures (Ref.1) and in various developmental stages (Ref. 2).

When dissolved in well water under natural sunlight, more than 90% of PCP was decomposed in a day. However, in a paddy, a part of the applied PCP was absorbed into soil particles. The concentration in paddy water and soil after application of 86% water soluble granules of PCP-sodium at a rate of 300 kg/ha is shown in Table 2. When it was consecutively cloudy, it took more than 5 days for PCP to be detected, and no remarkable decrease in its level in the soil occurred even after one week (Ref. 3).

Table 2. Concentration (ppm) of PCP in paddy water and soil after application

Date	Weather	Procedure	Concentration Water	Soil
June 24	Fine	Control samples taken.	nd.	0.1
27	Cloudy	Herbicide applied and first sampling made.	2.4	4.0
28	Cloudy	Second sampling made.	6.0	
29	Cloudy	Third sampling made.	0.24	1.6
30	Cloudy			
July 1	Cloudy			
2	Rain	Fourth sampling made.	0.02	3.1
3	Cloudy			
4	Cloudy	Fifth sampling made.	nd.	1.9

1). Dry weight basis.
2). Precipitation 51.1 mm.

From these toxicity and residue data, the detailed precautions for application were strictly observed. However, it was very troublesome for farmers to follow these instructions and the agencies concerned did not recommend the herbicide's use. Therefore, use had gradually decreased with development of low fish-toxicity herbicides such as nitrofen, chlornitrofen or dichlobenil, and PCP has not been practically used since 1980.

SUB-ACUTE TOXICITY OF MOLINATE TO CARP

Molinate, which was developed by Stauffer Chemical Co., was registered as an herbicide for paddy use in 1971 with a mixture containing symetrin. Since it is very effective against 3-leaved barnyard grass, producing no phytotoxicity to rice seedlings, it gained wide acceptance and within a few years became one of the leading herbicides. On the other hand, a series of massive kills of carp had been reported from the central and northeast parts of this country since 1975. Pronounced symptoms of hemorrhagic anemia were observed in the dead or dying fish. At first, suspicion fell on denatured feeds, deficiency of vitamine K and some kinds of parasites or infections diseases which had been reported to induce similar symptoms.

However, it was soon experimentally proved that the symptoms appeared when carp were exposed to higher concentrations of molinate for a few days or to low concentrations (about 10 ppb) for more than 10 days (Refs.4,5). The symptoms were characterized by a decrease of Hct, RBC and Hgb values, and an increase in the number of immature erythrocytes, and were concluded to be due to loss of blood resulting from the alteration of the gill-capillary wall (Ref. 6). Recently Nishiuchi et al. conducted the following experiment for confirmation (Ref. 7).

Carp (15 cm in length and 50 g in weight) were exposed to molinate for 29 days in a flow-through system at 25 C. At 1 ppm and 0.1 ppm, partial kills from anemia were observed after 11 and 12 days, and all the fish tested died after 15 and 25 days, respectively. At 0.01 ppm, first kills occurred after 15 days, but some fish survived the entire test period. Hematological analyses at the termination of the experiment are given in Table 3.

Table 3. Hematological analysis of carp after 29 day exposure to molinate

Item	Concentration				
	1 ppm	0.1 ppm	0.01 ppm	0.001 ppm	Control
RBC ($10^4/mm^3$)	-	-	169.7	236.5	227.8
Hgb (h/dl)	-	-	3.23	7.60	7.35
Hct (%)	-	-	24.37	39.10	37.40

Molinate is still in use as a leading herbicide because of its high effectiveness and lower price than other competitor herbicides. To prevent further hazards, the National Federation of Agricultural Cooperative Association (Zenno), which is the sole distributor of the herbicide, has voluntarily determined the use-restraint areas surrounding carp production ponds. This strategy is successful. Practically no hazard from molinate has been reported since 1979.

OCCURRENCE OF DEFORMED FISH

In the 1960s and 1970s, deformed fish were reported in every part of this country, and extensive studies were made on the possibility that pesticides cause these deformities. It was revealed that most of the organophosphorus and a part of phenylcarbamate insecticides caused curvature of the vertebrae column in yellowtail, *Seliola quinqueradiata*, carp, medaka and some kinds of marine and freshwater fish (Refs. 8-10). Of the herbicides, trifluralin caused similar defamities in carp and medaka (Ref. 10), and benthiocarb did so in yellowtail (Ref. 8). The symptoms developed mostly in short time exposures to concentrations near LC-50 values and involved internal hemorrhaging at the deformed sites. However, it is yet inconclusive whether or not these pesticides actually produced the deformed fish in the field.

DISCUSSION

From this and other data, hormone-type and photosynthesis inhibitor herbicides can be said to have a generally low toxicity to aquatic animals, probably because their targets do not exist in the heterotrophic organisms. The acute toxicity of biosynthesis inhibitor herbicides now in use is moderate. However, benthiocarb, molinate and trifluralin, which produce peculiar symptoms, also belong to this category. The relatively high toxicity of benthiocarb and pyperohos to Daphnia may be explained by the fact that they contain a group which probably has anti-cholinesterase activity, although no explanation can be made for the high toxicity of butachlor and pyrazolate to carp. PCP acts as an uncoupler of oxidative phosphorylation, inhibiting ATP synthesis. Dinitrophenol herbicides, such as dinoseb and ioxynil octanoate, which have never been used in paddies, have high toxicity to aquatic animals in general, and they are also uncouplers. The compounds falling into this category are therefore inappropriate herbicides for paddy use

REFERENCES

1. Y.Nishiuchi, *Aquiculture*. *24*, 140 (1977)
2. Y.Hashimoto et al., *Abstracts from the 5th Annual Meeting of Pesticide Sci. Soc. Japan*. 232 (1980)
3. S.Goto et al., *Bull. Agr. Chem. Inspect. Stn.6*, 19 (1965)
4. S.Fukatsu, Oral presentation at the Annual Meeting of Japan. Soc. Sci. Fish. in 1976
5. K.Suzuki et al., *Bull.Fukushima Inlandwater Fish. Exp. Stn*. No.1, 30 (1978)
6. H.Kawatsu, *Bull. Japan. Soc. Sci. Fish*. *43*, 905 (1977)
7. Y.Nishiuchi et al., *Abstracts from the 7th Annual Meeting of Pesticide Sci. Soc. Japan*. 318 (1982)
8. K.Baba et al., *Bull Shizuoka Pref. Fish. Exp. Stn*. No. 11, 51 (1977)
9. K.Hirose and M.Kisukawa, *Bull. Tokai Reg. Fish. Res. Lab*. No. 84, 11 (1976)
10. Y.Nishiuchi, *Aquiculture*. 19, 151 (1975)

ALTERNATIVE TECHNOLOGY AND ECONOMIC ASSESSMENT OF WEED CONTROL IN WETLAND RICE

S. K. De Datta and R. W. Herdt

Departments of Agronomy and Agricultural Economics, The International Rice Research Institute, P.O. Box 933, Manila, Philippines

Abstract - The introduction of fertilizer-responsive early-maturing semi-dwarf varieties and other aspects of modern rice technology in tropical Asia make early and timely weed control highly critical if high yields are to be obtained.

In transplanted rice, hand weeding is the most common weed control method in South and Southeast Asia. Phenoxy acid herbicides such as 2,4-D and MCPA and some selective herbicides such as butachlor and thiobencarb are used by a few rice farmers. As labor costs rise, chemical methods of weed control combined with cultural practices and other direct methods provide attractive alternatives to hand weeding. Furthermore, with area under wet seeding increasing in some places, chemical weed control will play a more important role. Countries with high cost of labor and good control over irrigation water such as Japan, Korea, and Taiwan, use herbicides on 75 to 100% of their rice.

INTRODUCTION

Yield losses caused by weeds in rice fields vary with the time of weed infestation, soil fertility, rice varietal type, and planting method (11).

Rice farmers are aware of the impact weeds have in reducing their yields and use a combination of methods to obtain the level of control they desire. The combination depends on the technology available, what farmers know, the prices of various weed control inputs, and the methods used to carry out the other functions of rice production.

Weed control takes a large fraction of the inputs used in rice production but because of the contribution of indirect control methods it is difficult to quantify the amount. In deciding on the level of weed control that is optimal, farmers compare its cost with the value of the yield increase resulting from control (7).

METHODS OF WEED CONTROL

Weed control is achieved through various combinations of direct methods within systems in which land preparation, water control, planting method, and even fertility management indirectly help control weed growth.

Hand weeding is the most common weed control method in transplanted rice systems of tropical Asia, even though it is one of the most labor-intensive operations (Table 1). Hand tools ranging from double bladed knives to hoes are used in a few locations, but these are not common.

Some simple weeding machines have been developed, but weeding by machine is feasible only where rice is planted in straight rows. The rotary weeder is by far the most efficient mechanical tool for controlling weeds in transplanted rice. Manual rotary weeders are used in some provinces in the Philippines (20), and modifications of the basic device are used by a few farmers in many countries of South and Southeast Asia.

Chemical weed control offers an alternative to mechanical means, and with increasing labor costs and improving water control, herbicides may become practical in tropical Asia. A number of herbicides are now available at reasonable costs. Many more are being tested and may contribute to effective and economical weed control for tropical Asian rice farmers.

TABLE 1. Labor use by farmers for various operations in producing rice in some countries of Asia.

Location	Year	Labor (days/ha)				
		Land preparation	Crop establishment	Fertility management, water, and insect control	Weed control	Harvest, postharvest
Bangladesh	1979	52	77	15	62	74
Nepal	1978	33	27	n.a.	18	46
Indonesia (Java)	1980[a]	31	45	7	41[b]	57
Taiwan (Central)	1972	9	14	25	19	17
Philippines (Laguna)	1978	14	10	7	27	28
Philippines (Central Luzon)	1979	19	22	14	5	26
Malaysia (West)	1979	16	55	18	20	80
Sri Lanka (Mid-country)	1974	43	51	19	5	40

[a]Assuming 6 hours/day.

[b]Weeding, guarding, and water management.

Source: Bangladesh (1), Nepal (12), Indonesia (4), Taiwan (22), Philippines (14), Malaysia (21), and Sri Lanka (3).

Chemical weed control

Chemical weed control has been extensively evaluated in many areas in South and Southeast Asia. Major findings on chemical control in wetland rice are reviewed here, details are discussed elsewhere (6).

Herbicides for transplanted rice. The chlorophenoxy herbicides 2,4-D and MCPA have been available throughout most of Asia for the past 30 years. Some growers have been using them for postemergence control of annual broadleaf weeds and sedges. Since 1968 it has been recognized that 2,4-D and MCPA are also effective herbicides for most annual weeds, including grassy weeds, if they are applied preemergence to the weeds (10).

Other selective herbicides available for rice in many tropical Asian countries are butachlor and thiobencarb. Butachlor controls many annual grasses, broadleaf weeds, and sedges and can be applied pre- or post-emergence to weeds. In tropical countries in South and Southeast Asia, it is available in granular and liquid formulations. Thiobencarb, similar to butachlor, is highly effective against most annual grasses, broadleaf weeds, and sedges.

Herbicides for direct-seeded flooded rice. Direct-seeded wetland rice culture will become an increasingly attractive alternative to transplanted rice as the cost of labor rises, as less expensive selective herbicides become available, and as water control improves (5).

Yields of transplanted and direct-seeded rice are presently comparable in many areas, and the switch is extensive in some provinces in the Philippines. The most common practice is to spray butachlor 4 to 8 days after seeding pregerminated rice followed by 2,4-D spray 15 to 20 days after seeding.

In the tropics, butachlor, piperophos/dimethametryn, and butralin control weeds in direct-seeded flooded rice (8). Among these, butachlor and thiobencarb are perhaps the most widely tested in direct-seeded rice, with some encouraging results (15) but by no means uniformly positive findings (2). In 9 trials during 1979 to 1981 in the Philippines, butachlor and thiobencarb with 2,4-D gave significantly higher yields than the untreated control (Table 2).

TABLE 2. Weed control in direct-seeded wetland rice at IRRI and at two Philippine Bureau of Plant Industry research stations, 1979-1981 wet seasons.

Treatment[a]	Rate (kg a.i.[b]/ha)	Grain yield[c] (t/ha)			Trials resulting higher yields[d]
		IRRI	Maligaya	Bicol	
Naproanilide/thiobencarb	1.0/0.7	2.2	5.4	4.0	7
Piperophos/2,4-D IPE	0.33/0.17	2.1	5.7	3.7	7
Butachlor + 2,4-D	0.75 + 0.5	2.5	4.5	4.4	9
Thiobencarb/2,4-D IPE check	1.0/0.5	2.5	5.1	4.5	9
Untreated check	-	0.9	2.6	2.7	

[a]IPE = isopropyl ester.

[b]Active ingredient.

[c]Av. of 3 years/site.

[d]Number of trials that resulted in significantly higher yields over untreated control. Total number of trials were 9.

Integrated weed control systems

Each weed control method has its advantages and disadvantages. None is applicable in all cases because weed species vary so much in growth habits and life cycles. There is a growing concern that continuous use of one method of weed control, whether land preparation, interrow cultivation, or herbicides, will build up weed species that are tolerant of the control method used. This has happened in rice fields in Japan (16) and in Korea (17).

In the Philippines, research data clearly suggest that continuous rice production with a single land and water management system leads to a buildup of one or more weeds -- mostly perennials (9). To avoid this buildup of perennial weeds, it is essential to combine various methods of weed control or to change from one system to another.

ECONOMICS OF WEED CONTROL PRACTICES

Hand weeding is the main method of direct weed control in tropical Asia. Table 3 illustrates the range of direct weed control inputs commonly reported in farm surveys in the 1970s. (Labor and herbicide inputs were converted at their farm level prices to equivalent value of rough rice.) At one extreme is Bangladesh where more than 60 days of labor are used for control of weeds and no chemicals are used. The data from Java, Indonesia, also show a high level of manual weed control, but only half that of Bangladesh. Taiwan and the Philippine studies show intermediate levels of both herbicide use and hand labor. The Sri Lanka and Thailand studies report little labor use or expenditure on chemicals for weed control.

Farmers seem to adjust their intensity of weed control in line with the potential productivity of the crop as grown under their conditions. As a result, one observes that weed control is much more intensive where yields are high, but intensive weed control by itself will not have much impact on yields where water control, variety, and other factors are limiting.

TABLE 3. Weed control inputs, yield, and value of output reported in selected surveys of Asian rice farmers.

Location	Year	Direct weed control inputs				Yield (t/ha)	Farm prices[a]	
		Labor (days/ha)	Value in kg rough rice/ha				Rough rice ($/kg)	Labor
			Labor	Herbicide	Total			
Thailand (Central)	1968	0	0	6	6	2.1	0.06	0.50
Philippines (Central Luzon)	1979	6	79	30	109	3.4	0.14	1.19
Indonesia (Java)	1980	36	108[b]	0	108	3.3	0.19	0.57
Bangladesh	1979	62	232	0	232	2.7	0.14	0.52
Malaysia (West)	1979	20	263	25[c]	288	2.3	0.18	2.38
Philippines (Laguna)	1978	27	294	39	333	3.5	0.14	1.73

[a]Domestic currency per US$: Bangladesh, Tk15/$; Japan, ¥314/$; Indonesia, Rp625/$; Taiwan, NT$40/$; Philippines, ₱7.4/$; Thailand, ฿20/$; Malaysia, M$2.15/$.

[b]Using a real wage of 2 kg rice/day (3 kg rough rice), Collier (4).

[c]Half of all chemicals -- insecticides plus herbicides.

Source: Thailand (13), Philippines (14), Indonesia (4), Bangladesh (1), and Malaysia (21).

Factors associated with farmers' choice of technology

Farmers choose the combination of weed control inputs that provide the desired degree of weed control at the lowest cost and, therefore, input prices are an important factor determining input use.

In 1950 more than 400 hours of manual labor was used per hectare in Japanese rice production, and herbicides were virtually unknown (Fig. 1). As farm wages began to rise, hand weeding was reduced and herbicide use increased dramatically. From 1962 to 1972, herbicide prices fell more than 6% per year relative to rice prices while weeding labor cost increased at about 5% per year relative to rice prices (19). By the 1970s, weeding labor was less than one-fourth its former level and every rice field received an average of 2.5 treatments of herbicides.

Similar response to economic incentives is illustrated for the Philippines in Figure 2, which shows that weeding labor in Laguna increased between 1970 and 1975 when herbicide prices increased sharply and wages declined. Between 1975 and 1978, weeding labor per hectare decreased when wage rates increased and herbicide prices remained unchanged.

The impact of the extreme diversity in prices facing Asian farmers is illustrated in Table 3. Rice prices during the study years ranged from US$0.06/kg to nearly $0.20/kg while labor costs ranged from $0.50/day to $2.38/day. In those areas with low cost labor, little or no herbicide expenditure was reported, while those areas with high labor costs reported the use of herbicide equal in value to 25-40 kg of rough rice/ha. This amount is small relative to Japan, but indicates that farmers are beginning to use chemicals.

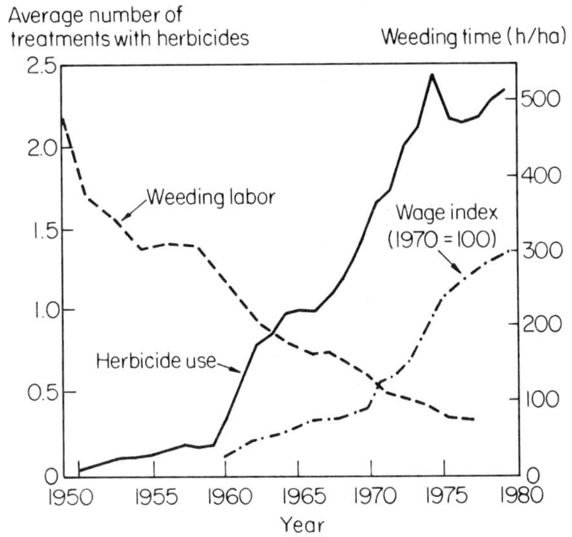

Fig. 1. Changes in area applied with herbicides in rice fields in Japan, 1950-1979 (16).

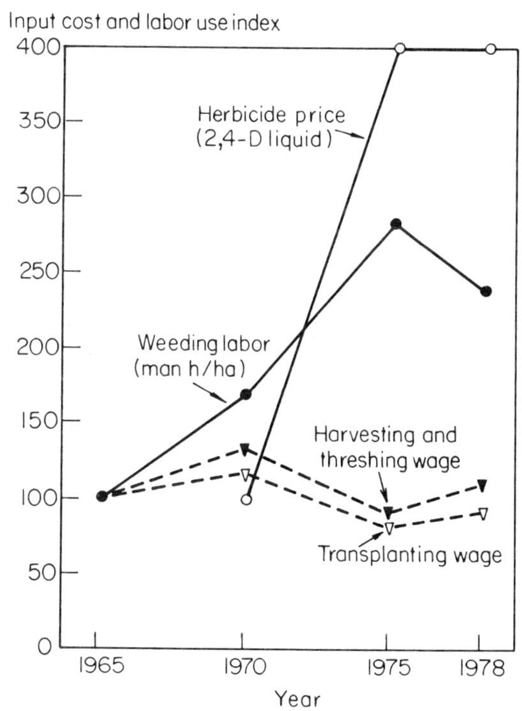

Fig. 2. Effect of relative input costs on weeding labor for 45 Laguna farmers, 1965-1978 (20).

The Philippine data illustrate the case of rising labor costs and improving growing conditions. As irrigation, fertilizer, and yields improved in Central Luzon between 1966 and 1979, the use of direct weed control methods increased on both irrigated and rainfed farms (Table 4). More of the farmers with irrigation used herbicides, both alone and in combination with hand weeding. By 1979, only 8% of irrigated farmers used no weed control compared to 22% of rainfed farmers.

TABLE 4. Use of four weed control methods as reported by farmers in the IRRI Loop Survey in Central Luzon, Philippines, 1966 and 1979 wet seasons.

Control method	Irrigated				Rainfed			
	1966		1979		1966		1979	
	No.	%	No.	%	No.	%	No.	%
No weed control	14	27	8	8	12	36	10	22
Hand weeding only[a]	31	61	26	26	23	63	21	47
Herbicide only[b]	2	4	25	25	0	0	8	18
Herbicide plus hand weeding	4	8	41	41	2	5	6	13
Total number surveyed	51	100	100	100	37	100	45	100

[a]In 1979, under hand weeding only, 3 farms have mixed type of irrigation.

[b]In 1979, under herbicide only, 1 farm has mixed type of irrigation.

Note: In 1966 four farms used rotary weeder, 3 rainfed and irrigated farms.

India continues to have low cost labor and a low price for rice. More than 75% of 2500 farm households in a nationwide survey reported some manual methods of weed control, while only 5% reported using herbicides. The region with the highest proportion of farmers reporting the use of herbicides was, as expected, the northern region of Punjab, Uttar Pradesh, Haryana, and Jammu and Kashmir, but even there only 9% used herbicides in 1977-78 (18).

The chosen combination of inputs is determined by their relative prices while the total expenditure on weed control is determined by its effectiveness and cost relative to the total value of the crop. Where technology is high and growing conditions are good, yields are high. Furthermore, if prices are also high, farmers put in high inputs. But where the level of technology is such that total output value is low, farmers do not exert much effort on weed control.

REFERENCES

1. Agro-Economic Research Unit. 1979. Costs and returns survey for Bangladesh, 1978-79. Crops. Vol. V, Boro Paddy, Ministry of Agriculture and Forests, Bangladesh.

2. Ahmed, N.U. and M.Z. Hoque. 1981. Weed control in dry-seeded rainfed bunded rice and its residual effect on weed growth of the subsequent transplanted rice. Int. Rice Res. Newsl. 6(2):13-14.

3. Amerasinghe, N. 1975. Economic resource use and decision making in paddy farming in some mid-country villages of Sri Lanka, Faculty of Agriculture, University of Sri Lanka, Peradeniya.

4. Collier, W.L., Soentoro, K. Hidayat, and Y. Yuliati. 1981. Background paper: Labor absorption in Javanese rice cultivation. For Technical Meeting on Labor Absorption in Agriculture organized by the Agriculture University, Bogor and the Asian Employment Programme (ILO), Bangkok.

5. De Datta, S.K. 1977. Approaches in the control and management of perennial weeds in rice. p. 205-226. In Proc. 6th Asian-Pac. Weed Sci. Soc. Conf., 11-17 July 1977, Jakarta, Indonesia.

6. De Datta, S.K. 1981. Principles and practices of rice production. John Wiley & Sons, Inc., New York. 618 p.

7. De Datta, S.K. and R. Barker. 1977. Economic evaluation of modern weed control techniques in rice. p. 205-288. In J.D. Fryer and S. Matsunaka (ed.) Integrated control of weeds. Univ. Tokyo Press, Tokyo.

8. De Datta, S.K. and P.C. Bernasor. 1973. Chemical weed control in broadcast-seeded flooded tropical rice. Weed Res. 13:351-354.

9. De Datta, S.K. and H.C. Jereza. 1976. The use of cropping systems and land and water management to shift weed species. Philipp. J. Crop Sci. 1:173-178.

10. De Datta, S.K., J.K. Park, and J.E. Hawes. 1968. Granular herbicides for controlling grasses and other weeds in transplanted rice. Int. Rice Comm. Newsl. 17(4):21-29.

11. De Datta, S.K., J.C. Moomaw, and R.T. Bantilan. 1969. Effects of varietal type, method of planting and nitrogen level on competition between rice and weeds. p. 152-153. In Proc. 2nd Asian-Pac. Weed Contr. Inter., Los Baños, Philippines.

12. Flinn, J.C., B.B. Karki, T. Rawal, P. Masicat, and K. Kalirajan. 1980. Rice production in the Tarai of Kosi Zone, Nepal. IRRI Res. Pap. Ser. 54. 15 p.

13. Green, B.A. 1970. Rate of adoption of new farm practices in the Central Plains, Thailand. USAID prices project, occasional paper no. 41, Dept. Agric. Econ., Cornell Univ.

14. IRRI (International Rice Research Institute). 1982. Annual report for 1981. Los Baños, Philippines. (in press)

15. Kannaiyan, S., K. Govindarajan, and H.D. Levin. 1981. Studies on the chemical control of weeds in dry-seeded wetland rice. Int. Rice Res. Newsl. 6(2):14.

16. Kataoka, T. 1980. Recent changes in rice culture methods and weed control methods. Jap. Pesticide Information 37:26-29.

17. Kim, K.U. 1981. Weed control in Korea. p. 37-50. In "Weeds and weed control in Asia." Food Fert. Tech. Cent., Asian Pac. Region, 6-9 October 1980, Tokyo, Japan.

18. NCAER (National Council of Applied Economic Research). 1981. Monitoring and evaluation of rice cultivation in India. New Delhi, India.

19. O'Brien, D.T. and M. Kikuchi. 1981. Impact of the changing energy situation on weed control technology. Paper presented at the IRRI/IWSS conference on "Weed control in rice", 31 August-4 September 1981. Int. Rice Res. Inst., Los Baños, Philippines. (in press)

20. Smith, J. and F.E. Gascon. 1979. The effect of the new rice technology on family labor utilization in Laguna. IRRI Res. Pap. Ser. 42. 17 p.

21. Taylor, D.C. 1981. The economics of Malaysian paddy production and irrigation. Agricultural Development Council, Bangkok.

22. Tsai, L.Y.S. 1976. Production costs and returns for rice farms in Central Taiwan, 1895-1976. M.A. thesis, Univ. Philipp., Diliman, Quezon City, Philippines.

AUTHOR INDEX TO VOLUME 2

SUBJECT INDEX TO VOLUME 2